Mental Health Nursing

Mental Health Nursing

Dimensions of Praxis

Third Edition

Edited by
Karen-leigh Edward, Ian Munro,
Anthony Welch and Wendy Cross

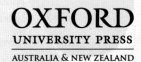

OXFORD
UNIVERSITY PRESS
AUSTRALIA & NEW ZEALAND

OXFORD
UNIVERSITY PRESS

Oxford University Press is a department of the University of Oxford.

It furthers the University's objective of excellence in research, scholarship, and education by publishing worldwide. Oxford is a registered trademark of Oxford University Press in the UK and in certain other countries.

Published in Australia by
Oxford University Press
253 Normanby Road, South Melbourne, Victoria 3205, Australia

© Karen-leigh Edward, Ian Munro, Anthony Welch and Wendy Cross 2018

First edition published 2010

Second edition published 2014

This edition published 2018

The moral rights of the author/s have been asserted.

National Library of Australia Cataloguing-in-Publication entry
   Title: Mental health nursing : dimensions of praxis / Karen-leigh Edward; Ian Munro; Anthony Welch; Wendy Cross.

   Edition: Third Edition

   ISBN: 9780190305222 (paperback)

   Notes: Includes bibliographical references and index.

   Subjects: Psychiatric nursing—Australia.
   Psychiatric nursing—New Zealand.

   Other Creators/Contributors:
   Edward, Karen-leigh, editor.
   Munro, Ian Leslie, editor.
   Welch, Anthony J., editor.
   Cross, Wendy, editor.

Edited by Pete Cruttenden
Cover image: Shutterstock
Cover design: OUPANZ
Text design: Watershed Design
Typeset by Newgen, Chennai, India
Proofread by Liz Filleul
Indexed by Jeanne Rudd
Printed in China by Leo Paper Products Ltd.

The Madwoman in this Poem

(After Bronwen Wallace)
For Gudrun
Yet how stupendous a psychosis
in which God is heard…
Gudrun Hinze
The madwoman in this poem
lives on the twenty-second floor
of a block of flats
her husband and children gone
each day she waits for a letter
that never comes
her wrists carry a flurry of scars
her arms are dotted with cigarette burns
every day she contemplates jumping.
The madwoman in this poem
walks the streets
reciting Shakespeare and Milton
she shelters in bus stops and doorways
scrounges through rubbish bins
drinks from discarded beer bottles
begs for money to buy cigarettes
and a moment's respite.
The madwoman in this poem
slumps into a ramshackle chair
hiding herself
her large torpid body founders
her heavy breasts gush
drug-induced lactation
her body grows
with each anti-crazy pill
she reluctantly swallows.
The madwoman in this poem
transfixes in front of the TV
absorbing its many messages
Ally McBeal is her daughter

Eddie McGuire can read her mind
Ridge and Brooke are talking to her
are going to come in a helicopter
take her to Venice to meet Brad Pitt.
The madwoman in this poem
lives in a holy grotto
awaiting the Pilgrims
she carries the burden of Eve
smells God in the toilet
sees the Virgin above the lintel
has given birth to the New Messiah
carries the secret of the Holy Grail in her heart
was raped by the Devil
sees maggots wriggling in her stigmata.
The madwoman in this poem
is sure Beethoven stole the
nine symphonies from her
cannot walk on the cracks of the pavement
can feel spiders eating her brain
fears her head is about to explode
is going to the firing squad next morning
is a character in a Bruegel painting
is an oracle of the dead.
The madwoman in this poem
is everywoman
is any woman
is a mother, daughter
sister, lover, friend —
the madwoman in this poem —
is me.

Reproduced with permission from *The Mad Poet's Tea Party* by Sandy Jeffs published by Spinifex Press.

Foreword

In Australia, mental health and mental illness are increasingly topics of significant concern.

A report commissioned by the World Economic Forum, undertaken by the Harvard University School of Public Health in 2011 indicated that 'the global cost of mental health conditions in 2010 was estimated at US $2.5 trillion with the cost to surge to $6.0 trillion by 2030'.

Consider suicide alone; the Australian Bureau of Statistics (2016) identified that in 2015, suicide was the leading cause of death among Aboriginal and Torres Strait Islander and non-Indigenous children and young people, and the second leading cause of death among those 45–54 years of age. The age-specific death rate is highest among males 85 years and over, but it should be noted that the number of suicides in this age group accounted for 3% of all male intentional self-harm deaths in 2015. There is no limit to the work that needs to be done.

Nurses and midwives encompass the largest professions in the health workforce, and are crucial to improving mental health outcomes for Australians—both now and in the longer term. This requires leadership from across the professions, to ensure that nurses and midwives are better skilled, more knowledgeable and more confident to address the mental health needs of the people they work with. It also requires the expansion and development of the mental health nursing workforce, to provide access to skilled mental health nursing interventions, and treatment and care coordination for people with mental health conditions.

The required knowledge around mental health and mental health nursing practice is ever expanding. As such, preparing to be a contemporary well-educated nurse, midwife or mental health nurse will mean a journey of lifelong learning. *Mental Health Nursing: Dimensions of Praxis* Third Edition, provides the perfect foundation from which knowledge, theory, and mental health nursing practice will flourish.

This text considers the roots of mental health nursing and remains steadfastly committed to many important foundational elements of mental health nursing practice. However, it does so with a focus firmly on the future and committed to contemporary ways of practice. Drawing from mental health nursing theorists and pioneers such as Hildegard Peplau and Joyce Travelbee, it assists with understanding the therapeutic relationship and focuses our attention on working *with* consumers and moving away from the more paternalistic approaches.

Throughout the text the important themes of relationship, partnership, communication, holistic care, and, above all, caring, emerge. The phrase within the text which describes caring as needing to be 'extended to encompass the additional expertise of emotional intelligence, praxis and resilience' has particular relevance. It also reminds us that in order to provide care that is meaningful and helpful to consumers, we need to ensure we engage with and understand the role that reflective practice plays in our role and in our own self-care, and why clinical supervision, which 'provides us opportunities to test our belief systems, and question and challenge our behaviours and the way we operate as mental health nurses', is such a fundamental requirement for mental health nurses.

This text prepares students and others to work with people across the age, service and illness-wellness spectrum, and provides an opportunity to develop understanding of the health care system. It is a timely text with a strong focus on contemporary service settings (such as primary care), ways of working (for example, co-design in research and practice) and targets for intervention (particularly, the physical health care needs of people with mental illness).

Our communities are not homogeneous and so to provide the best mental health nursing care we can, we need to be able to work with people from all walks of life, from all corners of the world, and responding in whatever capacity they choose to consult with us. Contributions to this text come from many national and internationally acclaimed mental health professionals and those with a lived experience. The consumer stories that link through the chapters reinforce the benefit of scaffolded opportunities for learning, thinking and reflection. Not only does this text address diagnostic issues, assessment and intervention skills, it prepares the neophyte nurse for the ethical, moral and legal conundrums they may face in the real world. The text is easy to read and digest, and the critical thinking questions and the reflections (including the self-tests) will be valuable points of learning for individuals or groups.

I recommend this text to those with a desire to enter the mental health nursing profession, and to all nurses and midwives who aspire to become more skilled, knowledgeable and confident in the provision of holistic care. Remember, our role is to hold the hope for consumers, carers, families and friends, and when the time is right, hand it back. This text will show you how.

Adjunct Associate Professor Kim Ryan
CEO Australian College of Mental Health Nurses
Credentialed Mental Health Nurse
Inaugural Australian Mental Health Prize Winner 2016

REFERENCES

Australia Bureau of Statistics (2016). *Causes of death in Australia 2015*, ABS cat no. 3303.0. Canberra: ABS. Retrieved from www.abs.gov.au/ausstats/abs@.nsf/Lookup/by%20Subject/3303.0~2015~Main%20Features~Intentional%20self-harm:%20key%20characteristics~8.

World Economic Forum and Harvard School of Public Health (2011). *The Global Economic Burden of Non-communicable Diseases*, Retrieved from www3.weforum.org/docs/WEF_Harvard_HE_GlobalEconomicBurdenNonCommunicableDiseases_2011.pdf.

Contents

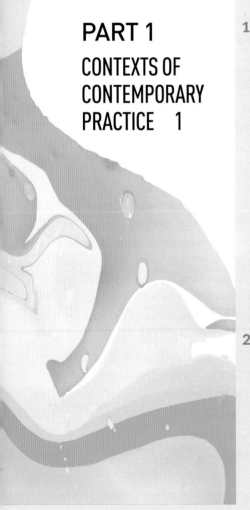

PART 1
CONTEXTS OF CONTEMPORARY PRACTICE   1

3 Physical and Mental Health 54

STEVE HEMINGWAY | JULIE SHARROCK |
GAGANPREET LEGHA

4 Promoting Mental Health 74

EILEEN PETRIE | EVAN BICHARA

5 Primary Mental Health Care 92

KATE COGAN | FREYJA MILLAR

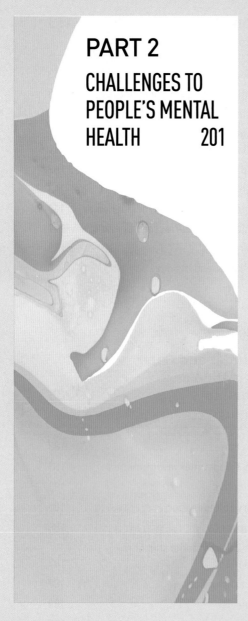

PART 2

CHALLENGES TO PEOPLE'S MENTAL HEALTH 201

13 Eating Disorders 271

LEANNE JAVEN | ALAN MOORE |
ALYSON MARCHESANI

14 Alcohol, Tobacco, Other Drugs and Co-occurring Disorders 285

NAOMI CRAFTI | VICTORIA MANNING

15 Psychopharmacology 316

CHRIS ALDERMAN | KAREN-LEIGH EDWARD

16 The Older Person 343

ROBYN GARLICK

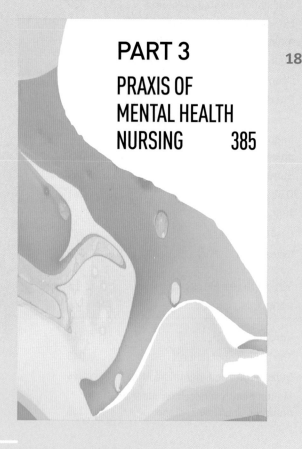

PART 3
PRAXIS OF MENTAL HEALTH NURSING   385

Acknowledgments

The author and the publisher wish to thank the following copyright holders for reproduction of their material.

Images: Alamy/Photos 12, figure 1.11; Alexander Turnbull Library, Porirua psychiatric hospital. Squires, D : Photographs of Porirua Hospital. Ref: 1/2-057695-F. Alexander Turnbull Library, Wellington, New Zealand. /records/22835420, figure 1.2; aturnofthekey.com, figure 1.5; Frederick Manning, figure 1.3; Getty/ David Lees, figure 1.10; National Library of Australia - nla.pic-an10698594-57-v, figure 1.4; National Library of Australia, figure 1.7; State Library of Queensland, figure 1.1.

Text: Anthony, W. for extract from 'Recovery from Mental Illness: The Guiding Vision of the Mental Health Service in the 1990s'. *Psychosocial Rehabilitation Journal*, 16(4), 1993; Brookes, N., Murata, L. & Tansey, M. (2008). for extract from 'Tidal Waves: Implementing a New Model of Mental Health Recovery and Reclamation'. Sourced from *Canadian Nurse*, August. p. 24; Department of Health for extract from *National Risk Management Program* (2007). Best Practice in Managing Risk. 11–13 Cavendish Square, London, UK; International *Journal of Eating Disorders* for table 13.1 from Berkman, N., Lohr, K. & Bulik, C. (2007). 'Outcomes of Eating Disorders: A Systematic Review of the Literature'. International Journal of Eating Disorders, 40(4), 293–309; *International Journal of Nursing Studies* for table 2.5 from Shuel, F., White, J., Jones, M. & Gray, R. (2010). 'Using the Serious Mental Illness Improvement Profile (HIP) to Identify Physical Problems in a Cohort of Community Patients: A Pragmatic Cases Series Evaluation'; *Psychiatric Rehabilitation Journal*, for extract from Rapp, C. A., & Goscha, R. J. (2004). The principles of effective case management of mental health services. Psychiatric Rehabilitation Journal, 27(4), 319–333; Random House Australia for extract from *The Essence of Health: The Seven Pillars of Wellbeing* by Dr Craig Hassed Copyright © Dr Craig Hassed 2008; RCPsych Publications for Sarkar, J, & Adshead, G. (2012). The nature of personality disorder. In J. Sarkar & G. Adshead (Eds.), *Clinical Topics in Personality Disorder* (pp. 3–20): rcpsych publications, p.7; Sage Journals for table 15.3 from Strand, L. M., P. C. Morley, et al. (1990). "Drug-related problems: their structure and function." *The Annals of Pharmacotherapy*, 24(11): 1093–1097; World health Organization for extract from Barry, M. M. & McQueen, D. V. (2005). 'The Nature of Evidence and its Use in Mental Health Promotion'. In Herrman, H., Saxena, S. & Moodie, R. (eds). *Promoting Mental Health Concepts, A Report of the World Health Organization* and extracts from *Measuring health and disability: manual for WHO Disability Assessment Schedule* (WHODAS 2.0), World Health Organization, 2010, Geneva.

Every effort has been made to trace the original source of copyright material contained in this book. The publisher will be pleased to hear from copyright holders to rectify any errors or omissions.

About the Editors

KAREN-LEIGH EDWARD

Professor Edward is internationally recognised for her work in resilience in chronic mental and physical health conditions. She has authored over 140 publications (90 in the past five years), including three books and eleven book chapters, in high-quality international nursing and health-care journals. She is Professor of Nursing and Practice-based Research, Faculty of Health Sciences, Swinburne University of Technology and Director of Research at St Vincent's Private Hospital Melbourne. She has been influential in engaging staff in research activities and has played a major role in the translation of research into practice and building research capacity in staff. She advises a staff of 1800 nurses, midwives, medical and allied health professionals on clinical and translational research matters related to acute and chronic conditions. She is an expert in translational research and her research interest also includes the use of technology to promote change in health behaviours. She also has extensive research experience in leading large clinical research projects as well as clinical trials.

IAN MUNRO

Dr Ian Munro has been a mental health nurse for over 40 years. He has had experience within acute hospital and community care, but his main interest is providing care within the community. Making the transition to academia in the mid 1990s, he has taught at a number of universities in Victoria. Currently he is a senior lecturer at Monash University, School of Nursing and Midwifery in Victoria. He is the postgraduate coordinator for postgraduate mental health nursing, and teaches in the undergraduate program. Ian has a long history working with consumers and carers, seeing the value in partnership for the ongoing care, and is passionate about nurses addressing client's poor physical health, substance misuse and improving the recovery focus as an approach to collaborative mental health care. Additionally, he supervises Honours, Masters and PhD students, mainly within the area of mental health nursing.

ANTHONY WELCH

Dr Anthony Welch is Associate Professor of Mental Health, Discipline Lead of Mental Health Nursing, and Strengths Research Lead for Health, Well-being and Community in the School of Nursing, Midwifery and Social Sciences, Central Queensland University, as well as Visiting Research Fellow, Sunshine Coast Hospital and Health Care Services, Queensland. Prior to commencing at Central Queensland University, he held senior academic positions at Queensland University of Technology, RMIT University, Australia Catholic University and was Foundation Deputy Head of School, Ballarat University. He has held a number of positions internationally including New Zealand, Hong Kong, Singapore and China. He has extensive experience in the supervision of higher degrees by research candidates (Honours, Masters and PhD). He is an internationally recognised Senior Parse Scholar and has published extensively in the areas of mental health and mental health nursing.

WENDY CROSS

Professor Wendy Cross is Professor of Mental Health Nursing at Monash University and is a National Mental Health Commissioner. Prior to commencing at Monash, she held senior executive and academic appointments in nursing at Monash Health, Deakin University and the University of Western Sydney. She was the National President of the Australian College of Mental Health Nurses (2012-2017) and is a Fellow of the Australian College of Nursing. She chaired the Council of Deans of Nursing and Midwifery (Australia and New Zealand) (2013-2017) and is a Board Director for the Australian Nursing and Midwifery Accreditation Council (ANMAC) and the Australian Osteopathy Accreditation Council (AOAC). Professor Cross contributes to a number of state and national committees, sits on several Editorial Boards and supervises many higher degrees by research students (Honours, Masters and PhD). She has authored more than 100 publications.

About the Contributors

CHRIS ALDERMAN

Dr Chris Alderman is a clinical pharmacist with more than 25 years of experience in clinical pharmacy. He holds specialty practice certifications in psychiatry and geriatrics and has a long-standing interest in the safe and effective use of psychotropic drugs. The author of over 130 peer reviewed publications, he is frequently sought as a speaker at national and international conferences, and as an expert witness in legal matters relating to psychotropic medications.

EVAN BICHARA

Evan Bichara arrived in Australia with his family of Greek-Egyptian background at the age of six. His promising academic career received a setback when he developed a mental illness in the first year of science at the University of Melbourne. He maintained, however, a profound determination to heal himself and contribute to others. Evan is now a tireless consumer advocate for those who have his condition—supporting individuals in crisis, building awareness in ethnic communities and advising government. His disability has become the means of expressing his passion to make a difference in the lives of other Australians.

LOUISE BYRNE

Dr Louise Byrne works within the mental health sector from the perspective of her own experience of significant mental health challenges, service use and recovery. Louise has worked from her lived experience in a variety of roles in government, non-government and tertiary settings since 2005, including a role as an expert advisor to the Queensland Mental Health Commission. Louise conducts research focused on the experiences and needs of the lived experience workforce. Louise has won numerous awards for her ground-breaking work. Louise believes firmly in the role of industry based and focused research in aiming for best practice.

KATE COGAN

Kate is a credentialed mental health nurse and a clinical family therapist with a Master's degree in conflict resolution, as well as a member of the Australian College of Mental Health Nurses. Her role as Manager of Mental Health at Outcome Health includes maintaining a clinical load, managing a team of credentialed mental health nurses delivering the Mental Health Nurse Incentive Program and suicide prevention, liaising and collaborating with primary health networks and overseeing other innovative mental health programs in a range of primary health-care settings.

NAOMI CRAFTI

Dr Naomi Crafti is a Senior Research/Education Fellow at Turning Point Alcohol and Drug Centre. She started at Turning Point in 2012 following 15 years at Swinburne University, where she coordinated the Graduate Diploma of Human Services (Counselling), and several years in community education at Eating Disorders Victoria (EDV). With a background in counselling psychology, Dr Crafti manages the Workforce Development area at Turning Point and is involved in the Master of Addictive Behaviours offered through Monash University.

SIMON DODD

Simon Dodd is a senior mental health nurse within a national mental health program in Melbourne. He has more than 25 years of experience in adult and youth clinical settings in Australia and the UK. Simon has worked as a senior clinician in acute mental health settings including hospital and community. Simon has a particular interest and experience in engagement and early intervention with young people with early psychosis. Simon has been an Honorary Fellow of the Department of Psychiatry and a Clinical Fellow of the Department of Post-Graduate Nursing at the University of Melbourne.

GERALD A. FARRELL

Gerald A. Farrell has clinical experience in general and psychiatric nursing and senior management experience both in health and tertiary education. Since leaving full-time university employment in 2012, Gerald has undertaken teaching and consultancy work for Melbourne's La Trobe University and other public and private organisations. His research has made him a leading international expert on problematic clinical relationships, including aggression management and bullying in health-care environments. His 1991 book was among the first to show that problems of aggression can be understood and managed by analysing the characteristics of the participants in their unique contexts.

ROBYN GARLICK

Robyn Garlick is a registered nurse and Senior Nurse—Aged Persons Mental Health Services at Melbourne Health. She has a passion for the delivery of safe and quality care for older people in acute, community and residential care mental health settings. Her research is focused on health and well-being outcomes for older people and she is currently involved in research on clinical decision making by nurses, Safewards, falls, nutrition screening and clinical handovers. She is also on a departmental steering committee for reducing restrictive interventions.

DON GORMAN

Don Gorman is Professor of Mental Health at the University of Southern Queensland. With a professional background in mental health nursing, he has for many years undertaken research into, and taught, cultural issues in health, especially mental health and Indigenous health, with an emphasis on research that builds capacity of communities to cope with adversity. Most of his past research has been in collaboration with health facilities, Divisions of General Practice and Aboriginal Medical Services, exploring ways that they can better provide care for clients and also work together to identify and address gaps in services.

KAREN HARDER

Karen Harder has bachelor's and master's qualifications in nursing. With more than 20 years' experience in mental health nursing, she has worked with some exceptional mental health clients and clinicians from across the lifespan. Karen currently works at Monash University's Peninsula campus, teaching in the Bachelor of Nursing & Midwifery courses as well as the Masters of Advanced Nursing (mental health stream). Karen's research areas include child and adolescent mental health nursing and clinical supervision.

STEVE HEMINGWAY

Dr Steve Hemingway is a Senior Lecturer in Mental Health at the University of Huddersfield and Senior Nurse within a memory clinic based in West Yorkshire, England. He has a longstanding interest in improving the services consumers receive from mental health nurses. His research interests include physical health, medicines management and nurse prescribing.

LEANNE JAVEN

Leanne Javen has bachelor's and master's qualifications in nursing and currently works in a city hospital emergency department and police response team. Leanne has worked overseas and in Australia in a variety of settings, including eating disorders, consultation liaison, primary mental health, crisis assessment teams, drug and alcohol services and community services. Leanne has also established private practice as a nurse practitioner in primary care. Leanne is a fellow of the Australian College of Mental Health Nurses (FACMHN), College of Australian Nurse Practitioners, Victorian Collaborative of Nurse Practitioners and Nurse Practitioners Special Interest Group.

SANDY JEFFS

Sandy Jeffs has lived with schizophrenia for 40 years and has been a human face to this often misunderstood condition. She was among the first wave of consumers in the late 1980s to speak publicly about living with schizophrenia. Sandy is the author of the best-selling *Poems from the Madhouse* and in 2010 her memoir, *Flying with Paper Wings: Reflections on Living with Madness*, was published. Sandy's latest poetry collections are *Chiaroscuro* with Black Pepper Publishing and *The Mad Poet's Tea Party* with Spinifex Press.

SUSAN JOHNSON

Susan Johnson has been a member of the Mental Health Nursing research team at Melbourne's Monash University. Susan has previously worked as a secondary school mathematics teacher and a registered nurse at the Alfred Hospital. Susan completed a Master of Public Health and has worked in the research areas of genetic epidemiology, cancer patient services and nursing. Susan has cared for a number of people close to her who have faced mental health challenges. Susan is a member of the International Society for the Psychological and Social Treatment of Psychosis (ISPS). Susan has developed and presented courses for MIND Recovery College.

GAGANPREET LEGHA

Gaganpreet Legha is a Nurse Practitioner endorsed in mental health and primary care specialising in physical health issues in mental health. Gagan commenced her nursing career in India after completing a Bachelor of Nursing degree. She later completed a Master of Advanced Nursing Practice (Nurse Practitioner) in 2010 in Australia. Gagan has worked across a variety of mental health and acute care settings. She is currently working as a Nurse Practitioner at an adult community mental health clinic, as well as delivering lectures and training graduate mental health nurses in her health organisation.

VICTORIA MANNING

Victoria is a Senior Researcher Fellow at Turning Point and Monash University. She is a chartered psychologist and holds a PhD on neurocognition and co-occurring disorders. She has worked as a clinical researcher for almost two decades in the UK, Asia and now Australia, where she leads the Treatment and Systems research team. Her research portfolio includes clinical trials, prevalence studies on co-occurring disorders and studies involving clinician training in screening and assessment mental health, addiction and related problems. Victoria is also a lecturer and unit co-coordinator on the Masters of Addictive Behaviours course at Monash University.

ALYSON MARCHESANI

Alyson is a registered Nurse Practitioner specialising in mental health and eating disorders at Monash Health in Melbourne. Alyson has completed Bachelor's and Master's degrees in nursing, and has worked across a variety of settings, including adult acute psychiatry, community, drug and alcohol, clozapine and consultation liaison psychiatry. Alyson currently works for a specialist tertiary eating disorder clinic for 12–65-year-olds, specialising in assessment and treatment. She is also a sessional lecturer for the Masters of Nursing (Nurse Practitioner) at Monash University.

MARGARET MCALLISTER

Margaret McAllister is Professor of Nursing at CQ University. Her research and teaching focus is in mental health and nursing education. She has co-authored several books including: *Solution Focused Nursing*, *The Resilient Nurse* and *Stories in Mental Health*. Over her career she has been the recipient of four awards for excellence in teaching, including in a national citation for outstanding contributions to student learning in Nursing. In 2017, she completed research evaluating the impact of universal mental health promotion in Queensland Schools.

FREYJA MILLAR

Freyja is a credentialed mental health nurse and primary care mental health nurse practitioner with Outcome Health. She has completed two Master's degrees in nursing practice (by research and Nurse Practitioner) and published research papers on cardio-metabolic monitoring and mental health, as well as service delivery options for people who experience co-occurring mental and physical health concerns. Freyja finds that working across primary and tertiary mental health services allows her to utilise her specialist advanced practice skill set to promote collaborative and recovery-oriented delivery of physical and mental health across all health-care sectors.

ALAN MOORE

Alan Moore is a registered nurse, credentialed mental health nurse and Fellow of the Australian College of Mental Health Nurses. He trained as a general and mental health nurse in the UK; in Australia he has worked as a clinical nurse in psychiatric in-patient and community settings. Currently he works as a Psychiatric Consultation Liaison Nurse at Monash Medical Centre in Melbourne, a role that includes promoting a close working relationship between the general hospital and mental health services in the care of consumers with eating disorders. He is the co-author of papers on mental health nursing and is an Adjunct Lecturer in Nursing at Monash University.

DANIEL NICHOLLS

Dr Daniel Nicholls is currently a senior lecturer at Western Sydney University and the advisor for postgraduate mental health nursing courses. He has worked for many years in clinical and academic settings in NSW, Victoria and the ACT, having a particular focus on clinical supervision. He applies his scholarly training in philosophy to problem solving with respect to mental health issues and human relationships. Through a number of publications in peer-reviewed journals and books he has been able to link deep philosophical reflection with everyday issues, applying principles derived from phenomenology and postmodern thinking.

HALEY PECKHAM

Dr Haley Peckham completed her mental health nursing training at the Florence Nightingale School of Nursing at King's College London in 2008 and has predominantly worked with adolescents and adults with borderline personality disorder. She has Master's degrees in Philosophy of Cognitive Science (Sussex) and Molecular Neuroscience (Bristol). In 2016, Haley completed her doctorate at the University of Melbourne where she researched a molecular mechanism of neuroplasticity. Haley has undertaken a number of courses in counselling and psychotherapy as well as engaging with her own personal therapy, and seeks to inspire nurses to collaboratively seek the sense and story underneath the symptoms.

EILEEN PETRIE

After qualifying in Basic Psychiatric Nursing at Mayday Hills Hospital, Beechworth, Victoria, Eileen has attained the degrees in: Post Graduate Diploma in Community Psychiatric Nursing (La Trobe University), Master of Nursing Science (La Trobe University), and PhD (Adelaide University). She has been employed in Academia since 2002. Eileen's area of research expertise is in Action Research. Using this methodology for her PhD, she examined the stressors in rural and remote Community Mental Health nursing that contribute to workplace burnout. Eileen is internationally and nationally published in both text books and Journal articles; and has presented at both international and national conferences.

CHRISTINE POOLE

Christine has worked in mental health nursing for more than 30 years, with the majority of this time spent in the speciality of child and youth. She has worked as a nurse unit manager in an inpatient adolescent unit, as a lecturer at Melbourne's RMIT University, and for 10 years in community infant mental health. Currently, she is a clinical nurse consultant in an Assertive Mobile Youth Outreach Service, working with youths with severe and complex needs.

CHRIS QUINN

Dr Chris Quinn is a clinical nurse consultant at Forensicare and an Adjunct Associate Professor with Synergy at the University of Canberra. His doctorate explored the sexual health practice of mental health nurses and he continues to explore this area of practice. He has extensive experience in mental health nursing in a variety of adult inpatient and community settings. He has a strong commitment to the promotion of best practice and education for nurses working in forensic settings. Chris coordinates the Post Graduate Nursing program at Forensicare, a role he is passionate about.

JO RYAN

Jo Ryan is the Director of Nursing at Forensicare. She has over 25 years of nursing experience in forensic mental health settings as a clinician, manager and educator. Jo is responsible for providing nursing leadership and creating a nursing culture that values professional standards and the delivery of high-quality evidence based care. Jo is also responsible for the management of the Nursing Practice Development Unit and is a co-author of Forensic *Mental Health Nursing: Standards of Practice*. Her clinical interests include improving patient care, the relationship between mental illness and offending, and risk assessment and management.

JULIE SHARROCK

Julie Sharrock's nursing career commenced in 1977 with 10 years' experience in general and intensive care nursing before beginning psychiatric nursing. Since then, Julie has worked in general and specialist psychiatry, drug dependence and nursing management and education. In 1997 Julie commenced work in consultation–liaison psychiatry, which has been her passion ever since. Julie's other passion is clinical supervision, which she has received and provided for 25 years.

GLENN TAYLOR

Glenn Taylor is a registered nurse and CEO of the Nursing & Midwifery Health Program, Victoria. His experience is in mental health nursing and in the area of addiction services. He is in the privileged position of directly supporting his nursing and midwifery colleagues with their individual health challenges, while working to influence the management and understanding of nurse and midwife health in Victoria. Glenn is keen to support and assist the industry in understanding the health challenges experienced by many in our profession and highlighting how these challenges are associated with the industry's work.

GRAEME THOMPSON

Graeme Thompson is of Māori descent and his iwi is *Ngati Awa*. A registered nurse with a postgraduate diploma in mental health, he holds a position as a Māori Health Manager, as well as an advisory role within a district health board mental health service and is a member of a child youth and mortality review group.

VERENA TINNING

Verena is a mental health nurse with over 30 years of experience in Australia's Top End and overseas. She worked across inpatient nursing, then many years in adult community mental health teams as case manager, followed by work in a triage, crisis and acute care team as clinician and team manager. She undertook nurse practitioner study and moved to the Remote Mental Health Team within the Northern Territory's Top End Mental Health Service, and is now consolidating her practice as an endorsed and credentialed nurse practitioner in remote communities, delivering holistic care in this novel role in the Northern Territory.

ROBERT TRETT

Robert is a registered nurse on secondment to University of Melbourne as a lecturer in nursing at the Centre for Psychiatric Nursing. His substantive position is with Eastern Health in Melbourne where he is Associate Clinical Director and a senior nurse consultant with Spectrum, the personality disorder service for Victoria. Robert holds a Master's degree in psychotherapy, but he considers the many service users and colleagues he has worked with over his 36 years, in both nursing and psychotherapy fields, to be his key teachers and informants. He is an enthusiast, teacher, supervisor and practitioner in psychotherapeutic nursing.

SCOTT TRUEMAN

Dr Scott Trueman is currently an academic at James Cook University with teaching and research interests in law and ethics, rural and remote health, and mental health. He has published and presented at national and international conferences on these topics. His formal academic grounding covers general and mental health nursing, law and commerce (accounting). Scott's doctoral thesis explored the delivery of remote mental health services by generalist nurses. Before entering academia Scott held numerous positions both in the private and public sectors in various clinical and management positions. He is currently a board member and treasurer of the Australian College of Mental Health Nurses.

KIM USHER

Kim is currently Professor and Head of School, School of Health, University of New England (UNE), Armidale, Australia. She is an experienced mental health nurse and researcher. Kim's research areas of interest focus primarily on issues related to mental health including the psychosocial impact of emergencies and disasters, psychopharmacology, adolescent substance use and the impact on the family, stress and substance withdrawal, alcohol related injuries, Indigenous health (especially mental health), and workforce issues. Kim has published extensively in the nursing and health related

literature, has been an invited keynote speaker at many national and international conferences, has served on Editorial Boards of many key journals and is the current Editor-in-Chief of the International Journal of Mental Health Nursing (IJMHN). Kim has conducted writing retreats with good outcomes for people at various levels.

PHILIP WARELOW

Dr Philip Warelow worked in nursing (practice and academia) across the lifespan, and more recently this focus has been extended into teaching across undergraduate/postgraduate degree programs. Dr Warelow has always been interested in service provision at both a practice and teaching perspective that is person-centred, grounded and provides service to clients/families that is accessible and usable. He has a strong belief in the core commitments that look at making a difference and advocating the provision of distinctive/humanistic values that encourage people to see mental illness differently. Dr Warelow has an interest in the history of nursing, which provided the catalyst for his doctoral study and his extensive publication range.

ROIANNE WEST

Dr Roianne West was born in Cloncurry and raised between Cloncurry and Mount Isa for the first half of her life. Dr West is Griffith University's Foundation Professor and Director of the First Peoples Health Unit. Professor West has over 20 years of experience in Indigenous Health where she commenced as an Aboriginal Health Worker in an Aboriginal Community Controlled Health Service, prior to completing a Bachelor of Nursing, Masters of Mental Health Nursing and a PhD. Dr West was the first Aboriginal member of the Australian College of Mental Health Nurses and recipient of the Stan Alchin award for Mental Health Excellence in 2003.

SUZANNE WILLEY

Suzanne has an extensive background in midwifery, maternal and child health nursing and refugee health nursing in primary health care. She joined the School of Nursing and Midwifery at Monash University in 2011 as a lecturer, developing and coordinating Refugee Health and Wellbeing education within the Master of Advanced Nursing. Suzanne teaches across both undergraduate and postgraduate nursing and midwifery curriculum. Her doctoral research will evaluate the implementation of a perinatal mental health screening program for women from a refugee background from both the women's and health professionals' perspective.

ANNETTE WOODHOUSE

Dr Annette Woodhouse has worked across a number of clinical and educational roles in Australia and New Zealand, including Senior lecturer/Discipline senior mental health, regional mental health promotion and manager of a professional development unit. She has specialised in child, adolescent and family mental health working in public mental health and private practice. Her doctorate was in rural family therapy and she is currently the Nursing Director of the Mental Health and Addictions Service, Queensland. She is the proud parent of three amazing young people and remains committed to the relentless pursuit of professional development of herself and others in nursing.

KRISTY YOUNG

Kristy Young is a mental health nurse and family therapist with 17 years' experience working in child, adolescent and youth mental health settings. She is currently employed as a senior clinician at the Child and Youth Mental Health Service at Eastern Health in a community outpatient team, providing assessment and treatment to children and youths aged 0–25 and their families. Kristy has also worked in an early intervention program for children at risk of developing conduct disorder, in child and adolescent inpatient settings, adult psychiatric inpatient settings, mental health triage and juvenile justice.

List of abbreviations and acronyms

AACAP	American Academy of Child and Adolescent Psychiatry	CALD	culturally and linguistically diverse
ABS	Australian Bureau of Statistics	CAM	complementary and alternative medicine
ACAS	aged care assessment	CAMDEX-DS	Cambridge Examination For Mental Disorders In The Older Adult
ACMHN	Australian College of Mental Health Nurses	CAMDEX-R	Cambridge Examination for Mental Disorders of the Elderly
ACT	acceptance and comittment therapy	CAMI	Confusion Assessment Method Instrument
ADHD	attention-deficit hyperactivity disorder	CAPE	Clifton Assessment Procedures for the Elderly
ADL	activities of daily living		
ADR	adverse drug reaction	CBT	cognitive behaviour therapy
AHMAC	Australian Health Ministers Advisory Council	CD	conduct disorder
		CDAMS	Cognitive, Dementia and Memory Services
AHPRA	Australian Health Practitioner Regulation Authority	CSDD	Cornell Geriatric Depression Scale
		CF	cultural formulation
AHW	Aboriginal health worker	CLN	consultation–liaison nurse
AIHW	Australian Institute of Health and Welfare	CLT	consultation–liaison team
AMHW	Aboriginal mental health worker	CMO	community management order
AN	anorexia nervosa	CO	conscientious objection
ANMC	Australian Nursing and Midwifery Council	COAG	Council of Australian Governments
AOD	alcohol and other drugs	CPA	*Community Protection Act 1990* (Cth)
APATT	aged persons assessment and treatment team	CRPD	*Convention on the Rights of Persons with Disabilities* (UN)
ASD	autism spectrum disorder	CTO	community treatment order
BASICs	behavioural assessment and specialist intervention consultations services	CVD	cardiovascular disease
		DAS	Depression Anxiety Scale
BD	twice a day	DASA	Dynamic Appraisal of Situational Aggression
BEHAVE-AD	Behavioral Pathology in Alzheimer's Disease Rating Scale	DBT	dialectical behaviour therapy
BMI	body mass index	DSM	*Diagnostic and Statistical Manual of Mental Disorders*
BN	bulimia nervosa		
BPD	borderline personality disorder	DSM-IV	*Diagnostic and Statistical Manual of Mental Disorders* (4th edition)
BPRS	Brief Psychiatric Rating Scale		
BPSD	behavioural and psychological symptoms of dementia	DSM 5	*Diagnostic and Statistical Manual of Mental Disorders* (5th edition)
BSL	blood sugar levels	EBM	evidence-based medicine
BVC	Broset Violence Checklist	EBP	evidence-based practice
CADE	confused and demented elderly	ECAT	emergency crisis assessment and treatment

ECT	electroconvulsive therapy
ED	emergency department
FEDNEC	feeding or eating disorder not elsewhere classified
FSP	forensic service patient
GAD	generalised anxiety disorder
GAF	Global Assessment of Functioning Scale
GAI	Geriatric Anxiety Inventory
GDS	Geriatric Depression Scale
GP	general practitioner
GSIS	Geriatric Suicide Ideation Scale
HELP	health enhancement lifestyle program
HIP	health improvement profile
HoNOS	Health of the Nation Outcome Scales
HREOC	Human Rights and Equal Opportunity Commission
IADL	Instrumental Activities Of Daily Living
ICD	*International Classification of Diseases*
ICT	intensive community treatment team
ICU	intensive care unit
IDP	internally displaced people
IMI	intramuscular injection
IPP	information privacy principle
IV	intravenous
K10	Kessler Psychological Distress Scale
MBT	mentalisation based treatment
MDD	major depressive disorder
MHADNP	mental health alcohol and drug nurse practitioner
MHN	mental health nurse
MHNP	mental health nurse practitioner
MMSE	mini-mental status examination
MSE	mental status examination
NCCAM	National Center for Complementary and Alternative Medicine (US)
NCNZ	Nursing Council of New Zealand (Te Kaunihera Tapuhi o Aotearoa)
NGO	non-government organisation
NHMRC	National Health and Medical Research Council
NICE	National Institute for Clinical Excellence
NMBA	Nursing and Midwifery Board of Australia
NP	nurse practitioner
NPCP	Nurse Practitioner Candidate Program
NPP	national privacy principle
NSP	needle and syringe program
OCD	obsessive-compulsive disorder
OCPD	obsessive-compulsive personality disorder
ODD	oppositional defiant disorder
OTC	over-the-counter (medications)
PAD	psychiatric advance directives
PANSS	positive and negative syndrome scales
PAS	psychogeriatric assessment scale
PD	personality disorder
PGAT	psycho-geriatric assessment team
PHAMS	personal health and mentor supervisor
PHARMAC	Pharmaceutical Management Agency of New Zealand
PHC	primary health care
PHCC	primary health care centre
PICO	Population, Intervention, Comparison, Outcomes
PND	postnatal depression
PRN	as needed
PTSD	post-traumatic stress disorder
PTT	primary treating team
QID	four times per day
QOL	quality of life
QT	the Q wave and the end of the T wave in the heart's electrical cycle
QUM	quality use of medicines
RAN	remote area nurse
RANZCP	the Royal Australian and New Zealand College of Psychiatrists
RCN	Royal College of Nursing
RCT	randomised controlled trial
RHN	refugee health nurse
RN	registered nurse
RSP	residential support program
SAD	separation anxiety disorder
SMI	severe mental illness
SNRI	selective serotonin and noradrenaline reuptake inhibitor
SSRI	selective serotonin reuptake inhibitor
START	Short-Term Assessment of Risk and Treatability
TCA	tricyclic antidepressant
TDS	three times a day
TIA	transient ischaemic attack
TPR	temperature, pulse and respirations
UNHCR	United Nations High Commission for Refugees
WHO	World Health Organization
WHODAS	WHO Disability Assessment Schedule
YLD	years lost because of disability
YLL	years of life lost

List of Figures

List of Tables

The Nursing Process – A framework for nursing practice

The nursing process guides nursing practice to assess the client's health status and healthcare needs (assessment stage).

The framework helps the nurse to then plan specific nursing interventions to meet those needs (planning stage).

Implementation of the specific interventions can then occur (implementation stage).

Finally, the framework helps the nurses in evaluating the outcomes of the interventions that have been implemented for the client (evaluation stage).

The nursing process can be easily remembered using the acronym APIE (Assessment, Planning, Implementation Evaluation), and by reminding yourself that the nursing process can be recalled as easy as A-PIE!

Assessment

- Psychiatric history
- Medical history
- Social history
- Family health history
- Major life events (e.g. losses); and response, coping, recovery and resilience factors
- Developmental history
- Substance use behaviours
- Risk potential
- Mental status examination

Planning for treatment

Treatment planning can help set goals, monitor progress, lead to better treatment and provide life-saving information.

- Perform an assessment of the client's needs.
- Identify risk factors.
- Generate a problems and goals list with the client and/or their significant other.
- Include other clinicians involved in the client's care. Interventions for care

Interventions for care

The treatment plan is a point of reference for treatment interventions.

- As soon as the plan is complete, ensure the client receives a copy of the treatment/care plan.
- People with an agreed role in the plan should have been involved in the planning stage. They should also receive a copy of the plan.
- Other services involved in the implementation of the treatment plan should also receive a copy as soon as practicable.

Evaluation

- Treatment planning is an ongoing, dynamic process. It involves the treating team, the client and their significant other in the client's treatment needs.
- Plans should be regularly revised and reviewed, i.e. as often as clinically relevant.

PART 1

Contexts of Contemporary Practice

Mental health is fundamental to holistic health, yet 20% of the population will experience a mental health problem at some point in their lives. Despite this striking number, we often view people with a mental heath problem as a problem themselves. We call them disparaging and pejorative names: 'schizo', 'mad' and 'wacky' to name a few. We think nothing of using these stigmatising words because they are so commonplace. However, for people with a mental health problem, they are alienating, isolating and demeaning.

Many of these harmful words originated from a time we mistreated people with a mental health problem. Society deems the parameters of acceptable behaviour and those who did not conform were incarcerated—in prison or insane asylum.

Asylum, that's another interesting word. The literal meaning is refuge, sanctuary, protection or haven but over time its meaning changed to that of 'nuthouse' or 'madhouse'. People needing refuge from the debilitating symptoms of mental illness were housed in appalling conditions that were eventually discarded for contemporary models of treatment and care that focus on community, recovery and capability. These modern models are based on evidence and embrace consumer involvement.

Part one of this textbook offers the reader explorations of the historical foundations of mental illness, treatment and care. It also examines the ways in which illnesses are manifested and diagnosed. It focuses on the positive aspects of resilience and coping with service delivery, based in ethical conduct and empowerment. Carl Jung embraced his madness and challenges everyone to examine his or her own. This part helps you do that.

CHAPTER 1

A Brief History: The Role of the Nurse in Caring for the Mentally Ill in Australia and New Zealand (Aotearoa)

PHILIP WARELOW

Acknowledgment

The authors would like to acknowledge the contribution of Gylo Hercelinskyj, who wrote this chapter in the previous edition.

KEY OUTCOMES

AFTER READING THIS CHAPTER, YOU SHOULD BE ABLE TO:

- understand that mental health nursing has always been fundamental to the care provided for people living with a mental illness in Australia and New Zealand (Aotearoa)

- examine more clearly the importance of mental health nursing history and how these understandings have shaped the public perceptions of mental illness

- identify some of the changes and challenges to the caring role of mental health nurses, especially those driven by the anti-psychiatry movement, along with deinstitutionalisation, mainstreaming and nurse training moving into the tertiary sector

- identify some of the major historical milestones in the treatment and care of people living with mental illness

- recognise how stigma is linked with mental illness and the role of the media

- understand the development of mental health nursing as a discipline and the caring role of mental health nurses.

KEY TERMS

- asylum
- case management
- deinstitutionalisation
- Dreaming (or Dreamtime)
- mainstreaming
- medical model
- mental health nursing
- psychiatry
- stigma
- Te Tiriti O Waitangi
- therapeutic alliance/relationship

Introduction

This chapter examines some of the complex issues of mental health as a topic, and more importantly the history of mental health nursing and the care provided to people who were mentally unwell in Australia and New Zealand (Aotearoa). First, the chapter examines aspects of the initial history of care for those deemed mentally unwell. This foundational history provides a context that will act as an introductory base to the care provided in more recent times, with a specific focus on mental health nursing care since the 1960s. Note that the terms 'psychiatric nurse' and 'mental health nurse', and the words 'psychiatric' and 'mental health' are terms that have historical perspectives, having been used at varying times across the history of the profession, depending on when and where staff were trained and the accepted terminology of the day. The terms used in this chapter endeavour to bridge these different historical perspectives. For example, the term 'patient' became accepted in the 1970s, while the term 'client' or 'consumer' is now being more readily used in contemporary mental health care.

Education and training have also fundamentally changed over the past 50 years. In recent years, educational preparation for nurses has moved away from an apprenticeship style of training to a tertiary education setting, with speciality degree programs or units for mental health nursing. Today, Australian and New Zealand nurses complete comprehensive degree programs, and on graduation are recorded on a single register, with no separate register for mental health nurses. Nurses interested in working in mental health are expected to undertake post-graduate studies in mental health nursing.

Though mental health nursing is now practised in a different way, with a shift from the institutionalised asylum care model into more community-based and recovery-oriented options, stigma regarding mental illness is still very much alive, and nurses choosing this speciality of nursing are often influenced by it. In fact, mental health nursing numbers are in serious decline (Holmes, 2006; Grant, 2006; Sabella & Fay-Hillier, 2014; Stuhlmiller, 2005) and the advent of this in Australia and New Zealand appears to coincide with the arrival of the comprehensive degree programs and the single nursing register. The movement of nursing education into the tertiary sector has meant the slow whittling down of mental health nursing courses/units into comprehensive degrees. This philosophy is built upon a misguided idea that the skills and expertise of mental health nursing can be easily incorporated into acute medical surgical pedagogical structures. The arguments that suggest that anxiety is the same illness in a person pre-surgery and someone who is constantly fearful and hyper-vigilant is misleading, fanciful and useful only to those who hold the purse strings. The nuances of any illness and the therapeutic relationship that nurses build and use towards recovery are significant to consumer care and philosophically important to mental health nursing's professional identity. These are matters that others will touch on or address in following chapters of this text.

History of care in Australia and New Zealand

The history of mental health nursing, and the care of those who are mentally ill in Australia and New Zealand, has not been well recorded or in any great depth. Psychiatry by its very nature, and by the picture it may conjure up to the general public, has remained a rather elusive, problematical, mythical and a consistently fascinating topic (Bostock, 1968). Those considered mentally ill were often institutionalised, with this care (as containment) taking place in large asylums that were often placed on the edges of larger towns, driven by an 'out of sight out of mind' philosophy. Nolan (1993) talks of the removal of the pauper insane from the community into institutions in England as having a practical utility in freeing others in their families from caring for them and thus allowing them to work. Nolan (1993) suggests that this arrangement was almost a win/win situation as it underlined the values of a bourgeois society where rationality came to be identified with work and irrationality with idleness

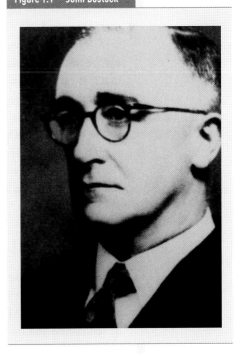

Figure 1.1   John Bostock

PHILIP WARELOW

and poverty. The subsequent lack of information about the early years of mental health nursing has resulted in an absence of founding fathers and mothers, and a lack of historical role models; hence, this type of nursing has been left in a state of almost professional obscurity (Nolan, 1993). Mental health nurses are distinctive professional people and much of the care provided to those deemed mentally ill has been provided by this dedicated group. Digby (1985) adds to this point, calling asylum keepers and attendants the hidden dimension of the asylum system. Russell (1983) adds to this, saying that attendants were the backbone of the system exercising considerable influence over the lives of patients.

Few authors have chosen to examine mental health nursing beyond that of a cursory glance. Many refer to a history of psychiatry rather than examine a history of psychiatric nursing, with Shorter (1997, p. ix) describing the history of psychiatry as being like an 'uncharted minefield' with both literary and anecdotal evidence, suggesting that the richness and rather abstract nature of the sources make it possible to demonstrate almost anything through the use of selective quotations. The lack of any clear defining (and often rather elastic) diagnostic boundaries tends to keep psychiatry and its linkage to mental health nursing shrouded in mystery and not really topics for any in-depth critique.

Over time, the number of people deemed mentally ill continued to increase and concern was raised about these growing numbers. Nolan (1993, p. 33) suggested that in 1890 there were 86,067 officially certified cases in England and Wales. Nolan (1993) also argued that history tends to confirm the legitimacy of the service one provides; yet mere inclusion in the history of another group implies one-down subordination. Under this benchmark, mental health nursing is seen as an integral yet subordinate part of psychiatry, having its contribution mostly painted and organised by another professional discipline (mostly medical), which tends to marginalise (and in many ways disenfranchise) nursing. Clearly, both the historical and contemporary roles played by mental health nursing in the care and recovery of those who are mentally ill are both substantial and significant and there are concerns that the current educational structure is not adequate to provide the future care that is required.

Given the relatively recent European settlement of Australia and New Zealand, the history of psychiatric and mental health nursing is not as extensive as its overseas counterparts. It is apparent that many of the foundational origins related to the care provided for 'the insane' in Australia and New Zealand had their beginnings in English and similar overseas institutions. Carpenter (1986, p. 15) described this English heritage by saying that the Victorian image of the asylum was still prevalent in the mid 1980s, with 'asylums likened to public sewers designed to cleanse cities of moral filth, unobtrusively removing it to a distant place where its threat to decent society could be contained'. Because of these views, asylums were seen by the general public as punishment-centred bureaucracies (Nolan, 1986) where 'mad' was often equated with 'bad' in the eyes of the community and treated in a similar fashion.

An ignorant general public

Unless directly involved in some aspect of psychiatry, the general public in countries around the world during this period tended to ignore mental illness or casually attach it to other more benevolent or charitable activities. Many chose to make fun of those who were mentally ill in the hope of hiding both its seriousness and the impact it may have on themselves, the sufferer and the sufferer's family. This, in many ways, is still done today despite how stigmatising this strategy is to those who are unwell. Along this same theme, 'madness' was often viewed in the nineteenth century as 'possession', usually by the Devil, but sometimes as the person being in some way touched by God.

People were often spoken of as being insane or as lunatics, thought of as idiots, invariably scorned and often tried by the courts or punished as witches or warlocks (Jones, 1972, pp. 4–9). This was probably the genesis of stigma and forms the basis of the stereotypical view in mental illness, whereby if we make fun of those who are mentally ill then it allows us to separate 'us from them' and this safeguard acts as a defence mechanism—labelling them rather than ourselves. Historians tended to record insanity based on these archetypal symbols and ideas, and were not especially interested in those who delivered the care nor the quality of care received by people with mental illness.

Understanding mental illness

Much of the literature depicts the history of psychiatry in Australia and New Zealand through the common view of the time, which tended to link mental illness to suspect metaphysical beliefs (Lewis, 1988). Insanity was often subsumed within larger disenfranchised groups, such as vagrants, petty criminals, the physically disabled and paupers: mentally ill people were often not recognised as a separate group that required special accommodation and care. As Lewis (1988) noted, the varieties of insanity from which they suffered were more easily defined as medical conditions, the preserve of a new type of medical specialist. These 'mad-doctors' (as they were called) not only provided specialist care but usually also administered the asylums that housed their patients (Scull, 1979). The adoption of the medical model in psychiatry across the world for the treatment of the insane was to remain dominant for the next hundred years (probably longer), and still sets the scene at varying levels today (Lewis, 1988). The mentally ill were physically isolated from the rest of the community in the belief that a combination of medicine and geographical distance and asylum could help to restore sanity and balance. Furthermore, insanity itself was conceptualised in a new way: moving from being thought of as being attached to metaphysical beliefs to a disease category or an entity with an underlying pathology, which would be better understood, and more accepted (it was assumed) with the advancement of medical science and when supported by nursing care (Lewis, 1988). Using a medical model to label illnesses also allowed the pathology of the problem to be more easily understood, and therefore the treatment and management of illnesses became possible with a range of pharmacological preparations. Today, the medical model is being harnessed to other theoretical inputs where models of care are tailored to the illness, and consumers are encouraged to take an active part and become more invested in their own treatment and recovery. Many of the more contemporary treatment strategies that are tailored to recovery have merit, although strategies such as consumer-centred therapy, solution-focused therapy, motivational interviewing, mindfulness, mentalisation, music therapy, drama therapy, aromatherapy and the strengths model need to be carefully selected and used by practitioners based on the contextual circumstances and needs of the individual person, rather than their catchy names or by cost constraints.

Nolan (1990, p. 3) suggests that in more recent years there has been a plethora of new ideas, fads and fashions about care in general, and provision for the mentally ill in particular. He rightly points out that 'it is easy to fall into the simplistic trap of adopting a condescending attitude towards the past as we view it from the enlightened theories of the present'. Hunter and McAlpine (1974, 1992) extend this point by arguing that to consider the past as wholly primitive and barbaric would be, and should be, considered erroneous, and that the history of the care of the insane has revealed many examples of good consumer care that were delivered on the back of profound and intelligent humanity. Anecdotal evidence from the 1960s and 1970s supports this view:

> Those old arrangements were so much better than how we practice psychiatric nursing today. At times it was a bit rough and ready, but we cared about our patients treating them as people rather than as the illness they suffered from.

An experienced nurse trained in the 1970s (Ward, 2001)

Clearly, not all the care provided by nursing staff was of the textbook variety (and arguably still isn't), with variations of some of the day-to-day micro-skills required for good consumer care built on the accumulated wisdom and experience gained over the life of the profession and modified for more contemporary practice settings. Many practitioners used a more eclectic model of care that incorporated many of the more recent strategies mentioned above. In addition, these interventions were built on the foundational wisdom learnt across generations of nurses who imparted their skills across the apprenticeship model of training and often followed on from one generation to another, as children often followed their parents into asylum work (Nolan, 1993).

English principles and practice in the Australian and New Zealand context

English principles and practice in the late eighteenth century and across the nineteenth century continued to be influential in the Australian and New Zealand context. However, the law, administration and systems of care were gradually shaped by the colonial experience—first, by the penal character and autocratic government of the early settlement, and later by the values of a more confident bourgeois society (Lewis, 1988). Lewis suggests that the 'principles and practice' and the 'law, administration and systems of care' were less intimately linked than one might have expected, arguing that the shaping of the approach, which was essentially English, was templated on the context of the colonial experience. However, the limited depiction in the literature regarding this shaping (Bostock, 1968) suggests that it could almost be the other way round. It appears that British laws and administration systems were quickly modified to suit the Australian and New Zealand situations, taking into consideration location, size, geography, environmental issues, climate and the local inhabitants. These changes were accepted in the absence of any suitable alternatives because there were no government officials to carry out the laws, or arbitrate their suitability in any way. There were limited physical facilities in which to detain prisoners or deal with the insane (criminals and the mentally ill were often housed in the same sites, promulgating the 'bad equals mad' maxim) and with no judiciary in rural areas, a country policeman was often the law and the mentally ill were at the mercy of local officials. On this basis, any care was dispensed on the premise that anything is better than nothing. Under these parameters there was also often a custodial basis or nature to this care.

Bostock (1968, p. 9) states that 'Australia began its life beset with some of the problems of the older world'. By implication, 'New Zealand fared under the same arrangements' (Elder, 2009, p. 47). According to records from the Porirua Hospital Museum (n.d.), the beginning of mental health services in New Zealand occurred in 1844 when an advertisement appeared in the *New Zealand Gazette* and *Wellington*

Spectator calling for tenders to construct temporary wooden buildings for the insane in Wellington. This signalled the building of a pauper lunatic asylum attached to the Wellington jail. However, there was a growing awareness that the mentally ill were a group needing special attention and that their care was not appropriate for a penal institution, and there developed a public demand that they be housed separately in an asylum, as a place of refuge, separate from jails and ordinary hospitals. The first legislation concerned with the mentally ill in New Zealand was the Lunatics Ordinance of 1846, which, among other considerations, provided that after certification a mentally ill person could be sent to a jail, house of correction or public hospital; or alternatively to a public colonial asylum, although no such institution existed at that time. This represented a step forward in the development of special services for the mentally ill in that it envisaged state provision of services and was available to every person in the community (Porirua Hospital Museum, n.d.).

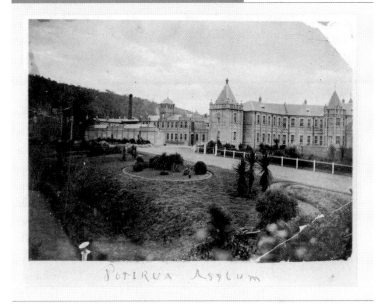

Figure 1.2   Porirua Psychiatric Hospital (1910)

Building different provisions for criminals and the mentally ill was also part of the development of care in both Australia and New Zealand, as evidenced by the design of Sydney's Tarban Creek Asylum (Gladesville Mental Hospital; see Figure 1.4) by William Lewis (1834–37), which was adapted from contemporary British plans. These British designs were significant across Australia, with the Yarra Bend

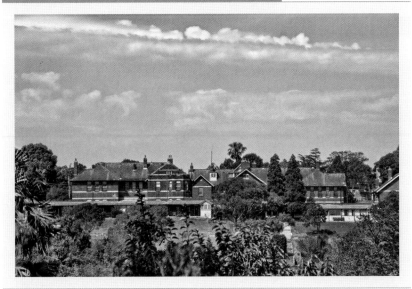

Figure 1.3   Tarban Creek Asylum (Gladesville Mental Hospital)

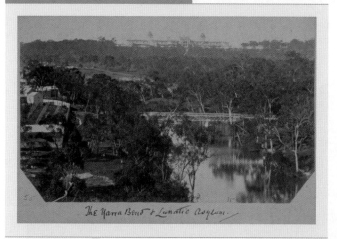

Figure 1.4   Yarra Bend Lunatic Asylum

Lunatic Asylum in Victoria (see Figure 1.5) exemplifying this point. The illustrations demonstrate how similar the structures of asylums in Australia and England actually were. Yarra Bend, Melbourne (Figure 1.5) and St Georges Hospital (Figure 1.6) in Stafford clearly have a similar design.

Another consideration is indigenous cultural issues; these are significant in both Australia and New Zealand, and are based on different understandings that fall outside the culture shaped by Anglo-centric colonisation. The approach to culturally sensitive practice in both Australia and New Zealand has evolved separately, reflecting different historical backgrounds to the relationships between indigenous peoples and settlers (Bradley & De Souza, 2013). Māori are the indigenous people of Aotearoa/New Zealand, whose relationship with Pakeha (non-Māori) is defined in Te Tiriti O Waitangi (the Treaty of Waitangi)—a document signed in 1840 by the British Crown and Māori chiefs. Te Tiriti forms the basis for biculturalism: an equal partnership between the two groups in which the Māori are acknowledged as tāngata whenua (people of the land/ Earth) and the Māori translation of Te Tiriti O Waitangi is acknowledged as the founding document of Aotearoa/New Zealand (Wood, Bradley & De Souza, 2009). Indigenous populations in both Australia and New Zealand go about their daily lives in a range of ways different from non-indigenous groups; because of this, and a host of other considerations, care delivered by mental health providers needs to consider these different beliefs and perspectives. Tāngata whenua for the Māori and the Dreaming (or Dreamtime) for Australian Aborigines need to be considered within any nursing care and/or medical treatment package provided (Awty, 2013). To avoid these considerations would be counter-productive and therapeutically unwise.

Figure 1.5   St Georges Hospital, Stafford

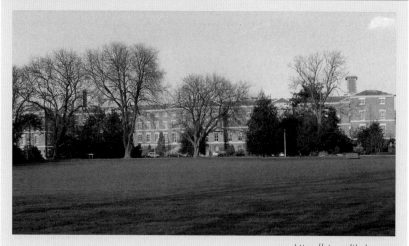

https://aturnofthekey.com

Psychiatry as a topic is often represented from an English perspective by examining the care delivered at the facility popularly known as 'Bedlam'—St Mary's of Bethlehem in London. Built in 1247, Bethlehem had a controversial history, but its practices and approaches were used as the blueprint for much of the Australian and New Zealand mental health systems. Bethlehem has always had its defenders and attackers. Since some of the early records of the hospital have now been destroyed, records are largely dependent on partisan accounts of the treatment at this time. *The Story of Bethlehem Hospital* (O'Donoghue, 1913) was written by the hospital chaplain, who outlined a range of disturbing issues related to hospital life. These issues included using Bethlehem inmates as a source of amusement for the general public, who paid for this entertainment. This payment probably went to the attendants. A poem, which was said to describe life at Bethlehem (Jones, 1972, p. 14), was written by J. Clark in 1744 and sold to visitors:

> … to our Governors, due praise be giv'n Who, by just care, have changed our Hell to Heav'n.
>
> A Hell on earth no truer can we find than a disturbed and distracted mind.
>
> … our learned Doctor gives his aid, and for his Care with Blessings ever paid, This all those happy Objects will not spare who are discharged by his Skill and Care.
>
> Our Meat is good, the Bread and Cheese the same, our Butter, … Beer and Spoon Meat none can blame. The Physic's mild, the Vomits are not such, But, thanks be prais'd, of these we have not much. Bleeding is wholesome, and as for the Cold Bath. All are agreed it many Virtues hath. The beds and bedding are both warm and clean, … Which to each comer may be plainly seen, Except those rooms where the most Wild do lie.

Excerpts such as these perhaps summarise how the general public felt about insanity, but did little except to deter them from being involved or to change their understandings of what it would be like to be ill in such a facility—they served only to make people wary of what insanity may mean or entail. Manning (1880) makes similar reference to conditions across the care offered in New South Wales in Australia, while Digby (1985, p. 4) takes up the issue of insanity having a marketable value:

> From the mid seventeenth century onwards, certain individuals began to make a living from insanity through the development of private madhouses. But it was not until the middle of the eighteenth century, when there was an appreciation that the mad could be managed, rather than brutalised, that different kinds of provision for the insane could develop.

Nolan (1993, p. 45) argues that the emergence of the asylum system in England was in response to threats posed by problems of the lower class, which involved both moral and paternalistic attitudes, and that there was an 'increasing power of the State over the lives of individuals in the mid-19th century. Although asylums wrapped their aims in medical rhetoric, as state-funded institutions their purpose was essentially social and lay in welfare administration'. Nolan (1993, p. 45) also stated

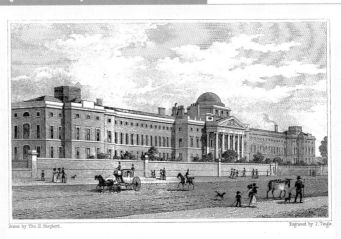

Figure 1.6   St Mary's of Bethlehem

Drawn by Tho. H. Shepherd.   Engraved by J. Tingle.

NEW BETHLEM HOSPITAL, ST. GEORGE'S FIELDS.

that the 'idealists who had hoped that the newly built institutions would be hospitals where mentally ill patients could be protected from the hostility of society, were rapidly disillusioned'. This idealist view went to the provision of care to those who were mentally ill in the 1800s and early 1900s in England. Scull (1979) proposes that social class may well have contributed to this issue, suggesting that humanitarian attitudes held by nineteenth-century upper-class Evangelicals and Benthamites were really the views that the dominant class had towards those lower down the social structure. Since the establishment of the asylums and the introduction of carers to work within them, attendant care (or nursing) has always found itself sandwiched between those in pursuit of scientific certainty in the diagnosis and treatment of mental disorder and those whose pragmatic approach to psychiatric institutions has seen them 'merely as centres for the dispensation of welfare [calling them workhouses]' (Nolan, 1993, p. 5) and the instigators of social control. These foundational benchmarks, whereby all institutions were locked and overseen by what were then called 'turnkeys' under the medical model regime, have probably set the scene for how mental health nursing is thought about and practised today in the UK, USA, Australia and New Zealand.

The role of the attendant from the start of the asylum system was determined initially by the medical profession who assumed responsibility for the selection, supervision and termination of employment of attendants, but also realised that the success of the asylum system was dependent on these attendants. In 1841, Dr Kirkbride from Pennsylvania Hospital for the Insane prepared a manual for attendants in which he spelt out the requirements for a good attendant. He spoke of a high moral character, a good education, strict temperance, kind and respectful manners, a cheerful and forbearing temper, with calmness under irritation, industry, zeal and watchfulness in the discharge of duty and above all sympathy that springs from the heart. Dr Kirkbride was forced to acknowledge that finding such upright individuals to work in asylums would not be easy. Further to these qualities for a good attendant came an interpretation of the role of attendant, which incorporated the attendant as a rule keeper, an enforcer, a servant to the patients, a spiritual guide and an intermediary between doctor and consumer.

Australian psychiatry was originally overseen by Frederic Norton Manning and written about by Tucker (1887). Manning sought advice from clinical practice overseas with the view of introducing to Australia what was thought to be good psychiatric practice. Good practice at that time was benchmarked on the medical control of asylums for the insane and was viewed by Lewis (1988, p. 27) as being instrumental in the setting up of 'specific training requirements of nursing staff'. Norton Manning, who was appointed as medical Superintendent of Tarban Creek Asylum in 1868, toured a range of asylums in Australia and internationally to see what was considered standard practice in psychiatric care in counterparts elsewhere.

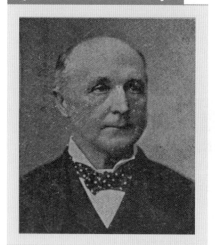

Figure 1.7   Frederic Norton Manning

Manning was particularly critical about the condition of the Parramatta asylum, suggesting that 'the buildings at Parramatta were utterly and completely unfit for the purpose for which they are at presently employed' (Manning, 1868, in Smith, 1999, p. 15). Manning argued further that no amount of money would render them adequate, and that the asylum should be abandoned and a new asylum be erected. Manning also suggested that many new asylums should be constructed in country areas and they should resemble what was on offer in England under the guidance of William Tuke at the York Retreat: a pioneering, more open, different, more recovery-based option that had the beginnings of a facility based on humanitarian principles.

1   How do you think psychiatry or mental illness as topics are represented in the media?

2   How do you think the past has contributed to the emergence of stigma experienced by people who are mentally ill?

3   What keeps that stigma alive and well today?

4   Did locked mental health facilities keep patients safe or were they designed to keep the general public safe?

By the end of the Second World War a range of pharmacological treatments had emerged, including a range of antipsychotics and antidepressants. The introduction of new pharmacological measures began gathering momentum in the 1950s and 1960s, and saw radical changes in the care and treatment of people with a mental illness. Pharmaceutical management meant that there was less reliance on physical restraint and increased opportunities for mental health nurses to engage with consumers therapeutically. The concept of the psychiatric hospital as a therapeutic community, where nurses took 'a personal interest in and formed a healthy relationship' with consumers (Sainsbury, 1968, p. 20), was incorporated into the education and training of mental health nurses. Education programs included the topics of psychology, psychiatric/mental health nursing, sociology and rehabilitation, as well as anatomy and physiology, medical and surgical nursing, and pharmacology. These programs moved away from what Sainsbury (1968) viewed as the previous authoritarian approach to the care of the mentally ill. The usage of medications allowed mental health care to emerge and complemented a range of skills given to mental health nurses through their specialist training. These centred on the therapeutic relationship and the development of working alliances with consumers, which assessed consumers along recovery-based principles that had improvement of overall functioning as its cornerstone. These new therapeutic strategies brought to the fore the theoretical approaches constructed by key mental health pioneers such as Hildegard Peplau and Joyce Travelbee, where mental health-care professionals began to see the merits of rapport building, empathy, understanding, keeping consumers safe, improving self-esteem, insight and milieu, plus employment-related activities as all foundational to recovery and moving consumers forward.

Aside from having a complementary relationship with the pharmacological regimes prescribed by the psychiatrist, these activities also added to the treatment options contained within the different Mental Health Acts (in both Australia and New Zealand), which included involuntary options for consumers that incorporated seclusion, or treatment strategies such as electro-convulsive therapy.

Peplau (1962) viewed mental health nursing as a therapeutic and interpersonal process, believing that the nurse–consumer relationship was the crux of mental health nursing. Through this relationship, the nurses use themselves as the therapeutic instrument or as travelling companions to consumers. That is, the nurse engages with

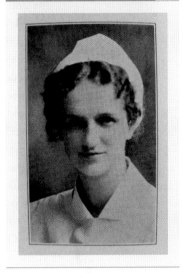

Figure 1.8   Hildegard Peplau

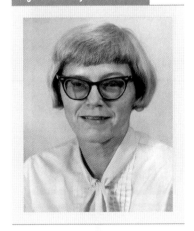

Figure 1.9   Joyce Travelbee

consumers through a variety of psychosocial interventions to facilitate personal growth on the part of the consumer. This concept moved the idea of nursing practice to one of 'being with' a consumer rather than 'doing things' to them. This last point implied a much more active and interactive dialogue between nurse and consumer (Barkway, 2009). Peplau (1962) also proposed the therapeutic relationship passed through a number of phases that evolved from the initial contact through to discharge. Peplau identified these phases as the orientation, working and resolution phases, and saw each stage as a building block to the consumer's recovery. In order to maximise their work with consumers, Peplau (1962) proposed that nurses assume a variety of roles at different times, in response to the emerging needs of the individual. The collective activities were arranged to produce the best possible outcome for the consumer despite, of course, not many consumers or their relatives enjoying some aspects of this treatment.

The anti-psychiatry movement came to the fore in the 1960s and was really a movement that questioned and challenged the fundamental claims and practice of mainstream psychiatry. This movement was promulgated on the basis that mental health treatments were thought to be ultimately more damaging than helpful to patients. Rather than being compassionate medical practice, it was seen as a coercive instrument of oppression and social control involving an unequal power relationship between doctor and consumer, and a highly subjective diagnostic process, leaving too much room for opinion and interpretation. R D Laing, Thomas Szasz and Michel Foucault all challenged the very basis of psychiatric practice and cast it as repressive and controlling. This movement incorporated a range of views promulgated via professional bodies, the mass media and myriad activist organisations. Laing, Szasz, Theodore Lidz and Franco Basaglia in varying ways argued that mental illness was best described as an inherently incoherent combination of medical and psychological concepts. These arguments opposed the use of psychiatry to detain and treat, or excuse what they saw as mere deviance from societal norms or moral conduct. Many other notable authors made contributions to this debate, including Erving Goffman, Gilles Deleuze and Félix Guattari, and Thomas Scheff, with these authors suggesting that

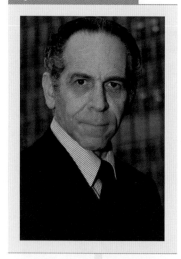

Figure 1.10 Thomas Szasz

psychiatry was variously stigmatising, an instrument of social control and an option that afforded the consignment of a label that people then often self-fulfilled, and was (because of these) morally wrong. The media influenced this movement and this influence was bolstered by the novel and film *One Flew Over the Cuckoo's Nest* (Kesey, 1962; Forman, 1975) where involuntary admission, involuntary treatment, lobotomy and shock therapy, plus the acerbic nature of Nurse Ratched, added weight to the arguments put forward by the anti-psychiatry movement. The image of Nurse Ratched (see Figure 1.13) as a jailor remains indelibly printed in the minds of many members of the public when they think about the role of mental health nurses.

Running concurrently with these issues was the increasing emphasis on the social rights of the individual, with statements regarding changes to health-care delivery generally—and mental health care in particular—being considered with an emphasis on every person suffering from a mental illness having their civil, political, economic, cultural and social rights recognised (as in the UN Universal Declaration of Human Rights) and protected by the various state and territory Mental Health Acts (*Mental Health Coordinating Council*, 2011). A range of authors alerted the mental health profession that change in mental health care was coming, with Holland (1978),

1 Is psychiatry an instrument of social control? Give two reasons to support your answer—agreeing or disagreeing.

2 When considering movies about mental illness, what role do you think this has in such things as stigma of, and discrimination towards mental illness and the mentally ill?

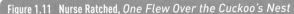

Figure 1.11 Nurse Ratched, *One Flew Over the Cuckoo's Nest*

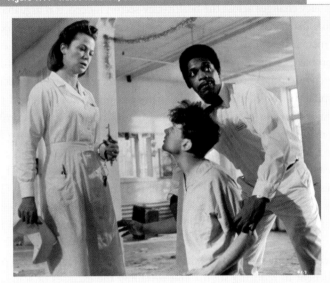

Habibis and colleagues (2003) and many others suggesting that mental health-care services outside hospitals was the future. The primary focus for mental health nurses at that time was perceived as containment and being focused on the behaviour of consumers as a response to the emotional and personality changes resulting from mental illness. Alchin and Weatherhead (1976) developed their text on mental health nursing with the premise that 'psychiatric nurses in training needed to know/ have a range of skills about what to do in specific situations which they would be confronted with in the ward environment and similarly, in the community' (Shea, 1976, p. i). The caring role of the mental health nurse was grounded in helping consumers deal with their reactions to the symptomatology of their illness (Alchin & Weatherhead, 1976).

The approach to care and the roles of mental health nurses continued to develop through deinstitutionalisation, the advent of nurse–independent practitioner roles, the prescribing options afforded some practitioners and the modifications made to the various Mental Health Acts (Australia and New Zealand), which endorsed a more community and recovery orientation to care. Case management and mainstreaming were both policy initiatives of the 1980s and 1990s, while a range of mental health strategies and the Burdekin and Richmond reports in Australia shifted the practice of mental health nursing care away from the traditional institutions. The promise of the Burdekin report was that the dollars would follow the consumer from institution to the community. Those in clinical practice at the time know that this wasn't the case and many patients moved from the asylum to unsupported bedsits or makeshift shelters. This shift for some did provide what might be described as reasonable acute care in medically oriented services within a few hospital settings as part of their deinstitutionalisation, and embodied the rhetoric of what Burdekin called improved community oriented and supported service provision. However, this was not the trajectory for far too many who tried to fend for themselves once this health reform came into place. Many nurses also found these changes difficult, which slowed the acceptance of these policy changes across the health-care sector; indeed, it is arguable that they still have some way to go before being totally accepted by current practitioners (Sharrock & Happell, 2000) as this push by public mental health services to 'mainstream' the care of individuals experiencing mental illness has had its problems. This health reform means the provision of services for people who are mentally ill are treated within the current general health system rather than in a specialist mental health, publicly funded hospital. In consideration of this, many comprehensively trained nurses who provide care to these individuals tend not to have a wide-ranging understanding of the problems and needs of people experiencing mental health problems (Sharrock & Happell, 2000; Fleming & Szmukler, 1992). Consequently, many nurses tend to avoid in-depth contact with people/patients experiencing mental health problems because of fear and a sense of powerlessness due to a knowledge gap. This feeling of powerlessness goes to preparation of skills (Happell & Platania-Phung, 2004; Gillette, Bucknell & Meegan, 1996). This is obviously an area for improvement in the current health-care system and not what the architects of deinstitutionalisation and mainstreaming had in mind when these schemes were introduced.

While these policies initially promulgated the role of the general practitioner in providing treatment, and also had some benefit in reducing stigma and curtailing the excesses of some treatment practices in the older, more isolated, stand-alone mental health facilities, more broadly they have been a failure. 'Mainstreaming' as a term is full of rhetorical promise, but the reality produces a range of what might be described as unintended consequences. The mainstreaming of mental health service reform in the 1990s tends to miss the unique needs of individuals suffering mental illness and does not fully appreciate and provide for these people with regard to access to services. This last point has led to a secondary marginalisation of mentally ill people in general health services.

CRITICAL THINKING OPPORTUNITY

1   What do you think nursing care contributes to reducing discrimination against people with mental illness?

2   What are the factors to consider in your assessment of this question?

Caring and the mental health nurse

As Happell (2007) points out, the history of mental health nursing differs significantly from that of other branches of nursing. For example, there is the clear influence of iconic figures such as Florence Nightingale and Lucy Osborne on the development of nursing services in the colonies (Bessant, 1999). Historically, the care of people with mental illness has been a completely different matter. Caring attitudes and actions cannot be specifically defined or prescribed—they depend on the unique circumstances surrounding each event because caring is always/should always be understood within a context (Warelow, 1996). For example, if technical expertise is needed, then knowledgeable technical care is experienced as caring. Similarly, curative methods of practice can and should be harnessed under a more caring framework, because before caring behaviours can be displayed there must be a combination of the personal values, ideas and beliefs to which the carer is committed, as well as his/her cognitive and technical competencies (Shiber & Larson, 1991). For mental health nursing, this means that personal qualities must be fused with nursing skills.

Benner (1984) emphasises the ability of the expert nurse to be able to combine these components in daily practice. Her premise is that experience allows nurses to move through stages from novice to expert based on developing experience (using an intuitive base), rather than relying on formal theoretical models. Benner advocates that a mental health nurse should be able to notice problems, suggest solutions and implement strategies, with each case cared for on the merits and contextual circumstances at play. Some might call this intuition, but others say it is a learnt or constructed skill (Peck, 2013).

The mental health nurse must then, as part of nursing care, evaluate the effectiveness of the strategies used; that is, the nurse's 'commitments to the client as a person could/should take precedence over the nurse's commitment to the client's treatment goals' (Morse et al., 1990, p. 10). Another difficulty for the mental health nurse in forming an interpersonal relationship with consumers is the call by peers to avoid personal involvement. For many health-care professionals, personal involvement conflicts with the traditional view of remaining objective and is therefore considered unprofessional in some quarters. Health professionals share the concept that failure of objectivity decreases the accuracy of diagnosis, the correctness of treatment decisions and the success rate of procedures (Curzer, 1993). Looking at the concept from the consumer's perspective, a transpersonal or interpersonal relationship could still present problems, such as in a situation where the consumer dislikes the nurse, as this must be preclusive to developing rapport and moving into successful nurse–consumer relationships. Some consumers are embarrassed by the intrusive invasion of privacy often necessary in nursing treatments, and for their own self-esteem prefer the mental health nurse to focus on the task rather than themselves. These consumers may resent the need to become an object of significant emotional attachment in order to receive care (Curzer, 1993).

When a person is asked what they do for a living, it is common to hear them refer to their position title; for example, 'I am a nurse'. Explaining what a nurse does is usually described in terms of their place of employment, specific tasks or functions, who they work with and perhaps examples of their work. What people are actually describing is their role (Hercelinskyj, 2010). Caring is argued to be an activity that is central to the role of nurses generally (Henderson et al., 2007; Watson, 1988) and the term 'caring' could almost be said to be interchangeable with the term 'nursing'. The caring role of nurses in mental health has also been explored, with Warelow and Edward (2007) suggesting that the demands of mental health nursing today extend well beyond the more traditional skills of care and caring; and that in order to meet mental health needs in the twenty-first century, caring should be extended to encompass the additional expertise of emotional intelligence, praxis and resilience. Emotional intelligence, praxis and resilience have the potential to assist individuals to transcend negative experiences and transform these experiences into positive self-enhancing ones. This has implications for improved consumer outcomes through role-modelling and educational processes, but also may hold implications in supporting a strong workforce in mental health nursing into the future.

PHILIP WARELOW

Generally speaking, caring in nursing is in itself not that hard to do. However, with changes to the nurse role, educational preparation and the effects of community-based care—which means dealing with more acutely mentally ill consumers and having a quicker turnover of consumer numbers—the caring role is becoming more complicated and confounded by myriad day-to-day circumstances that come into play related to the context of the care required. Some argue that the ability to care is inherited and then often built on via parents and other close loved ones; others suggest consistency in caring; while still others suggest caring can be taught (Dunlop, 1986). I suggest here that caring is not simply a set of identifiable attitudes or rules such as sympathy or support; nor does it comprise all that nurses do. Instead, as Morse and colleagues (1990) suggest, caring combines both attitudes with action in the carer's commitment to maintaining a person's dignity and integrity. Nursing care is determined by the way a nurse is able to use knowledge and skills to appreciate the uniqueness of the consumer, and physically and emotionally assist and apply this knowledge and skill to the individual merits and intricacies of the particular circumstances. For example, if someone is unconscious we physically care for and about the consumer and/or their family and friends. Similarly, if our consumer is anxious we care for them and their family in a more emotionally supportive way to overcome their anxiety. In this sense, caring will always be fundamentally variable across a range of differing yet similar themes.

Florence Nightingale advanced the view that nurses needed to assist patients and put them in the best place to allow nature to work and heal (Nightingale, 1863). Orem (1991) also encouraged nurses to promote self-care and to help people to help themselves—working with patients instead of for them. This shift is significant from the traditional approaches. Barker and Buchanan-Barker (2006) likewise suggest that we should begin recovery from day one of treatment and that consumers need to be instrumental in their own care; and thus nursing care along these lines is more 'doing with' than 'doing to'. This type of care invests in the consumer and this investment empowers the consumer throughout the illness–health continuum. This would mean that the many different theories attached to the formats in which care takes place actually change how care is delivered—with care also being modified on multiple perspectives outside of the practitioners who deliver it (Stockdale & Warelow, 2000). McCormack and colleagues (2002) suggest that we all should blend these types of care options and base the delivery of care within the context of the circumstances in which people and their nurses find themselves.

By not responding to the relationship, will consumers compromise the care they receive or deny themselves good-quality care? The concern here is that if a relationship is not built, or seen as important by the consumer, the nurse or the educational sector, then surely this has implications for therapeutic potential in consumer outcomes. Caring for another involves a level of emotional labour on the part of the carer—in this case, the mental health nurse. A study undertaken by Sourdif (2004) suggests that satisfaction at work and satisfaction with administration are the best predictors of intent to stay at a particular nursing job. Use of self, including the emotional self, is important in establishing a therapeutic nurse–consumer relationship, but carries the risk of burnout or vicarious trauma if prolonged or intense (Sabin-Farrell & Turpin, 2003). Caring in mental health nursing is complex and requires clear boundaries while forging an alliance with consumers to facilitate an intimate dialogue of often extremely sensitive personal information.

The modern mental health nurse uses the self and their history in therapeutic interactions. We call this using emotional intelligence, which in many ways is what we encourage our consumers to adopt in relation to their mental health issues (Warelow, 2005; Sánchez-Álvarez et al., 2016). The therapeutic use of self involves using aspects of yourself—such as your personality, experience, knowledge of mental illness, and life skills—as a way of developing and sustaining the therapeutic relationship with consumers. A consumer needs to feel trust and safety in order to disclose sensitive information about himself or herself to another person; importantly, the consumer may not have spoken about this sensitive material to another person before. Therefore, the beginnings of the therapeutic alliance/relationship are critical to the establishment and maintenance of the caring relationship. This therapeutic alliance between the mental health nurse and the consumer is one that can be emotionally charged and often challenging for the mental health nurse. The modern demands of mental health nursing requires nurses to draw on the skills of resilience to meet the needs of direct consumer care within the framework of a therapeutic alliance (Edward & Warelow, 2005; McQueen, 2004; Cleary, Jackson & Hungerford, 2014).

The research literature also demonstrates that consumers value the therapeutic potential of the nurse–consumer partnership. Key elements are identified as clear communication, empathy, trust and cultural sensitivity. Concerns are also raised with regard to consumer autonomy; notably, that there be an absence of any coercion (Gilburt, Rose & Slade, 2008; Langley & Klopper, 2005; Williams & Irurita, 2004). While it appears that consumers share a similar view as to the importance of the mental health nurse's caring role, Norman and Ryrie (2009) believe that the caring role and identity of the mental health nurse has been shaped by two distinct and at times conflicting traditions in relation to their caring role. These arguments centre on the 'artistic interpersonal relations tradition' of mental health nursing—in which the therapeutic relationship assumes the central position in relation to how mental health nurses enact their role—and the 'scientific tradition with the delivery of evidence-based interventions that can be applied with good effect' (Norman & Ryrie, 2009, p. 1537). Within mental health nursing, Gournay (1995, 1996) dismissed psychoanalytic understandings and nursing knowledge, such as Peplau's ideas (1962), as outdated relics, presumably because they were not supported by empirical evidence. Gournay argued that community mental health nurses needed to embrace specific knowledge, such as information processing theory, neuropsychology and attribution theory, to meet local context needs, and simultaneously be 'sensitive and responsive to the needs of individual users and their carers and families' (Gournay, 1995, p. 14). However, he appeared to qualify his remarks regarding the biological model when he stated that the biological approach is one approach to the care and treatment of people living with mental illness and cannot be divorced from other models, but that 'a humane approach to all patients, regardless of the problem, must be paramount' (Gournay, 2006, p. 345).

There are also a number of other factors that create or perpetuate tensions in relation to the caring role of mental health nurses. These factors relate to the stigma attached to mental illness and the association of nurses with such an area of health, the perceived image of mental health nurses and the overreliance on the medical model at the expense of broader psychosocial responses (Hazelton et al., 2011). Another factor is role conflict created by the tension between legislative requirements related to the treatment of people experiencing mental ill health and the expectations of mental health nurses based on their professional socialisation and education.

Authors such as Halter (2002) and Humble and Cross (2010) suggest that the role and identity of mental health nursing is inextricably linked to psychiatry and public perceptions of mental illness, which remain largely stigmatised (Adewuya & Oguntade, 2007; Halter, 2002; Overton & Medina, 2008). Additionally, health professionals are no less likely to share stigmatising views than the general population towards people living with mental illnesses (Björkman, Angelman & Jonnsen, 2008; Rao et al., 2009). The public does hold perceptions about who nurses are and what they do. Some researchers have hypothesised that these social perceptions, together with media representations and professional attitudes, converge and stigmatise mental health nurses through a negative association with mental illness (Aber & Hawkins, 1992; Bridges, 1990; Brodie et al., 2004; Fiedler, 1998; Gordon, 2001; Kalisch, Kalisch & McHugh, 1980; Takase, Maude & Manias, 2006).

Morrall (1998) and Morrall and Muir-Cochrane (2002) have drawn attention to what they describe as the fundamental issue that impacts on the caring role of mental health nurses. This is the constant tension between the therapeutic intent of the mental health nurse's role and interaction with consumers, and the legislative demands that govern involuntary admission and enforced treatment of the seriously unwell. Continuous changes to the economic policy and legislative mandates of varying governments and, increasingly, better-informed health-care consumers (Hardy & Hardy, 1988) can create role conflict for the nurse because there is a dissonance between the professional nursing role and competing organisational requirements, fiscal considerations and legislative demands (with one often getting in the way of the others).

Hazelton and colleagues (2011) also argue that the medical model remains the dominant focus of health-care policy. This dominance on curing and concomitant reliance on pharmaceutical treatments relegates broader approaches to working with consumers to a more marginal or adjunct status (Hazelton et al., 2011). This view is reinforced by an experienced mental health nurse who argues that mental health nurses are all working with a narrower skill and knowledge base, fewer role models and more of a focus on the medical model that is the predominant paradigm in the world of mental health; further, there's been a huge shift away from anything that's psychotherapeutic (Hercelinskyj, 2010).

Clearly, mental health nurses need to learn from history or in some ways be cognisant of what it means and entails. In this, history needs to inform what we do now, where mental health nursing learns by its mistakes. Further, those who hold the purse strings and those who make uninformed policy decisions that have no relevance to contemporary practice need to recognise errors made and move this profession in a new direction. This new direction needs to learn from history and provide quality care for those it is there to help.

CRITICAL THINKING OPPORTUNITY

1   Why is it important to learn about the history of caring in mental health nursing's development as a discipline?

2   Is care the same for an anxious consumer as someone anxious about a fractured neck or femur?

3   How does this knowledge assist you in developing an understanding of the mental health nurse's caring role and any tensions within this role?

Some commentators have argued that mental health nursing has been experiencing an identity crisis (Holmes, 2006). This crisis has been brought about by a whole series of factors, including bio-medicalisation and education issues, and these have led to a steady decline in graduate numbers of those showing interest in mental health nursing and the subsequent recruitment and retention of staff. History clearly demonstrates that the significant decline in numbers of graduates coming into this speciality area of nursing practice, with 6434 females in clinical practice and 6058 males in Victoria in 2002 (Nurses Board of Victoria, 2002). These figures, which have not improved over the intervening years, clearly highlight that in Australian and New Zealand there have been significant and poorly thought-out changes to the ways in which mental health nurses are recruited and educated. The trajectory of these changes was sealed over 25 years ago, when professional nursing organisations expressed support for a change to 'comprehensive' courses located in the tertiary education sector. With the benefit of hindsight, these decisions have been instrumental in the deleterious position of mental health nursing today.

The future for mental health nursing is to clearly define and take ownership of nursing's contribution to the treatment and recovery of people who are mentally ill. This should be done by demonstrating this contribution through professional, empathic and informed in-depth practice and research to provide evidence for practice (Beaton, Mann & Grigg, 2011). Also important is to harness assessment and care practice to an obligation and responsibility for each nurse to improve both the quality of the person-to-person care that is such a hallmark of nursing, as well as to positively influence the system that delivers it. History allows us to look back at what has gone before with the hope that we collectively learn from past experience and grow in this process. We suggest that changes need to be made to how we recruit, educate, promote and retain mental health nurses, and to acknowledge that their skills are vital in the care offered to those who are ill. Change can be difficult, but inputs from consumer movements in both Australia and New Zealand are offering new conceptualisations of what is mental illness and, because of this, different ideas about how to treat those who are mentally ill. History itself may be used to the overall advantage of nursing in mental health care. Using the words of Churchill: the further backward you can look, the further forward you can see.

SUMMARY

The history of care for people diagnosed with mental illness is poorly recorded and therefore poorly understood. The contribution that nurses have made, and continue to make, to the care of people with mental illnesses in Australia and New Zealand has largely been ignored. The literature that does exist primarily relates to the history of psychiatric services, with nursing only considered in a subsidiary capacity. Historical notions of madness were associated with deviance and punishment. These views had a significant impact on the attitudes towards the mentally ill, their treatment and their recovery.

Contemporary public perceptions of the role of the mental health nurse have been shaped by media representations, together with prevailing social attitudes towards mental illness. These views can stigmatise those who are mentally ill and those who nurse the mentally ill through their association with mental ill health.

Regardless of clinical context, caring in nursing is both an attitude and an active interpersonal process between the nurse and consumer. Tensions between the therapeutic intent of mental health nursing practice and factors such as legislative demands, government policy and fiscal imperatives continue to challenge the way in which mental health nurses practise. Changes to mental health nursing education, recruitment and retention are required to improve the deleterious position of mental health nursing today. Nolan (1993, 4) suggests the biggest issue of all for mental health nursing is whether it can survive.

PHILIP WARELOW

DISCUSSION QUESTIONS

1 Traditionally, 'out of sight and out of mind' appears to have been a major consideration in the containment and treatment of people who were deemed to be mentally ill. Why was this?

2 Australian and New Zealand institutions were carbon copies of treatment sites from other countries, particularly Great Britain. Was this a good strategy for these colonies?

3 If mental illness can be effectively treated, shouldn't this mean that stigma should also disappear in line with successful treatment options? Think about the role of stigma—does it serve more than one purpose?

4 What progress in regard to mental health care have we made in the last two hundred years? Reflect on your insights.

5 What progress in regard to mental health care have we made in the last ten years? Reflect on your insights.

TEST YOURSELF

1 What skills do you feel best reflect the role of a nurse in treating someone presenting at an emergency department with a mental illness?

  a Cool, calm and collected

  b Inquisitive, insistent and detached

  c Friendly and warm

  d Understanding, reassuring and knowledgeable

2 Who initially oversaw building up of Australian psychiatry?

  a Frederic Norton Manning

  b William Tuke

  c Henry Maudsley

  d Thomas Szasz

3 In what year was St Mary's of Bethlehem built in London?

  a 1434

  b 1247

  c 1286

  d 1178

4 In what year were the documents known as Te Tiriti O Waitangi signed by the British Crown and the Māori Chiefs?

  a 1852

  b 1799

  c 1865

  d 1840

USEFUL WEBSITES

20/20 Hindsight—A history of the Mental Health Legal Centre: www.communitylaw.org.au/clc_mentalhealth/cb_pages/images/20_20_Hingsight_Final.pdf

ABC Adelaide—Inside Glenside: A history of mental health in Adelaide: www.abc.net.au/local/photos/2011/05/11/3213910.htm

The Porirua Hospital Museum—History: http://www.poriualibrary.org.nz/Heritage/History-of-Porirua-City-Centre--Elsdon-and-Takapuwahia/History-of-health-care-in-Porirua

The Time Chamber—The history of the asylum: http://thetimechamber.co.uk/beta/sites/asylums/asylum-history/the-history-of-the-asylum

REFERENCES

Aber, C. S., & Hawkins, J. W. (1992). Portrayal of nurses in advertisements in medical and nursing journals. *IMAGE Journal of Nursing Scholarship*, *24*(4), 289–293.

Adewuya, A. O., & Oguntade, A. A. (2007). Doctors' attitudes towards people with mental illness in Western Nigeria. *Social Psychiatry & Psychiatric Epidemiology*, *42*(11), 931–936.

Alchin, S. C., & Weatherhead, R. G. (1976). *Psychiatric nursing: A practical approach*. Sydney: McGraw-Hill Book Company.

Awty, P. (2013). Personal conversation. Federation University, Ballarat, Victoria, Australia.

Barker, P., & Buchanan-Barker, P. (2006). *The tidal model: A guide for mental health professionals*. New York: Routledge.

Barkway, P. (2009). Theories on mental health and illness. In R. Elder, K. Evans & D. Nizette (Eds.), *Psychiatric and mental health nursing* (2nd ed.) (pp. 119–133). Sydney: Elsevier.

Beaton, T., Mann, R., & Grigg, M. (2011). Future directions. In K-L Edward, I. Munro, A. Robins & A. Welch (Eds.), *Mental health nursing: Dimensions of praxis*. Melbourne: Oxford University Press.

Benner, P. (1984). *From novice to expert: Excellence and power in clinical nursing practice*. Menlo Park: Addison-Wesley.

Bessant, B. (1999). Milestones in Australian nursing. *Collegian*, *6*(4), i–iii.

Björkman, T., Angelman, T., & Jönsson, M. (2008). Attitudes towards people with mental illness: A cross-sectional study among nursing staff in psychiatric and somatic care. *Scandinavian Journal of Caring Sciences*, *22*(2), 170–177.

Bostock, J. (1968). *The dawn of Australian psychiatry*. Glebe: Australasian Medical Publishing Company Ltd.

Bradley, P., & De Souza, R. (2013). Mental health in Australia and New Zealand. In R. Elder, K. Evans & D. Nizette (Eds.), *Psychiatric and mental health nursing* (3rd ed.). New South Wales: Mosby, Elsevier Australia.

Bridges, J. M. (1990). Literature review on the images of the nurse and nursing in the media. *Journal of Advanced Nursing*, *15*(7), 850–854.

Brodie, D. A., Andrews, G. J., Andrews, J. P., Thomas, G. B., Wong, J., & Rixona, L. (2004). Perceptions of nursing: Confirmation, change and the student experience. *International Journal of Nursing Studies*, *41*(7), 721–733.

Carpenter, M. (1986). Asylum nursing before 1914: The history of labour. In C. Davies (Ed.), *Rewriting Nursing History*. London: Croom Helm.

Cleary, M., Jackson, D., & Hungerford, C. L. (2014). Mental health nursing in Australia: Resilience as a means of sustaining the specialty. *Issues in Mental Health Nursing*, *35*(1), 33–40.

Curzer, H. (1993). Is care a virtue for health care professionals? *Journal of Medicine and Philosophy*, *18*, 51–69.

Digby, A. (1985). *Madness, morality and medicine: A study of the York Retreat, 1796–1914*. Cambridge: Cambridge University Press.

Dunlop, M. (1986). Is a science of caring possible? *Journal of Advanced Nursing*, *11*(6), 661–670.

Edward, K. L., & Warelow, P. (2005). Resilience: When coping is emotionally intelligent. *Journal of the American Psychiatric Nurses Association*, *11*(2), 101–102.

Elder, R. (2009). Settings for mental healthcare. In R. Elder, K. Evans & D. Nizette (Eds.), *Psychiatric and mental health nursing*. Sydney: Elsevier.

Fiedler, L. A. (1998). Images of the nurse in fiction and popular culture. In A. H. Jones (Ed.), *Images of nurses, perspectives from history, art and literature* (pp. 100–112). Philadelphia: University of Pennsylvania Press.

Fleming, J., & Szmukler, G. I. (1992). Attitudes of medical professionals towards patients with eating disorders. *Australian and New Zealand Journal of Psychiatry*, *26*, 436–443.

Forman, M. (Writer) (1975). *One flew over the cuckoo's nest*. M. Douglas (Producer). USA: United Artists.

Gilburt, H., Rose, D., & Slade, M. (2008). The importance of relationships in mental health care: A qualitative study of service users' experiences of psychiatric hospital admission in the UK. *BMC Health Services Research*, *8*(92). Retrieved from www.biomedcentral.com/1472–6963/8/92.

Gillette, J., Bucknell, M., & Meegan, E. (1996). *Evaluation of psychiatric nurse consultancy in emergency departments project*. Victoria: RMIT Bundoora, Faculty of Nursing.

Gordon, S. (2001). Nurses speaking out about what they do. *Australian Nursing Journal*, *9*(3), 46–47.

Gournay, K. (1995). Training and education in mental health nursing. *Mental Health Nursing*, *15*(6), 12–15.

Gournay, K. (1996). Mental health nursing: Issues and roles. *Advances in Psychiatric Treatment*, *2*(3), 103–108.

Gournay, K. (2006). Psychiatric/mental health nursing: Biological perspectives. In J. R. Cutcliffe & M. F. Ward (Eds.), *Key debates in psychiatric/mental health nursing* (pp. 344–355). Edinburgh: Churchill Livingstone, Elsevier.

Grant, A. (2006). Undergraduate psychiatric nursing education at the crossroads in Ireland. The generalist vs. specialist approach: Towards a common foundation. *Journal of Psychiatric and Mental Health Nursing*, *13*(6), 722–729.

Habibis, D., Hazelton, M., Schneider, R., Davidson, J., & Bowling, A. (2003). Balancing hospital and community treatment: Effectiveness of an extended-hours community mental health team in a semi-rural region of Australia. *Australian Journal of Rural Health*, *11*(4), 181–186.

Halter, M. J. (2002). Stigma in psychiatric nursing. *Perspectives in Psychiatric Care*, *38*(1), 23–29.

Happell, B. (2007). Appreciating the importance of history: A brief historical overview of mental health, mental health nursing and education in Australia. *International Journal of Psychiatric Nursing Research*, *12*(2), 1439–1445.

Happell, B., & Platania-Phung, C. (2004). Mental health issues within the general health care system: Implications for the nursing profession. *Australian Journal of Advanced Nursing*, *22*(3), 41–47.

Hardy, M. E., & Hardy, W. L. (1988). Role stress and role strain. In M. E. Hardy & M. E. Conway (Eds.), *Role theory: Perspectives for health professionals* (Vol. 2). Connecticut: Prentice Hall.

Hazelton, M., Rossiter, R., Sinclair, E., & Morrall, P. (2011). Encounters with the 'dark side': New graduate nurses' experiences in a mental health service. *Health Sociology Review*, *20*(2), 172–186.

Henderson, A., Van Eps, M. A., Pearson, K., James, C., Henderson, P., & Osborne, Y. (2007). 'Caring for' behaviours that indicate to patients that nurses 'care about' them. *Journal of Advanced Nursing*, *60*(2), 146–153. doi: 10.1111/j.1365–2648.2007.04382.x.

Hercelinskyj, G. (2010). Professional identity in mental health nursing and the implications for recruitment and retention. Unpublished PhD thesis, Charles Darwin University.

Holland, J. (1978). New health body to take over. *The Age*, 6 December. Retrieved from Google News.

Holmes, C. A. (2006). The slow death of psychiatric nursing: What next? *Journal of Psychiatric and Mental Health Nursing*, *13*(4), 401–415.

Humble, F., & Cross, W. (2010). Being different: A phenomenological exploration of a group of veteran psychiatric nurses. *International Journal of Mental Health Nursing*, *19*(2), 128–136.

Hunter, R., & McAlpine, I. (1974). *Three hundred years of psychiatry*. London: Oxford University Press.

Hunter, R., & McAlpine, I. (1992). Trained for what? A history of mental nursing and its training. *History of Nursing Journal*, *4*, 131–142.

Jones, K. (1972). *A history of the mental health services*. London: Routledge & Kegan Paul.

Kalisch, B. J., Kalisch, P. A., & McHugh, M. (1980). Content analysis of film stereotypes of nurses. *International Journal of Women's Studies*, *3*(6), 531–558.

Kesey, K. (1962). *One flew over the cuckoo's nest*. New York: Viking.

Langley, G. C., & Klopper, H. (2005). Trust as a foundation for the therapeutic intervention for patients with borderline personality disorder. *Journal of Psychiatric and Mental Health Nursing*, *12*(1), 23–32.

Lewis, M. (1988). *Managing madness: Psychiatry and society in Australia 1788–1980*. Canberra: Australian Government Publishing Service, Dordrecht.

Manning, F. N. (1880). The causation and prevention of insanity. *Journal of the Royal Society of NSW*, *14*, 340–355.

McCormack, B., Kitson, A., Harvey, G., Rycroft-Malone, J., Titchen, A., & Seers, K. (2002). Getting evidence into practice: The meaning of 'context'. *Journal of Advanced Nursing*, *38*(1), 94–104.

McQueen, A. C. H. (2004). Emotional intelligence in nursing work. *Journal of Advanced Nursing*, *47*(1), 101–108.

Mental Health Coordinating Council, (2011) *Mental Health Rights Manual: a consumers guide to the legal and human rights of people with mental illness in NSW*. Retrieved from http://www.healthinfonet.ecu.edu.au/key-resources/promotion-resources?lid=22624.

Morrall, P. (1998). Speaking out … when psychiatrists and nurses refuse to acknowledge their role as agents of social control they fuel public resentment and media panic. *Nursing Times*, *94*(19), 15.

Morrall, P., & Muir-Cochrane, E. (2002). Naked social control: Seclusion and psychiatric nursing in post-liberal society. *Australian e-journal for the Advancement of Mental Health*, *1*(2), 101–112.

Morse, J. M., Solberg, S. M., Neander, W. L., Bottorff, J. L., & Johnson, J. L. (1990). Concepts of caring and caring as a concept. *Advances in Nursing Science*, *13*, 1–14.

Nightingale, F. (1863). Looking back. Taken from 'Notes on Hospitals' by Florence Nightingale, 1863. *The Lamp*, *36*(8), 39–43.

Nolan, P. (1986). Mental nurse training in the 1920s: The history of a Nursing Group at the Royal College of Nursing. *Bulletin*, *10*, 17–23.

Nolan, P. (1990). The servant, the poet and the doctor: An example of 18th century psychiatric care. *History of Nursing Journal*, *3*(2), 3–13.

Nolan, P. (1993). A *history of mental health nursing*. London: Chapman and Hall.

Norman, I., & Ryrie, I. (2009). The art and science of mental health nursing: Reconciliation of two traditions in the cause of public health. *International Journal of Nursing Studies*, *46*(12), 1537–1540.

Nurses Board of Victoria (2002). *Review of Mental Health/Psychiatric Nursing: Components of the Undergraduate Nursing Program*. Discussion Paper. Melbourne.

O'Donoghue, E. G. (1913). *The story of Bethlehem Hospital from its foundation in 1247*. London: T. Fisher Unwin.

Orem, D. E. (1991). *Nursing: Concepts of practice* (4th ed.). St. Louis: Mosby-Year Book Inc.

Overton, S. L., & Medina, S. L. (2008). The stigma of mental illness. *Journal of Counseling and Development*, *86*(2), 143–151. Electronic version, retrieved 25 January 2008 from EBSCOHost Database.

Peck, B. (2013). Hermeneutic constructivism: An ontology for qualitative research. Unpublished PhD thesis, University of Ballarat.

Peplau, H. E. (1962). Interpersonal techniques: The crux of psychiatric nursing. *American Journal of Nursing*, *62*(6), 50–54.

Porirua Hospital Museum (n.d.). *The origins of mental health care in New Zealand and Wellington*. Retrieved from www.poriruahospitalmuseum.org.nz/history.

Rao, H., Mahadevppa, H., Pillay, P., Sessay, M., Abraham, A., & Luty, J. (2009). A study of stigmatized attitudes towards people with mental health problems among health professionals. *Journal of Psychiatric and Mental Health Nursing*, *16*(3), 279–284.

Russell, R. (1983). Mental physicians and their patients. Unpublished PhD thesis, Sheffield University, England.

Sabella, D., & Fay-Hillier, T. (2014). Challenges in mental health nursing: Current opinion. *Nursing: Research and Reviews*, *4*, 1–6.

Sabin-Farrell, R., & Turpin, G. (2003). Vicarious traumatization: Implications for the mental health of health workers? *Clinical Psychology Review*, *23*(3), 449–480.

Sainsbury, M. J. (1968). *Psychiatry for students* (vol. 1). Sydney: Shakespeare Head Press.

Sánchez-Álvarez, N., Extremera, N., & Fernández-Berrocal, P. (2016). The relation between emotional intelligence and subjective well-being: A meta-analytic investigation. *Journal of Positive Psychology*, *11*(3), 276–285.

Scull, A. (1979). *Museums of madness: The social organization of insanity in nineteenth century England*. London: Allen Lane.

Sharrock, J., & Happell, B. (2000). The role of the consultation-liaison nurse in the general hospital. *Australian Journal of Advanced Nursing*, *18*, 34–39.

Shea, P. (1976). Foreword. In S. C. Alchin & R. G. Weatherhead, *Psychiatric nursing: A practical approach*. Sydney: McGraw-Hill Book Company.

Shiber, S., & Larson, E (1991). Evaluating the quality of caring: Structure, process, and outcome. *Holistic Nursing Practice*, *5*(3), 57–66.

Shorter, E. (1997). *A history of psychiatry: From the era of the asylum to the age of Prozac*. New York: John Wiley & Sons, Inc.

Smith, T. (1999). *Hidden heritage: 150 Years of public mental health care at Cumberland Hospital, Parramatta 1849–1999*. Sydney: Western Sydney Area Health Service.

Sourdif, J. (2004). Predictors of nurses' intent to stay at work in a university health center. *Nursing & Health Sciences*, *6*(1), 59–68.

Stockdale, M., & Warelow, P. (2000). Is the complexity of care a paradox? *Journal of Advanced Nursing*, *31*(5), 1258–1264.

Stuhlmiller, C. (2005). Rethinking mental health nursing education in Australia: A case for direct entry. *International Journal of Mental Health Nursing*, *14*(3), 156–60.

Takase, M., Maude, P., & Manias, E. (2006). Impact of the perceived public image of nursing on nurses' work behaviour. *Journal of Advanced Nursing*, *53*(3), 333–343.

Tucker, G. A. (1887). *Lunacy in many lands*. Sydney: Charles Potter, Government Printers.

Ward, I. (2001). Registered Psychiatric Nurse, personal interview, 24 May.

Warelow, P. (1996). Is caring the ethical ideal? *Journal of Advanced Nursing*, *24*, 655–661.

Warelow, P. (2005). The significance of gender to Australian psychiatric nursing. Unpublished PhD thesis, James Cook University.

Warelow, P., & Edward, K. L. (2007). Caring as a resilient practice in mental health nursing. *International Journal of Mental Health Nursing*, *16*, 132–135.

Watson, J. (1988). *Nursing: Human science and human care: A theory of nursing*. New York: National League for Nursing.

Williams, A. M., & Irurita, V. F. (2004). Therapeutic and non-therapeutic interactions: The patient's perspective. *Journal of Clinical Nursing*, *13*, 806–815.

Wood, P., Bradley, B., & De Souza, R. (2009). Mental health and wellness in Australia and New Zealand. In R. Elder, K. Evans & D. Nizette (Eds.), *Psychiatric and mental health nursing* (pp. 93). Sydney: Elsevier.

CHAPTER 2

Diagnostic Systems Used in Clinical Assessment

KAREN HARDER, IAN MUNRO AND ANNETTE WOODHOUSE

Acknowledgment

The authors would like to acknowledge Alan Robins who co-wrote this chapter in the first edition. We would also like to acknowledge Nick Gaynor who passed away during the writing of this chapter.

KEY OUTCOMES

AFTER READING THIS CHAPTER, YOU SHOULD BE ABLE TO:

- describe the classification systems used to diagnose mental illness
- identify the clinical features of mental illness identified in a mental status examination
- describe the factors incorporated into a psychiatric assessment
- identify the clinical features of risk in psychiatry
- identify therapeutic interventions for assessment in a multicultural society
- define the skill set required by the assessing mental health nurse.

KEY TERMS

- complementary alternative medicine (CAM)
- comprehensive psychiatric assessment
- *Diagnostic and Statistical Manual of Mental Disorders* (DSM)
- diagnostic overshadowing
- Health of the Nation Outcome Scales (HoNOS)
- *International Classification of Diseases* (ICD)
- mental status examination (MSE)
- risk
- risk assessment
- risk management
- risk plan
- WHO Disability Assessment Schedule (WHODAS)

Introduction

This chapter introduces you to the classification categories and diagnostic instruments used to assess the mental health or illness of a consumer. Within the scope of this chapter we focus on the clinical features of mental illness, and the instruments and skills required by the mental health nurse to undertake a comprehensive psychiatric assessment.

The clinical context

The predominant clinical roles of the mental health nurse are to assess consumers' mental health needs and offer therapeutic support. Mental health nurses conduct their practice in myriad clinical settings, including:

- general practice surgeries
- crisis assessment and treatment teams
- emergency response teams
- community mental health teams
- forensic services
- aged persons' mental health services
- acute hospital settings
- speciality services for consumers with eating disorders or postpartum difficulties
- child and adolescent mental health services.

To ensure optimum service provision for each consumer, the mental health nurse conducts an initial mental status examination (MSE) to assess immediate needs and risks before undertaking a comprehensive biopsychosocial assessment (that is, an assessment of the biological, psychological and social domains of the person's life). A comprehensive psychiatric assessment allows the mental health nurse to formulate a holistic care plan (Varcarolis & Halter, 2010), which informs the basis of the multidisciplinary team approach to assist the consumer over the course of recovery (Barker, 2009). An examination of a consumer's mental state is undertaken when a consumer has initial contact with any mental health service and at each therapeutic encounter. It can occur within a variety of settings, such as an accident and emergency department, a general surgical ward, the office of a case manager working within a community mental health team or in the consumer's own home.

There are two different classification systems that mental health nurses use to assist in the diagnosis of mental disorders: the *International Classification of Diseases* (ICD) and the *Diagnostic and Statistical Manual of Mental Disorders* (DSM). These systems of diagnosis and classification are based upon the understanding of the symptomatology, pathophysiology, natural history of the human condition, neurosciences and genetic linkages, allowing mental health practitioners to identify discrete disorders (American Psychiatric Association, 2013; Saunders, 2006).

Sadock and Sadock (2007) suggest that the signs and symptoms of mental illness have changed; they make the point that in the DSM various disorders have altered and diagnostic categories have changed over various editions. The fifth edition of the DSM (DSM 5), which is produced by the American Psychiatric Association (APA), is commonly used in the USA, Australia and New Zealand, while the ICD 10 is produced by the World Health Organization (WHO) and is mainly used in Europe. Historically, the lack of uniformity between the DSM and the ICD classification systems has contributed to confusion with regard to the terms used and diagnosis generated. To ease this situation, collaboration between the DSM task force and the collaborators for ICD 11 (due to be published in 2017) has aligned key areas with regard to organisational structure and coding of disorders to assist in promoting clarity in the assessing and diagnosing process (American Psychiatric Association, 2013).

It is important for students and clinicians to have an awareness of how these two systems work, given that both systems can be encountered in the clinical environment.

International Classification of Diseases

The International Classification of Diseases (ICD) is divided into 'blocks' of disorders; these blocks of disorders have subdivisions to further define the disorders. To illustrate this point, consider the blocks indicated below (Videbeck, 2009, p. 5).

- F00–F09 Organic, including symptomatic, mental disorders
- F10–F19 Mental and behavioural disorders due to psychoactive substance use
- F20–F29 Schizophrenia, schizotypal and delusional disorders
- F30–F39 Mood (affective) disorders
- F40–F48 Neurotic, stress-related and somatoform disorders
- F50–F59 Behavioural syndromes associated with physiological disturbances and physical factors
- F60–F69 Disorders of adult personality and behaviour
- F70–F79 Mental retardation
- F80–F89 Disorders of psychological development
- F90–F98 Behavioural and emotional disorders with onset usually occurring in childhood and adolescence
- F99 Unspecified mental disorders.

Diagnostic and Statistical Manual of Mental Disorders

The fifth edition of the *Diagnostic and Statistical Manual of Mental Disorders* (known as DSM 5) was published in June 2013 after a lengthy review and consultation with key stakeholders. Sadock and Sadock (2007) highlight the fact that the DSM's various disorders and diagnostic criteria have altered over each edition; the reallocation of diagnostic labels from DSM-IV to DSM 5 can be observed in Table 2.1.

The DSM 5 has taken a broad approach to dividing the disorders to include *externalising* and *internalising clusters*. Externalising clusters can include 'disorders with predominant impulsive, disruptive conduct and substance use symptoms', while internalising clusters are 'disorders predominant with anxiety, depression and somatic complaints' (American Psychiatric Association, 2013, p. 13). Additional changes observed in DSM 5 include a lifespan approach across each diagnostic category that aims to facilitate a more inclusive approach to diagnosis, so co-morbid risk factors—including age, gender, culture, and social and lifestyle practices—can be included to inform the assessment process (American Psychiatric Association, 2013). The multiaxial system that was observed in DSM-IV has now been removed, with the American Psychiatric Association (2013) suggesting the 'multiaxial system was not required to make a … diagnosis' (p. 16).

The American Psychiatric Association (2013) indicates that the Z codes from the ICD-10 CM (Clinical Modification) should be used by clinicians when problems in the consumer's psycho-social and environmental domains are identified. Therefore, clinicians should continue to utilise a broad range of assessment tools (as discussed in this chapter) to identify the consumer's diagnosis and document any co-morbid medical conditions. They should also utilise the WHO Disability Assessment Schedule (WHODAS), which is a standard method for assessing the overall level of disability for the consumer (American Psychiatric Association, 2013); this is discussed later in this chapter. The WHODAS replaces the Global Assessment Functioning (GAF) scale used in the DSM-IV.

TABLE 2.1 A DIAGNOSTIC CLASSIFICATION COMPARISON BETWEEN DSM-IV AND DSM 5

DSM-IV	DSM 5
Disorders usually first diagnosed in infancy, childhood and adolescence	Neurodevelopmental disorders
	Elimination disorders
Delirium, dementia and amnestic and other cognitive disorders Mental disorders due to a general medical condition	Neurocognitive disorders
Substance-related disorders	Substance-related and addictive disorders
Schizophrenia and other psychotic disorders	Schizophrenia spectrum and other psychotic disorders
Mood disorders	Bipolar-related disorders
	Depressive disorders
Anxiety disorders	Anxiety disorders
	Obsessive-compulsive and related disorders
Somatoform disorders	Somatic symptoms and related disorders
Factitious disorders	Somatic symptoms and related disorders
Dissociative disorders	Dissociative disorders
Sexual and gender identity disorders	Gender dysphoria
	Sexual dysfunctions
	Paraphilic disorders
Eating disorders	Feeding and eating disorders
Sleep disorders	Sleep–wake disorders
Impulse control disorders not elsewhere classified	Disruptive, impulsive-control and conduct disorders
Adjustment disorders	Trauma and related stressor-related disorders
Personality disorders	Personality disorders
Other conditions that may be the focus of clinical attention	

Mental status examination

The mental status examination (MSE) is a process designed to assess objectively the mental state of a consumer, and is defined by Elder, Evans and Nizette (2013) as a 'semi-structured interview … to assess a person's current neurological and psychological status using several domains, such as perception, affect, thought content, thought form and speech' (p. 528). Obtaining a comprehensive assessment depends on the interview skills of the mental health nurse. These skills are influenced by each nurse's personality, level of skill and knowledge base, and when combined with the consumer's individual concerns, each interview becomes unique in context, timing and sequencing.

The MSE highlights the consumer's current difficulties while informing the provision of collaborative care and treatment planning (Gamble & Brennan, 2006). When used within the continuum of care, it provides a baseline for identifying the presence, acuity and impact of symptoms on the consumer's ability to complete their daily activities. It also assists in the formulation of a diagnosis, the monitoring of the consumer's fluctuating mental state in the presence of psychosocial stressors, and the evaluation of the consumer's responsiveness to treatments (Sadock & Sadock, 2007).

Essential components of the MSE

The Australian national competency standards for the registered nurse (Australian Nursing and Midwifery Council, 2006) supports the use of multiple assessment techniques to ensure accuracy of assessment (see Table 2.2).

TABLE 2.2 MSE ASSESSMENT FOR THE REGISTERED NURSE

MSE component	Method of assessment	Associated terminology
Appearance	Observation/interview	Dishevelled, unkempt
General behaviour	Observation	Restless, agitated, hostile, guarded, catatonic, cooperative
Speech	Observation/interview	Pressured, poverty of speech, mute, stuttering
Mood	Interview	Depressed, anxious, euphoric, labile, euthymic
Perception	Observation/interview	Hallucinations, illusions
Memory	Interview	Long- and short-term memory
Orientation	Interview	Oriented to the right time/place/person
Thought	Interview/observation	Delusions/thought insertions/poverty of thought
Judgment	Interview/observation	Disinhibition/compulsions
Insight	Interview	Concordance/adherence
Motor activity	Interview/observation	Mania/depression
Intelligence	Interview	Education/knowledge/IQ

Each of the MSE components is now discussed in turn.

- *Appearance.* The mental health nurse assesses the consumer's overall appearance. Is the consumer dressed appropriately for the climate or circumstance and/or for their stated age? Does the consumer look dishevelled, childlike or bizarre? Posture, grooming and attention to hygiene are noted.
  For example: The male consumer is dishevelled, wearing stained, torn clothing, unkempt facial hair, with body odour evident, and with matted greying hair.

- *General behaviour.* Both quality and quantity of movement are assessed by the mental health nurse. Are there any tics, or is there hyperactivity, agitation, restlessness, wringing of hands or evidence of psychomotor retardation?
  For example: The consumer is slumped in the chair, with evidence of psychomotor retardation on entering the room.

- *Speech.* The quality, rate, volume and tone of speech are assessed. Speech may be rapid, pressured, slow, monotonous or whispered. Accents and stuttering may also be evident.
  For example: The consumer's speech is slow and monotonous.

- *Mood.* The consumer's enduring emotional state is described. The term 'affect' is the external expression of the consumer's emotional state. Mood may be described as happy, sad, depressed, euphoric, anxious or angry. Mood can be labile: rapidly changing from laughter one moment to tearfulness and distress the next.

  For example: The consumer's mood is depressed.

- *Thought content and process.* Do the consumer's stated thoughts make any sense? Are the ideas linked and can you follow the consumer's interactions easily? Common terms used to describe thought content and process include delusions, flight of ideas, thought blocking, poverty of thought and tangential.

  For example: The consumer has a firm and false belief that he is the 'son of God'.

- *Perception.* This refers to the presence of illusions and/or hallucinations. Common terms include derealisation and depersonalisation.

  For example: The consumer reports hearing voices.

- *Cognition.* The mental health nurse assesses the consumer's intelligence, abstract thought, insight and judgment. Factors assessed include alertness; orientation to time, place and person; concentration; memory; general knowledge; abstract reasoning; and arithmetical abilities.

  For example: When assessing cognition it is usually assessed across the domains of short-term memory (STM) and longer-term memory (LTM). When assessing STM the three-item recall test is used. For example, when a consumer aged 80 years old was assessed, she was unable to identify and accurately recall two items, indicating to the clinician that further advanced cognitive testing was required to assist assess her area of cognitive decline.

- *Insight.* The mental health nurse assesses the consumer's understanding of their illness and recommended treatments.

  For example: This is usually assessed across the areas of good, partial or poor (also referred to as being 'insightless'). An example of poor insight is when the consumer refuses to accept their diagnosis while frequently being non-adherent to associated treatment recommendations to assist in their recovery.

- *Judgment.* Can the consumer establish the likely consequences resulting from their actions or adapt to a new environment?

  For example: If a consumer has bipolar affective disorder and is in the manic phase with grandiose beliefs, their judgment is significantly impaired. Due to the consumer's grandiose beliefs, they cannot understand that when they stand on the train tracks, the train will not stop for them. The likely consequence of the consumer's impaired judgment is that they will be killed upon impact.

The psychiatric assessment

A comprehensive psychiatric assessment encompasses the areas given in detail below. When combined with the mental status examination (Epstein et al., 2007; Sadock & Sadock, 2007), it forms a holistic assessment of the consumer to identify areas of unmet needs, symptoms of mental illness and supports to be utilised in collaborative care and treatment planning.

The comprehensive psychiatric assessment

- *Reason for referral.* Why is the consumer here now? Who referred the consumer? What assessments have already been completed? What are the consumer's, family's and carer's reasons for seeking assessment?
- *Current living situation.* Who lives with the consumer? What is the location of residence and type of residence (owned, rented or no fixed abode)?
- *Presenting problem.* What are the consumer's presenting problems? The consumer will describe their experiences and associated distress. The mental health nurse will acknowledge, paraphrase, reflect, validate, clarify and summarise the consumer's concerns, leading to a hypothesised diagnosis, which is confirmed via the completed MSE and associated specialised screening tools.
- *History of the presenting problem.* The consumer describes the duration and impact of their difficulties in social, educational or occupational areas. The mental health nurse obtains a chronological order of symptom presentation where possible. Has the consumer experienced similar difficulties before and, if so, what strategies worked? What were the previous treatments? When and by whom were they finished?
- *Family history.* Is there a family history of mental illness, drugs and/or alcohol abuse or other serious medical conditions? If so, which family members were affected, what was the illness, were there any periods of hospitalisations, what was the treatment, and what was the impact upon the other family members? The use of genograms will illustrate the quality of the relationship: is the relationship between the consumer and their parent or parents a positive influence, characterised by closeness, support and understanding? Or is it distant, hostile and frequently demanding?
- *Personal history:*
  - *Preschool.* Was there any delay in the consumer's developmental history; any separation difficulties? What is the consumer's earliest memory of preschool?
  - *Schooling and education.* What is the consumer's highest level of achievement? Were there any incidences of bullying? What has been the consumer's ability to form and maintain friendships? Were there attendance and/or behavioural difficulties? Were there any suspensions, expulsions or multiple changes of schooling?
  - *Occupational history.* What is the consumer's current occupation and the duration of that position? Have they undergone job changes or disruptive experiences in the work environment? If the consumer is not employed, how do they utilise the day?
  - *Sexual history.* Does the consumer have a current partner or spouse? Has the consumer had multiple sexual partners? Is the consumer using safe sexual practices or at increased risk of sexually transmitted infections (STIs) and associated conditions?
- *Children and parenting.* Does the consumer have any children? What are the ages of the children? What is the consumer's experience of parenting children? Have there been any miscarriages or deceased children? Is there shared parenting? If so, is it a cooperative arrangement? Are there access arrangements or protection orders?
- *Forensic history.* Is the consumer engaged in any criminal activity? Does the consumer have any convictions, pending charges or upcoming court appearances?
- *Previous or current illness.* Does the consumer have any previous or current medical conditions and/ or associated treatments that may have an impact on the current presentation? Review the pathology

results and other organic testing results. Does the consumer have any previous psychiatric diagnosis and/or treatment? Did the consumer adhere to treatments recommended? Access previous medical records if available.

- *Personality.* Does the consumer have a premorbid personality? How does the consumer describe themselves? How do members of the family or carers describe the consumer?
- *Safety and risks.* Does the consumer have cuts or scars that have been caused by deliberate self-harming behaviours? These may often be observed on the forearms, thigh or chest area of the consumer. Does the consumer have a stated suicide plan to harm themselves or others? Does the consumer have direct access to means to harm himself, herself or others? Is the consumer displaying slurred speech and have they potentially overdosed before assessment?
- *Substance use or misuse.* Is the consumer intoxicated by alcohol and/or drugs or other substances? Have they an unsteady gait, slurred speech or signs of withdrawal, or are puncture marks evident from intravenous use? Complete a urine drug screen (UDS), blood alcohol concentration (BAC) and pathology screening to confirm assessment findings.

See Table 2.3 for a method to record a psychiatric history and MSE systematically.

TABLE 2.3   HOW TO MAKE A SYSTEMATIC RECORD OF A PSYCHIATRIC HISTORY AND MSE
Introducing (consumer's name and age) .... years old of .... background *(assessment of English or use of interpreter required)* admitted at ...... hours under section ...... of the *Mental Health Act*. *(Copy of rights given and explained in appropriate language)*
Arrived via .... *(ambulance or police or accompanied by family or friends)*
Presenting problems or symptoms .... *(Document MSE and symptom duration)*
Symptoms exacerbated by .... *(Assessment of stressors, precipitating factors or non-adherence to treatment, and drug and alcohol use)*
Risk assessment .... *(Suicidal/self-harm/aggression/drug or alcohol withdrawal/AWOL)*
Previously admitted to .... *(Name of hospital, when, diagnosis and context)*
Previous or current case manager .... *(Name of clinician, service name and contact number, previous and current treatments)*
Consumer lives with .... *(Significant others, work associates, and education activities)*
Physical conditions, allergies and/or pathology results .... *(Treatments)*
Current medication(s) .... *(Assess adherence and attitude towards role of medications, side effects and past medications)*
Level of nursing observations required .... *(Rationale for same)*
Immediate nursing plan .... *(F/up next shift)*
Next of kin notified of admission..

Clinical risk assessment, management and positive therapeutic risk

Recognising and managing clinical risk is an essential component of mental health nursing practice (Downes et al., 2016; Higgins et al., 2015a; Higgins et al., 2015b; Muir-Cochrane et al., 2011) and one of the critical tasks of a mental health service. The significance role of managing clinical risk is reflected in national mental health protocols, polices and standards (New South Wales Government, 2016; Stokes, 2012; Victorian Department of Health, 2010; Western Australia Department of Health, 2008). Table 2.4 is a suicide risk assessment guide offered as an example of a clinical tool used in the assessment of suicide risk from the state of New South Wales, Australia.

While documents such as these offer relevant guidance to clinicians, there is a wide variation in approaches to managing risk (Higgins et al., 2016). Mental Health Professional Online Development (MHPOD) is a Commonwealth-funded, evidence-based online learning resource that offers an excellent introduction to risk assessment and management for beginning clinicians and workers in mental health (see the 'Useful websites' section at the end of this chapter).

MHPOD provides a succinct definition of risk assessment and management:

- A risk assessment typically has several components, and focuses on identifying the type of harm that may occur, the time frame and circumstances in which it may occur, and the likelihood that it may occur.
- Risk management aims to identify appropriate steps to reduce risks, action these steps, and review the outcomes (MHPOD, 2016).

Approaches to understanding risk

There are three main approaches to understanding risk (Higgins et al., 2015a, Higgins et al., 2015b):

- *Unstructured clinical judgement.* Based upon nurses' 'intuition' or 'gut feeling' (Doyle & Dolan, 2002) or clinicians' experiences (Harris & Lurigio, 2007).
- *Actuarial approaches.* Include the use of widely used validated assessment tools, such as the Historical-Clinical-Risk-20 scale (HCR 20), the Violence Risk Appraisal Guide (VRAG) and the Psychopathy Checklist-Revised (PCL-R) to predict risk (Jaber & Mahmoud, 2015).
- *Structured clinical judgment.* Combines the previous two approaches and is considered by many as the preferred method (Higgins et al., 2016).

Research highlights the imperative to not only undertake risk assessments but also to translate these into practical nursing approaches. This includes communicating and documenting the management of risk with consumers and, wherever possible, family, carers or significant others and interdisciplinary team members (Higgins et al., 2015a; Higgins et al., 2015b; Higgins et al., 2016). Similar to nursing care planning and management being based upon prior nursing assessment processes, clinical risk management needs to be assessed, planned and reviewed on an ongoing basis with consumers to reflect the complexities of their needs and the dynamic nature of risk. A risk plan is the integration of our clinical risk assessments and consultation processes with consumers, family, carers or significant others, interdisciplinary team members and other relevant people (such as general practitioners and non-government support services) to create, communicate and implement specific strategies to manage risk within a collaborative approach. This plan includes a set of actions, allocates responsibilities to specified clinicians and defines the time frames or frequencies for this to occur.

KAREN HARDER, IAN MUNRO AND ANNETTE WOODHOUSE

TABLE 2.4 SUICIDE RISK ASSESSMENT GUIDE

Suicide Risk Assessment Guide

To be used as a guide only and not to replace clinical decision-making practice.

Issue	High risk	Medium risk	Low risk
'At risk' Mental State - depressed - psychotic - hopelessness, despair - guilt, shame, anger, agitation - impulsivity	Eg. Severe depression; Command hallucinations or delusions about dying; Preoccupied with hopelessness, despair, feelings of worthlessness; Severe anger, hostility.	Eg. Moderate depression; Some sadness; Some symptoms of psychosis; Some feelings of hopelessness; Moderate anger, hostility.	Eg. Nil or mild depression, sadness; No psychotic symptoms; Feels hopeful about the future; None/mild anger, hostility.
Suicide attempt or suicidal thoughts - intentionality - lethality - access to means - previous suicide attempt/s	Eg. Continual/specific thoughts; Evidence of clear intention; An attempt with high lethality (ever).	Eg. Frequent thoughts; Multiple attempts of low lethality; Repeated threats.	Eg. Nil or vague thoughts; No recent attempt or 1 recent attempt of low lethality and low intentionality.
Substance disorder - current misuse of alcohol and other drugs	Current substance intoxication, abuse or dependence.	Risk of substance intoxication, abuse or dependence.	Nil or infrequent use of substances.
Corroborative history - family, carers - medical records - other service providers/sources	Eg. Unable to access information, unable to verify information, or there is a conflicting account of events to that of those of the person at risk.	Eg. Access to some information; Some doubts to plausibility of person's account of events.	Eg. Able to access information / verify information and account of events of person at risk (logic, plausibility).
Strengths and Supports (coping & connectedness) - expressed communication - availability of supports - willingness / capacity of support person/s - safety of person & others	Eg. Patient is refusing help; Lack of supportive relationships / hostile relationships; Not available or unwilling / unable to help.	Eg. Patient is ambivalent; Moderate connectedness; few relationships; Available but unwilling / unable to help consistently.	Eg. Patient is accepting help; Therapeutic alliance forming; Highly connected / good relationships and supports; Willing and able to help consistently.
Reflective practice - level & quality of engagement - changeability of risk level - assessment confidence in risk level.	Low assessment confident or high changeability or no rapport, poor engagement.		- High assessment confidence / low changeability; - Good rapport, engagement

No (foreseeable) risk: Following comprehensive suicide risk assessment, there is no evidence of current risk to the person. No thoughts of suicide or history of attempts, has a good social support network.

Is this person's risk level changeable? **Highly Changeable** ☐ Yes ☐ No

Are there factors that indicate a level of uncertainty in this risk assessment? Eg: poor engagement, gaps in/or conflicting information. **Low Assessment Confidence** ☐ Yes ☐ No

Framework for Suicide Risk Assessment and Management for NSW Health Staff NSW Health

Included with permission. ©NSW Department of Health 2004

The dynamic nature of risk assessment and management

Management plans must take into account the consumer's changing circumstances over time, and therefore incorporate the following parameters of risk:

- *Static risk factors (past).* These factors inform clinicians about a consumer's baseline functioning or long-term risk and include historical factors that don't change over time, such as personal history, past history of risk or violence, substance use problems, relationship instability, mental illness and family history.
- *Dynamic risk factors (present).* These factors focus on a consumer's ability (or that of their environments) to manage risk. These factors can be internal or external to consumers, are more dynamic, tend to fluctuate and move the risk from a consumer's baseline functioning—for example, clinical acuity or stability, irritability, lack of insight, being unresponsive to treatment, impulsivity, threats, active substance abuse, confusion, violent thoughts, agitation, treatment adherence and therapeutic alliance, active psychotic symptoms and current psychosocial stressors (Allnutt et al., 2010).

As stated, risk is dynamic and is directly connected to consumers' lives, their circumstances and unforeseen events. Therefore, risk assessment needs to take into account both short-term and long-term time frames and be reviewed in an ongoing basis as part of regular nursing care. For example, consumers at moments of transition—such as moving from one part of a mental health service to another (an inpatient setting to community follow-up) or being discharged from the mental health service to other follow-up (general practitioner or a non-government organisation)—are particularly vulnerable, and therefore at risk, at these times (Higgins et al., 2016). Engagement with consumers (and their families where possible), careful collaborative monitoring of previous risk management plans for effectiveness, and assessing any changes in risk and the need for new strategies is required to individualise care and minimise risk during times of transition.

Risk is also contextual. Mental health nurses practise in a variety of clinical settings that influence the degree of autonomy the consumer has in decision-making. The onus is on the mental health nurse, via duty of care, to ensure safety and the management of risk. The clinical assessment and management of risk are core competencies required of the mental health nurse, and must be adapted to the social context of the consumer. Caring for someone in their own home environment poses a different set of risks and responsibilities than those posed when caring for a hospitalised consumer in a locked ward, an emergency department or a staffed residential facility.

While there is debate about the use of risk assessment tools in relation to their potential negative impact on engagement with consumers (Downes et al., 2016), applicability to a consumer's needs (Webb, 2012), role in the control of consumers (Clancy, Happell & Moxham, 2015; Crowe & Carlyle, 2003) and suggested lack of research evidence (Wand, Isobel, & Derrick, 2015), their use has been shown to be effective alongside clinical judgment (Woods, 2013). Higgins and colleagues' (2016) statement that, 'Risk assessment tools are there to support, rather than replace, clinical judgements' (p. 391) succinctly summarises contemporary thinking in nursing risk assessment. In addition, it is acknowledged that no risk assessment is flawless (Allnutt et al., 2013; Webb, 2012) and risk itself will never be completely eliminated (Allnutt et al., 2010; Wrycraft, 2015).

CRITICAL ⁂ THINKING OPPORTUNITY

One of the authors of this chapter has practised as a mental health nurse practitioner in a rural child, adolescent and family mental health service. This context created many complexities for practice in relation to geographical isolation, and limited access to professional development and clinical supervision. Consultation with interdisciplinary colleagues was essential to support professional accountability and responsibility—including risk management, clinical decision making and reflective practice—to ensure the delivery of the best practice nursing care for consumers and their families. This interdisciplinary consultation process with colleagues is considered best practice in the management of risk (Higgins et al., 2016).

Recovery-oriented nursing practice: Positive therapeutic risk

The assessment and management of risk is complex (Gilbert, Adams & Buckingham, 2011). Higgins and colleagues (2016) propose traditional approaches to assessing risk have primarily focused only on harm by a consumer to themselves or others by suicide, self-harm or violence. Higgins and colleagues (2015a) suggest expanding these traditional understandings of risk to consider additional factors, such as sexual vulnerability, partner violence, financial exploitation, victimisation, harassment from the public, self-neglect, adverse drug reactions and '"iatrogenic risks" or risks posed to service users as a result of their engagement with the mental health service' (Higgins et al., 2015a, p. 166).

An attitudinal shift is also called for in national framework documents for recovery-oriented mental health services (Commonwealth of Australia, 2013) to embed recovery principles into clinical practices. In addition, the need to embrace the recovery paradigm has been highlighted. Implications for nursing practices to become recovery-oriented have been discussed (Clancy et al., 2015; Lemon, Stanford & Sawyer, 2016; Muir-Cochrane et al., 2011; Wand et al., 2015), suggesting a shift in traditional thinking about clinical risk to ensure:

- That consumers themselves are involved in risk assessment processes (Woods, 2013).
- The vital role family members play in supporting consumers in managing their own risk is recognised (Higgins et al., 2015a).
- The language we use in talking about and documenting risk is recovery-oriented and does not alienate consumers. For example, embracing new terminology and replacing the language of clinical risk with positive risk or therapeutic risk (Higgins et al., 2016).

Downes et al. (2016) offer useful guidance for the overall focus of recovery-oriented nursing practices:

> the role of the nurse in this context [recovery-oriented mental health practice] is to work with risk, in ways that balance risks with opportunities and support service users to actively participate in making informed decisions about risk in ways that enable their personal development, learning, autonomy and self-determination while minimizing harmful consequences (p. 194).

TOPIC LINK ■

See Chapter 6 for more on the recovery paradigm.

Recovery-oriented approaches for the clinician undertaking a comprehensive risk assessment

Best practice principles for risk assessment and safety planning for nurses (Higgins et al., 2015b), detailed below, provide a recovery-oriented approach that is inclusive of protective factors for consumers. It is suggested that this approach be used by clinicians to complete a risk assessment with consumers—and, wherever possible, family, carers or significant others—at the points of:

- initial assessment/admission to an inpatient unit
- clinical review
- transfer
- discharge
- as clinically indicated, such as when a consumer is showing signs of clinical deterioration in mental or physical health status.

The following risk factors should be considered when assessing the level of risk, noting that these prompts are neither prescriptive nor exhaustive.

Risk classification and protective factors

According to Higgins and colleagues (2015b), risk can be classified into the four categories, which can be mitigated by three types of protective factors.

Risk classification and examples

- Risk the person experiencing the mental health issue may pose to themselves.
- Risk the person experiencing the mental health issue may pose to others.
- Risk others may pose to the person experiencing the mental health issue.
- Risk to the person from engaging with the mental health system or what can be termed 'iatrogenic risks'.

Examples of risk to self:

- Deliberate or unintentional harm to self-suicide, self-harm (including repetitive self-injury), self-neglect and substance misuse.
- Loss of social and financial status arising from mental health status such as loss of employment, loss of accommodation, loss of supports (family/friends/other relationships), loss of custody of children, loss of reputation.
- Risks to physical, psychological and sexual health as a result of engaging in risk behaviours, such as substance misuse, sexual risk behaviours.

Examples of risk to others:

- Violence, aggression, verbal or physical assault.
- Sexual assault or abuse, harassment, stalking or predatory intent.
- Property damage including arson.
- Neglect or abuse of children or adults for whom care is being provided.
- Behaviour that could be thought of as reckless or high risk to others, such as drink driving.

Examples of risk from others:

- Physical, sexual and emotional abuse by others.
- Financial abuse or neglect by others.
- Victimisation and harassment (in own home and public: name calling, having objects thrown, having offensive graffiti written on the walls).
- Being treated unfairly in the workplace.
- Losing accommodation or having difficulty getting accommodation.

Examples of iatrogenic risk:

Risk to the person from engaging with the mental health service may be associated with:

- Diagnosis and labelling.
- Erosion of identity and self-esteem, loss of autonomy and voice, institutionalisation.
- Stigma and discrimination.
- Emotional trauma associated with detention, seclusion, restraint.
- Negative attitudes and controlling behaviours of staff.
- Violation of human rights.
- Health problems associated with side effects of medication.
- Experiencing harassment within the service.

Protective factors

- Personal: Capacity and willingness to understand distress; sense of potential to change; level of optimism, self-esteem, sense of personal control; ability to use adaptive coping mechanisms; communication and assertiveness skills; willingness to talk about emotions and feelings; previous positive experience of managing crisis and risk potential; collaboratively agreed crisis plan.
- Support networks: Family support (and willingness/ability to access such support); friends and other networks (eg., work colleagues/religious groups/social media/volunteering); interests and activities; involvement in the community; other important attachments (eg., pets, gardening); engagement with mental health services; previous positive experiences of engaging with services during periods of crisis.
- Environmental: Living in stable accommodation; having financial security; availability, acceptability, diversity and flexibility of mental health service; availability and accessibility of informal mental health supports (eg., peer support, advocacy groups etc.).

Higgins, A., Morrissey, J., Doyle, L., Bailey, J., & Gill, A. (2015b). *Best Practice Principles for Risk Assessment and Safety Planning for Nurses working in Mental Health Services*. Reproduced with permission.

Professional development, education and training

Training in risk assessment, particularly related to suicide, is essential. One example of such training is the Applied Suicide Intervention Skills Training (ASIST; see the 'Useful websites' section at the end of this chapter), which has been utilised by many public mental health services and other relevant organisations, such as the police force within Australia. This is an evidence-based, in-depth, two-day training workshop developed in Canada. It is designed to develop skills in risk recognition, intervention and management.

Research indicates education and training on clinical risk needs to include an understanding of how to approach risk assessment, the tools involved, protective factors for consumer and how to teach nurses skills to engage with families while including them in the process (Higgins et al., 2015b). In addition, an understanding of positive risk-taking practices, and addressing concerns related to perceived conflicts between the use of risk assessment tools and our therapeutic engagement with patients, has been identified as important in training (Downes et al., 2016).

Organisational support in managing risk

Organisational support, via training, policy, procedures and guidelines, underpins all risk management activity. A variety of tools and training has been designed to assist organisations and clinicians in policy formulation when assessing degrees of risk via clinical practice guidelines. In addition, services often design their own tools to align practice guidelines to localised policies. Many have built-in prompts for the clinician that ensure relevant questions are asked and further details established as risks are identified or diminish. Accurate documentation and communication of risk to all concerned are crucial, and form part of the management plan.

While an emphasis has been placed on risk assessment in relation to the consumer's needs, there is also an essential requirement under occupational health and safety (OH&S) legislation for mental health nurses to practise in safe work environments. The prevention of the risk of aggression and violence in the workplace is an issue that requires constant attention, vigilance and commentary from our profession. Again, all organisations are mandated to develop supporting policies and procedures that guide mental health nurses' practice, based on the parameters of risk. Adherence by all staff to all measures designed to identify, eliminate and manage risk in the workplace is mandated by the OH&S legislation.

■ TOPIC LINK
See Chapter 20 for more on managing consumers' aggression, de-escalation skills and staff training.

ABOUT THE CONSUMER Cari's story

You are working in the accident and emergency department, and have been given the following triage information on the consumer that you are about to assess:

> Cari is a 28-year-old female and parent of two children, Benji and Samantha aged eight and four years. She has been living in a women's refuge centre after recently leaving her partner in the context of a long history of domestic violence. Cari reports this history included multiple physical, emotional and sexual assaults on her. Cari attempted suicide at the refuge, which was witnessed by her two children. She has limited social support apart from the refuge worker who has brought her to the assessment. Cari was previously admitted to an interstate mental health service with a diagnosis of depression and anxiety, and does not have a current general practitioner. She is nervous about the assessment and feels guilty about the impact of her suicide attempt upon her children.

REFLECTION QUESTIONS

1   What are the legal and ethical issues that the mental health nurse needs to address for Cari and her family?

2   What issues do you imagine you would encounter when assessing Cari, given her recent suicide attempt, history of domestic violence and feelings of nervousness and guilt?

3   Which areas of the psychiatric assessment, MSE and risk assessment might require further investigation?

4   What preliminary diagnosis would you make, given Cari's presentation?

5   What initial nursing interventions would you recommend for Cari? Her children? Her refuge worker as an identified support person?

6   What issues and risks might you encounter in assessing and developing a management plan for Cari and her family?

KAREN HARDER, IAN MUNRO AND ANNETTE WOODHOUSE

Therapeutic skills in the assessment process

Mental health nursing has a rich history of the therapeutic use of self, built upon the seminal work of nursing theorist Hildegard Peplau (D'Antonio, 2014; Peplau, 1952; Shattell, Starr & Thomas, 2007). The importance of developing a good working therapeutic relationship or alliance with consumer and, where relevant, their families is essential to all aspects of nursing care. A strong therapeutic relationship with the consumer enhances treatment outcomes and facilitates a shared understanding of the situation, while identifying strengths and potential barriers to treatment (Happell et al., 2008).

The first step in meeting a consumer is to engage with them to begin developing a therapeutic relationship to work collaboratively together through the issues they have presented with. Without this engagement, any attempts to assess aspects of nursing care—including clinical risk—are limited, as an alliance with the consumer has not yet been formed.

Consumers presenting to mental health services are often in distress. The role of the mental health nurse is to alleviate this distress by offering care and compassion in addition to specialised skills in the assessment and treatment of clinical risk. Essential skills of empathy, genuineness and unconditionally accepting a person, as taught by the influential psychologist Carl Rogers (Rogers & Dorfman, 1951), allow the therapeutic relationship to develop and enhance the assessment and management of a consumer's care, including clinical risk. MHPOD offers further information and resources on developing a therapeutic relationship (MHPOD; see 'Websites' at the end of this chapter).

Mental health nurses are in a privileged position of working closely with a vulnerable and marginalised consumer group while joining with families and carers on a journey of finding meaning from this experience. Adherence to professional standards also aids therapeutic engagement by providing a safe and consistent approach to service delivery.

Clinical risk within the wider context of mental health nursing

Clinical risk assessment and management sits within the wider context of mental health nursing knowledge and skills; for example, establishing a therapeutic relationship with consumers, assessing, planning and implementing consumer care (inclusive of physical and mental health needs) and utilising evidenced-based treatments. Recent work by the Victorian Department of Health (2013) on nursing observation provides a valuable guide for care that is trauma-informed, and gender and culturally sensitive to supplement skills previously outlined.

In addition, the Australian Commission on Safety and Quality in Health Care (2012) standards on clinical handover and recognising and responding to deterioration in mental state offers practical guidance and resources for nurses dealing with these issues in their everyday practice. Best practice clinical handover and recognising the deteriorating in a consumer's mental state is a critical component of nursing care and linked to understanding and assessing clinical risk within a comprehensive assessment process.

Figure 2.1 illustrates the richness of this nursing context.

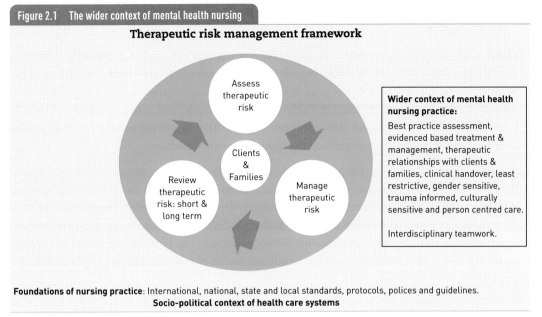

Figure 2.1   The wider context of mental health nursing

Therapeutic risk management framework

Wider context of mental health nursing practice:
Best practice assessment, evidenced based treatment & management, therapeutic relationships with clients & families, clinical handover, least restrictive, gender sensitive, trauma informed, culturally sensitive and person centred care.

Interdisciplinary teamwork.

Foundations of nursing practice: International, national, state and local standards, protocols, polices and guidelines.
Socio-political context of health care systems

Note: for the full schedule, visit www.who.int/classifications/icf/whodasii/en.

Potential barriers influencing the MSE and the mental health nurse response

There are many variables affecting the outcome of the MSE and the mental health nurse response to the consumer's situation, including:

- *the physical environment*, which may not be conducive to the completion of the MSE. For example, if the MSE is conducted in a busy emergency department, a consumer displaying symptoms of paranoia may become increasingly agitated. The physical environment needs to be safe for both the consumer and the mental health nurse; it needs to have adequate space, lighting and exits, with emergency response support should the consumer's condition deteriorate.
- *the consumer's age or the presence of intellectual or cognitive impairment*, which will affect the mental health nurse's selection and use of a communication style, including the avoidance of complex medical terminology and utilisation of picture cues (Boggs, 2007). Specialist cognitive screening tools—such as the Mini-Mental Status Examination (MMSE) and the clock drawing test—can also be used to support the assessment findings when delirium or dementia is suspected (Jett, 2008).
- *the acuity of the consumer's presentation*, which will govern the immediacy and implementation of the mental health nurse's response, and may include the use of psychotropic medications or implementation of the Mental Health Act relevant to the state, territory or country to refer the consumer for admission to an acute hospital environment.
- *the consumer's culture and command of the English language*, which will also affect their ability to articulate and comprehend the experience. Many non-English-speaking consumers, and their families, will not accept that the family member has a mental illness. Some cultural groups view psychotic phenomena within the context of culturally bound syndromes, such as *shenkui*, which is observed in the Chinese community (American Psychiatric Association, 2000). To reduce these barriers, the mental health

■ TOPIC LINK

See Chapter 22 for more on consumers from culturally and linguistically diverse backgrounds.

nurse can access an accredited interpreter service to provide information in the consumer's or carer's preferred language.

TOPIC LINK

See Chapter 14 for more on alcohol, tobacco and other drugs.

- *alcohol, drugs and psychoactive substances such as inhalants*, which can mask a consumer's underlying mental state. The amount of substance ingested and frequency of use can cloud formulation of the MSE assessment, as a consumer can present with impaired judgment, or increased impulsivity with associated risk taking or exacerbation of psychotic and/or depressive and anxiety symptoms (Moore & Dietze, 2008). The mental health nurse must ensure that pathology testing and the use of adjunctive drug and alcohol screening tools are used to support assessment findings.

- *co-morbid physical conditions*, which can be identified or excluded through medical screening and the assessment of the consumer's physical status. Review of test results and liaison with medical staff are crucial in the assessment process; for example, depression and anxiety symptoms have been observed in consumers with diabetes mellitus (Balhara & Sagar, 2011). Family members or carers can be a reassuring and supportive presence for the consumer, and can be a rich source of information, particularly when the consumer is acutely unwell and unable to take an active role in the assessment process.

The *National Standards for Mental Health Services* (Commonwealth of Australia, 2010) states that 'consumers are partners in the management of all aspects of their treatment and care and recovery planning' (p. 14), while mental health professionals are to encourage and support the participation of consumers and carers in determining the consumer's care; however, concerns have been raised about this taking place in practice. Wilkinson and McAndrew (2008) found that families and carers frequently feel isolated and excluded during the assessment and admission process. Clarke, Dusome and Hughes (2007) established that families and carers desire to be more involved, and suggest that it is a crucial component of the care continuum that they are supported and informed of the assessment process, that they are invited to contribute to consumer care and that collaborative relationships are established with respect to the consumer's rights to confidentiality.

The WHO Disability Assessment Schedule

The WHO Disability Assessment Schedule (WHODAS) is a standard method for assessing the consumer's overall level of disability for the last 30 days. It has thirty-six assessment points across six domains, including 'understanding and communicating, getting around, self-care, getting along with people, life activities and participation in society' (American Psychiatric Association, 2013, p. 745).

The WHODAS replaces the use of the previously used Global Assessment Functioning (GAF), with the American Psychiatric Association (2013) recommending version two of the schedule as it produces the more comprehensive information. The WHODAS schedule is available in a variety of languages and can be conducted within 20 minutes as a self-administered schedule, via interview or with family members or carers that have intimate detail of the consumer's condition (American Psychiatric Association, 2013).

The WHODAS is 'based on the International Classification of Functioning, Disability and Health (ICF) for use across all of medicine and health care' (American Psychiatric Association, 2013, p. 16). The WHODAS can be used to assess the consumer's level of disability on admission and can be used at regular intervals to reassess the consumer's level of disability in response to treatment and nursing interventions (American Psychiatric Association, 2013). The World Health Organization and American Psychiatric Association (2013) have recommended using both 'average scores for each domain and the general disability score' as markers to identify areas of clinical concern assisting clinicians to target their interventions (American Psychiatric Association, 2013, p. 746). Directions for calculation of the domains can be sought from the DSM 5 manual on page 745.

Health of the Nation Outcome Scales

The initial aim of these scales was to provide a means of recording progress towards the Health of the Nation target to significantly improve the health and social functioning of mentally ill people. Meadows, Singh and Grigg (2007) state that the Health of the Nation Outcome Scales (HoNOS) is one tool recommended for routine review of the outcomes that mental health services provide to consumers.

Development and testing of the HoNOS was conducted over three years, resulting in an instrument with twelve items measuring behaviour, impairment, symptoms and social functioning (Wing, Curtis & Beevor, 1996). The scales are completed after routine clinical assessments in any setting, and have a variety of uses for clinicians, researchers and administrators (see Royal College of Psychiatrists, 2013).

These twelve scales are used to rate mental health consumers who are working-age adults. There are differing sets of scales for children, adolescents and older-age people. The scales consider different aspects of mental and social health, each on a scale of 0–4. The scales are designed to be used by practitioners before and after interventions, so that changes attributable to the interventions (outcomes) can be measured.

The HoNOS scales for working-age adults are as follows:

1. Overactive, aggressive, disruptive or agitated behaviour
2. Non-accidental self-injury
3. Problem drinking or drug-taking
4. Cognitive problems
5. Physical illness or disability problems
6. Problems associated with hallucinations and delusions
7. Problems with depressed mood
8. Other mental and behavioural problems
9. Problems with relationships
10. Problems with activities of daily living
11. Problems with living conditions
12. Problems with occupation and activities

Each scale is rated as follows:

1. No problem
2. Minor problem requiring no action
3. Mild problem but definitely present
4. Moderately severe problem
5. Severe to very severe problem (Wing, Curtis & Beevor, 1996).

König and colleagues (2009) undertook research to explore various scales—the GAF and HoNOS being two—using what they called a 'time trade-off (TTO) procedure'. Research respondents expressed

Figure 2.2 Part of the WHODAS 2.0 (World Health Organization Disability Assessment Schedule 2.0): thirty-six-item version, self-administered.

WHODAS 2.0
World Health Organization Disability Assessment Schedule 2.0
36-item version, self-administered

Patient Name:_____ Age:_____ Sex: ☐Male ☐Female Date:_____

This questionnaire asks about <u>difficulties due to health/mental health conditions</u>. Health conditions include **diseases or illnesses, other health problems that may be short or long lasting, injuries, mental or emotional problems, and problems with alcohol or drugs.** Think back over the **past 30 days** and answer these questions thinking about how much difficulty you had doing the following activities. For each question, please circle only **one** response.

		1	2	3	4	5	Raw Item Score	Raw Domain Score	Average Domain Score
Numeric scores assigned to each of the items:							_Clinician Use Only_		
In the <u>last 30 days</u>, how much difficulty did you have in:									
Understanding and communicating									
D1.1	<u>Concentrating</u> on doing something for <u>ten minutes</u>?	None	Mild	Moderate	Severe	Extreme or cannot do			
D1.2	<u>Remembering</u> to do <u>important things</u>?	None	Mild	Moderate	Severe	Extreme or cannot do			
D1.3	<u>Analyzing and finding solutions</u> to problems in day-to-day life?	None	Mild	Moderate	Severe	Extreme or cannot do			
D1.4	<u>Learning</u> a <u>new task</u>, for example, learning how to get to a new place?	None	Mild	Moderate	Severe	Extreme or cannot do		30	5
D1.5	<u>Generally understanding</u> what people say?	None	Mild	Moderate	Severe	Extreme or cannot do			
D1.6	<u>Starting and maintaining</u> a <u>conversation</u>?	None	Mild	Moderate	Severe	Extreme or cannot do			
Getting around									
D2.1	<u>Standing</u> for <u>long periods</u>, such as <u>30 minutes</u>?	None	Mild	Moderate	Severe	Extreme or cannot do			
D2.2	<u>Standing up</u> from sitting down?	None	Mild	Moderate	Severe	Extreme or cannot do			
D2.3	<u>Moving</u> around <u>inside your home</u>?	None	Mild	Moderate	Severe	Extreme or cannot do		25	5
D2.4	<u>Getting out</u> of your <u>home</u>?	None	Mild	Moderate	Severe	Extreme or cannot do			
D2.5	<u>Walking a long distance</u>, such as a kilometer (or equivalent)?	None	Mild	Moderate	Severe	Extreme or cannot do			
Self-care									
D3.1	<u>Washing</u> your <u>whole body</u>?	None	Mild	Moderate	Severe	Extreme or cannot do			
D3.2	Getting <u>dressed</u>?	None	Mild	Moderate	Severe	Extreme or cannot do			
D3.3	<u>Eating</u>?	None	Mild	Moderate	Severe	Extreme or cannot do		20	5
D3.4	Staying <u>by yourself</u> for a <u>few days</u>?	None	Mild	Moderate	Severe	Extreme or cannot do			
Getting along with people									
D4.1	<u>Dealing</u> with people <u>you do not know</u>?	None	Mild	Moderate	Severe	Extreme or cannot do			
D4.2	<u>Maintaining a friendship</u>?	None	Mild	Moderate	Severe	Extreme or cannot do			
D4.3	<u>Getting along</u> with people who are <u>close</u> to you?	None	Mild	Moderate	Severe	Extreme or cannot do		25	5
D4.4	<u>Making new friends</u>?	None	Mild	Moderate	Severe	Extreme or cannot do			
D4.5	<u>Sexual</u> activities?	None	Mild	Moderate	Severe	Extreme or cannot do			

their preferences by trading a reduction of life time in a given health state for an improvement to perfect health. The respondents were three differing consumer groups:

- consumers with a diagnosis of affective disorders
- consumers with a diagnosis of schizophrenia spectrum disorders
- consumers with a diagnosis of alcohol-related mental disorders.

The sample consisted of 172 consumers with affective disorders, 166 consumers with schizophrenia and 160 consumers with alcohol-related mental disorders. The researchers explored respondents' quality of life (QOL) and their psychopathology, and symptoms were assessed subjectively using the Symptom Checklist 90R (SCL-90R), and objectively using the Clinical Global Impression Severity of Illness Scale (CGI-S), as well as the Positive and Negative Syndrome Scale (PANSS) for consumers with schizophrenia, and the Bech-Rafaelsen Melancholia Scale (BRAMES) for consumers with affective disorders. Functioning was assessed objectively by the GAF, the Global Assessment of Relational Functioning Scale (GARF) and the Social and Occupational Functioning Scale (SOFAS), as well as the HoNOS.

The researchers' findings produced interesting results, in that consumers with affective and alcohol-related disorders had TTO utility scores that were moderately correlated with theoretically related measures used for comparison, indicating reasonable construct validity. However, in consumers with schizophrenia spectrum disorder, TTO utilities showed only weak correlation with subjective measures, and no correlation with objective measures when used for comparison, indicating insufficient validity in this consumer group.

Physical health and mental illness

While the subject of physical and mental health is explored in more detail in the next chapter, the physical well-being of people who experience mental illness has been the focus of care considerations for many decades. Since the 1920s, reports have linked both bipolar disorder and schizophrenia with abnormal glucose metabolism. This was before the existence of modern psychotropic medication (Fagiolini & Goracci, 2009). Fagiolini and Goracci drew upon a large British study ($n = 626$) in the 1950s that explored both inpatients and outpatients, where they found consumers with a psychiatric illness had more physical illness than the general population, and consumers who had schizophrenia had higher rates of somatic disease, which included cardiovascular disease (CVD), than other groups. These health-care concerns have also been identified by many other authors (Bowers et al., 2008; Bushe et al., 2008; Kilbourne et al., 2008; Scott et al., 2008). A decade later, in the 1960s, Roessler and Greenfield (in Fagiolini & Goracci, 2009) undertook a medical records audit of severely mentally ill consumers ($n = 951$), all of whom were outpatients, and found that more individuals experienced physical illness, except they did not experience skin or endocrine disorders, when compared with others who didn't have a mental illness.

Wand and Murray (2008) identified other physical illnesses that have been seen as having a reciprocal relationship with mental illness: diabetes, chronic obstructive pulmonary disease, cancer, CVD, hypertension, osteoporosis, HIV and hepatitis C.

Fagiolini and Goracci (2009) argue that consumers with severe mental illness (SMI) have a substantially shorter lifespan than the general population in the developed world. They go on to examine the US population, where the average life expectancy is about 78 years, yet the lifespan for someone with a mental illness is at least 30 per cent shorter. Given the psychiatric world has been aware of the nexus between SMI and physical illness for over 90 years, it is a sad indictment that we still are debating this issue and not doing much to improve the quality of life for people with SMI. Maj (2009, p. 1) argues:

> If we are really concerned about the quality of life of our consumers with severe mental disorders and with the protection of their civil rights, we cannot ignore that physical health is a crucial dimension of quality of life in these persons, and that the access to a physical health care of the same quality as that available to the rest of the population is a basic right of these persons as human beings and as citizens.

Maj (2009) cites De Hert and colleagues (2009), who argue that the gap between SMI and the rest of the population concerning the prevalence of some of these diseases (most importantly, type 2 diabetes mellitus) has been increasing in the past few decades. The consequence of under-recognition and treatment of physical illness is that the coexistence of one or more physical diseases has a significant impact on many quality-of-life and psychopathological variables in persons with SMI. This problem has not yet been addressed and the access to quality physical health care of people with SMI is reduced compared with the rest of the general population.

Given the growing body of evidence that supports the poorer general health of those with a SMI, the question becomes: why has this not been addressed? Why do we health-care workers continue to overlook the physical health of people with a mental illness? In the next section we examine one of the reasons for this, and look at some areas of general health that need to be explored with consumers. The exploration of various illnesses that many of our consumers of mental health care are potentially exposed to is examined, and it is hoped that through this illumination health-care workers will be spurred into action to ensure that those with SMI can have improved health care.

ABOUT THE CONSUMER   Juanita's story

Juanita is a 24-year-old woman who is experiencing depression, and has been receiving ongoing counselling from her psychologist. Juanita works at the local grocery shop and has been experiencing ongoing conflict with her manager, which has resulted in Juanita taking 'sick days' from her place of employment. Juanita has recent stressors including the death of a grandparent, a relationship break-up with her girlfriend and a recent diagnosis of endometriosis. Juanita is estranged from her parents, who do not support her relationship with her girlfriend.

REFLECTION QUESTIONS

1   When conducting a risk assessment, what do you think are the static, dynamic and future risk factors in relation to Juanita's situation?

2   What are other risk factors that could influence the provision of care and identify services that would be appropriate for Juanita's ongoing care?

Diagnostic overshadowing

Diagnostic overshadowing, a term first used in 1982, refers to the tendency for clinicians to attribute symptoms or behaviours of a person with a learning disability or SMI to their underlying cognitive deficits.

Jones, Howard and Thornicroft (2008) argued that diagnostic overshadowing led to underdiagnosing the presence of co-morbid physical health issues. Fleischhacker and colleagues (2008) highlight the same damning statistics as Fagiolini and Goracci (2009): that the life expectancy of someone with a SMI is 30 per cent shorter than that of the general population. Fleischhacker and colleagues drew upon conference attendees' experience in 2006, exploring some of the barriers to health for people with a SMI. Some of the key problems they saw included:

- the stigmatisation of mental illness, which leads to discrimination against people with mental illness in all areas of life, including gaining access to health care
- the suboptimal integration of general health care with mental health care
- a lack of consensus between health-care professionals about who is responsible for the prevention and management of co-morbid somatic illness in people who have a SMI
- in some countries, a lack of funding for people with co-morbid problems and mental illness.

Fleischhacker and colleagues (2008) argue that, even when somatic health care is provided, it tends to be of a lower quality; also there is a deficiency in health service delivery and treatment for conditions such as diabetes, CVD and other illnesses people with SMI may acquire. Fleischhacker and colleagues draw upon a 2003 World Health Organization survey that showed that 32 per cent of 191 countries across the world do not have specified budgets for mental health, whereas 21 per cent of the countries spend less than 1 per cent of their total health-care budget on mental health. This low funding clearly limits not only the mental health care, but also any access to general health care that people with SMI might require.

Fagiolini and Goracci (2009) suggest that the main contributor to the development of physical illness may be the side effects associated with the treatment of SMI. For instance, the use of atypical antipsychotics increases the likelihood of developing obesity, diabetes, hyperglycaemia, hyperlipidemia and CVD.

Adding to this research, Allison and colleagues (2009) focused upon second-generation antipsychotics or atypicals, along with other psychotropic medication such as mood stabilisers and antidepressants. While they found that most users gained weight, they also found that some antidepressants, such as bupropion, had been associated with weight loss. Allison and colleagues argue that metabolic risk factors, such as obesity and type 2 diabetes, were 1.5–2 times more common in people with schizophrenia when compared with the general population. Drawing on the largest US study, from more than fifty sites, the Clinical Antipsychotic Trials of Intervention Effectiveness (CATIE), Allison and colleagues highlight the weight gain over a 10-week period of treatment from antipsychotics: clozapine, 4.5 kg; olanzapine, 4.2 kg; risperidone, 2.1 kg; and ziperasidone, 0.4 kg. The CATIE study reported that the mean weight gain for consumers who received olanzapine was 12 kg (they received the common dose of 12.5–17 mg per day).

Allison and colleagues emphasise that there are now more than 1000 reports in the literature on antipsychotics and metabolic risks. They indicate that treatment with certain antipsychotics is associated with increased risk of insulin resistance, hyperglycaemia and type 2 diabetes, compared with no treatment. They make the valid point that most clinical trials are too short to identify most occurrences of diabetes. Citing the second phase of the CATIE study, Allison and colleagues stress that olanzapine was associated with increases in overall cholesterol and triglyceride levels, compared with risperidone and ziperasidone, which showed a decrease in these indices.

While Allison and colleagues (2009) point to the fact that while there are other factors that do increase weight gain, such as a sedentary lifestyle or limited access to low-calorie food, what is clear is that there is a need to find metabolicly safe and effective antipsychotic medications. As a guide, Allison and colleagues suggest that weight-gain-sparing antipsychotic medications may be a more reasonable first-line approach with new consumers, or a preferred treatment option when a medication change is required.

Screening tools

There are various health screening tools available. We have chosen to review two comprehensive tools that allow for holistic assessment of a consumer. We believe that the mind–body dichotomy should be avoided, as it is detrimental to good consumer care. Added to this, there is strong evidence that supports the concept that mental health care should be comprehensively holistic, so that consumers who have difficulty accessing general health care can gain a review of their general health, as well as good mental health care.

Health improvement profile (HIP)

The health improvement profile (HIP) tool, which was developed by Shuel and colleagues (2010; see Table 2.5), was used to examine a cohort of 31 community outpatients with SMI in Scotland. Remarkably, they identified 189 health issues in the small cohort of participants, using the screening tool in a session with community outpatients who were mostly on some form of medication to treat their mental illness. They found no one refused to complete the HIP. The items that were most frequently 'flagged', using a traffic light colour system, were increased BMI ($n = 24$), breast self-examination problems ($n = 23$), increased waist circumference ($n = 21$), pulse irregularities ($n = 14$) and dietary problems ($n = 13$). The researchers found there was a high prevalence of obesity and poor diet, especially related to eating fresh fruit and vegetables, and a lack of exercise. Added to this, breast self-examination was not routinely done, and they found that a tachycardia was common. An interesting finding in relation to waist measurements was that while these did indicate obesity, there were average lipid and glucose levels. Along with this, smoking, alcohol and cannabis use was recorded in smaller numbers than expected, but this might reflect the small number of participants in the study. One clear omission in terms of questions from the HIP was that the safe sex and sexual satisfaction items were not regularly asked by mental health nurses. The potential for drug interactions having an impact upon sexual satisfaction and the lack of understanding about safe sex practices by people with a SMI makes this an essential line of enquiry for holistic health-care planning by mental health nurses.

Metabolic syndrome screening tool (MSST)

The metabolic syndrome screening tool (MSST) provides the nurse with a validated tool that can track various general health-care changes over time, and can alert the treating team to the potential risks associated with mental health treatment, where health-care action can be initiated in conjunction with the consumer. Brunero and Lamont (2009) have used this tool with consumers, finding that compliance with screening was high. They rightly point out that Usher (2006, in Brunero & Lamont, 2009) argues that the mental health nurse is ideally placed to undertake screening and implement interventions to ameliorate the risks associated with mental illness or treatment.

Complementary alternative medicine

One growing area that mental health nurses must endeavour to have an understanding of is the use of many forms of complementary alternative medicine (CAM), as many consumers of mental health services do use alternative medication to assist in treating their illness. Lovell (2009) argues that alternative

TABLE 2.5 HEALTH IMPROVEMENT PROFILE (HIP) ITEMS	
1 Body mass index	15 Breast check (female and male)
2 Waist circumference	16 Menstrual cycle (female)
3 Pulse	17 Smoking status
4 Blood pressure	18 Exercise
5 Temperature	19 Alcohol intake
6 Liver function tests	20 Diet: 5-a-day
7 Lipid levels	21 Diet: fat intake
8 Glucose	22 Fluid intake
9 Cervical smear (women only)	23 Caffeine intake
10 Prostate and testicles check (men only)	24 Cannabis use
11 Sleep	25 Safe sex
12 Teeth	26 Urine
13 Eyes	27 Bowels
14 Feet	28 Sexual satisfaction

Shuel et al. (2010)

medicine is often based in culture, which then has an impact on health beliefs and practices. Culturally based alternative medicines are forms of traditional medicine, indigenous healing beliefs and practices of a particular culture or society, predating contact with Europeans and inseparable from concerns with spiritual issues (Lovell, 2009).

There can be harmful interactions between herbal medicines and allopathic drugs, which have been well documented, in particular for CAMs that are ingested, smoked, inhaled or injected.

The inability to achieve a shared understanding and acceptance of each other's beliefs inhibits the therapeutic relationship between the nurse and the consumer (Lovell, 2009). The consequence is that consumers feel disclosing usage of traditional therapies might result in lower quality of care or hinder the carer–consumer therapeutic relationship (Lovell, 2009).

Cultural assessment

Individuals who experience mental health problems are embedded in cultural systems that have a variety of beliefs, opinions and attitudes towards mental health, as well as a variety of treatment options (Olafsdottir & Pescosolido, 2009). Sociologists in the 1990s began to rethink models to explain why individuals either did or didn't access treatment services. Olafsdottir and Pescosolido argue that, while we have built a better understanding of how social networks structure pathways to care, and how disadvantaged sociocultural groups face substantial barriers to treatment, we have less understanding of the larger cultural context in which individuals recognise and respond to symptoms. Therefore, it is essential that nurses have an understanding of the health care and the context in which we practise, so that others who have a culture different from our own are not stereotyped or marginalised in gaining health care.

KAREN HARDER, IAN MUNRO AND ANNETTE WOODHOUSE

Olafsdottir and Pescosolido (2009) used data from the 1996 Mental Health Module of the *General Social Survey* to compare Americans' willingness to recommend providers in the general medical and speciality mental health sectors. Their results indicated that, despite unrealistically high levels of endorsement, individuals do discriminate between providers based on their evaluation of the problem. This perceived severity leads individuals to suggest care attributed to biological causes be directed to general or speciality medical providers (that is, doctors, psychiatrists and hospitals). By contrast, for symptoms such as schizophrenia or violence, individuals are allocated to the speciality mental health sector (that is, psychiatry or a mental hospital); and if the problem is being seen as caused by stress, they are sent to non-medical mental health providers (Olafsdottir & Pescosolido, 2009), such as a chiropractor or acupuncturist, highlighting the use of alternative methods of health care.

Therefore, it is especially important to have an understanding of the cultural context for mental health problems. Olafsdottir and Pescosolido (2009) highlighted issues of stigma, the lack of public understanding, the near absence of physical symptoms and the use of legal coercion, which make the attitudes, values and predispositions embedded in cultural systems critical in terms of service use for mental health problems. While Olafsdottir and Pescosolido (2009) draw upon American culture in its broadest sense, suggesting that it appears supportive of medical solutions to mental health problems (Pescosolido et al., 1999), they draw the conclusion that research offers little help in understanding the role that cultural beliefs and attitudes play in low utilisation rates. The same point could well be made in multicultural Australia.

One way of incorporating an individual's culture into your practice is the use of both a cultural formulation (CF) tool and the DSM 5 for assessment of psychopathology and treatment needs. Roholf, Knipscheer and Kleber (2009) report that consumers find it difficult to define their own culture and provide explanations of illness; this leads to a difficulty for practitioners in identifying culturally based problems in the clinical relationship. To help overcome this problem, Roholf and colleagues (2009) devised the CF tool to help practitioners and their consumers bridge the gap between their different cultures. The four main areas of inquiry that Roholf and colleagues identified in the CF were cultural identity, cultural explanation of the illness, cultural factors related to the psychosocial environment of the consumer, and cultural elements of the relationship between the individual and the clinician. They argue that the CF is an important contribution to clinical work with psychiatric consumers from different cultures. They make the point that the CF was also meant to facilitate a dialogue among clinicians about a less static culture, and gain a deeper understanding of culture in the processes of assessment and treatment (Kleinman & Benson, 2006). They also believe that the CF is useful in making therapists more culturally sensitive.

TOPIC LINK

See Chapter 22 for more on consumers from culturally and linguistically diverse backgrounds.

ABOUT THE CONSUMER   Fadi's Story

My name is Fadi. I came as a female refugee from Turkish Kurdistan. I am a Muslim. I see my headache and the feeling of heaviness in my head as the effect of brain diseases. My backache is surely due to heavy beatings and torture in a police cell. I don't want to talk to other people (besides the clinician) about the group rape by policemen. I am afraid that my husband will leave me when he hears of it. My lack of sleep and energy come from a curse by my mother who feels abandoned by me: she swore that I would not feel better until I have returned to her. During the night I hear her voice. I feel unable to change anything about my situation. I feel alone in this asylum centre; I don't have any friends. All is in the hands of Allah. My prayers just do not help.

Roholf, Knipscheer and Kleber (2009)

REFLECTION QUESTIONS

1   What elements of Fadi's story relate to her being a refugee?

2   What disorder do you think Fadi presents with?

3   How does this differ from someone else presenting with this disorder?

4   How would you as a nurse address Fadi's problems?

Interpreters and assessment

One method to assist in the assessment of people whose first language is not English is the use of interpreters. While this is a valuable tool, there are some important points for nurses to be aware of when incorporating interpreter services into the treatment plan. Recent research has shown that when working with interpreters, the personality of the interpreter and their influence on the therapeutic process should be taken into account (Bot, 2005; Bot & Wadensjö, 2004). The use of an interpreter brings a third person into the interview, which has both positive and negative aspects. The interpreter can be of great assistance in a clinical setting because of their accepting attitude and non-verbal signs of support to the consumer. Roholf and colleagues (2009) assert that the consumer considers interpreters to be important, and relationships can be built with the particular use of the same interpreter; sometimes consumers may refuse another interpreter, as they may not trust the individual or they may come from a different geographical area or class. Roholf and colleagues (2009) argue that translations by telephone should be avoided—although this is not always possible, especially if the consumer presents in an emergency and there is no interpreter present. Careful consideration should to be given to the use of family members as interpreters, as the meaning or intended meaning may be compromised by the bias or concerns of the relative involved. Often this is a poor choice; it is far better to use a health-care worker who speaks the language of the consumer rather than a family member.

■ TOPIC LINK
See Chapter 22 for more on the use of interpreters.

Documentation

The mental health nurse is required to document the findings of investigations noted in this chapter in a timely and systematic manner to ensure consumer safety, adherence to legal and professional standards, promotion of continuity of care within the multidisciplinary team, and optimal consumer outcome (Poole & Higgo, 2006).

The documented assessment findings are a legal record of the consumer's presentation and reported concerns, and also form a baseline for treatment interventions should a consumer's mental state fluctuate in response to the presence of symptoms or the environment in which assessment occurs (Videbeck, 2009). Documentation on paper, or in electronic format, is a legal requirement for all mental health nurses. Despite this requirement, Blair and Smith (2012) found that common barriers to accurate and timely documentation included staff attitude towards documenting and staff allocation of resources. Taylor (2003) also raised concerns regarding nurses' documentation of accurate records, finding that nurse apathy and the time taken to document was felt to be excessive, and played a role in poor record keeping, despite nurses' understanding that such entries inform consumer care. Despite the introduction of electronic records being sporadic around Australia, a study conducted by Munyisia, Yu and Hailey (2011) indicated the use of 'electronic documentation system did not reduce the time that staff spent on documenting' (p. 782).

Irrespective of documentation format, all nursing entries ought to include any education given to the consumer and their family or carers; responsiveness to interventions; therapeutic effects of medications administered; and support services to assist the multidisciplinary team to provide continuity of care. Requirements for all nursing entries include the following:

- They should be written or documented in blue or black ink.
- The entry should have the correct day, month and year entered.
- It should also include time of entry, designation, name and signature of the entrant.
- Entries should be legible, systematic and sequential in recording.
- Information should be relevant to the consumer, and recorded in the appropriate section and on the correct form within the file or electronic record, without excessive space.
- Whiteout is not permitted in the medical record; in the event of an error, the entry must have a diagonal line placed through the entry, 'in error' recorded, and it must be signed and dated by the author (Barker, 2009).

SUMMARY

There are two predominant systems of classification used in Australia and New Zealand to aid in the formulation of diagnosis for persons presenting with mental illness: the *International Classification of Diseases* (ICD) and the *Diagnostic and Statistical Manual of Mental Disorders* (DSM). The mental health nurse aims to provide a multifaceted assessment of a consumer to design and operationalise a holistic plan for ongoing care, including identifying any potential elements of risk to the consumer and taking into account the relationship between their mental health and physical health. Cultural factors also ought to be considered, with interpreters used where necessary, and all plans and treatments should be made in collaboration with consumers and their carers, where appropriate, and professionally documented. The therapeutic relationship the mental health nurse builds with the consumer is paramount to obtaining assessment information and continuance of ongoing care, and all plans and treatments should be professionally documented.

The relationship the mental health nurse builds with the consumer is paramount to obtaining assessment information and continuance of ongoing care.

DISCUSSION
QUESTIONS

1 What are some of the risk factors a mental health professional may look for when assessing a consumer?

2 Why is risk management one of the critical tasks of mental health professionals?

3 What are the key differences between ICD and DSM?

4 What does it mean when we say it is important that health-care professionals take a holistic approach when caring for those who experience mental illness?

5 Given that mental health consumers might not always present with a clearly defined set of symptoms, what are some of the ways a health professional might attempt to identify the issues affecting a consumer and how best to treat them?

6 As a class, read Fadi's story and discuss how a mental health professional could best address Fadi's problems in this situation.

7 What could be some of the ramifications of not appropriately documenting the assessment and care of a consumer with mental illness?

TEST YOURSELF

1 Mental status examination includes:

a appearance and behaviour

b affect, mood and perceptions

c cognitive and thought processes

d all of the above

2 Which of the following are risk factors that a mental health nurse may look for?

a ICD 10 and DSM 5

b GAF and HoNOS

c psychiatric and medical history

d mood

3 A suicide risk assessment includes:

a family history

b use of substances

c previous self-harm

d all of the above

4 HoNOS refers to:

a scoring outcomes for people with mental health problems

b determining need for medication

c scoring overall social functioning

d making a psychiatric diagnosis

USEFUL WEBSITES

Applied Suicide Intervention Skills Training (ASIST): www.livingworks.net/programs/asist

Australian Commission on Safety and Quality in Health Care: www.safetyandquality.gov.au

Global Assessment of Functioning Scale (GAF): https://www.ncbi.nlm.nih.gov/pmc/articles/PMC3036670/

Mental Health Professional Online Development (MHPOD): www.mhpod.gov.au

Royal College of Psychiatrists—Health of the Nation Outcomes Scale (HoNOS): www.rcpsych.ac.uk/quality/honos/whatishonos.aspx

World Health Organization—International Classification of Diseases (ICD): www.who.int/classifications/icd/en

REFERENCES

Allison, D. B., Newcomer, J. W., Dunn, A. L., Blumenthal, J. A., Fabricatore, A. N., Daumit, G. L., Cope, M. B., Riley, W. T., Vreeland, B., Hibbeln, J. R., & Alpert, J. E. (2009). Obesity among those with mental disorders: A National Institute of Mental Health meeting report. *American Journal of Preventive Medicine, 36*(4), 341–350.

Allnutt, S., O'Driscoll, C., Ogloff, J. R., Daffern, M., & Adams, J. (2010). *Clinical risk assessment and management: A practical manual for mental health clinicians*. Retrieved from www.justicehealth.nsw.gov.au.

Allnutt, S., Ogloff, J., Adams, J., O'Driscoll, C., Daffern, M., Carroll, A., & Chaplow, D. (2013). Managing aggression and violence: The clinician's role in contemporary mental health care. *Australian and New Zealand Journal of Psychiatry, 47*(8), 728–736.

American Psychiatric Association (2000). *Diagnostic and statistical manual of mental disorders* (4th ed.; DSM-IV-TR). Arlington: American Psychiatric Association.

KAREN HARDER, IAN MUNRO AND ANNETTE WOODHOUSE

American Psychiatric Association (2013). *Diagnostic and statistical manual of mental disorders* (5th ed.; DSM 5). Arlington: American Psychiatric Association.

Australian Commission on Safety and Quality in Health Care (2012). *National Safety and Quality Health Service Standards*. Sydney: ACSQHC. Retrieved from https://www.safetyandquality. gov.au/wp-content/uploads/2011/09/NSQHS-Standards-Sept-2012.pdf.

Australian Nursing and Midwifery Council (2006). *Australian national competency standards for the registered nurse*. Canberra: Department of Health and Ageing.

Balhara, Y. P. S., & Sagar, R. (2011). 'Correlates of anxiety and depression among patients with type 2 diabetes mellitus'. *Indian Journal of Endocrinology and Metabolism*, 15(1), 50–54.

Barker, P. (2009). *Psychiatric and mental health nursing: The craft of caring* (2nd ed.). London: Edward Arnold.

Blair, W., & Smith, B. (2012). Nursing documentation: Frameworks and barriers. *Contemporary Nurse*, 41(2), 160.

Boggs, K. U. (2007). Communication with clients experiencing communication deficits. In E. C. Arnold & K. U. Boggs (Eds.), *Interpersonal relationships: Professional communication skills for nurses* (pp. 382–394). Philadelphia: Saunders Elsevier.

Bot, H. (2005). *Dialogue interpreting in mental health*. New York: Rodopi.

Bot, H., & Wadensjö, C. (2004). The presence of a third party: A dialogical view on interpreter-assisted treatment. In J. P. Wilson & B. Drozdek (Eds.), *Broken spirits* (pp. 355–378). New York. Brunner-Routledge.

Bowers, A. R., Novelli, S., Morris, L., Knott, M., Freedman, J. E., Lousley, W., Farrow, J., & Burnett, F. E. (2008). Mental health and wellbeing review for severe mental illness register patients: A feasibility study. *Primary Care & Community Psychiatry*, 13(4), 162–167.

Brunero, S., & Lamont, S. (2009). Systematic screening for metabolic syndrome in consumers with severe mental illness. *International Journal of Mental Health Nursing*, 18(2), 144–150.

Bushe, C., Yeomans, D., Floyd, T., & Smith, S. M. (2008). Categorical prevalence and severity of hyperprolactinaemia in two UK cohorts of patients with severe mental illness during treatment with antipsychotics. *Journal of Psychopharmacology*, 22(2), 56–62.

Clancy, L., Happell, B., & Moxham, L. (2015). Perception of risk for older people living with a mental illness: Balancing uncertainty. *International Journal of Mental Health Nursing*, 24(6), 577–586.

Clarke, D. E., Dusome, D., & Hughes, L. (2007). Emergency department from the mental health client's perspective. *International Journal of Mental Health Nursing*, 16(2), 126–131.

Commonwealth of Australia (2010). *National standards for mental health services*. ACT: Commonwealth of Australia.

Commonwealth of Australia. (2013). *A national framework for recovery-oriented mental health services. Guide for practitioners and providers*.

Crowe, M., & Carlyle, D. (2003). Deconstructing risk assessment and management in mental health nursing. *Journal of Advanced Nursing*, 43(1), 19–27.

D'Antonio, P., Beeber, L., Sills, G., & Naegle, M. (2014). The future in the past: Hildegard Peplau and interpersonal relations in nursing. *Nursing Inquiry*, 21(4), 311–317.

Downes, C., Gill, A., Doyle, L., Morrissey, J., & Higgins, A. (2016). Survey of mental health nurses' attitudes towards risk assessment, risk assessment tools and positive risk. *Journal of Psychiatric and Mental Health Nursing*, 23(3–4), 188–197. doi:10.1111/jpm.12299.

Doyle, M., & Dolan, M. (2002). Violence risk assessment: Combining actuarial and clinical information to structure clinical judgements for the formulation and management of risk. *Journal of Psychiatric and Mental Health Nursing*, 9(6), 649–657.

Elder, R., Evans, K., & Nizette, D. (2013). *Psychiatric and mental health nursing* (3rd ed.). Chatswood: Elsevier Mosby.

Epstein, M., Fossey, E., Leggatt, M., Meadows, G., & Minas, H. (2007). *Assessment: Essential skills*. In G. Meadows, B. Singh & M. Grigg (Eds.), *Mental health in Australia: Collaborative community practice* (2nd ed.) (pp. 277–318). Melbourne: Oxford University Press.

Fagiolini, A., & Goracci, A. (2009). The effects of undertreated chronic medical illnesses in patients with severe mental disorders. *Journal of Clinical Psychiatry*, 70(3), 22–29.

Fleischhacker, W. W., Cetkovich-Bakmas, M., De Hert, M., Hennekens, C. H., Lambert, M., Leucht, S., Maj, M., Lieberman, J. A. (2008). Comorbid somatic illnesses in patients with severe mental disorders: Clinical, policy, and research challenges. *Journal of Clinical Psychiatry*, 69(4), 514–519.

Gamble, C., & Brennan, G. (2006). Assessments: A rationale for choosing and using. In C. Gamble & G. Brennan (Eds.), *Working with serious mental illness: A manual for clinical practice* (2nd ed.) (pp. 111–131). London: Elsevier.

Gilbert, E., Adams, A., & Buckingham, C. D. (2011). Examining the relationship between risk assessment and risk management in mental health. *Journal of Psychiatric and Mental Health Nursing*, 18(10), 862–886.

Happell, B., Cowin, L., Roper, C., Foster, K., & McMaster, R. (2008). Mental health and illness assessment. In B. Happell, L. Cowin, C. Roper, K. Foster & R. McMaster (Eds.), *Introducing mental health nursing: A consumer-orientated approach* (pp. 101–126). Sydney: Allen & Unwin.

Harris, A., & Lurigio, A. J. (2007). Mental illness and violence: A brief review of research and assessment strategies. *Aggression and Violent Behavior*, 12(5), 542–551.

Higgins, A., Doyle, L., Downes, C., Morrissey, J., Costello, P., Brennan, M., & Nash, M. (2015a). There is more to risk and safety planning than dramatic risks: Mental health nurses' risk assessment and safety-management practice. *International Journal of Mental Health Nursing*, 25(2), 159–170.

Higgins, A., Morrissey, J., Doyle, L., Bailey, J., & Gill, A. (2015b). *Best practice principles for risk assessment and safety planning for nurses working in mental health services*. Dublin: Office of the Nursing & Midwifery Services Director.

Higgins, A., Doyle, L., Morrissey, J., Downes, C., Gill, A., & Bailey, S. (2016). Documentary analysis of risk-assessment and safety-planning policies and tools in a mental health context. *International Journal of Mental Health Nursing*, 25(4), 385–395.

Jaber, F., & Mahmoud, K. (2015). Risk tools for the prediction of violence: 'VRAG, HCR-20, PCL-R'. *Journal of Psychiatric and Mental Health Nursing*, 22(2), 133–141.

Jett, K. (2008). Health assessment in gerontological nursing. In P. Ebersole, P. Hess, T. A. Toughy, J. Jett & A. S. Luggen (Eds.), *Toward healthy aging human needs and nursing response* (7th ed.) (pp. 104–119). St Louis: Mosby Elsevier.

Jones, S., Howard, L., & Thornicroft, G. (2008). 'Diagnostic overshadowing': Worse physical health care for people with mental illness. *Acta Psychiatrica Scandinavica*, 118(3), 169–171.

Kilbourne, A. M., Post, E. P., Nossek, A., Drill, L., Cooley, S., & Bauer, M. S. (2008). Improving medical and psychiatric outcomes among individuals with bipolar disorder: A randomized controlled trial. *Psychiatric Services*, 59(7), 760–768.

Kleinman, A., & Benson, P. (2006). Anthropology in the clinic: The problem of cultural competency and how to fix it. *PLoS Medicine*, 3, 1673–1676.

König, H. H., Günther, O. H., Angermeyer, M. A., & Roick, C. (2009). Utility assessment in patients with mental disorders: Validity and discriminative ability of the time trade-off method. *Pharmacoeconomic*, 27(5), 405–419.

Lemon, G., Stanford, S., & Sawyer, A.-M. (2016). Trust and the Dilemmas of Suicide Risk Assessment in Non-government Mental Health Services. *Australian Social Work*, 69(2), 145–157.

Lovell, B. (2009). The integration of bio-medicine and culturally based alternative medicine: Implications for health care providers and patients. *Global Health Promotion*, 16(4), 65–68.

Maj, M. (2009). Physical health care in persons with severe mental illness: A public health and ethical priority. *World Psychiatry; Official Journal of the World Psychiatric Association*, 8(1), 1–2.

Meadows, G., Singh, B., & Grigg, M. (2007). *Mental health in Australia: Collaborative community practice* (2nd ed.). Melbourne: Oxford University Press.

MHPOD (2016). *Mental Health Professional Online Development.* Retrieved from https://www.health.qld.gov.au/qcmhl/mhpod.

Moore, D., & Dietze, P. (2008). *Drugs and public health: Australian perspectives on policy and practice.* Melbourne: Oxford University Press.

Muir-Cochrane, E., Gerace, A., Mosel, K., O'Kane, D., Barkway, P., Curren, D., & Oster, C. (2011). Managing risk: Clinical decision-making in mental health services. *Issues in Mental Health Nursing, 32*(12), 726–734.

Munyisia, E. N., Yu, P., & Hailey, D. (2011). Does the introduction of an electronic nursing documentation system in a nursing home reduce time on documentation for the nursing staff? *International Journal of Medical Informatics, 80,* 782–792.

New South Wales Government (2012). *Mental Health Triage Policy.* New South Wales Ministry of Health. (pp. 17–19). Retrieved from http://www1.health.nsw.gov.au/pds/ActivePDSDocuments/PD2012_053.pdf

New South Wales Government (2016). *Care of people who may be suicidal.* Sydney: New South Wales Government.

Olafsdottir, S., & Pescosolido, B. A. (2009). Drawing the line: The cultural cartography of utilization recommendations for mental health problems. *Journal of Health and Social Behavior, 50,* 228–244.

Peplau, H. E. (1952). *Interpersonal relations in nursing.* New York: G. P. Putnam & Sons.

Pescosolido, B. A., Monahan, J., Link, B. G., Stueve, A., & Kikuzawa, S. (1999). The public's view of the competence, dangerousness, and need for legal coercion of persons with mental health problems. *American Journal of Public Health, 89,* 1339–1345.

Poole, R., & Higgo, R. (2006). *Psychiatric interviewing and assessment.* New York: Cambridge University Press.

Queensland Government (2016). *Mental Health Professional Online Development.* The State of Queensland (Queensland Health): Queensland Government. Retrieved from https://www.health.qld.gov.au/qcmhl/mhpod.

Rogers, C. R., & Dorfman, E. (1951). *Client-centered therapy: Its current practice, implications, and theory:* ICON Group International.

Roholf, H., Knipscheer, J. W., & Kleber, R. L. (2009). Use of the cultural formulation with refugees. *Transcultural Psychiatry, 46,* 487.

Royal College of Psychiatrists (2013). *What is HoNOS?* Retrieved from www.rcpsych.ac.uk/quality/honos/whatishonos.aspx.

Sadock, B. J., & Sadock, V. A. (2007). *Kaplan and Sadock's synopsis of psychiatry: Behavioural sciences/clinical psychiatry* (10th ed.). Philadelphia: Lippincott Williams & Wilkins.

Saunders, J. B. (2006). Substance dependence and non-dependence in the Diagnostic and Statistical Manual of Mental Disorders (DSM) and the International Classification of Diseases (ICD): Can an identical conceptualization be achieved? *Addiction, 101*(1), 48–58.

Scott, K., McGee, M. A., Schaaf, D., & Baxter, J. (2008). Mental–physical comorbidity in an ethnically diverse population. *Social Science & Medicine, 66*(5), 1165–1173.

Shattell, M. M., Starr, S. S., & Thomas, S. P. (2007). 'Take my hand, help me out': Mental health service recipients' experience of the therapeutic relationship. *International Journal of Mental Health Nursing, 16*(4), 274–84.

Shuel, F., White, J., Jones, M., & Gray, R. (2010). Using the serious mental illness improvement profile (HIP) to identify physical problems in a cohort of community patients: A pragmatic cases series evaluation. *International Journal of Nursing Studies, 47*(2), 136–145.

Stokes, B. (2012). *Review of the admission and discharge and transfer practices of public mental health facilities/services in Western Australia.* Perth: Mental Health Commission.

Taylor, H. (2003). An exploration of the factors that affect nurses' record keeping. *British Journal of Nursing, 12*(12), 751–758.

Varcarolis, M., & Halter, M. J. (2010). *Foundations of psychiatric mental health nursing: A clinical approach* (6th ed.). Missouri: Elsevier.

Victorian Department of Health (2010). *Working with the suicidal person. A summary guide for emergency departments and mental health services.* Melbourne: Mental Health, Drugs and Regions branch, Department of Health.

Victorian Department of Health (2013). *Nursing observation through engagement in psychiatric inpatient care.* Department of Health guideline. Melbourne: Mental Health, Drugs and Regions Division, Department of Health.

Videbeck, S. L. (2009). Assessment approaches. In S. L. Videbeck (Ed.), *Mental Health Nursing* (pp. 139–155). London: Arnold.

Wand, T., Isobel, S., & Derrick, K. (2015). Surveying clinician perceptions of risk assessment and management practices in mental health service provision. *Australasian Psychiatry, 23*(2), 147–153.

Wand, T., & Murray, L. (2008). Let's get physical. *International Journal of Mental Health Nursing, 17*(5), 363–369.

Webb, L. (2012). Tools for the job: why relying on risk assessment tools is still a risky business. *Journal of Psychiatric and Mental Health Nursing, 19*(2), 132–139.

Western Australia Department of Health (2008). *Clinical risk assessment and management (CRAM) in Western Australian services. Policy and standards.* Perth: Mental Health Division, WA Department of Health.

Wilkinson, C., & McAndrew, S. (2008). 'I'm not an outsider, I am his mother!' A phenomenological enquiry into carer experiences of exclusion from acute psychiatric settings. *International Journal of Mental Health Nursing, 17*(6), 392–401.

Wing, J. K., Curtis, R. H., & Beevor, A. S. (1996). *HoNOS: Health of the Nation Outcome Scales: Report on research and development July 1993–December 1995.* London: Royal College of Psychiatrists.

Woods, P. (2013). Risk assessment and management approaches on mental health units. *Journal of Psychiatric and Mental Health Nursing, 20*(9), 807–813.

Wrycraft, N. (2015). *Assessment and care planning in mental health nursing.* Open University Press.

CHAPTER 3

Physical and Mental Health

STEVE HEMINGWAY,
JULIE SHARROCK AND
GAGANPREET LEGHA

Acknowledgment

The authors would like to acknowledge the contribution of Gail Kohrsen who co-wrote this chapter in the second edition. The authors would also like to thank Jacque White, Associate Dean Learning Teaching and Quality, Faculty of Health and Social Care, University of Hull (UK), for help in using the health improvement profile, and Rebecca Burgess-Dawson, Placement Development Manager, Health Education England (UK), for preparing the basic observation and physiological test content.

KEY OUTCOMES

AFTER READING THIS CHAPTER, YOU SHOULD BE ABLE TO:

- identify the importance of providing physical status assessment and related interventions for consumers diagnosed with severe mental illness

- discuss barriers and challenges in service provision in non-psychiatric settings and why it has not met the obvious care need

- identify an appropriate tool to undertake physical health screening

- describe potential interventions that can be utilised to promote well-being and health

- identify the skill set appropriate to undertaking physical health interventions in all care contexts.

- describe the role of a CLN.

KEY TERMS

- co-morbidity
- consultation–liaison nurse (CLN)
- delirium
- diagnostic overshadowing
- iatrogenic
- lifestyle choices
- mental health
- physical health
- recovery
- severe mental illness (SMI)

Introduction

This chapter examines the physical and mental health of those consumers with diagnoses of severe mental illness (SMI). These diagnoses include schizophrenia, major depressive disorder and bipolar affective disorder. It also considers the mental health needs of consumers within the general hospital setting. In every clinical setting of nursing practice, the nurse has been educated to view the consumer holistically—to be alert and sensitive to the psychological impact of physical illness on an individual. Conversely, this awareness must also extend to the impact of physical illness on those who have severe mental health issues and include a comprehensive assessment of the consumer's physical, psychological and social needs (Happell, Davies & Scott, 2012; Lambert, 2012). This chapter also introduces the reader to the role of the Consultation Nurse in the acute care setting and, also importantly, the roles of mental health nurses working in general health-care settings in addressing the mental health needs of people with physical illnesses.

Physical health problems in people diagnosed with mental illness

The causes of physical health problems are related to physiological (Mitchell et al., 2012), psychological (Nocon, 2004) and sociological determinants (Allen et al., 2014; Nash, 2010), as well as lifestyle choices (Happell, Scott & Platania-Phung, 2012). Co-morbidity of physical illness and mental illness is also a longstanding concern (Muir-Cochrane, 2006). The population with SMI is vulnerable for a number of reasons due to the nature of the illness—many have a number of co-morbid conditions such as obesity, poor nutrition, smoking and poor oral health (Edward, Felstead & Mahoney, 2011; Happell et al., 2012). Iatrogenic side effects from taking psychotropic medication have also been identified as a major cause of physical health problems for the mental health consumer (Happell, Scott & Planania-Phung, 2012).

Complications that have been highlighted as experienced by people diagnosed with a severe mental illness include diabetes, respiratory problems, infections, cancer, cardiovascular diseases, stroke, other neurological disorders, sexual health problems and other health problems such as HIV and hepatitis B and C (Happell, Scott & Planania-Phung, 2012; Robson & Gray, 2007).

In Australia it is estimated around 3 per cent of the adult population will experience a severe mental illness (National Mental Health Commission, 2012, p. 14). The health-care system is increasingly faced with the need to address the management of individuals with multiple coexisting diseases (Valderas et al., 2009). Co-morbidity of physical illness and mental illness has long been identified, and certain behaviours associated with those with severe mental illness are considered to be high risk, such as smoking, and abuse of alcohol and other substances (WHA, 2009). A longitudinal study carried out in Western Australia from 1990 to 2006 found that the incidence of diabetes was significantly higher in those participants with severe mental illnesses (SMI) compared with participants without SMI. This included a higher rate of hospitalisation for diabetes-related physical complications (Qun et al., 2010).

■ TOPIC LINK

See Chapter 15 for more on psychopharmacology.

Physical health intervention: a pressing priority

Individuals with mental illness have increased risk of physical health problems when compared with the general population (Happell et al., 2011; Robson & Gray, 2007). It is estimated that individuals with mental illness die as much as 25 years earlier than the general population (Brown et al., 2010; Manderscheid et al., 2010; Parks et al., 2006). In addition, people with psychiatric disorders have higher rates of physical disorders than the general population (Happell, Davies & Scott, 2012). Psychiatric consumers have a death rate two-and-a-half times greater than the general population, a 30 per cent greater rate of death once diagnosed with cancer, and increased risk of complications post surgery resulting in readmission. There are also increased rates of injuries, infectious diseases such as hepatitis C, and vascular, respiratory and gastrointestinal problems (Robson & Gray, 2007). Some of this might be explained by higher levels of smoking, alcohol and substance use, decreased levels of self-care and adherence to treatment for physical problems, the effects of the disorder itself and the effects of psychotropic medication (Happell et al., 2011). Although Australia and New Zealand have universal health-care systems, not everyone with a SMI avails themselves of these services on a regular basis. Some people with a SMI may not have strong links or a relationship with their GP or with other health professionals due to the nature of their illness—for example, social withdrawal, isolation and lack of motivation—which may prevent them from having regular health checks to address lifestyle issues (Happell et al., 2011). For consumers with SMI, experiences of physical health provision are often poor and, when appropriate treatments are accessed, the outcomes are often less successful than for the rest of the community (World Federation for Mental Health, 2010). Consumers in Australia have echoed this issue, stating that due to the complexity of their needs (including physical health) they need appropriate support from a wide range of services (Townsend et al., 2006).

There are also added complications of access to services in rural areas (Happell, Davies & Scott, 2012). In addition, Howard and Gamble (2011) suggest that individuals with SMI experience poorer physical health outcomes and earlier mortality than the general population, despite having more frequent contact with GPs (Colton & Manderscheid, 2006; Qun et al., 2010).

Governmental response

There is a nationally recognised need to address high mortality rates due to physical illness for people with SMI. A National Summit on Addressing the Premature Death of People with a Mental Illness (2013) affirmed the need for reforms in the existing Australian health system to meet the physical health-care needs of people with mental health issues. In 2016, a draft consensus statement was developed by the National Mental Health Commission after seeking views of various stakeholders to address this gap of providing physical health care to people with mental illness. The statement highlighted six essential elements to address this issue:

- capacity building for all health-care professionals and empowering consumers to make decisions about their health
- improving equity of access to primary care services by flexible funding models
- improving quality of care by incorporating the physical health-care checks and management of physical health co-morbidities in the routine care of people with mental illness
- promoting healthy lifestyle education and early detection and intervention by all health-care clinicians
- improving care coordination, referral pathways and integration of primary care services and specialist mental health services and promoting development of integrated physical and mental health plans
- introducing targets and indicators to monitor compliance with standards of physical health care for people with mental illness (National Mental Health Commission, 2016).

In Australia, clinical algorithms and structured monitoring forms for assessing physical health issues and cardiovascular risk factors have been developed in Victoria, NSW and Western Australia (Mental Health Commission of NSW, 2016). Furthermore, Duggan (2015) discussed the benefits of integrated and collaborative interventions, but also proposed a shift towards developing population health systems through integrating primary and specialist services, shared learning, peer support, education and support systems for people with mental illness to assist them in managing their physical health.

Collins, Tranter and Irvine (2012) advanced the idea that mental health nurses have a major role to play in improving accessibility to specialist health services for people with mental illness, by improving existing services for their consumers and by proactively collaborating with other health-care providers.

Victoria's Ministerial Advisory Committee on Mental Health (2010) emphasised strengthening and supporting the existing roles and services like mental health nurses working in GP practices, consulatation liaison nurses, case managers in community mental health services, psychiatric disability rehabilitation and support services (PDRSS), GPs and the Hospital Admission Risk Program (HARP), as well as developing specialist roles such as nurse practitioners and clinical nurse specialists, for addressing the complex physical health and mental health needs of these consumers.

All government policies and documents support targeted health interventions and health promotion activities such as smoking cessation, drug and alcohol services and safe sex education to encourage positive health behaviours and reduce the common risk factors.

Physical status screening: a care gap

The ability to screen for physiological health conditions is therefore of fundamental importance to the mental health nurse, yet there is evidence that such conditions go largely unnoticed, and if identified may be poorly managed (Phelan, Stradins & Morrison, 2001). The seriousness of physical symptoms being identified as psychosomatic cannot be underestimated when one considers the number of people with severe and enduring mental illness being at risk of, and suffering from, long-term physiological conditions where the issue of diagnostic overshadowing is present (Nash, 2013). Qun and colleagues (2010) found those with more severe mental illness visited GPs more often than those with less severe mental illness. The results were similar in metropolitan, rural or remote areas, so the opportunity is there to screen for physical health problems. Other researchers found that, despite being frequent attenders at the GP surgery, mental health consumers are less likely to be offered routine screening that the general population would expect; for example, cholesterol, urine or weight checks and opportunistic advice regarding smoking cessation (Happell et al., 2011, Peckham et al., 2015).

Case note reviews have also found serious problems with the assessment and recording of the physical health status of consumers with mental health needs (Disability Rights Commission, 2006; Happell et al., 2014; Howard & Gamble, 2011), and this group appears to be less successfully targeted by health promotion efforts than the general population (Happell, Davies & Scott; Happell, Scott & Platania-Phung, 2012).

Jordan, Philpin and Davies (2000) and latterly Edward, Felstead and Mahoney (2011) posited that the physical health-care needs of the consumer diagnosed with a SMI was a 'care gap' where neither primary care nor secondary mental health services were being provided.

Physical health knowledge and skills

There are many reasons why mental health consumers' long-term physical condition may not be identified, and one of these is a lack of confidence or ability in relation to physical health monitoring by mental health staff (Happell et al., 2011). It has been suggested that mental health nurses are in an ideal position to assess service consumers' physical health needs and to promote healthy living (Happell, Davies & Scott, 2012; Howard & Gamble, 2011). Gray, Hardy and Anderson (2009) have asked: if the mental health nurse does not intervene to improve the physical health needs of mental health consumers, then who will? In the Australian and New Zealand context of holistic training of undergraduate nursing, this provides an opportunity for those who develop their career in mental health to have the knowledge and skills to meaningfully address these issues (Wand & Murray, 2008). Therefore it would appear that part of the duty of the mental health practitioner is to have greater awareness of the signs and symptoms of physical illness, long-term physical conditions and also local service provision, so that they can guide consumers to the most appropriate care and support (Gray, Hardy & Anderson, 2009; Hardy, 2008). This would suggest that, in providing holistic care to the service consumer and their carers, mental health nurses need some basic knowledge in relation to screening and management of long-term conditions. Thus the mental health nurse has a dual role in promoting both mental and physical health, as it would appear that a person cannot have one without the other (Gray, Hardy & Anderson, 2009; Happell et al., 2011; Hardy & White, 2013; Howard & Gamble, 2011; Lawn, 2012; Nash, 2010; White, Gray & Jones, 2009).

Finally, it has been suggested that mental health consumers should feel respected, be treated as equal partners and be informed in the choices they have about their physical health (Lawn, 2012). This has been mirrored in the mental health nursing literature with the message that mental health nurses need the knowledge and skills to be able to meaningfully engage in interactions that allow transfer of information that keeps the mental health consumer at the heart of their physical needs (Happell et al., 2012; Happell, Scott & Platania-Phung, 2012).

Basic vital monitoring and general investigations

Basic tests are done because they're a good general measure of physiological functioning and they're not particularly invasive. They are also routine and commonplace, so people usually understand the procedures and their usefulness. Monitoring and recording them over time can give us an indication of how someone's health is progressing (see Table 3.1 and Table 3.2).

Specific physiological tests are available to screen for and diagnose a condition, as well as monitor treatment of a condition. Richards and Gurr (2000) found that emergency physicians regularly attend to consumers presenting with acute psychosis, and 20 per cent are found to have a purely medical aetiology—and this is still very much the case today. Thus, physical causation should never be discounted. Table 3.3 provides an indication of some general investigations that may be undertaken if a problem is suspected and more specific pathological investigations for specific conditions are required.

TABLE 3.1 ROUTINE PHYSICAL OBSERVATIONS

Observation	Comments
Blood pressure	This is now often measured using electronic sphygmomanometers, although there is suggestion that irregular heart rhythms and other warning signs may be missed, which may indicate the possibility of stroke or transient ischaemic attack (TIA).
Pulse	Resting pulse rates can vary widely, often showing greatest differences between sedentary individuals and those with active lifestyles that include exercise. As well as the rate of the pulse, other indicators such as rhythm, volume and tone can be obtained by palpating the radial pulse.
Respiration	Often accompanying the respiratory rate itself, measurements of oxygen saturation using portable devices can add detail to this assessment of functioning.
Temperature	Baseline normal limits can vary widely depending on the site of measurement and its distance from 'core' temperature, as well as environmental variables.

TABLE 3.2 ROUTINE OBSERVATION RANGES

Observation	Normal range	Risk area
Blood pressure	120/80	<100/60, >160/90
Pulse	60–99 beats per minute	<45, >100
Respiration	10–19 breaths per minute	<8, >20
Temperature	36–37.5°C	<35.0, >38.0

TABLE 3.3 GENERAL AND PATHOLOGICAL INVESTIGATIONS

Pathological investigations	General Diagnostic investigations
Haematological testing	Diagnostic X-rays
Biochemical testing	Anatomical imaging (MRI/CT)
Other tests (for example, prolactin levels, levels of various tests)	Electrocardiography (ECG)
	Neurological examinations
	Electroencephalography (EEG)
	Nuclear medicine imaging (PET scans)

CRITICAL THINKING OPPORTUNITY

1 When have you undertaken basic vital monitoring and why?

2 Should temperature, pulse and respirations (TPR) be used as a regular part of the role of the mental health nurse? If so, why?

3 What other basic health monitoring can nurses do to identify physical health issues or risk of medical co-morbidities for people with SMI?

4 Research each specific physiological test. Why would these relate to people who are diagnosed with a SMI?

5 Think of possible occasions when a consumer would present with psychiatric symptoms, but may actually have an underlying physical illness that requires treatment.

ABOUT THE CONSUMER Bradley's story

Bradley is a 39-year-old man brought into an emergency department (ED) by police and ambulance officers. He had been reported by a passer-by as wandering in traffic at risk of being run over. Bradley is a tall, obese man with long greasy hair, and on arrival at the ED he was in an agitated and disoriented state. He was dressed in an overcoat, even though it was a hot day, and was malodorous. He appeared to mutter to himself, possibly responding to internal stimuli, suggesting that he may have been experiencing auditory hallucinations. His manner was threatening and guarded, and he was shouting obscenities at the police, displaying disinhibited behaviour.

ADMISSIONS

From past discharge summaries from the ED, Bradley had been seen a number of times over the previous few months. These past reports mentioned that he was an intravenous drug user of amphetamines, that he had been treated previously for cellulitis on his arm, and alcohol intoxication. He had been under the care of mental health services with a diagnosis of bipolar affective disorder and had been prescribed a mood stabiliser and an antipsychotic medication Olanzapine 10mg to help regulate his mood. However, he'd had no contact with these services or his GP for three months. He had not appeared mentally ill at these ED visits and had refused a mental health services assessment. He had also refused any contact to be made with his mother, stating that they had a tenuous relationship due to his substance use.

STEVE HEMINGWAY, JULIE SHARROCK AND GAGANPREET LEGHA

A report by the paramedics who were the first contact point for Bradley reported that his vital signs showed that he had an elevated temperature, his blood pressure was raised and he appeared to be dehydrated. He was thought to be substance-affected and psychotic.

During the assessment and engagement process with the ED mental health nurse, he was concurrently examined by a resident medical officer, who found Bradley to be pyrexic and dehydrated, with his left arm swollen and inflamed, so the possibility of cellulitis was questioned. An intravenous saline and glucose drip was ordered and various pathology and diagnostic tests were performed. The ED mental health nurse continued to liaise with the medical team about managing Bradley's mental health issues.

The findings from Bradley's blood test results showed a raised cholesterol level, raised glucose levels and some abnormalities in urea and electrolytes suggestive of dehydration. His liver function levels were also raised, with a blood alcohol level of 0.18 indicating intoxication, while urine testing showed levels of amphetamines and marijuana in his system. ECG showed tachycardia. His full blood examination didn't show any significant changes.

Bradley's next of kin was his mother, who lived some 100 kilometres away in a rural country town, and he had no clear links with a GP.

A picture was emerging of a man with a co-morbid diagnosis of a mood disorder and substance abuse, combined with major stressors of homelessness, unemployment and estrangement from his family of origin. He was in a debilitated physical condition, with factors such as dehydration, infection and amphetamine and alcohol intoxication contributing to his behavioural disturbance. The potential for longer-term complications such as diabetes and ischaemic heart disease had also been identified.

With the treatment of intravenous rehydration, and close monitoring while Bradley's body detoxified from the acute intoxication of alcohol and amphetamine, his mental state improved and he became more rational. He was able to cooperate with a full mental status examination by the ED mental health nurse and this highlighted a lowered mood, with no suicidal ideation and no cognitive impairment or psychotic symptoms present. He showed insight and stated that he had continued to be adherent with his prescribed mood stabiliser. With Bradley's permission contact was made with his mother, who was prepared to provide him with a place to stay. The ED medical officer prescribed him a course of oral antibiotics for the cellulitis in his arm. He was agreeable to follow up with the family GP who would monitor his possible indicators of diabetes and ischaemic heart disease, and continue treatment for cellulitis as required. He was referred to other appropriate pathways of care, such as a community mental health clinic for assessment for case management, and drug and alcohol counselling for lifestyle choices.

1 What would be your first impression of Bradley's presentation?

2 Would you be influenced by his past history of mental illness and illicit drug use? What else may be influencing his behaviour?

3 What other physical complications may be influencing his behaviour?

4 Would you be confident in identifying symptoms of delirium?

5 What arrangements or referral on Bradley's discharge would assist him to maintain stability and meet his health needs?

Mental health care of people who have physical health problems

Increased psychiatric co-morbidity in general hospital consumers has been demonstrated (Giandinoto & Edward, 2014; Slade et al., 2009) that results in increased suffering, morbidity and mortality, causes significant distress for relatives and staff, and increases resource usage (Zolnierek, 2009). One of many examples is in relation to ischaemic heart disease, where depression has been established as an independent risk factor for myocardial infarction (Lichtman et al., 2014). It is also clear that people with SMI are at a higher risk of medical co-morbidities and thus may require medical treatment in acute care settings like the emergency department, intensive care units or medical-surgical wards.

Mental disorders most commonly seen in general hospitals are mood (particularly depression), anxiety, somatoform, cognitive (particularly delirium and dementia), substance-related, personality and psychotic disorders. These mental disorders could be pre-existing, coexisting or arising in response to consumers' deteriorating physical health. In any case, there is a need to address all health concerns to ensure holistic care.

ABOUT THE CONSUMER Margaret's story

Margaret is a 75-year-old woman admitted to a medical ward for treatment and management of hyperglycaemia and diabetic ketoacidosis. She has been on the ward for five days and the nursing staff noticed that she is forgetful, has poor dietary intake and becomes tearful easily. She was medically stable and her diagnostic tests didn't suggest any acute organic issues. The CLN was on the ward reviewing another consumer when a nurse discussed her symptoms with the CLN, but said that other staff didn't think a psychiatric review was necessary at this point. The CLN advised the nurse to discuss this within the multidisciplinary team and consider referral.

Margaret was initially reluctant to receive a psychiatric review, but later agreed after advice by her 35-year-old daughter. She requested for her daughter to be present at time of review.

The CLN arranged for the assessment in the ward's family room. (Psychiatric assessments in a medical ward can be challenging as the focus is on the consumer's medical condition. This could be the person's first psychiatric contact/ assessment. All efforts should be made to maintain the consumer's privacy and comfort.)

BACKGROUND

Margaret lives independently a two-bedroom unit. She was married for 38 years and her husband passed away last year. He had various medical conditions and had been on dialysis for two years prior to his death. Margaret has three children (two sons and a daughter). Her daughter lives close to her house, but both her sons live interstate. She used to be a primary school teacher and retired at 62; she says that she felt physically fit and able to continue work but had to retire as she had to look after her husband.

Margaret was diagnosed with diabetes mellitus type II at age 65, which worsened over a period of time and she has been on insulin therapy for the last two years. She is also on treatment for hypertension and increased cholesterol. She manages her own medication. She stated that for the last six months she has often forgotten to take her medication. Prior to admission she hadn't checked her blood sugar levels (BSL) for a few days. Her daughter noticed that she looked more unwell and so took her to her GP, who checked her BSL and ketones and advised her to take Margaret to the emergency department, leading to this medical admission. Margaret doesn't have history of any psychiatric illness or contact with psychiatric services.

STEVE HEMINGWAY, JULIE SHARROCK AND GAGANPREET LEGHA

ASSESSMENT

On assessment Margaret presented with a low mood and was tearful on many occasions. She expressed ongoing grief over her husband's death. She talked about significant factors affecting her, like her sons moving interstate, difficulties and changes in her life while caring for her husband, and guilt over feeling this way. She reported low energy levels, poor motivation and poor-quality sleep. She denied any suicidal or self-harm thoughts, but admitted to feeling hopeless and helpless. She expressed fear about her own medical issues as her diabetes seems to be getting worse and had started to affect her renal function. She admitted to poor concentration and attention that had emerged over the previous three months and coincided with the drop in mood, low energy levels, poor sleep and guilt. This resulted in her forgetting to take her medication.

INTERVENTION

The CLN felt that Margaret was depressed and needed treatment for the same. She also identified the need for psychological and social support for her. In liaison with the medical team she found that Margaret was planned for discharge on the same day, so it was difficult to arrange a review with a psychiatrist or psychiatric registrar. The CLN then liaised with Margaret's GP to arrange a referral to a community mental health centre for brief intervention, with a view for them to work with the GP for ongoing follow-up and to arrange psychological support.

The CLN also identified that Margaret required some more assistance with her medical co-morbidities and so advised ward staff to arrange community nursing services for supervision of her medication at home for some time. The nurse also requested a diabetes educator to speak to Margaret regarding her concerns about her health. The ward arranged this through the outpatient diabetes clinic and the CLN suggested that the appointment might be more beneficial if scheduled after treatment of her depression had commenced.

The CLN also provided education to Margaret and her daughter around depression and its treatment. They were receptive to psychiatric community team support.

After this case the CLN felt the need to educate the ward staff about identifying mental health needs for their consumer and the value of early referral. The CLN arranged these sessions with assistance from the nurse unit manager.

REFLECTION QUESTIONS

1 Have you had experience of accessing the expertise of a CLN? Reflect on whether this has helped in consumer care and improved your understanding.

2 In this case scenario, what role did the CLN play in consumer care, education and liaison with different teams?

3 The CLN role is considered to be an advanced nursing role. Do you agree with this and can you identify the advanced practices in the above scenario?

Mental health care in physical health-care settings: The role of a consultation–liaison nurse

Non-psychiatric acute care settings are complex places where staff are busy and often task oriented, and thus lack either the time or confidence to manage consumers with psychiatric co-morbidities. The attitudes and perceptions of staff towards mental health problems also influences their ability to identify and respond to the mental health needs of the people in their care. There has been considerable evidence to suggest the availability of skilled mental health nurses to health professionals working in general health services can positively influence the care of consumer with mental health problems in that setting (Brinkman et al., 2009; Clarke et al., 2005; Cullum et al., 2007; de Jonge, Latour & Huyse, 2003; Happell & Sharrock, 2002; Harvey, Fisher & Green, 2012; Johnston & Cowman, 2008; Koekkoek, van Baarsen & Steenbeek, 2015; McDonough et al., 2004; Sharrock & Happell, 2001, 2002; Sharrock et al., 2006; Sinclair et al., 2006; Wand & White; Wand et al., 2011a, 2011b; Wand et al., 2012, 2015; Wood, Middleton & Leonard, 2010).

There is also evidence that the Consultation–Liaison Nurse (CLN) can have an impact on resource usage (Fossey & Parsonage, 2014), in particular in relation to the rationalisation of one-to-one nursing for at-risk consumers. Improving processes in relation to assessment, documentation, review and supervision of one-to-one nurses and other colleagues not only reduces costs but also improves the quality of care to consumers (Wood & Wand, 2014).

There is no universally agreed upon term to describe advanced mental health nurses working in general hospitals, including emergency departments. Various titles are used including Mental Health Nurse Consultant, Consultation–Liaison Nurse, Liaison Nurse and Emergency Department Mental Health Nurse. Consultation–Liaison Nurse (CLN) is used in this chapter.

A request for consultation from the CLN is made when staff are uncertain if symptoms presenting in a consumer warrant attention from a mental health specialist (Sharrock & Happell, 2006). Nursing staff are more likely to require assistance in cases where the mental health needs of the consumer are beyond the expertise of the staff. This is particularly so where the symptoms (particularly behavioural) interfere with treatment; have implications for nursing care; present risks to consumer, staff and others; are disturbing or perplexing for staff; or have a significant impact on the ward system (Sharrock et al., 2006). Sometimes all that is required is a brief consultation that provides staff with an opportunity to clarify concerns, receive advice or guidance, receive assistance to decide on a course of action and/or be linked with relevant resources and information. It may also be that this type of conversation uncovers a person and/or a staff team that requires more extensive involvement by the CLN.

In these circumstances, the CLN gathers all the available information, including a consumer assessment. The CLN continues to maintain regular contact and provide feedback to the staff during the consultation. This is important in order to do a comprehensive assessment, translate the mental health assessment for the staff, monitor the progress of the consumer and the effectiveness of the management plan, answer questions, respond to concerns, and provide guidance and support to staff. Throughout the consumer assessment and review process, the CLN pays particular attention to the impact of the presenting problems on nursing staff and the delivery of care.

Each interaction with the consumer is an opportunity for role modelling and informal education of staff. The CLN is mindful of the goals of improving the care of the consumer and supporting mental health expertise development in the staff. Formal education sessions in the care of the consumer can be provided with written resources to support the sessions, and for staff who are unable to attend. Care-planning meetings with staff are also very useful, particularly for complex care issues, providing staff with an opportunity to reflect on the care they are providing (Sharrock & Happell, 2006).

The consultation remains active until there is satisfactory resolution or containment of the issues that precipitated the request, and this is evaluated through discussion between the CLN and the staff. The CLN seeks feedback from the staff to review and evaluate the strategies undertaken within the consultation, especially what was and was not helpful, and to check if the expectations of the staff were met (Antai-Otong & Krupnick, 2003). The consumer's feedback is also incorporated and the CLN pays attention to the ending of this relationship.

ABOUT THE CONSUMER Bradley's story (continued)

Two weeks following discharge from hospital, Bradley attended the clinic and as well as agreeing to the need for case management he stated he wished to change his lifestyle and improve his fitness and health overall. The community mental health nurse conducted a comprehensive physical assessment.

1   What physical health assessments have you seen used in clinical practice?
2   Does the nurse need to have sophisticated knowledge and skills in physical health interventions to carry out such assessments?

Physical health assessments

There are comprehensive assessments available for the mental health nurse and allied practitioners to assess and inform clinical decision-making regarding a mental health service consumer's physical needs (Eldridge, Dawber & Gray, 2011; White, Gray & Jones, 2009). One such assessment tool is the health improvement profile (HIP), which is designed to guide mental health practitioners towards assessing and implementing care that comprehensively addresses the consumer's physical health status (Hardy, White & Gray, 2015; White, 2015). The HIP has a female and male version. Each consists of twenty-eight items relating to the physical health of the consumer, and is completed by the mental health nurse interviewing the consumer. The HIP, in turn, guides the intervention as related to the presenting health need (Happell et al., 2012). 'Flags' are used to signpost relevant interventions as appropriate. A green flag indicates normal presentation with no intervention necessary. A red flag indicates action necessary and the HIP guides the mental health nurse to the appropriate intervention. This may include advice and referral for lifestyle choices, and liaison between the mental health nurse and GP and/or psychiatrist, with the danger to health indicating how immediate this needs to be. As a baseline measure, the HIP also can inform annual reviews of consumers' physical health status and subsequent treatment plans (Happell et al., 2011).

The HIP has been designed to be readily used in clinical practice and is available online (see 'Useful websites' at the end of this chapter). It has been developed to use in typical secondary care mental health settings (White, Gray & Jones, 2009) as well as in primary care by non-mental health nurses (Hardy & Gray, 2010). Randomised controlled trials are underway in the UK to determine the effectiveness of the HIP on clinical practice and outcomes for consumers (White et al., 2011). Happell and colleagues (2012) have discussed its development and use in Australia and it does seem to be promising in its potential applicability to both metropolitan and rural areas to detect and manage health problems for an optimum outcome.

Some health organisations have developed comprehensive physical health assessment, metabolic monitoring tools and algorithms for assessment and management of physical health issues of mental health consumers. Readers are encouraged to research which specific assessments of mental health consumers' physical status are used and implemented.

ABOUT THE CONSUMER Bradley's story (continued)

As a result of Bradley's assessment using the HIP, and although he was in the green range indicating no intervention was necessary, he was found to have a BMI of 32 and waist circumference of 99 cm. His lipid levels were elevated. His dietary fat intake was high and fruit and fibre intake low. Bradley's exercise activity was also assessed as minimal. These areas are listed in the red flag column of Table 3.4, along with recommended actions.

TABLE 3.4 HEALTH IMPROVEMENT PROFILE ASSESSMENT SCORES

Parameter	Level	Green	Red	Recommended action for red group
BMI	32	18.50–24.9	<18.50 ≥25.00	• BMI <18.50—refer for further investigations • BMI ≥25.00—advice and support on diet and exercise, referral to local weight/exercise management program, consider medication review
Waist circumference	99 cm	<94 cm	≥94 cm	• Advice and support on diet and exercise, referral to local weight/exercise management program, consider medication review
Lipid levels				
TC	7.2	TC <5.1 mmol/L	TC ≥6.2 mmol/L	• Refer to GP for appropriate treatment
LDL	3.6	LDL–C <4.1 mmol/L	LDL–C ≥4.1 mmol/L	
HDL	0.8	HDL–C > 1.0 mmol/L	HDL–C <1.0 mmol/L	
TG	5.5	TG <2.2 mmol/L2	or TG ≥2.2 mmol/L2	
Diet: Fruits and vegetables	1–2 a day	5 portions a day	<2 portions a day	• Offer recommendations on reduction of health risks with 5 servings of fruit and vegetables a day • Address potential barriers to accessing and eating fruit/vegetables • Agree and implement a plan with the consumer (and carers if appropriate) • May include referral to other members of the MDT; for example, occupational therapist for meal planning, shopping and cooking skills
Diet: fat intake	4–5 a day	≥1 portion a day	≥3 portions a day	• Advice on reducing fat intake and achieving a well-balanced diet • Agree and implement a plan with the consumer (and carers if appropriate) • May include referral to other members of the MDT; for example, occupational therapist for meal planning, shopping and cooking skills
Exercise	10 minutes a day	30 minutes a day	None	• Recommend 30 minutes of activity 5 days a week • Follow up on a 3–6-monthly period • Refer to exercise referral scheme if required

Adapted from Hardy and Gray (2012)

As a result of the HIP assessment, the community mental health nurse liaised with Bradley's GP and the primary care team. Subsequently, Bradley was prescribed a statin due to his raised lipid profile and his existing olanzapine medication was stopped because his mood was well controlled and the dose may have been one of the factors causing his increased lipid profile. In discussion about transport, Bradley stated he took the bus, or a taxi when he could afford it. He was encouraged to exercise by walking more, starting with walking to the shops. For a change in dietary intake Bradley was referred to the weekly cooking club, which was facilitated by the local community mental health team's occupational therapist. This was socially positive for Bradley and exposed him to ways in which he could increase healthy living options in his diet.

DRUG AND ALCOHOL COUNSELLING

Bradley attended drug and alcohol counselling sessions, gradually reduced his alcohol intake and now has not used intravenous drugs for some time, with the encouragement of his girlfriend. He now states he would like to take up sport to get fit again. He used to play Aussie Rules football for his local team and would like to pursue this as an option.

REFLECTION QUESTIONS

1 How would you progress the interview with Bradley?
2 What is a realistic plan that will support Bradley towards his goal of achieving fitness?
3 What are the agencies that can be involved in facilitating sport and exercise as an option for people diagnosed with a SMI?

Exercise and lifestyle factors that promote wellness

An extensive body of evidence regarding the effectiveness of lifestyle interventions in the general population already exists, but the challenge facing mental health services is to adapt such programs for the unique needs of people living with mental illness (Mental Health Commission of NSW, 2016). Physical activity can have a positive impact on physical status and subsequently mental health and well-being (Happell et al., 2011; Hirst & Hemingway, 2012). Besides knowing the benefits of physical activity, it can often be hard to motivate the general population to engage in regular physical activity (Mental Health Commission of NSW, 2016). This is further compounded in people with mental illness due to ongoing symptoms, poor motivation, side effects of medication, access to exercise equipment, and cost and knowledge (Stanton, Reaburn & Happell, 2015). Mental health nurses are in an ideal position to introduce physical activity into the lives of mental health consumers (Happell et al., 2011). The ideal physical activity program for people with mental illness is the one they are likely to do with a consistent message of 'move more, sit less' (Vancampfort et al., 2015).

Adjunct or alternative considerations are lifestyle changes in diet (Eldridge, Dawber & Gray, 2011; Park, Usher & Foster, 2011) and reducing or quitting smoking (Robson, 2010), both of which could have a positive impact on the health status of the mental health consumer. In a review of research literature, Happell, Davies and Scott (2012) found that mental health nurses can also make a difference in helping consumers change their health behaviours; for example, through physical exercise, nutrition, reduction in smoking and alcohol misuse interventions. Research into sexual risk behaviour among people with 'severe' mental illness suggests that they are likely to engage in high-risk sexual behaviour and therefore screening and education about consumers' sexual health should also be a part of healthy lifestyle education (Higgins, Barker & Begley, 2006).

Ideally, multifaceted interventions incorporating lifestyle education on diet, exercise and behavioural modification components promoting healthy behaviours are more effective (Ward, White & Druss, 2015). These should become a normal part of the mental health nurse role as they could make a significant contribution to lessening the high rates of physical morbidity and resultant mortality.

ABOUT THE CONSUMER   Bradley's story (continued)

Bradley previously suffered sexual dysfunction, seemingly from the consumption of a cocktail of intravenous drugs and alcohol. In a discharge session with the drug and alcohol counsellor, he disclosed he and his girlfriend would now like to make their relationship more intimate. However, Bradley's girlfriend is worried she is at risk due to his past intravenous drug use. The HIP screening (see Table 3.5) identified that Bradley was at risk, and it was now felt to be appropriate to refer him to a specialist sexual health nurse to screen for sexually transmitted diseases.

TABLE 3.5 HEALTH IMPROVEMENT PROFILE ASSESSMENT SCORES (SAFE SEX)

Parameter	Level	Green	Red	Recommended action for red group
Safe sex	Inconsistently	Always	Inconsistently/never	• Identify if consumer is in high risk group for STIs • Identify if consumer is engaging in behaviours that increase risk of STIs • Provide sexual health advice • If STI suspected, refer to GP or sexual health practice nurse

Adapted from Hardy and Gray (2012)

REFLECTION QUESTIONS

1   Discussing issues to do with sexual behaviour is sometimes seen as taboo. Would you be comfortable in this situation?

2   What is the mental health nurse's role when consumers engage in behaviours that put them at risk?

Primary, secondary and tertiary interventions for physical health

Nash (2014) gives examples of where mental health nurses can provide education and promotion of all aspects of physical health as part of their assessment and interventions. Primary intervention prevents the condition occurring before it happens; as discussed in this chapter, mental health consumers are highly likely to develop certain physical health problems. Therefore, a review of any physical risks and how to minimise these literally could be a life-saving intervention. Secondary intervention involves working with a condition in the early onset period and reducing complications that may arise as the condition progresses. Tertiary intervention is when the physical health condition is already well advanced. The mental health nurse's role here is to improve the quality of life and reduce the impact of the condition on daily life. In all areas of physical health, the mental health nurse can make a fundamental difference in improving the consumer's physical health status and their chances of a longer, fulfilling life.

Mental health nurses work in many roles where physical health is as much a priority as mental health. We have discussed one such role; that is, the psychiatric clinical liaison nurse. Most mental health nurse practitioners roles in Australia have been developed to provide an integrated health approach. Nurses working in Hospital Admission and Risk Programmes (HARP) manage people with complex health needs and provide care coordination and education on all related matters.

The carer's perspective

The carers of people with SMI face a Herculean task in, first, coming to terms with this diagnosis for their loved ones; and, second, processing how it will impact on their lives. The importance of the carer's role is further acknowledged in the *2012 National Report Card on Mental Health and Suicide Prevention* (National Mental Health Commission, 2012, p. 39), which suggests that mental health service professionals need to rethink their approaches in an inclusive way in order to assist the carers' 'need to recover', as well as that of the individuals with the SMI.

Carers play an important role in supporting and managing the general health and wellbeing of those suffering with SMI. They support people with SMI in routine activities like meal preparation, assistance with shopping, supervising medication, escorting to appointments etc. They can also support a consumer in making healthy lifestyle choices. Clinicians should understand and acknowledge the role of carers and involve them, with permission from the consumer, in planning care and providing education to their consumers.

ABOUT THE CONSUMER   Bradley's story (continued)

Bradley's mother has remained involved in his care, and has requested support in her role as his carer. Her needs will also be addressed through the local area mental health service, through an integrated service model. This model entails not only her inclusion in Bradley's ongoing treatment and recovery, but also in assessing her ongoing needs for services to safeguard her own emotional and psychological health. Appropriate referrals to lessen her burden may include a peer education program conducted by the Mental Illness (MI) Fellowship of Australia. The MI fellowship has also created a *Physical Health and Wellbeing* handbook for consumers, carers and support workers.

Recovery

Jacobson and Greenley (2001) encapsulate the concept of recovery as a 'healing process, in defining a self apart from illness and control'. The guiding principles of recovery-oriented practice include the notions of 'self determination, personal growth, choice and meaningful social engagement' for those with a SMI

(Victorian Department of Health, 2011). The recovery model promotes the principles of choice for the consumer with a SMI from a holistic perspective, instilling hope, encouraging autonomy and providing assistance to the consumer in navigating their own individual journey. Boardman and Shephard (2011) emphasise the importance of self-determination and optimism in 'sustaining motivation and supporting expectations' for this consumer group. The need for the consumer to 'identify their own strengths and preferences' is also acknowledged by Davidson and colleagues (2006). Recurring themes emerge in the literature on recovery-oriented practice, integrating concepts to assist those consumers with a SMI. They include the need for social inclusion 'provided through participation in community life' (Le Boutillier et al., 2011).

These overarching principles reflect the rights of the consumer for self-determination in fashioning and fine-tuning their own individual recovery process. The mental health nurse, by working in collaboration with the consumer, should have a vision of recovery, incorporating all the goals and preferences of the consumer. To assist with recovery and integration of the consumer into meaningful, fulfilling activities, the mental health nurse needs to have a broad knowledge of the range of community and health-related services available.

■ TOPIC LINK

See Chapter 6 for more on recovery.

SUMMARY

Nurses in all clinical settings have the responsibility to implement and use tools to identify potential health issues for the population of the seriously mentally ill, and to work in partnership with mental health services, GPs and other community services. The issues highlighted in this chapter should raise the awareness of all mental health clinicians of the need to closely monitor and to be proactive in working with their clientele to ensure the best possible physical care to this already disadvantaged population. The discrepancies in health-care provision to those with a SMI raised in this chapter highlight the need for systemic, organisational and governmental interventions to provide the resources to address this growing trend in co-morbidity by improving services to those with a SMI. Nurses in every clinical setting will deal with people with a SMI, be it at a GP's surgery, the medical-surgical ward, outpatient services or nursing homes. It is hoped that awareness of this population's complex needs will be viewed holistically with an integrated health-care response.

This chapter has also highlighted some the issues that those with a severe mental illness have to contend with, including:

- a poor prognosis in terms of their physical health if timely interventions do not occur
- co-morbid conditions associated with their treatment and lifestyle choices

Service issues that impact on the care of people with both physical and mental health problems include:

- the need for mental health nurses to take a leading role in identifying potential or existing health issues in those with a SMI
- establishment of stronger linkages between agencies that provide a service to those with a SMI
- ongoing education in using the tools that assist in identifying potential or existing health issues in those with a SMI.

STEVE HEMINGWAY, JULIE SHARROCK AND GAGANPREET LEGHA

DISCUSSION QUESTIONS

1 Are the physical health needs of consumers diagnosed with a severe mental illness given sufficient emphasis in the clinical contexts you have experienced?

2 Given barriers between and within organisations in implementing physical health interventions for the seriously mentally ill, how do you think these can be overcome?

3 Is the type of intervention the MHN undertakes contextualised to where they work?

4 How do you realistically work with a consumer who is not motivated to deal with their health needs?

5 Does the mental health nurse have the requisite knowledge and skills to undertake physical health interventions?

TEST YOURSELF

1 It is estimated that when compared to the general population people with a serious mental illness die:

a 2 years younger

b 10 years younger

c 25 years younger

d 46 years younger

2 Diagnostic overshadowing is:

a a shadow on the lungs related to cancer

b mixing up a diagnosis between anxiety and depression

c too much emphasis on diagnosis rather than a consumer's recovery

d when practitioners focus on the mental health diagnosis rather than physical health needs of the consumer

3 Mental disorders most commonly seen in general hospitals are:

a mood (particularly depression), anxiety, somatoform, cognitive (particularly delirium and dementia), substance-related, personality and psychotic disorders

b co-morbid disorders such as diabetes and schizophrenia

c iatrogenic side effects from mental health medication

d PTSD, AN, bulimia and panic disorder

4 The role of the consultation nurse is required when:

a mental health symptoms (particularly behavioural) interfere with treatment; have implications for nursing care; or present risks to consumer, staff and others

b psychotherapy is needed on the ward units

c mental health medication is needed to be prescribed

d general nursing staff need to be positively educated about mental illness

USEFUL WEBSITES

Health improvement profile: www.trialsjournal.com/content/12/1/167

Physical health checks for people with severe mental illness: A primary care guide: http://physicalsmi.webeden.co.uk

Psychiatry Positive Cardio Metabolic Algorithm—www.heti.nsw.gov.au/cmalgorithm

Wellways—Peer education programs: www.mifellowship.org/content/well-ways

Wellways— Information and resources: www.mifellowship.org/content/physical-health-wellbeing-resource-guide

REFERENCES

Allen, J., Balfour, R., Bell, R., & Marmot, M. (2014). Social determinants of mental health. *International Review of Psychiatry, 26*(4), 392–407.

Antai-Otong, D., & Krupnick, S. L. W. (2003). Psychiatric consultation-liaison nursing. In D. Antai-Otong (Ed.), *Psychiatric nursing: Biological and behavioral concepts* (pp. 923–947). Cengage Learning.

Boardman, J., & Shephard, G. (2011). Putting recovery into practice: Organisation change and commissioning. *Journal of Mental Health Training, Education and Practice, 6*(1), 7–16.

Brinkman, K., Hunks, D., Bruggencate, G., & Clelland, S. (2009). Evaluation of a new mental health liaison role in a rural health centre in Rocky Mountain House, Alberta: A Canadian story. *International Journal of Mental Health Nursing, 18*(1), 42–52.

Brown, S., Kim, M., Mitchell, C., & Inskip, H. (2010). Twenty-five year mortality of a community cohort with schizophrenia. *British Journal of Psychiatry, 196*(2), 116–121.

Clarke, D. E., Hughes, L., Brown, A.-M., & Motluk, L. (2005). Psychiatric emergency nurses in the emergency department: The success of the Winnipeg, Canada experience. *Journal of Emergency Nursing, 31*(4), 351–356.

Collins, E., Tranter, S., & Irvine, F. (2012). The physical health of the seriously mentally ill: An overview of the literature. *Journal of Psychiatric and Mental Health Nursing, 19*(7), 638–646.

Colton, C. W., & Manderscheid, R. W. (2006). Congruencies in increased mortality rates, years of potential life lost, and causes of death among public mental health clients in eight states. *Preventing Chronic Disease, 3*(2), A42.

Cullum, S., Tucker, S., Todd, C., & Brayne, C. (2007). Effectiveness of liaison psychiatric nursing in older medical inpatients with depression: A randomised controlled trial. *Age and Ageing, 36*(4), 436–442.

Davidson, L., Golan, S., Lawless, M. S., Sells, D., & Tondora, J. (2006). Play, pleasure and other positive life events: 'Non specific' factors in recovery from mental illness? *Psychiatry, 69*(2), 151–163.

de Jonge, P., Latour, C. H. M., & Huyse, F. J. (2003). Implementing psychiatric interventions on a medical ward: Effects on patients' quality of life and length of hospital stay. *Psychosomatic Medicine, 65*(6), 997–1002.

Disability Rights Commission (2006). *Equal treatment: Closing the gap—a formal investigation into physical health inequalities experienced by people with learning disabilities and/or mental health problems.* London: Disability Rights Commission.

Duggan, M. (2015). *Beyond the fragments: Preventing the costs and consequences of chronic physical and mental diseases.* Australian Health Policy Collaboration Issues Paper No. 2015–05. Melbourne: Australian Health Policy Collaboration.

Edward, K., Felstead, B., & Mahoney, A. M. (2011). Hospitalized mental health patients and oral health. *Journal of Psychiatric and Mental Health Nursing, 19*(5), 419–425.

Eldridge, D., Dawber, N., & Gray, R. (2011). A well-being support program for consumers with severe mental illness: A service evaluation. *BMC Psychiatry, 11*, 46.

Fossey, M., & Parsonage, M. (2014). *Outcomes and performance in liaison psychiatry: Developing a measurement framework.* Centre for Mental Health.

Giandinoto, J. A. & Edward, K. L. (2014). Challenges in acute care of people with co-morbid mental illness. *British Journal of Nursing. 23*(13), 728–32.

Gray, R., Hardy, S., & Anderson K. H. (2009). Physical health and serious mental illness: If we don't do something about it who will? *International Journal of Mental Health Nursing, 18*, 299–300.

Happell, B., & Sharrock, J. (2002). Evaluating the role of a psychiatric consultation-liaison nurse in the Australian general hospital. *Issues in Mental Health Nursing, 23*(1), 43–60.

Happell, B., Davies, C., & Scott, D. (2012). Health behaviour interventions to improve physical health in individuals diagnosed with a mental illness. *International Journal of Mental Health, 21*(3), 236–247.

Happell, B., Platania-Phung, C., Gray, R., Hardy, S., Lambert, T., McAlister, M., & Davies, C. (2011). A role for mental health nursing in the physical health care of consumers with severe mental illness. *Journal of Psychiatric and Mental Health Nursing, 18*(8), 706–711.

Happell, B., Platania-Phung, C., Scott, D., & Nankivell, J. (2014). Communication with colleagues: Frequency of collaboration regarding physical health of consumers with

mental illness. *Perspectives in Psychiatric Care, 50*(1), 33–43.

Happell, B., Scott, D., & Platania-Phung, C. (2012). Rural physical health care services for people with serious mental illness: A nursing perspective. *Australian Journal of Rural Health, 20*(5), 248–253.

Happell, B., Scott, D., Platania-Phung, C., & Nankivell, J. (2012). Nurses' views on physical activity for people with serious mental illness. *Mental Health and Physical Activity, 5*(1), 4–12.

Hardy, S. (2008). Integrating models of care for mental illness. *Practice Nurse, 36*(3), 38–40.

Hardy, S., & Gray, R. (2010). Adapting the severe mental illness physical health improvement profile for use in primary care. *International Journal of Mental Health Nursing, 19*, 350–355.

Hardy, S., & Gray, R. (2012). The health improvement profile for primary care (HIP-PC). In *Primary care physical health checks for people with severe mental illness (SMI)—Best practice guide* (3rd ed.). Northamptonshire: The Northampton Physical Health and Wellbeing Project (PhyHWell).

Hardy, S., & White, J. (2013). Why are people with serious mental illness still not getting their physical health checked? *Mental Health Nursing, 33*(1), 14–18.

Hardy, S., White, J., & Gray, R. (2015). *The Health Improvement Profile: A manual to promote physical wellbeing in people with severe mental illness.* Keswick: M&K Publishing.

Harvey, S. T., Fisher, L. J., & Green, V. M. (2012). Evaluating the clinical efficacy of a primary care-focused, nurse-led, consultation liaison model for perinatal mental health. *International Journal of Mental Health Nursing, 21*(1), 75–81.

Higgins, A., Barker, P., & Begley, C. M. (2006). Sexual health education for people with mental health problems: What can we learn from the literature? *Journal of Psychiatric and Mental Health Nursing, 13*(6), 687–697.

Hirst, C., & Hemingway, S. (2012). Exercise and older people who are diagnosed with depression: Reviewing the evidence. *Mental Health Nursing, 32*(3), 12–16.

Howard, L., & Gamble, C. (2011). Supporting mental health nurses to address the physical health needs of people with serious mental illness in acute inpatient settings. *Journal of Psychiatric and Mental Health Nursing, 18*(2), 105–112.

Jacobson, N., & Greenley, D. (2001). What is recovery? A conceptual model and explication. *Psychiatric Services, 52*(4), 482–485.

Johnston, M. L., & Cowman, S. (2008). An examination of the services provided by psychiatric consultation liaison nurses in a general hospital. *Journal of Psychiatric and Mental Health Nursing, 15*(6), 500–507.

Jordan, S., Philpin, S., & Davies, S. (2000). The biological sciences in mental health nursing: Stakeholders' perspectives. *Journal of Advanced Nursing, 32*(4), 881–891.

Koekkoek, B., van Baarsen, C., & Steenbeek, M. (2016). Multidisciplinary, nurse-led psychiatric consultation in nursing homes: A pilot study in clinical practice. *Perspectives in Psychiatric Care, 52*, 217–223.

Lambert, N. (2012). Understanding and supporting the physical health needs of clients. *Mental Health Practice, 15*(10), 14–19.

Lawn, S. (2012). In it together: Physical health and well-being for people with mental illness. *Australian and New Zealand Journal of Psychiatry, 46*(1), 14–17.

Le Boutillier C., Leamy, M., Bird, V. J., Davidson, L., Williams, J., & Slade M. (2011). What does recovery mean in practice? A qualitative analysis of international recovery-oriented practice guidance. *Psychiatric Services, 62*(12), 1470–6.

Lichtman, J. H., Froelicher, E. S., Blumenthal, J. A., Carney, R. M., Doering, L. V., Frasure-Smith, N., Vaccarino, V. (2014). Depression as a risk factor for poor prognosis among patients with acute coronary syndrome: Systematic review and recommendations. A scientific statement from the American Heart Association. *Circulation, 129*(12), 1350–1369.

Manderscheid, R. W., Ryff, C. D., Freeman, E. J., McKnight-Eily, L. R., Dhingra, S., & Strine, T. W. (2010). Evolving definitions of mental illness and wellness. *Preventing Chronic Disease, 7*(1), A19.

McDonough, S., Wynaden, D., Finn, M., McGowan, S., Chapman, R., & Hood, S. (2004). Emergency department mental health triage consultancy service: An evaluation of the first year of the service. *Accident and Emergency Nursing, 12*(1), 31–38.

Mental Health Commission of NSW (2016). *Physical health and mental wellbeing: Evidence guide*. Sydney: Mental Health Commission of NSW.

Ministerial Advisory Committee on Mental Health (2010). *Improving the physical health of people with severe mental illness*. Retrieved from http://docs.health.vic.gov.au/docs/doc/20C06D82E2C17401CA2578B700253D49/ $FILE/improving-the-physical-health-of-people-with-severe-mental-illness-no-mental-health-without-physical-health.doc.

Mitchell, A. J., Delaffon, V., Vancampfort, D., Correll, C. U., & De Hert, M. (2012). Guideline concordant monitoring of metabolic risk in people treated with antipsychotic medication: Systematic review and meta-analysis of screening practices. *Psychological Medicine, 42*(1), 125–147.

Muir-Cochrane, E. (2006). Medial co-morbidity risk factors and barriers to care for people with schizophrenia. *Journal of Psychiatric and Mental Health Nursing, 13*(4), 447–452.

Nash, M. (2010). *Facilitating physical health and wellbeing in mental health nursing: Clinical skills for practice*. Milton Keynes: Open University Press.

Nash, M. (2013). Diagnostic overshadowing: A potential barrier to physical health care for mental health service users. *Mental Health Practice, 17*(4), 22.

Nash, M. (2014). *Physical health and well-being in mental health nursing: Clinical skills for practice*. Maidenhead: McGraw-Hill Education.

National Mental Health Commission (2012). *A contributing life: The 2012 national report card on mental health and suicide prevention*. Sydney: NMHC.

National Mental Health Commission (2016). *Draft consensus statement on the physical health needs of people with a mental illness*. Retrieved from https://consultations.health.gov.au/national-mental-health-commission/594530eb/user_uploads/national-consensus-statement---online-consultation-draft.pdf.

National Summit on Addressing the Premature Death of People with a Mental Illness (2013). *Communiqué*. 24 May, Sydney. Retrieved from www.health.nsw.gov.au/mhdao/summit/Documents/Physical-mental-healthcare-summit.pdf.

Nocon, A. (2004). *Background evidence for the DRC's formal investigation into health inequalities experienced by people with learning difficulties or mental health problems*. London: Disability Rights Commission.

Park, T., Usher, K., & Foster, K. (2011). Description of a healthy lifestyle intervention for people with serious mental illness taking second generation antipsychotics. *International Journal of Mental Health Nursing, 20*(6), 428–437.

Parks, J., Svendsen, D., Singer, P., & Foti, M. (2006). Foreword. *Morbidity and mortality of people with serious mental illness*. Alexandria: National Association of State Mental Health Program Directors (NASMHPD) Medical Directors Council.

Peckham, E., Bradshaw, T. J., Brabyn, S., Knowles, S., & Gilbody, S. (2015). Exploring why people with SMI smoke and why they may want to quit: Baseline data from the SCIMITAR RCT. *Journal of Psychiatric and Mental Health Nursing, 23*(5), 282–289.

Phelan, M., Stradins, L., & Morrison, S. (2001). Physical health of people with severe mental illness, *British Medical Journal, 322*(7284), 443–444.

Qun, M. C., Holman, D. J., Sanfilippo, F. M., Emery, J. D., & Stewart, L. M. (2010). Do users of mental health services lack access to general practitioner services? *Medical Journal of Australia, 192*(9), 501–506.

Richards, C. F., & Gurr, D. F. (2000). Psychosis. *Emergency Medical Clinics of North America, 18*(2), 53–62.

Robson, D. (2010). Mental health and smoking: Effects on wellbeing. *British Journal of Wellbeing, 1*(9), 22–26.

Robson, D., & Gray, R. (2007). Serious mental illness and physical health problems: A discussion paper. *International Journal of Nursing Studies, 44*(3), 457–466.

Sharrock, J., & Happell, B. (2001). The role of the psychiatric consultation-liaison nurse in the improved care of patients experiencing mental health problems receiving care within a general hospital environment. *Contemporary Nurse, 11*(2–3), 260–270.

Sharrock, J., & Happell, B. (2002). The psychiatric consultation-liaison nurse: Thriving in a general hospital setting. *International Journal of Mental Health Nursing, 11*(1), 24–33.

Sharrock, J., & Happell, B. (2006). Competence in providing mental health care: A grounded theory analysis of nurses' experiences. *Australian Journal of Advanced Nursing, 24*(2), 9–15.

Sharrock, J., Grigg, M., Happell, B., Keeble-Devlin, B., & Jennings, S. (2006). The mental health nurse: A valuable addition to the consultation-liaison team. *International Journal of Mental Health Nursing, 15*(1), 35–43.

Sinclair, L., Hunter, R., Hagen, S., Nelson, D., & Hunt, J. (2006). How effective are mental health nurses in A&E departments? *Emergency Medicine Journal, 23*(9), 687–692.

Slade, T., Johnston, A., Teesson, M., Whiteford, H., Burgess, P., Pirkis, J., & Saw. S. (2009). *The mental health of Australians: 2. Report on the 2007 National Survey of Mental Health and Well-being*. Canberra: Department of Health and Ageing.

Stanton, R., Reaburn, P., & Happell, B. (2015). Barriers to exercise prescription and participation in people with mental illness: The perspectives of nurses working in mental health. *Journal of Psychiatric and Mental Health Nursing, 22*(6), 440–448.

Townsend, C. E., Pirkis, J. E., Pham, A. T. N., Harris, M. G., & Whiteford, H. A. (2006). Stakeholder concerns about Australia's mental health care system. *Australian Health Review, 30*(2), 158–163.

Valderas, J. M., Starfield, B., Sibbald, B., Salisbury, C., & Roland, M. (2009). Defining comorbidity: Implications for understanding health and health services. *Annals of Family Medicine*, 7(4), 357–363.

Vancampfort, D., Stubbs, B., Ward, P. B., Teasdale, S., & Rosenbaum, S. (2015). Why moving more should be promoted for severe mental illness. *The Lancet Psychiatry*, 2(4), 295.

Victorian Department of Health (2011). *Framework for recovery-orientated practice*. Retrieved from www.vic.gov.au/mentalhealth.

Wand, T., & Murray, L. (2008). Let's get physical. *International Journal of Mental Health Nursing*, 17(5), 363–369.

Wand, T., D'Abrew, N., Barnett, C., Acret, L., & White, K. (2015). Evaluation of a nurse practitioner-led extended hours mental health liaison nurse service based in the emergency department. *Australian Health Review*, 39(1), 1–8.

Wand, T., White, K., Patching, J., Dixon, J., & Green, T. (2011a). An emergency department based mental health nurse practitioner outpatient service: Part 1—Participant evaluation. *International Journal of Mental Health Nursing*, 20, 392–400. doi:10.1111/j.1447–0349.2011.00744.x.

Wand, T., White, K., Patching, J., Dixon, J., & Green, T. (2011b). An emergency department based mental health nurse practitioner outpatient service: Part 2—Staff evaluation. *International Journal of Mental Health Nursing*, 20, 401–408. doi:10.1111/j.1447–0349.2011.00743.x.

Wand, T., White, K., Patching (Nee Redenbach), J., Dixon, J., & Green, T. (2012). Outcomes from the evaluation of an emergency department-based mental health nurse practitioner outpatient service in Australia. *Journal of the American Academy of Nurse Practitioners*, 24(3), 149–159.

Ward, M. C., White, D. T., & Druss, B. G. (2015). A meta-review of lifestyle interventions for cardiovascular risk factors in the general medical population: Lessons for individuals with serious mental illness. *Journal of Clinical Psychiatry*, 76(4), e477–e486.

WHA (2009). Duty of care document. Retrieved from www.dph.uwa.edu.au. Accessed 9 September 2016.

White, J. (2015). *Physical health checks in serious mental illness: A programme of research in secondary care*. Doctoral thesis, University of East Anglia. Available at https://ueaeprints.uea.ac.uk/56777/.

White, J., Gray, R., & Jones, M. (2009). The development of a serious mental illness physical health improvement profile. *Journal of Psychiatric and Mental Health Nursing*, 16(3), 493–498.

White, J., Gray, R. J., Swift, L., Barton, G. R., & Jones, M. (2011). The serious mental illness health improvement profile [HIP]: study protocol for a cluster randomised controlled trial. *Trials*, 12(1), 167.

Wood, A., Middleton, S., & Leonard, D. (2010). When it's more than the blues: A collaborative response to postpartum depression. *Public Health Nursing*, 7(3), 248–254.

Wood, R., & Wand, A., (2014). Quality indicators for a consultation-liaison psychiatry service. *International Journal of Health Care Quality Assurance*, 27(7), 633–641.

World Federation for Mental Health (2010). *Mental health and chronic physical illnesses: The need for continued and integrated care*. Retrieved from www.wfmh.org/2010DOCS/WMHDAY2010.pdf.

Zolnierek, C. D. (2009). Non-psychiatric hospitalization of people with mental illness: Systematic review. *Journal of Advanced Nursing*, 65(8), 1570–1583.

STEVE HEMINGWAY, JULIE SHARROCK AND GAGANPREET LEGHA

CHAPTER 4

Promoting Mental Health

EILEEN PETRIE AND
EVAN BICHARA

KEY OUTCOMES

AFTER READING THIS CHAPTER, YOU SHOULD BE ABLE TO:

- describe the concepts underpinning health promotion
- describe preventative measures designed to interrupt the disease process
- identify health promotion interventions
- define mental health promotion.

KEY TERMS

- consumer advocate
- health promotion
- mental health
- mental health promotion
- mental illness
- public health

Introduction

In this chapter we explore mental health promotion as an emerging area of health that includes research, policy development, community action and program activity. Public health, characterised by concern for the health of the population as a whole, makes it necessary for health professionals to develop an understanding of mental health promotion. Adopting a public-health-focused approach and related understandings should assist policy-makers and practitioners in the development and implementation of effective interventions in mental health promotion, aligning the physical and psychosocial environments (VicHealth, 2006).

Mental health promotion accounts for the mental health of populations. Currently in the field of mental health, public health principles are utilised in the promotion of mental health and well-being and the prevention of mental illness. Ensuring that values, systems, structures and processes operating at all levels of society are included in the promotion of mental health and well-being permits the inclusion of biopsychosocial perspectives. It is important that consumer participation is seen as a significant part of an agency's overall organisational ethos in working with the individuals they constantly support. Consumer–carer participation provides further opportunities for recovery for people with a mental illness.

There are fundamental universal rights identified as determinants of mental health and well-being, including freedom from racism and sexism and other forms of discrimination. Other considerations identified as determinants of mental health include: violence and lack of safety, poverty and unemployment, poor employment conditions, lack of access to education and needed health services, lack of support for parents and carers, and homophobia. Failure to address major issues can contribute to the global burden of disease related to mental illness and co-morbidities, which has serious human, social and economic consequences.

Definitions of health promotion

In 1958, the World Health Organization (WHO) introduced the broad concept of protecting the health of people, based on the input from member nations. The WHO definition of health promotion (WHO, 1958, cited in Wass, 2000, p. 7) states that health extends beyond the physical realm: 'Health is a complete state of physical, mental and social well-being and not merely the absence of disease or infirmity.' In its definition of health promotion, VicHealth (2006, p. 12) states that it represents a comprehensive social and political process, not only embracing actions directed at strengthening the skills and capabilities of individuals but also action directed towards changing social, environmental and economic conditions so as to alleviate their impact on public and individual health.

Definitions of mental health have been jargonistic and have predominantly focused on the individual's capacity to incorporate external factors into their lives. The emergence of a definition that encompasses not just the absence of symptoms but also positive constructs permits a definite distinction between mental illness and mental health. VicHealth (2006, p. 13) defines mental health as: 'A state of well-being in which the individual realises his/her own abilities, can cope with the normal stresses of life, can work productively and fruitfully and is able to make a contribution to his/her community.' In the definition of mental illness, VicHealth (2006, p. 13) states that a mental disorder is 'a diagnosable disorder that significantly interferes with an individual's cognitive, emotional and/or social abilities. Mental disorders are of different types.'

Incorporating the concept of mental illness as described by VicHealth, we can say that the promotion of mental health occurs within the social, economic, emotional and cognitive domains. In Australia, the *Fourth National Mental Health Plan* (Australian Health Ministers, 2009) identified key priorities for action in the prevention and promotion of mental health. The *National Action Plan for Promotion, Prevention and Early Intervention for Mental Health* (Department of Health and Aged Care, 2000) reflects a population health approach to develop strategies addressing the needs and mental health status of populations. VicHealth's definition of mental health promotion (2006, p. 13) includes the criterion that it 'contributes to general health promotion by taking action to ensure social conditions and factors create positive environments for the good mental health and well-being of populations, communities and individuals'. The draft Fifth National Mental Health Plan for 2017–2022 was released for consultation in October 2016 and has targeted priority areas that include coordinated treatment, suicide prevention, stigma reduction, physical health, safety and quality, the mental health of Aboriginal and Torres Strait Islander peoples, and the integrated regional planning and service delivery of mental health services.

Establishing public health policies

An international congress of member nations in Alma Ata, Kazakhstan, in 1978 agreed to reflect a philosophy of the social model of health in the delivery of health care. The Ottawa Charter, founded in 1986, which arose out of the Alma Ata Declaration, set an agreement among member nations around the world that action was required to achieve health for all by 2000 (World Health Organization, 1986). The charter stated that health promotion is more than telling people to change their behaviour. It includes prerequisites for health, advocacy, equity control and the involvement of all. In the context of the Ottawa Charter (see Box 4.1), this description of health promotion influences public health policy—that is, health and equity in all sectors to address environmental concerns, which include products, resources, unhealthy environments and poor nutrition—to ensure responses to health gaps between societies, acknowledge people as the key resource and move health resources to health promotion (Guzys et al., 2014; McMurray & Clendon, 2015).

There is an obligation for nurses to recognise health and its maintenance as a major social investment and to address the overall ecological issues of our ways of living. Fundamental conditions are recognised as being key determinates of health, such as peace, shelter, education, food, income, a stable ecosystem, sustainable resources, social justice and equity. This philosophy underpins the provision of health care to address the social determinants of health.

BOX 4.1 THE OTTAWA CHARTER

The building of health promotion policies must be built on the five principles set out in the Ottawa Charter of 1986:

1. Building public policies that support health: policy-makers are to be aware of and responsible for the health consequences of their decisions.

2. Creating supportive healthy living environments: a socio-ecological approach to health should ensure a positive benefit to health while protecting the natural and built environments.

3. Strengthening community action: this requires empowerment of communities,

giving ownership and control of their destinies.

4. Assisting people to develop personal skills: this means informing and educating individuals in health to enhance life skills, permitting them control to make choices conducive to good health.

5. Reorienting health-care services: this means the sharing of responsibility for health promotion among individuals, community groups, health professionals and service providers, and governments (Barry & McQueen, 2005; Wass, 2000; World Health Organization, 1986).

The development of public health policies has been described as requiring a 'decisive, ethical, fair and strategic' approach (McMurray & Clendon, 2015, p. 442; Baum, 2016). Key stakeholders involved in policy development should include members of the community, political representatives and the media. This combination provides a reasonable representation of those required in order to be fair and equitable. The ability to critically influence public policy development is provided through social advocacy that is socially acceptable and scientifically sound (McMurray & Clendon, 2015). It is essential that equity is demonstrated in policy development to ensure that all members of any population receive the health benefits associated with social change.

More recently, the trend in Australia has been to develop policy that reflects the philosophy of the Ottawa Charter, which promotes integration to enable actions and interventions of greater efficacy that facilitate mentally healthy lifestyles, the reduction in the possibility of developing mental illnesses and the lessening of the impact of mental illness on society. This would include the reaffirmation of the national mental health policies in Australia and New Zealand, assurance of adherence to continuity of care, access to the mental health system of effective primary and secondary interventions, addressing the access to all populations so as to include rural, remote and Indigenous populations, upskilling of the mental health workforce and a greater intersectoral collaborative approach to care (Baum; 2016; Elder, Evans & Nizette, 2005).

1   'Disease prevention strategies can prevent or interrupt the disease process.' Give an example of an intervention strategy in mental illness that is related to this statement.

2   How does this relate to the Ottawa Charter?

Prevalence of mental illness

The World Health Organization (WHO, 2008) identified mental illness as accounting for 13 per cent of the global burden of disease (Hungerford et al., 2015; Thyloth, Singh & Subramanian, 2016), with an estimated 25 per cent of the population in any given year affected by mental health disorders. Within an Australian context, the statistics surrounding mental health and well-being indicate that one in five Australians will experience a mental disorder at some stage of their life (Australian Bureau of Statistics, 2013), with depression constituting the most significant mental health issue as there is a correlation of multifactorial causes of depression (Hungerford et al., 2015).

These alarming statistics identified in Australia demonstrate the prevalence of mental health disorders (Keleher & MacDougal, 2016) and mental illness, and their impact on society. The implications of this for government policy-makers becomes challenging as they attempt to reduce the burden of disease and ensure the wellness of populations. The establishment of models based on public health principles originating from the Ottawa Charter form frameworks in which health services can develop mental health promotion policies (Guzys et al., 2014; McMurray & Clendon, 2015).

Health promotion

Health promotion is based on the assumption that the health status of individuals or communities may be influenced purposefully by both a knowledge base and resource availability. In understanding health promotion, you will need to consider the theoretical underpinnings of health promotion as well as health promotion goals.

Theoretical basis of health promotion

There are two predominant perspectives: persuasive strategies and new patterns of behaviour that assist rather than persuade people to change (Guzys et al., 2014). In the health behaviour change concept, it is understood that health behaviour is a complex choice. Understanding the reasons a person adopts a particular lifestyle must be acknowledged with the concept of a possibility for modification of health-related behaviours. An example could be the issue of harm minimisation associated with illicit drug usage. Change in this instance requires a significant departure from normal behaviour. Failure to change should not be viewed as a fault of the consumer or organisation, or irrational behaviour, but rather as the result of failing to address pertinent issues. This may be a result of inadequate assessment, unrealistic expectations or failure to account for complex circumstances.

The *theory of reasoned action* identifies a person's attitude towards certain behaviours informed by their beliefs; that is, a person's ideas of what others will think of his or her behaviour. The *value expectancy theory* emphasises human motivation based on the value of the outcome to the individual. The person will engage in behaviour to the extent that positive value is released, and the person's later behaviour is based on the subjective expectancy of success: prior knowledge of success emulating the success of others.

Social cognitive theory is strongly affected by self-efficacy, experience, perception of personal competencies, reaction to persuasion and response to present situations, and also influenced by past experience, present motivation, future goals and judgment of personal capabilities (McMurray & Clendon, 2015). It suggests that behaviour arises out of previous experience, anticipation of the future, learning, being able to set one's own standards, and evaluating the behaviour of others.

The theory predicts goals people set for themselves and their performance attainment. It is an integral part of motivation and the self-regulation of motivation, and includes cognitive–perceptual factors and modifying factors as preliminary to participating in health behaviours, including:

- personal goals
- capacity for self-reflection
- value of positive growth and behavioural regulation
- relationship to and interaction with the environment.

Under this theory, change is believed to occur through:

- pre-contemplation
- contemplation
- preparation
- action
- maintenance
- termination.

The *transtheoretical model* provides a stage-based progression through the behavioural change process. It identifies the stages as being sequential but cyclic, allowing for behavioural regression and multiple attempts to change, and relates behavioural change to changes in environment and/or life experiences (McMurray & Clendon, 2015).

Therefore health promotion is dynamic. Initially, it requires identification of what is the health problem. Who defines it? One size does not fit all. It focuses on a view of quality of life and well-being and perception of need. All participants have specific needs as well as the collective needs of the group. An assessment of need is essential to effective health promotion. There is a need for planned educational intervention aimed primarily at the voluntary actions people can take on their own or as citizens to look after their own health or health of others. Financial support for the individual or community engaging in the health behaviour is required. Laws and regulatory guidelines that contribute to the health of the population are required, and strategies must be set in place for the support of those engaging in healthy behaviours. Health promotion, then, is a process of personal development towards health, and an organisational development involving political development towards health.

Enabling people to manage their health through health promotion

To understand how mental health promotion works, we must first realise that health promotion is about enabling people to increase control over their own health. An example of this is preventing skin cancer. Having such control requires individual skills and knowledge and a supportive environment. These are identified through:

- screening and assessment, such as skin checks
- health education and skills development, such as Sun Smart education in school
- social marketing and health information, such as the 'Slip, Slop, Slap' television advertisements

- community actions, such as lobbying against solariums
- positive health settings and supportive environments, such as shaded environments.

Therefore, we can identify the following:

- Health promotion is aimed at stopping people from getting sick in the first place and is termed *primary prevention*.
- Health promotion is designed to enable people to take control of their lives, and requires providing people with skills, knowledge and environments that are supportive of good health.
- Health promotion works in a variety of ways to assist populations to good health (Guzys et al., 2014; McMurray & Clendon, 2015).

Health promotion is an interactive process aimed at enhancing the quality of life in the human environment. It incorporates interventions that encompass all aspects of those activities that seek to improve the health status of individuals and communities, including educational, environmental and legislative changes to improve health. The priorities identified for the twenty-first century are to promote social responsibility for health, increase investments for health development, consolidate and expand partnerships for health, increase community capacity and empower the individual, and secure infrastructure for health promotion (Guzys et al., 2014; McMurray & Clendon, 2015).

Health education within health promotion is a multifaceted activity employing a variety of means and strategies. It specifically transmits information, motivates the inner resources of people, and helps people to adopt and maintain healthy practices and lifestyles (Guzys et al., 2014; McMurray & Clendon, 2015). Nurses are instrumental in the promotion of healthy environments that optimise the well-being of individuals, families and communities. People should be given sufficient knowledge concerning alternative behaviour so that they can make intelligent choices themselves. A person's motivation and culture should be considered, as well as immediate needs and longer-term goals, such as attending to a sick child, then educating the mother.

Goals of health promotion

Health promotion results are improved if the goals relate to the person and the context; clear goals and benefits are identified; and immediate, intermediate and long-term outcomes are well defined. Examples of these outcomes are:

- reduction of risk factors
- enhancement of well-being, such as promoting stamina, energy, concentration and stress management
- increase in performance
- improvement of fitness
- increasing self-confidence
- improving self-esteem
- reducing visits to the doctor or chemist
- reduction of illness
- extension of life
- improvement of the quality of life (Guzys et al., 2014; McMurray & Clendon, 2015).

In order to address health promotion there must be significant partnerships in organisational development (Keleher, 2016a). This would mean reorienting the organisation to ensure the fluent and effective coordination of health promotion initiatives and practice. Practical examples of organisational development include:

- health promotion embedded into health service mission statements
- health promotion considered a core business of any health service
- health promotion embedded into department plans
- health promotion as part of quality procedure
- mapping of health promotion initiatives
- health promotion signage and promotion
- health promotion in position descriptions
- policies developed in response to health promotion needs (Guzys et al., 2014; McMurray & Clendon, 2015).

Increasing employees' ability to effectively promote health in their roles requires education, support from management and resources. Therefore, it requires workforce redevelopment to include:

- health promotion in-services for staff
- health promotion to be valued in staff recruitment
- health promotion as part of orientation to departments
- integrated health promotion to be valued by management
- opportunities to identify health promotion in statistics
- professional development opportunities to enhance specific health promotion skills (Guzys et al., 2014; McMurray & Clendon, 2015).

Mental health promotion

As with general health promotion, mental health promotion must be multilevel and intersectorial in action. Policies guiding mental health promotion must support social conditions and factors that create positive environments and are consistent with the philosophy of the Ottawa Charter in promoting health conducive to good mental health and the well-being of populations, communities and individuals. Therefore, mental health promotion policies must be based on a collaborative, biopsychosocial, multisectorial approach that incorporates the participation of not only services but also individuals and communities (Guzys et al., 2014)

Government and non-government agencies have the responsibility to develop and implement policies at the appropriate levels (Guzys et al., 2014; McMurray & Clendon, 2015) in order to establish a framework for the guidance of understanding the determinants of mental health, as applied to populations and the expected immediate and longer-term outcomes. The three key categories of mental health determinants are social connectedness, freedom from discrimination and violence, and access to economic resources (Guzys et al., 2014; McMurray & Clendon, 2015).

Determinants approach to mental health promotion

In a determinants approach to mental health promotion there must be an understanding of what contributes to the health of a community, including the effects of behaviours on social processes and disease risks, and the social and structural conditions that have an impact on that community (Baum, 2016; Guzys et al., 2014; McMurray & Clendon, 2015). Keleher and Murphy (2004) identify four complex interactions among determinants of health across social, environmental, economic and biological dimensions. Actions to address both positive and negative influences on mental health and well-being for intermediate outcomes involve the strengthening of individuals, organisations, communities and whole societies, including the reduction of barriers to mental health (Guzys et al., 2014; McMurray & Clendon, 2015; VicHealth, 2006).

The primary objectives of the federal Department of Health and Aged Care's *National Action Plan for Promotion, Prevention and Early Intervention for Mental Health* (2000) were to 'ensure the enhancement of social and emotional well-being among populations and individuals, reduce the incidence, prevalence and effects of mental health problems and mental disorders, improve the range, quality and effectiveness of population health strategies to promote mental health, and prevent and reduce the impact of mental health problems and mental disorders among the Australian population' (VicHealth, 2006, p. 19).

The National Mental Health Plan 2003–2008 built on the previous objectives to reduce barriers to obtainment of mental health services to include 'promoting mental health and the prevention of mental health problems and mental illness, increase service responsiveness, strengthen quality and foster research, innovation and sustainability' (VicHealth, 2006, p. 19). The new *National Mental Health Strategy* (2014) is a commitment by Australian governments to continue to support and promote the improvement of mental health for populations across Australia. Under this strategy the focus of recovery from mental health problems and mental illness is empowerment for the individual to assume control of how they would like treatments and interventions to evolve. The promotion of de-stigmatisation and the rights of the individual are prominent in this strategy, providing a platform for the individual to have a meaningful contribution to society (Baum, 2016; Gordon & Gray, 2015).

There are multiple interacting determinants of health in mental health and mental illness, including social, psychological and biological factors. Research supports the conclusion that the greatest factors influencing mental illness are low levels of education and income, and poor housing. These present a great vulnerability for those experiencing insecurity and feelings of hopelessness, social change and the risk of violence and physical harm (Guzys et al., 2014; Hungerford et al., 2015; McMurray & Clendon, 2015; Patel & Klienman, 2003).

The VicHealth (2006) framework identified three overarching social and economic determinants of mental health that reflect the philosophy and principles of the Ottawa Charter:

- *social inclusion*—meaning that each member within the community is concerned about social and community connection, stable and supportive environments, diversity of social and physical activity, and a valued social position
- *freedom from violence and discrimination*—reflecting the value of diversity, physical security and an opportunity for self-determination and control of one's own life
- *access to economic resources and participation*—enabling access to work, meaningful engagement, education and adequate housing and finances (Barry & McQueen, 2005; Guzys et al., 2014; Hungerford et al., 2015; McMurray & Clendon, 2015; VicHealth, 2006).

Social inclusion and connectedness allow individuals to feel a sense of belonging, permitting them to feel valued and respected within supportive relationships and community engagement. Marginal and vulnerable members of a community have reduced opportunities to contribute to and participate in economic and social dimensions within their community, because of economic deprivation—lack of material necessities and opportunity deprivation—and loss of substantive freedoms for social inclusion.

Examples include a lack of access to economic resources and employment opportunities, service exclusion and discrimination. Social relationships and networks can buffer the effects of or reduce the onset of mental illness, and enhance recovery from mental disorders. Social support can directly contribute to mental health (Barry & McQueen, 2005; Guzys et al., 2014; Hungerford et al., 2015; McMurray & Clendon, 2015).

Individuals diagnosed with mental disorders are easily marginalised and socially excluded. High rates of marginalised populations within a community result in the disintegration of that community. This is a reduction of social capital, which is central for a community to function effectively. Because of mental disorders, social participation becomes complex and requires a supportive environment in homes, schools, workplaces and communities. Mental health promotion programs must embrace an empowering philosophy to engage active participation, building on existing skills; and must enhance a sense of control, employing a combination of intervention methods functioning at different levels (Barry & McQueen, 2005; Baum, 2016; Guzys et al., 2014; Hungerford et al., 2015; McMurray & Clendon, 2015).

CRITICAL THINKING OPPORTUNITY

What are the primary objectives of the National Action Plan for Promotion, Prevention and Early Intervention for Mental Health?

Mental health promotion and the prevention of mental disorders

The prevention of mental disorders and mental health promotion have common overarching properties. However, they have significantly differing conceptual principles and frameworks. Mental health promotion is focused on building competencies, resources and strengths, but it is not primarily related to the prevention of mental disorders; by contrast, the primary concern in the prevention of mental disorders is the reduction of incidence and prevalence or seriousness of the targeted disorder (Barry, 2001; Guzys et al., 2014). The enhancement of individual human potential rather than the emphasising of the prevention of mental disorders reflects a competence enhancement approach that promotes programs built on strengths, abilities and feelings of efficacy.

Community competence is linked to community empowerment. Powerlessness is associated with a sense that the identified problems were not caused by that community, or that members of the community perceive themselves to have reduced knowledge and skill levels to address the issues that may or may not have a degree of complexity. Identification of community resources, social processes, communication patterns and economic networks, along with the edification of key stakeholders, including marginalised populations, are central to empowering the community, thus giving ownership of future changes (Baum, 2016; Talbot & Verrinder, 2005).

Models of community empowerment exist, and assist in understanding the process of influencing conditions that are of concern to people who share in a society, whether in neighbourhoods, workplaces, experiences or other concerns. These frameworks permit improved collaborative partnerships for community health and development in an interactive model (Baum, 2016; Keleher, 2016b). Mental health promotion permits positive and dynamic concepts that can be implemented in communities to enhance community wellness. A multidisciplinary approach maintains the basic concepts and principles of health promotion. Participation, empowerment and equity are the processes of enabling people to increase control over their health and the determinants of health. A systems approach of involving the individual, communities, policy-making, environments and organisations allows mental health promotion to become a socio-ecological model (Baum, 2016; Guzys et al., 2014; Hungerford et al., 2015; McMurray & Clendon, 2015).

Program planning for mental health promotion

To be successful, program development should be based on underpinning theory, research principles of efficacy and needs assessment. There should be a targeted approach to planning, implementation and evaluation that addresses a range of protective and risk factors. This is undertaken within the socio-environmental approach, fostering community action for social change towards health enhancement (Talbot & Verrinder, 2005), while remaining within the economic resources that can support the developed program. The primary health-care approach within a multidisciplinary framework permits an acceptable outcome for environmental and social change, while giving effect to underpinning social justice, efficiency and efficiency principles.

The process involved in successful programs should ensure that there is a collaborative and participatory approach, including the key stakeholders, that gives a clear outline as to what the need is, the types of interventions that would best suit an effective outcome, available resources (physical and social), available cognitive and social cooperation skills or training that is required to facilitate the program, and communication of the core components of the program.

One of the generic principles of mental health promotion is to embrace an *empowerment philosophy*. Under this philosophy, it is critical to engage the active participation of the program participants, building on their existing strengths and skills. This promotes a sense of control over their lives and addresses a system of socialisation and control (that is, poverty, social injustice and discrimination) (Barry & McQueen, 2005; Shaw, Welch & Williamson, 2015). Engaging in consultation and collaboration reflects community-based collaboration. Working in partnership and participation in all stages promotes greater ownership and facilitates capacity building. This supports the development of intersectoral structures, and facilitates improved chances of sustainability.

The global burden of mental illness requires an international resolution; the fact that persons who have a long-term mental illness have a higher probability of dying at a younger age than persons with other chronic disorders (Ivbijaro, 2012) and encounter poorer physical health (Chadwick et al., 2012). The *Global Mental Health Action Plan 2013–2020* (World Health Organization, 2012) proposed core principles to underpin universal access and equity. If adopted these principles would see the delivery of mental health service provision changed to reflect greater input and consideration to the mental health consumer and their families/carers. Closing the inequity gap requires a more effective collaborative partnership; applying what does work in meeting the needs of persons with mental illnesses and service providers in a systematic approach levering strengths and understanding all people's needs (Kidd, Kenny & McKinstry, 2015).

Global health promotion must be underpinned by evidenced-based practice, health system reform, and acknowledgement and respect of human rights. While policy-makers need to ensure that there is sufficient research data available to support the changes required for equity to mental health, they also should be cognisant of whether there is appropriate high-quality materials and support systems availability for such implementation and sustainability.

Mental health promotion: a consumer advocate perspective

Health promotion is a powerful and relevant promoting strategy for social development; in particular, as an important set of promoting strategies to address the factors influencing inequalities in health. These main prerequisites for health, which are considered to be fundamental needs, must always remain core goals for all action directed towards health, social and economic development. We know that health is a vital resource for life that allows people to lead individually, socially and economically productive lives. It is a positive concept emphasising social and personal resources—physical, mental or spiritual. These are strategies for reducing inequalities and therefore improving the health and well-being of individuals.

Some of these key strategies of this consumer advocate perspective are:

- reducing relative poverty
- increasing opportunities in education, employment and wages
- participating in the political and economic spheres.

These are strategies for reducing inequalities and therefore improving the health and well-being of individuals.

It can be tempting to define mental health as an emotional well-being state, rather than the absence of mental illness—particularly if your audience is people with a mental illness, who see their illness as an indefinite state. Because mental illness is often stigmatised, you will also need to consider the feelings of those with mental illness when developing promotional materials. You will need to strike a balance between developing materials that promote good mental health and materials that inform your audience about mental illness. Developing an alliance with mental health service consumers, families and/or carers and clinical professionals is critical, as their participation and feedback can inform how the promotional material can be improved in a cost-effective and precise way. This is essential as the mental health professional's target audience is mainly those who have been touched by mental illness in one way or another. This development of alliance between consumer, carer and clinician is of primary importance when dealing with health promotion activities, particularly in mental health. Much may be learned from each another that may benefit each participant of the alliance.

Mental health promotion also has the potential to empower consumers and their carers to embrace a better lifestyle and create better coping mechanisms, while simultaneously improving overall mental health and community services. There are five steps when preparing for a mental health promotion activity:

1 Define the mental health promotion activity.
2 Target your intervention to a specific audience.
3 Reach your population through a community-based intervention.
4 Create an interactive program that will enhance the social functioning (building autonomy, optimism and self-confidence, self-esteem and positive thinking).
5 Ask consumers whether they would be willing to provide an account, testimonial or story as success stories during mental health promotion.

Recognising that there are challenges in encouraging consumer participation is one thing—meeting them is another. Nurses committed to the concept of consumer participation in health promotion activities have a responsibility to ensure that effective strategies are used, and that these strategies are evaluated against effectiveness criteria. Each site and service conducting mental health promotion exercises that include consumers and carers as decision makers and planners will need to determine how best to engage the consumers and carers in the shaping of the health promotion exercise, as well as the overall culture of the service providing it.

Such decisions need to be based on available evidence, and nurses need to be prepared to search for new alternatives. Merely endorsing the value of consumer participation in health promotion strategies is insufficient—we must ensure that it is pursued in a meaningful way. There is no right way to enable consumers and carers to participate in their services. However, it is important that consumer participation is seen as a significant part of an agency's overall organisational ethos in working with the individuals they support.

Consumer and carer participation provides further opportunities for recovery for people with a mental illness. Its strengths include the following:

- It allows services to have greater scope to be more responsive to the needs of the people it supports.
- It is an ethical and a democratic rights process.
- It is one means to equalise the power relationship between the service and the people within it.
- It can improve service quality and therefore should be an integral part of most services.
- It is a way of enhancing consumer confidence to express opinions and viewpoints.
- It fosters a working relationship that opens opportunities for consumer engagement in a crucial event or activity organised via services.
- It creates a level of respect, integrity and rapport between consumers within the services they utilise.
- It may change the balance of decision making and control, expanding essential knowledge to everyone.

The community development approach for consumer participation is known to be most successful if it is driven and built from the bottom up. Community engagement can only occur at the grass-roots level—from where the momentum for the issues can be generated. Consumer and carer participation should be integrated into a service's core business because it:

- builds community capacity
- enhances reciprocal relationships
- generates motivation, knowledge bases, values, resources and commitment
- helps to prevent obstacles and difficulties that hinder projects
- allows service evaluations to be aired
- incorporates further opportunities for further growth and better reform processes
- brings a different perspective of a lived experience of using the service.

A consumer seeking treatment within the consumer participation model should be encouraged to be involved in their assessment and treatment, and the organisation of their treatment plan. They can further contribute to the mental health service though participation in surveys and consumer advisory groups, and representation on committees.

Ultimately, consumer and carer participation activities aim to make the invisible more visible, deliver sustainable improvements in mental health care and make quality mental health care more accessible to everyone.

New areas of work in the Australian consumer movement

The areas of work that have been expanded within the consumer movement in health promotion are co-designing, recovery colleges and peer support.

EILEEN PETRIE AND EVAN BICHARA

Co-designing

Co-designing is the new buzz word, but what does it mean? Co-designing new initiatives with people experiencing vulnerabilities engages professionals to begin health promotion initiatives working with consumers and using these people's experiences, perspectives, values, challenges and understandings as a foundation for the design of these initiatives. It involves finding ground-up or bottom-up solutions to many dilemmas or problems prevalent in the community. Co-designing involves coming alongside the many vulnerable people experiencing mental health issues and working with them to create genuine effective interventions and services or programs that will work in the context of their lives. These interventions and services or programs will also help to facilitate their individual goals and reflect their values in life. For clinicians, this involves letting go of professional assumptions about the consumer's perspectives or experiences and, more importantly, to actively learn from what people say or do.

Expertise and professional knowledge can then be considered in relation to consumer input to add depth to the possibilities of approaching social problems with specific groups. This is, however, different from traditional feedback methods that ask end-user groups to comment on their use of and satisfaction with services that have already been planned or implemented. Co-designing looks beyond people's vulnerabilities, thus challenging professionalism and the way professionals work with people experiencing vulnerabilities.

Co-designing mental health promotion alters the way professionalism conceptualises or approaches vulnerabilities in the pursuit of social change. Most of the time, identifying someone as vulnerable leads us to focus on their weaknesses and the need to protect them from possible harm. This intention is important and is rightly reflected in ethical protocols and guidelines for working with these people. However, an overemphasis on vulnerability may underestimate the degree to which people can determine their own well-being or participate in decision-making processes.

Focusing on vulnerabilities can also underestimate resilience: the capacity to grow in the face of adversity, using skills and abilities to self-manage risk and learning to employ coping strategies. That is, to move forward in life, actively influencing one's own environment to suit one's needs. Co-designing initiatives allow resilience to progress and offer people dignity and the opportunity to be valued in becoming productive citizens. Many people who have experienced profound trauma and/or disadvantage have clearly demonstrated significant resilience and skills, which need to be recognised and respected in engagement initiatives in relation to mental health promotion. Health professionals need to drop the idea that being a professional with expertise means getting it right straightaway or knowing all the answers. Health-care professionals need to be inclusive and in so doing use mental health consumers' lived experience of illness to inform initiatives for mental health promotion. This approach of designing services is currently defined as the way forward within Australia and now stands firm and better defined to produce better initiatives for mental health promotion in the community.

Recovery colleges

Recovery colleges (or recovery education centres) allow people to reinforce and focus on their strengths; that is, they empower, enhance and facilitate people to develop their defined strengths rather than adding attention on what is wrong with them (as many practitioners currently do with the intention of getting people better). The first recovery college opened in 2010 in London. Recovery colleges use an education model for approaching the notion of recovery. Within these recovery colleges people discover who they are, learn skills and tools to promote recovery, find out what they can be, and realise the unique contribution they have to offer.

Moving from a treatment approach to an educational approach carries with it a number of caring changes in the focus of relationships with people that are central to promoting effective recovery. These are:

- helping people recognise and make use of their talents and resources rather than defining their problems, deficits or dysfunctions, as therapy usually does
- assisting people to explore their possibilities and develop their skills beyond the therapy sessions
- supporting people to achieve their goals and ambitions rather than transforming all activities into therapies
- placing staff as coaches who help people find their own solutions, rather than defining problems and applying professional therapy.

Recovery colleges are still in their infancy in Australia so evaluative processes and the evidence is limited; however, they have certainly proved popular among those who have used them. That said, recovery colleges are not meant to replace specialist mental health assessment and treatment services, or non-specialist mental health outreach support. However, as an adjunctive to mental health services they offer the opportunity to reduce costs by providing services in the form of co-produced seminars or courses that decrease isolation and increase peer support, while at the same time offering a broad range of professional expertise, offering the potential to deliver a win–win situation for both the consumer and the health-care organisation. Recovery colleges also create a network of social opportunities among peers and the general community, which reduces the social isolation people experience when struck by mental illness.

Peer support

Peer support services follow the belief that individuals who have lived experience of mental illness, or an addiction or problem behaviour, can better relate to individuals experiencing the same condition and who are trying to deal with similar problems. The use of the peer support model has proven to be successful in mental health services, but has been greatly undervalued in the past. Peer support has played an important role in the lives of individuals who have been impacted by events, incidents or issues that have disrupted their well-being, including having a mental illness. Everyone living with or experiencing a mental health issue has the right to access avenues to share their lived experience in a confidential and safe environment where they are heard, respected, honoured and understood. Peer support allows this to happen. It provides an opportunity for individuals to benefit from the collective wisdom of other people in similar circumstances. It allows for opportunities to understand and to de-stigmatise mental illness using the power of sharing information. It provides a renewed sense of self-respect, understanding and belonging through being part of a circle of a caring community. It also allows people to help another person in similar circumstances—to rediscover themselves and to activate their own personal resources.

1 Referring to the latest literature, define:
- mental health
- mental illness and mental disorders
- mental health promotion.

2 After you have written these definitions, describe the steps in program planning for mental health promotion.

Needs assessment for health promotion

A needs assessment clarifies the issue that a project is planning to address, then provides for the exploration of the most effective approach to address that issue. It is tailored to the needs of the participants and the local setting: it is an ecological fit. It is essential when determining a need that you explore the evidence for your assumption that this is an important issue for your area or community (Baum, 2016). In this determination, consider who is most affected by this issue. This will assist with beginning to identify the target groups for a project or program.

A component of the needs assessment is to explore the *capacities and opportunities* that exist in the community, and how nurses will engage with these groups. Evidence supports the concept that strategies are often more effective if they explore the positives and abilities in a group situation rather than the problems. This approach will require an in-depth understanding of the communities involved in health promotion, and often involves a series of discussions over a period of time with a reference group.

Evidence is required in the needs analysis; this can be obtained through the review of reports, anecdotal evidence, waiting lists, data sources, consultations and other documents to demonstrate that this is an important issue for the area or community.

Categories of need include the following:

- *Comparative need* compares the similarities of services offered in one area with a particular population to the services required in another area with a similar population.
- *Felt need* identifies the community's beliefs of what it wants, or what it considers to be the health problem (or problems) that needs addressing. Some approaches of assessing felt needs are household surveys, phone-ins and public meetings and submissions.
- *Expressed need* reflects what you can determine about the health needs of a community by observation of their use of services. For example, long waiting lists at child guidance clinics may indicate there are more problems in the psychological and social adjustment of children than can be catered for by existing services.
- *Normative need* is what expert opinion defines as a need; for example, the immunisation of adolescent teenagers against measles as recommended by the National Health and Medical Research Council (Guzys, 2014: QIPPS, 2006).

A needs assessment will indicate particular health or social issues—that is, priority issues—that need to be addressed. There are current priority issues compiled by various governing departments and relevant sector stakeholders. These should be identified before any health promotion activity to facilitate appropriate interventions. It is critical to provide a rationale for selecting the target group. This assists in determining precisely where the proposed intervention is required. To achieve this accurately, it is imperative to draw on the experience of the target group and related people connected with that population (Baum, 2016; Hawe, Degeling & Hall, 1998).

Sustainability of programs

When using the term 'sustainability', do we mean sustainability of effort or sustainability of effect (Hawe, Ghali & Riley, 2005)? There are two components to sustainability of effect. The first component determines if the initial effects in the original target group are maintained over time. The second component refers to the continued effect of a program on subsequent cohorts (Hawe, Ghali & Riley, 2005; McMurray & Clendon, 2015).

Sustainability of effort is focused on the potential of an intervention that continues in effectiveness beyond the initial funding and program design. This is related to capacity building in health promotion. The continuance of a program, which is based on the initial program development, depends on the presence of a 'champion' higher up in the host organisation—it is imperative to have someone who could advocate for the program in the key decision-making forum. Program sustainability can be established and maintained if:

- there is evidence that the program is effective
- consumers, funders and decision-makers are involved in its development
- the host organisation provides real or in-kind support from the outset
- the potential to generate additional funds is high
- the host organisation is 'mature' (that is, stable and well resourced)
- the program and host organisation have compatible missions
- the program is not a separate 'unit', but rather its policies, procedures and responsibilities are integrated into the organisation
- someone in authority (other than the program director) is a champion of the program at high levels within the organisation
- the program has few 'rival providers' that would benefit from the program discontinuing
- the host organisation has a history of innovation
- the value and mission of the program fit well with the broader community
- the program has community champions who would decry its discontinuation
- other organisations are copying the innovations of the program (Baum, 2016; McMurray & Clendon, 2015; Shediac-Rizzkallah & Bone, 1998, in Hawe, Ghali & Riley, 2005, p. 254).

SUMMARY

Mental health promotion is an enormous domain that encompasses the biopsychosocial and spiritual dimensions of the lifespan. Mental health and well-being are encompassed in all aspects of an individual's life, and must be addressed at all levels to ensure quality of life and social well-being. Central to this is the need for autonomy, human rights and freedom from stigma and discrimination. Evidence supports that mental health promotion building on the strengths of an individual enhances the ability to cope with adversities, particularly if the individual is empowered through the use of consumer and carer participation programs.

Disease prevention provides interventions to prevent or interrupt the disease process. Mental health promotion, on the other hand, goes beyond the physical symptoms to the social aspects of health. Mental health promotion action requires public policy initiatives, supportive environments and interrelationships, strengthening of community action, identified personal skills and a reorientation of health care towards health promotion.

To strengthen the science of mental health promotion, there must be knowledge and a research base for mental health promotion, including enabling and creating positive mental health, empowerment and a participative and collaborative process. Mental health promotion should address the broader determinants of mental health. An important aspect of mental health promotion is that policy, research and practice need to be mediated through political process. This engagement will promote mental health at a government policy level that can stimulate public demand for a society that has mental health and well-being as a primary requirement.

EILEEN PETRIE AND EVAN BICHARA

DISCUSSION QUESTIONS

'**Health** promotion interventions encompass all aspects of those activities that seek to improve the health status of individuals and communities, including educational, environmental and legislative changes to improve health.'

1 How should the above statement be considered in relation to health promotion and capacity-building strategies?

2 How would you reorient health services towards health promotion, and how might this process be achieved?

3 Reflect on six areas that healthy public policy should include. List six environments conducive to healthy behaviours.

4 Reflect on three areas that would strengthen community action.

5 List six other disciplines that could be involved in mental health promotion.

TEST YOURSELF

1 The WHO definition of health promotion states that:

a Health is a complete state of physical, mental and social well-being and not merely the absence of disease or infirmity.

b Health is an incomplete state of physical, mental and social well-being and not merely the absence of disease or infirmity.

c Health is a complete state of mental and social well-being and not merely the absence of disease or infirmity.

d Health is a complete state of physical and mental well-being and not merely the absence of disease or infirmity.

2 The Ottawa Charter (1986) has:

a ten principles

b five principles

c seven principles

d one principle

3 The transtheoretical model:

a doesn't allow for multiple attempts at change

b is not based upon the individual's intentional behaviour

c doesn't have a sequential order to the stages for change

d identifies the stages as being sequential, allowing for behavioural regression and multiple attempts to change, and relates behavioural change to changes in environment and/or life experiences

4 Health education within health promotion:

a communicates information, encourages the inner resources of people, and helps people adopt and maintain healthy practices and lifestyles

b communicates information about what resources are available and how much these cost

c is provided only by nurses who communicate information helping people adopt and maintain healthy practices and lifestyles

d communicates information about lifestyles

USEFUL WEBSITES

Australian Bureau of Statistics: www.abs.gov.au

Australian Institute of Health and Welfare: www.aihw.gov.au

Health.vic–Composite data and reports on the health of Victorians: https://www2.
health.vic.gov.au/public-health/population-health-systems/health-status-of-victorians/
composite-data-and-reports-on-the-health-of-victorians

VicHealth—Capacity building for health promotion: https://www.vichealth.vic.gov.au/media-and-resources/
publications/capacity-building-for-health-promotion

REFERENCES

Australian Bureau of Statistics (2013). *Australian social trends 2009*, ABS cat. no. 4102.0. Canberra: ABS.

Australian Health Ministers (2009). *Fourth national mental health plan: An agenda for collaborative government action in mental health 2009–2014*. Canberra: Department of Health.

Barry M. M. (2001). Promoting positive mental health: Theoretical frameworks for practice. *International Journal of Mental Health Promotion*, *3*(1), 25–34.

Barry, M. M., & McQueen, D. V. (2005). The nature of evidence and its use in mental health promotion. In H. Herrman, S. Saxena & R. Moodie (Eds.), *Promoting mental health concepts; emerging evidence; practice: A report of the World Health Organization*. Melbourne: Department of Mental Health and Substance Abuse, with Victorian Health Promotion Foundation and University of Melbourne.

Baum, F. (2016). *The new public health: An Australian perspective* (4th ed.). Melbourne: Oxford University Press.

Chadwick, A., Street, C., McAndrew, S., & Deacon, M. (2012). Minding our own bodies: Reviewing the literature regarding perceptions of service users diagnosed with serious mental illness on barriers to accessing physical health care. *International Journal of Mental Health Nursing*, *21*, 211–219.

Department of Health and Aged Care (2000). *National action plan for promotion, prevention and early intervention for mental health*. Canberra: Mental Health and Special Programs Branch, Department of Health and Aged Care.

Elder, R., Evans, K., & Nizette, D. (2005). *Psychiatric and mental health nursing*. Sydney: Elsevier.

Gordon, S., & Gray, M. (2015). Rural and remote inclusive practice. In J. Davis, M. Birks & Y. Chapman (Eds.), *Inclusive Practice for Health Professionals*. Melbourne: Oxford University Press.

Guzys, D. (2014). Community needs assessment. In D. Guzys & W. Petrie (Eds.), *An introduction to community and primary health care*. Melbourne: Cambridge University Press.

Guzys, D., Robertson, V., Canfield G., & Petrie, E. (2014). Health promotion. In D. Guzys & W. Petrie (Eds.), *An introduction to community and primary health care*. Melbourne: Cambridge University Press.

Hawe, P., Degeling, D., & Hall, J. (1998). *Evaluating health promotion: A health worker's guide*. Sydney: MacLennan & Petty.

Hawe, P., Ghali, L., & Riley, T. (2005). Developing sustainable programmes: Theory and practice. In H. Herrman, S. Saxena & R. Moodie (Eds.), *Promoting mental health concepts; emerging evidence; practice: A report of the World Health Organization*. Melbourne: Department of Mental Health and Substance Abuse, with Victorian Health Promotion Foundation and University of Melbourne.

Hungerford, C., Hodgson, D., Clancy, R., Monisse-Redman, M., Bostwick, R., & Jones, (2015). *Mental health care: An introduction for health professionals in Australia* (2nd ed.). Australia: Wiley.

Ivbijaro, G. (2012). The case for change: The Global Mental Health Action Plan 2013–2020. *Mental Health in Family Medicine*, *9*, 135.

Keleher, H. (2016a). *Health Promotion*. In H. Keleher & C. MacDougal (Eds.), *Understanding health* (4th ed.). Melbourne: Oxford University Press.

Keleher, H. (2016b). *Health education for empowerment*. In H. Keleher & C. MacDougal (Eds.), *Understanding health* (4th ed.). Melbourne: Oxford University Press.

Keleher, H., & MacDougal, C. (2016). *Concepts of health*. In H. Keleher & C. MacDougal (Eds.), *Understanding health* (4th ed.). Melbourne: Oxford University Press.

Keleher, H., & Murphy, B. (Eds.) (2004). *Understanding health: A determinants approach*. Melbourne: Oxford University Press.

Kidd, S., Kenny, A., & McKinstry, C. (2015). *The meaning of recovery in a regional mental health service: an action research study*. Journal of Advanced Nursing, 71(1), 181–192.

McMurray, A., & Clendon, J. (2015). *Community health and wellness: Primary health care in practice* (5th ed.). Chatswood: Elsevier.

National Mental Health Strategy (2014). Accessed 18 January 2017 at www.health.gov.au.

Patel, V., & Klienman, A. (2003). Poverty and common mental disorders in developing countries. *Bulletin of the World Health Organization*, *81*, 609–615.

QIPPS (2006). *The quality improvement program planning system (QIPPS)*. Retrieved 9 November 2009 from www.qipps.com/tools/demo/planning/needs/index.php?program_id=4023.

Shaw, J. Welch, T., & Williamson, M. (2015). *Inclusion and health literacy*. In J. Davis, M. Birks & Y. Chapman (Eds.), *Inclusive Practice for Health Professionals*. Melbourne: Oxford University Press.

Talbot, L., & Verrinder, G. (2005). *Promoting health: The primary health care approach* (3rd ed.). Sydney: Elsevier.

Thyloth, M., Singh, H., & Subramanain, V. (2016). Increasing burden of mental illnesses across the globe: Current status. *Indian Journal of Social Psychiatry*, *32*(3, July–September).

VicHealth (2006). *Evidence-based mental health promotion resource*. Melbourne: Public Health Group, Department of Human Services.

Wass, A. (2000). *Promoting health: The primary healthcare approach* (2nd ed.). Sydney: Harcourt Saunders.

World Health Organization (1986). *Ottawa charter for health promotion*. Geneva: World Health Organization. Retrieved 2 November 2009 from http://who.dk./AboutWHO/Policy/20010827_2.

World Health Organization (2008). *Integrating mental health into primary care: A global perspective*. Geneva: WHO.

World Health Organization (2012). *Global Mental Health Action Plan 2013–2020*. Accessed 18 January 2017 at www.who.int/mental_health/mhgap/consultation_global_mh_action_plan_2013_2020/en.

CHAPTER 5

Primary Mental Health Care

KATE COGAN AND
FREYJA MILLAR

Acknowledgment

The authors would like to acknowledge the contribution of Janet Akehurst who co-wrote this chapter in the second edition.

KEY OUTCOMES

AFTER READING THIS CHAPTER, YOU SHOULD BE ABLE TO:

- describe the nurse–consumer relationship in primary health-care settings
- identify professional boundaries in the primary health-care setting
- describe professional autonomy
- identify work-related stressors and collegial support
- discuss future directions of the field.

KEY TERMS

- boundaries
- collaborative care
- collaborative-recovery model
- consumer
- credentialed mental health nurse
- primary care
- primary health care
- primary health-care team
- stepped care model
- Primary Health Network

Introduction

The prevalence of mental illness within our community is on the increase. A 2012 report by Community Mental Health Australia (p. 12) states: 'Mental illness has enormous health and social impacts in Australia. Every year, one in five Australians experience some form of mental illness … this figure is even higher for young people. Millions of other people are also affected: families, carers, co-workers and neighbours. It goes on to discuss that at some point in their lives almost half of all Australians experience a mental health-related illness. This increase in prevalence, along with an increase in community awareness and increased levels of consumer psychoeducation, has escalated the demand for services and changed the way in which we deliver mental health care.

In most cases, people present to their general practitioner (GP) for treatment, help and cure. If we look at the global figures, mental illness accounted for 11.7 per cent of the total burden of disease in 2008 (WONCA, 2008, p. 71) and this has now increased to 23 per cent (Whiteford, Ferrari & Degenhardt, 2016). Psychiatric syndromes make up four of the top ten global conditions: unipolar depression, alcoholism, schizophrenia and obsessive-compulsive disorder. 'Mental illness as a whole will account for 15 per cent of the total burden of disease worldwide; by 2030, depression alone is likely to be the second highest cause of disease burden' (WONCA, 2008, p. 24). Unipolar depression has risen from the eleventh leading cause of global disease burden to the ninth in twelve years (World Health Organization, 2016b). The *National Survey of Mental Health and Well-being* (Australian Bureau of Statistics, 1999) found that in Australia, the most common mental health disorders were anxiety, substance abuse and affective disorders. It also highlighted that one in four suffered from co-morbidity (suffering from more than one illness at a time). Only one-third of those suffering actually sought treatment, and the majority of those seeking treatment initially presented to their GP for help. The Council of Australian Governments (Martin, 2009) report that 2.1 million adult Australians suffering a mental health disorder in the previous 12 months did not access services, and perceived that their needs were not met by the health services industry.

More recent studies indicate an increase in GP encounters for psychological problems by 20 per cent in the last decade. This breaks down to approximately two million more GP presentations for depression, making depression the fourth most common reason for presentation to a GP in the 2014–15 period (Britt et al., 2015). These two conditions often occur in combination and can also precipitate physical symptoms. Generally, the cause of the presenting problem is complex, and assessment, diagnosis and treatment can be a protracted process. This places an increased burden on the general practice setting. GPs often report having difficulty in accessing mental health services, and are often not informed about community-based treatment options. Many consumers suffering from mental health issues fall within economically compromised groups and are unable to access private treatment options due to cost. The complexity of these cases often makes time-limited therapy (for example, a maximum of six sessions) not a viable option. Many of these consumers need multilayered collaborative–recovery model with treatment plans that address biological, psychological, social, cultural and spiritual needs (Oades et al., 2005). Clinical practice guidelines also recommend that recovery plans incorporate domains such as early intervention, physical health, psychosocial treatments, cultural considerations and vocational opportunities (NICE, 2014; RANZCP, 2016).

The placement of mental health nurses within the general practice setting provides access to high-quality advanced mental health assessment services and allows nurses to navigate and facilitate care pathways for this group of consumers, who are often immobile, vulnerable, disorganised, isolated, amotivated, economically compromised and unsure of how to access other community services. The mental health nurse placed within the primary care setting offers the GP access to specialist knowledge and advice, as well as a collaborative approach to managing consumer care (that is, collaborative care), thus easing the burden of risk and time for GPs. Due to these service changes in Australia, consumer care is enhanced, improving outcomes for consumers and carers (Lakeman, 2013).

---

1 Approximately one-third of people visiting a GP suffer from mental health issues. What types of illnesses would these people be presenting with?

2 'GPs often report having difficulty in accessing mental health services.' Discuss.

※ CRITICAL
THINKING
OPPORTUNITY

New directions in primary mental health nursing

Community mental health nursing developed in the mid 1970s, and the Mental Health Nurse Incentive Program—which employs only credentialed mental health nurses (discussed later in this chapter)—developed as an extension of this service.

As the need for services expanded, along with the knowledge that community-based supports and rehabilitation reduce the time required for inpatient bed stays, the role of the mental health nurse also expanded. Mental health care in the primary sector is under-resourced, as evidenced by the fact that the general practice health-care clinic is often the first port of call for all health-care needs and GPs struggle to meet demand in terms of time and clinical expertise. Therefore, in relation to mental health issues and psychotropic pharmacology, the profession began to look for other ways to develop the scope of practice for mental health nursing and the delivery of consumer care. The result has been the development of the primary health care mental health nurse practitioner.

Primary health care defined

The World Health Organization defines primary health care (PHC) as 'care that brings promotion and prevention, cure and care together in a safe, effective and socially productive way at the interface between the population and the health system' (WHO, 2008, p. 41). It goes on to say that 'the PHC movement [aims] to put people at the centre of health care, so as to make services more effective, efficient and equitable' (WHO, 2008, p. 43).

The Australian Medical Association (2006, p. 1) states that care is:

> socially appropriate, universally accessible, scientifically sound first level care provided by a suitably trained workforce supported by integrated referral systems and in a way that gives priority to those most in need, maximises community and individual self-reliance and participation, and involves collaboration with other sectors. It includes the following:

- health promotion
- illness prevention
- care of the sick
- advocacy
- community development.

The Primary Health Care Research and Information Service (www.phcris.org.au) provides a more comprehensive description of primary health care in Australia and draws significantly on the definitions as described above. It is worthwhile accessing their website for more information (Lunnay, McIntyre & Oliver-Baxter, 2014).

The primary health-care setting is the consumer's first point of contact with a health professional and the health-care system. Usually this contact is with a GP and will involve comprehensive history and data gathering, an assessment of presenting problems, education in relation to current health status, treatment options and recommendations, and, in some cases, referral to specialist practitioners. The GP is often conveniently located to where the consumer lives, and in many cases has an ongoing health-related relationship with the consumer and extended family members. It is expected that the GP will take responsible action in relation to health matters. As a result of this, the GP is well placed to address the ongoing health-related needs of consumers, and is entrusted with a high degree of credibility and trust from the consumer.

The breadth of primary care service delivery from within general practice encompasses nine levels of health care, framed around developmental stages of the illness experience:

1 prevention
2 pre-symptomatic detection of illness
3 early diagnosis or provisional diagnosis
4 diagnosis of established illness
5 management of illness
6 management of complications in relation to treatment
7 rehabilitation

8 terminal care

9 counselling.

Primary health care sits at the bottom of the health-care pyramid (see Figure 5.1), and is the entry level to all other health-care services. The primary health-care team is made up of professional practitioners who practise from the general practice setting. The collaborative approach in the primary setting is expanding and, along with a medical practitioner, primary settings may also have a practice nurse, diabetes clinic, mental health nurse clinic and allied health clinicians, such as a psychologist, podiatrist and administrative staff. For optimal care standards to be maintained and best practice protocols followed, it is imperative that excellent and rigorous communication channels exist between involved clinicians, GPs and consumers. This communication process involves establishing clear boundaries, defined areas of responsibilities and feedback loops.

Department of Health and Aged Care (2000)

An Australian Bureau of Statistics survey (2007) showed that the number of Australians with mental health-related illnesses not receiving adequate care had risen by 3 per cent. A staggering 2.1 million adult Australians in the year 2008–09 stated they had not received treatment for their mental illness (Martin, 2009). Figure 5.1 shows where primary care sits within the pyramid of health care.

Figure 5.1 The position of primary care within the health care pyramid

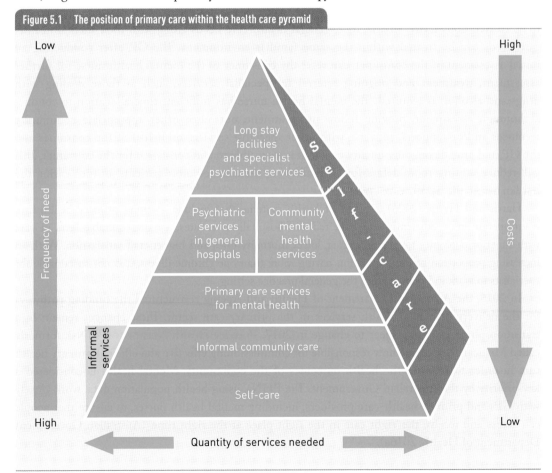

KATE COGAN AND FREYJA MILLAR

Delivery of mental health care in the primary health-care setting

As demand increases and the national mental health workforce decreases across the health-care sector, the need for innovative programs to meet consumer needs and improve the delivery of care is fundamental to ensuring the health-care needs of the community are met. Data collected by the Australian Bureau of Statistics (2009) show that more than one in ten GP consultations are related to consumers' mental health issues, and that more than ten million consultations for mental health-related issues are conducted each year by GPs.

If adequate time is not allocated to consumers with mental health needs, the quality of care can be seriously compromised, and the consumer will no longer feel valued, or will feel that the system can no longer provide the support required to address their needs. Over time, this will exacerbate the consumer's illness, placing an enormous burden on the GP and the administrative staff, and undue pressure on external support systems, such as family and carers, which ultimately places undue demand on the entire health system.

By placing experienced credentialed mental health nurses within the primary care setting and establishing them as part of the primary care team, the current gap in the provision of care to mental health consumers can be addressed. It will also allow for consumers with co-morbidities to be treated holistically: that is, their general health-care needs along with their mental health-care needs can be treated within the same familiar environment. The GP, after conducting an initial assessment of the consumer, can refer the consumer to the mental health nurse for further assessment, treatment and ongoing referral to specialist services, such as those dealing with drugs and alcohol, as required. The mental health nurse has sufficient time allocation to conduct a thorough assessment, provide follow-up treatment, outsource other appropriate community recourses and/or supports, converse with other specialist services on behalf of the consumer and the GP, and provide ongoing quality care that is accessible to and consistent for the consumer. This will reduce waiting-room delays for GPs, allowing them to see more patients, in turn easing the burden across the health-care system.

Harris and Harris (2006) advise that health systems that include a strong primary health-care team operate more efficiently and have reduced hospitalisation rates, a more equitable level of care with superior outcomes for the consumer, lower mortality rates and higher staff satisfaction. With an increasing proportion of the population having more than one chronic illness, it is not sustainable for specialists to work in isolation from the general practice setting.

In 2015, the Australian Department of Health and Ageing restructured the funding pathways for the delivery of mental health services in the primary care sector. These changes remain in a transition phase and are subject to change in 2017. Primary Health Networks (PHNs), formerly called Medicare Locals, are now responsible for commissioning effective and efficient primary health care in order to improve the health outcomes of the community. Mental health is considered a key priority by the Australian Government. The PHNs, using health population data, work closely with GPs and primary health-care providers, including mental health nurses, to ensure that people can access and receive the 'right care in the right place at the right time' (Australian Government Department of Health, 2016a).

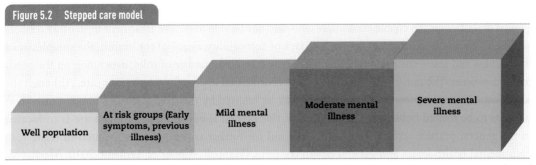

Figure 5.2 Stepped care model

Well population | At risk groups (Early symptoms, previous illness) | Mild mental illness | Moderate mental illness | Severe mental illness

Australian Government Department of Health (2016b)

The PHN model of care for mental health services delivery across Australia is called the stepped care model (see Figure 5.2).

Mental health nurses are capable of working across all of these steps in a variety of services and programs including health promotion and community engagement, primary, secondary and tertiary and acute programs. While many mental health nurses working in primary-care settings work with people who are at risk of, or living with, a mild or moderate mental illness, they also work with those who live with and experience severe and enduring mental illness, such as schizophrenia or major mood disorders with ongoing psychosocial disability.

CRITICAL THINKING OPPORTUNITY

1   What is your understanding of the effectiveness of clinical care, and the effectiveness of interpersonal care?

2   Are both of these concepts essential for effective health-care delivery? Discuss with reference to best evidence.

Role of the mental health nurse in general practice

The role and scope of practice of a mental health nurse is varied and complex, and involves some of the following areas of professional practice:

- assessments: including mental state assessment and safety
- collaborative: recovery-oriented goal planning
- interventions and treatments: including pharmacotherapy, psychotherapy and education
- regular monitoring of interventions
- evaluation and collaborative review of recovery plans.

Assessment and screening tools that have been accredited by Medicare for this program include the Kessler Psychological Distress Scale (K10) and the Health of the Nation Outcome Scale (HoNOS).

The Australian College of Mental Health Nurses has published a *Standards of Practice in Mental Health Nursing* and *Mental Health Nurses in Australia Scope of Practice*, and it is worth accessing these documents via their website (www.acmhn.org) and comparing these to the professional standards published by the Nursing and Midwifery Board of Australia (www.nursingmidwiferyboard.gov.au/Codes-Guidelines-Statements/Professional-standards.aspx).

The role of the mental health nurse is to provide specialist mental health care to consumers referred by general practitioners. To enable consumers who may not be able to receive treatment from other services because of a number of constraints—such as lack of accessibility, financial constraints, the complexity of their illness and fear—the mental health nurse may take on a number of roles, depending on the needs of the consumer. The nurse will aim to provide a coordinated approach to consumer care. Although the main focus is on consumers' mental health issues, as referred by the GP, it remains in consumers' best interests to be treated holistically. In many cases, this process is enhanced when the nurse is co-located in the general practice setting. The GP is on hand for further consultation as required in relation to both mental health issues and general health concerns (Happell, Palmer & Tennent, 2010; Meehan & Robertson, 2013).

Typically, the mental health nurse program provides the general practice clinic with sessional times consisting of 3.5 hours per session. The assessment session is booked in by the GP referral process, and consists of an initial appointment with the consumer of 1.5 to two hours. The time frames of subsequent sessions are negotiated between the nurse and the consumer, but are generally 45–50 minutes of face-to-face contact, and 15–30 minutes of non-face-to-face follow-up. There are always exceptions, whereby follow-up times can be extended.

The assessment entails taking a detailed history of the consumer's life (using a lifespan approach) and presenting concerns about their health and well-being; a mental status examination; risk assessment; HoNOS; a K10; and at times the Depression Anxiety Scale (DAS) and/or mood disorder questionnaire (see Figure 5.3). The assessment also entails an evaluation of the consumer's lifestyle and physical health; for example:

- Does the consumer have diabetes?
- Is there a family history of diabetes?
- Does the consumer smoke? If so, how much?
- What is the consumer's nutritional intake and dietary habits?
- What is the consumer's weight and BMI?
- How much and how often does the consumer exercise?
- What alcohol and or other substances does the consumer use, if any?
- What is the consumer's menstrual cycle regularity?
- What is the state of the consumer's libido?

TOPIC LINK

See Chapter 2 for more on diagnostic systems used in clinical assessment

See Chapter 3 for more on physical and mental health

Collaboration in the primary health-care setting

Collaboration is the process in which two or more people or organisations work together for a common goal. In the primary care setting, the process of collaborative care involves a holistic approach that takes into consideration the consumer's biopsychosocial, cultural and spiritual needs. This process involves the GP, mental health nurse, the consumer and consumer-identified carers. It can also involve information about the systems from which the consumer comes, including their family, surrounding culture, schools, universities, employment, mental health services and community support services.

As discussed above, the initial process involves the consumer and the GP identifying that there are mental health issues. The GP then refers the consumer to the mental health nurse for a full assessment and a clear diagnosis is made. This is done in a collaborative manner with the GP, who supplies background information on the consumer, the reason for referral and a provisional diagnosis. Strengths are identified and possible pathways for treatments are discussed (incorporating consumer strengths and skills training).

Figure 5.3   Mental health nurse clinic assessment

To claim MBS item 2710, must be completed with the GP plan (plan completed by GP)

GP	DR			Date	/	/
Practice				Allergies		
Patient						
D.O.B.	/ /	Gender	M ☐ F ☐			
HoNOS	Score/Type	K10	Score			

Recall Reminder (3 months) Set? ☐

PRESENTING ISSUES	
1	4
2	5
3	6
Family histroy of mental illness: genogram	

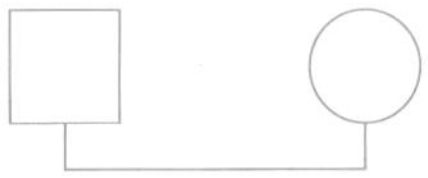

From this, in conjunction with the GP an individualised *mental health care plan* that is specific to the consumer's needs is developed. This approach is empowering for the consumer as they work collaboratively with the nurse and the GP in identifying the consumer's needs, setting recovery-oriented goals and identifying strengths. The plan can involve referral to other agencies, the use of medication, monitoring of side effects, efficacy of treatment, and ongoing counselling by the mental health nurse.

The nurse acts as a facilitator, promoting recovery by helping consumers to identify what they want to work on, acting as an advocate to support access to appropriate services and providing holistic feedback to the GP on consumers' physical and mental well-being during treatment. This is one of the ways in which the collaborative process assists the GP to understand more fully the consumer's needs. It establishes a pathway of care and support for the GP in providing treatment for their consumers. The burden on the GP is eased as the mental health nurse engages in collaborative and shared care practices with a broad range of other agencies, including hospital-based services, community health agencies as well as homelessness services, and other government organisations. For the primary care setting, especially in the climate of GP workforce shortages, this is an essential service designed to assist both the GP and the consumer in maintaining an optimal level of wellness, which in turn assists in relieving pressure on the acute care sector.

The mental health nurse's role also provides collaboration and support for the GP by supplying psychoeducation to the GP, the consumer and the consumer's significant others. The mental health nurse further assists this process by ensuring that the GP stays up to date on evidence-based treatment modalities, including pharmacology, community supports, resources and referral pathways, along with regular participation in peer support and clinical supervision.

1　What is meant by the term 'collaboration'?

2　Who constitutes members of a primary health-care team?

3　What is the role of a mental health nurse in a primary health-care team?

Treatment modalities

In the past, treatment modalities available to people with a mental illness have involved mental health inpatient facilities within acute care services, community care units, day patient programs and outpatient treatment services, such as community care. Accessing these facilities usually meant that the consumer was suffering an acute episode of a major mental illness, and therefore at risk of harm to self and/or others, requiring hospital-based treatment. Once the acute phase of the illness subsided, the consumer was referred to other agencies as required. Access to outpatient treatment modalities was—and remains—extremely difficult to achieve without first becoming in an inpatient of either the public or private system.

With the implementation of the Mental Health Nurse Incentive Program (discussed later in this chapter), advocacy meant that services became more available to consumers with chronic mental health issues or acute presentations prior to an episode that required hospitalisation. That is, this model supported a more preventative approach to mental health care. As distinct from traditional models, treatment was geographically available and affordable (it was bulk billed and offered within the consumer's normal health care setting), and the number of treatment sessions was not time limited.

Treatment modalities used by the mental health nurse involve psychological, physical, spiritual, cultural and social considerations in formulating a treatment program. Nurses require excellent observational and communication skills to enhance their ability to assess risk and engage with the consumer group. As the care is aimed at providing a holistic approach to care, these nurses are required to be able to assess a consumer both mentally and physically. The physical care relates to managing vital signs, assessing level of activity of the illness, and reviewing sleep, hygiene and dietary-related issues. The nurse requires a high level of training in interviewing techniques to assist with historical information gathering. It is important to understand what has or has not worked in the past and why this is so. What are the consumer's strengths and weaknesses? The more information that is made available about the consumer's life, illness and experiences of previous treatments, the more effective treatment planning will be.

The mental health nurse must have skills and training in the use of evidence-based treatment modalities such as cognitive behaviour therapy (CBT), brief solution-focused therapies, narrative therapy, family systems therapy, couples counselling, play and art therapy, psychotherapy, mindfulness therapy, acceptance and commitment therapy, grief counselling, motivational coaching and life skills modelling. The nurse requires a degree of flexibility along with the ability to provide structure to the sessions. There will be times when the sessions are focused wholly on activities of daily living, information delivery, psychoeducation, skills training and stress reduction strategies. The nurse must also have a sound understanding of the fifth edition of the American Psychiatric Association's (2013) *Diagnostic and Statistical Manual of Mental Disorders* (DSM 5) and its use in diagnosis, psychiatric disorders, and psychotropic medications and their interactions, benefits and side effects. An awareness of where and how to access relevant information is vital.

The nurse, the GP and the consumer should work together to develop a recovery-oriented treatment plan using the modalities most effective and acceptable for each individual consumer. The treatment plan and modalities used are reviewed at three-monthly intervals. This process, as well as the initial assessment and plan, provides direction, understanding and empowerment for the consumer in their treatment and journey of recovery. The review process helps the consumer, the nurse and the GP to identify gains made: what is working and what is not working. From this process appropriate adjustments to the treatment modalities can be made to further enhance recovery and eventual consumer autonomy.

Treatment modalities can involve many pathways, depending on the needs of the consumer. The systems they come from—such as family, school, university, social, employment and economic background—can have a significant impact on the treatment modalities to be used. As part of the treatment plan, referral to other agencies or allied health professionals may be required to address some of these issues. For example, many consumers, because of their mental health problems, become isolated and withdrawn from their community, so they may need a referral to a psychiatric disability support service in order to enhance recovery and improve self-esteem. A referral to a social worker for support with finances, or a referral to Centrelink support services, may be appropriate as the consumer works towards the goal of finding meaningful employment.

Many of the pathways and treatment modalities that can be used to enhance a consumer's journey of recovery are not limited to medication and psychotherapies. It is the mental health nurse's role to be aware of as many of them as possible in order to help consumers on their journey of recovery.

CRITICAL THINKING OPPORTUNITY

1 'The mental health nurse role requires a degree of flexibility along with the capability to provide structure to the sessions.' Discuss.

2 The mental health nurse must have skills and training in the use of evidence-based best practice in regards to treatment modalities. Why is this required? Review the literature in this area to inform your discussion.

The nurse–consumer relationship in the primary health-care setting

The nurse–consumer relationship is the primary therapeutic tool of the mental health nurse. It has been argued that this alliance is central to the delivery of effective care (Elder, Evans & Nizette, 2009).

The role of the mental health nurse in the primary health-care setting differs in many ways from that of the mental health nurse in acute mental health. The nurse in the primary health-care setting is able to provide continuity of care throughout the consumer's treatment cycle. This continuity allows the mental health nurse the opportunity to get to know consumers as people, and how their life stories and backgrounds interact to make them who they are. Consumers treated within the primary health-care setting often include people who have never had contact with the public mental health system; they often have preconceived ideas of what this means and harbour fears of being labelled as 'mental'. This requires the nurse to provide a non-judgmental climate that promotes trust, establishes engagement and allows psychoeducation to begin.

The establishment of trust, which empowers the consumer, is the basis for establishing an understanding of the consumer's needs when determining health-care goals. The goals direct the course of the relationship and the treatment outcomes. The balance of power, as much as is possible, should be in the consumer's hands, with the nurse providing education, support and facilitation of the therapeutic relationship. It is the role of the nurse to validate the consumer's experiences and feelings. For example, consumers may choose not to have medication, and instead use the nurse–consumer relationship and counselling as the pathway to better health and life outcomes. The mental health nurse has a strong role in promoting preventative medicine within the primary health-care system, providing health promotion and psychoeducation on mental health issues and advocating for the consumer on a needs basis.

In the primary health-care setting it is very important that the nurse remains self-aware. Self-awareness and attention to one's feelings, thoughts and experiences contribute to the therapeutic use of self in the effective provision of mental health nursing care.

TOPIC LINK

See Chapter 7 for more on self-care.

Although these practices are also true of the nurse–consumer relationship in the acute public sector, acute sector nursing is different in that it is team-based to cover shift work. The balance of power is more in the nurse's hands, and the sector is guided more by the medical model. In the acute sector, consumers can also be held involuntarily under various Mental Health Acts to have treatment imposed on them. The acute care nurse is often working shifts, and may be sent from an agency to fill in for a day; therefore, continuity of care from a single nurse often cannot be provided. Because of the workload and demand for public services, nurses in the acute setting are also often responsible for a number of consumers at any given time. This can leave inpatients who do not 'rock the boat' to manage by themselves while the nurses deal with the more pressing issues arising in a ward of mixed in consumers with diverse presentations at various stages of treatment.

Hildegarde Peplau's (1952) work on the nurse–consumer relationship laid the foundation of nursing practice that emphasises the give and take of the relationship. She developed an interpersonal model of care in which the consumer and nurse form a relationship that enables the consumer to become an empowered partner in the treatment (Stein-Parbury, 2005). Peplau identified three stages of the nurse–consumer relationship:

1   orientation phase
2   working, identification and exploitation phase
3   termination/resolution phase.

Peplau's model involved six nursing roles:

1   *Stranger role*—the nurse receives the consumer as if they were meeting a stranger in other life situations, and provides an accepting non-judgmental climate that engenders trust.
2   *Resource role*—the nurse answers questions, interprets clinical treatment data and gives information.
3   *Teaching role*—the nurse gives instruction, and provides training and education; this involves analysis and synthesis of the learner's experience.
4   *Counselling*—the nurse helps the consumer to understand and integrate the meaning of their current life, and provides guidance and encouragement to make changes.
5   *Surrogate role*—the nurse helps the consumer to clarify domains of dependence, interdependence and independence, and acts on the consumer's behalf as advocate.
6   *Active leadership role*—the nurse helps the consumer to assume maximum responsibility for meeting treatment goals in a mutually satisfying way.

Peplau's model is an effective framework from which to examine and understand the nurse–consumer relationship in the primary health-care setting. The mental health nurse in the primary care setting can be guided by this framework to establish a therapeutic relationship with their consumer that empowers the consumer, guides change and supports the healing process.

'The nurse–consumer relationship is the primary therapeutic tool of the mental health nurse.' Discuss, with reference to best evidence.

Professional boundaries in the primary health-care setting

Boundaries can be described as limits within professional relationships that allow safe connections based on the needs of individuals (Dawson & MacMillan, 1993). Professional boundaries guide nursing practice, and are underpinned by expert knowledge in the field of mental health nursing. Professional relationships involve the use of expert knowledge to underpin therapeutic interventions. Professional boundaries provide a framework within which we can develop therapeutic and beneficial relationships with our consumers; that is, they protect both the consumer and the nurse.

The nurse–consumer relationship within the primary health-care setting requires the nurse to have clear boundaries around their practice, expert knowledge to underpin therapeutic interventions, the ability to self-reflect, and recognition of the issues of transference and counter-transference. Clearly defined boundaries are one of the most important therapeutic tools of a mental health nurse working within the primary health-care setting.

Professional boundaries provide a framework for a trusting and therapeutic relationship to be established. People experiencing mental illness are, by the very nature of their disorder, possibly the most politically powerless and vulnerable group within society (Australian Human Rights Commission, 1993). Consumers come to the nurse in the belief that the nurse has the professional skills and knowledge to help them, and they often disclose personal information that they would not normally tell to others. This results in a power imbalance between the mental health nurse and the consumer. The nurse needs to be aware of their consumer's vulnerability and avoid anything in the relationship that may cause the consumer harm, at all times providing a safe environment for the consumer and the nurse so as to pursue consumer goals.

The mental health nurse in the primary care setting must also provide consumers with clear information and an assurance of confidentiality. All consumers must be informed of treatment options, the potential risks and benefits of this treatment, and alternative treatments available. This is a legal requirement. The consumer must be assessed as being able to make competent decisions and agree to treatment voluntarily. A mental status examination conducted by the mental health nurse establishes the consumer's level of competency. It is the mental health nurse's responsibility to outline the framework of care and ensure the relationship is maintained within the standards of professional practice.

Boundary and limit setting also provide structure for the nursing team and help to prevent workload burnout and stress-related issues. This also provides positive modelling by the nurse to the consumer, who has often experienced inadequate role modelling in the past.

1   What is the reason for the need to practise within the realm of professional boundaries?
2   Discuss the professional boundaries of a mental health nurse working in a primary health-care setting.

Professional autonomy

For nurses in the primary health-care setting, autonomy not only applies to their role in the clinical treatment of the consumer but also to consumers. *Professional autonomy* in mental health nursing requires nurses to have a good understanding of a unique body of knowledge and scope of practice, a set of required skills and educational understandings, a knowledge of professional boundaries, self-awareness, respect for consumers' autonomy in accepting treatment and the ability to make decisions that are in the best interests of their consumers.

The mental health nurse needs to be able to make judgments and act on these in the context of their professional knowledge within a clear moral, ethical and legal framework. Nurses need to know and understand their own morality: what they bring to the workplace and the therapeutic relationship. The nurse must be able to take responsibility for the decisions they make, and be able to practise in a collaborative manner, recognising the input and skill sets of other professions.

The credentialed mental health nurse is also guided by the Australian College of Mental Health Nurses (ACMHN). The ACMHN offers an added framework for support, education and research opportunities.

Professional autonomy in this light recognises the mental health nurse as a professional with a unique set of skills. This recognition increases the nurse's feelings of self-value and thus enhances their role in health promotion, preventative health, psychoeducation, rehabilitation and delivery of care in a holistic manner, ensuring greater job satisfaction. Assurance of professional autonomy will, in turn, attract more nurses into this challenging and rewarding specialist area of nursing, promoting greater opportunities for personal and professional development and helping to retain people in the profession.

ABOUT THE CONSUMER   John's story

John is a 35-year-old male referred for treatment for a major depressive episode. On assessment it was found that there was a strong family history, both paternal and maternal, of depression and substance abuse. The death of John's mother six months ago was brought on by longstanding alcohol-related abuse and illness.

John has a strong history of substance abuse and is hepatitis C positive. He left school at 15, and has been in and out of the family home since the age of 12. John had been placed in numerous foster care settings as a result of family conflict. John has a younger brother who is managing life 'well'. John has been living at home with his father since the death of his mother; he is also unemployed. John has presented with chronic thoughts of suicide; however, he has not acted on these thoughts for some time. He has no prior experience of counselling or medication, and has limited knowledge regarding the impact of mental illness. John reported poor sleep and a lack of energy and motivation, and was becoming increasingly isolated.

REFLECTION QUESTIONS

1   What are the main issues confronting John and his family?

2   What supports may be needed for John and his family?

3   Does medication have a role to play in John's recovery? Discuss with reference to best practice guidelines.

4   What clinical domains may a collaborative recovery-oriented care plan for John and his family include?

Credentialing and the Mental Health Nurse Incentive Program

According to the World Health Organization Depression Fact Sheet, depression is the leading cause of disability worldwide, and is a major contributor to the overall global burden of disease (WHO, 2016b). As the average person consults their GP at least once per year, GPs are well suited to screen and provide preliminary assessment in relation to a consumer's mental health. This places great pressure on the primary care system. To begin to address this, the Mental Health Nurse Incentive Program (MHNIP) was introduced to provide specialist mental health nursing care to this sector. For a nurse to be able to work as a mental health nurse clinician in the primary health-care setting within the Mental Health Nurse Incentive Program, they needed to be credentialed by the ACMHN.

Credentialing is a core component of clinical and professional governance or self-regulation whereby members of a profession set standards for practice and establish a minimum requirement for entry. The purpose of credentialing is to ensure that nurses working in this area have the required knowledge, skills, expertise and experience to work in this much specialised field. Credentialing also advises other health professionals and consumers that the mental health nurse has successfully met a particular standard and is authorised to practise as an accredited mental health nurse. This assessment needs to be supported by authentic documentation and, once completed, is assessed by independent auditors or assessors. The successful candidates are allocated a credentialing number, which is current for three years, during which time the mental health nurse needs to maintain a degree of development, along with a high standard of professional practice, to go forward into the next round. Being a credentialed mental health nurse also provides the nurse with important current information on evidenced-based treatments and ongoing collegiate support (discussed later in this chapter).

The MHNIP was funded by Medicare. The program funded community-based general practices and private psychiatric practices to engage mental health nurses to assist in the provision of coordinated clinical care for consumers with severe mental health disorders. The services were provided both in the clinics and in the community setting, such as the consumer's home. From January 2010, Medicare provided funding only for nurses who were credentialed until the program was discontinued in 2016. Primary Health Networks continue to provide mental health care through other funding.

1   What is your understanding of the term 'credentialing'?

2   What is the purpose of credentialing?

3   Discuss the relevance of credentialing to the primary health-care setting. Support your position with best evidence.

※ CRITICAL THINKING OPPORTUNITY

Work-related stressors and collegial support

Mental health nursing is a rewarding and challenging profession. It carries with it great responsibilities to provide the most up-to-date evidence-based treatments and best practice for consumers, while at the same time allowing them to make informed choices about their journey of recovery and supporting them in those choices. On the one hand we must maintain professional boundaries, yet on the other hand one of our most useful treatment tools is the therapeutic use of self. Maintaining this equilibrium is a challenging process requiring collegiate peer support, supervision and stress management.

Mental health nurses see people at their most vulnerable and often when they are behaving inappropriately. The mental health nurse holds the hope for recovery, displays caring, advocates on behalf of consumers and manages various systems, all with the intention of providing the best possible care guided by best practice. This level of involvement can at times require an enormous supply of energy and a heightened degree of self-restraint on the part of the mental health nurse. Every case has its own degree of complexity and distress, and requires the mental health nurse to display empathy towards consumers in order to enhance the engagement process. At times mental health nurses can feel deeply for their consumers; however, to be effective within the role mental health nurses must maintain professional boundaries and containment lines to protect their own emotional well-being. This means mental health nurses must be aware of their own physical, mental, social and emotional needs. Mental health nurses must take time to reflect on their practice to ensure their self-care is adequate. Clinical supervision, regular opportunities to debrief, ongoing education programs supported by management structure, appropriate program management support, peer support and self-care are ways in which the mental health nurse can guard against stress and burnout. An appropriate balance of exercise, pleasurable activities, regular vocational breaks, positive workplace communication and feedback loops can ensure the effective management of stress.

Mental health nursing is a stressful and demanding profession that can lead to burnout and nurses leaving the profession or becoming less effective in their practice. Interventions such as clinical supervision, debriefing and peer support provide effective ways of supporting mental health nurses to function at their optimum level, and these are discussed now.

Clinical supervision

Clinical supervision refers to a formal, structured process of professional support. Supervision assists members of staff to understand issues associated with their practice, gain new insights and perspectives, and develop their knowledge and skills while supporting staff and improving consumer and carer outcomes. Clinical supervision may involve individual, group or peer approaches, and can be informed by a variety of theoretical perspectives. The process of clinical supervision is different from management or administrative supervision, emphasising professional development, exploring treatment modalities and challenging the way a clinician views a consumer, and providing staff support rather than monitoring work performance.

TOPIC LINK ■
See Chapter 7 for more
on clinical supervision.

The purpose of clinical supervision is to assist mental health nurses to reflect on their practice, and to learn from this reflective process to develop skills and expertise and further enhance their practice. Supervision allows mental health nurses to talk about their practice and to access professional advice and support on aspects such as treatment modalities and medication. Talking with colleagues about their practice and any concerns they might be experiencing helps mental health nurses to debrief and gain a fresh view on life in general, and professional development in particular.

Debriefing

Debriefing is a process by which nurses who have experienced a traumatic event are encouraged to talk individually or in a group setting about their reactions and feelings about the event. This is a supportive process, which is usually conducted 24–48 hours after the event. In general terms, the aim of debriefing is to assist recovery in normal people experiencing normal reactions to abnormal events. Debriefing can be conducted individually, although it is frequently carried out with a group to reinforce the normality of the individual's reactions and to facilitate the provision of support from group members (MacLochlainn, Ryan & O'Mara, 1994).

Peer support

Peer support is normally less formal than supervision and is generally provided on a regular basis, such as once a month. Peer support is provided in a collegiate manner between colleagues and generally takes the form of an informal discussion to learn and share insights from professional events and learnings from reading, conferences and professional development seminars. The group can consist of two or more participants. It can be an open-invitation event, open to colleagues who are available, or a closed-group event (that is, invitation only), by agreement among the participants.

Along with forums to help manage stress, each workplace has access to independent counsellors to assist staff to manage workplace trauma. To access this service, the mental health nurse should contact their manager, human relations department or union.

Future directions

The initial phase of placing mental health nurses in the general practice setting has focused on the process of supporting GPs and psychiatrists with their existing caseloads, along with trying to bridge the gap for the cohort of consumers with mental health issues who are unable to access treatment. The initiative, which commenced in 2011, has demonstrated a range of benefits to consumers, carers and GPs and the acute sector through the potential reduction for hospital admissions (Happell, Palmer & Tennent, 2010; Lakeman & Bradbury, 2014). There is provision to further develop shared-care arrangements with private psychiatrists, outpatient clinics (such as hepatitis C clinics) and outpatient departments of public hospitals, and to look at providing group work. Further to this is the introduction of endorsed mental health nurse practitioners into the primary care setting. This new and innovative direction for mental health nurses in primary care is in its infancy in Australia and the potential benefits are currently being explored (Theophilos, Green & Cashin, 2015; WONCA, 2008).

To this end, discussions are already in place to explore these options, and the hope is that the service will continue to expand and further meet the needs of this vulnerable group of consumers.

SUMMARY

Mental health-related illnesses are on the increase, and pressure on all avenues of health care—both general practice and acute sectors—is at a premium. There is an urgent need to look at innovative ways of providing care to this vulnerable group. Case management as a method of delivering care is aimed at a target population that would generally fall through the gaps and not be able to access mental health care. Such consumers would perceive themselves as having mental health issues but are not being treated for the illness. If this target population continues to not receive adequate treatment, this will place greater stress on the health-care system—in particular, the mental health-care system.

Inability to access services because of geographical constraints, sessional limitations, fear of treatment modality, and inability to trust external health professionals leads members of this group to trust GPs and nurses, but results in them remaining unsure about other disciplines, such as psychiatrists and psychologists.

The Mental Health Nurse Initiative Program has benefited both consumers and GPs, who perceive the program or service as easing the burden on the primary health-care sector. The flow-on benefits are many, taking pressure off the public health-care system. One of the more positive effects is the ability to manage the consumer in a holistic manner from one site.

KATE COGAN AND FREYJA MILLAR

A more collaborative approach to care not only provides a more efficient level of care but also increases clinician satisfaction. The long-term benefit will be a strengthened workforce. Providing strong career pathways will encourage clinicians to take up the challenges of expanding their scope of practice through further education, which will in turn have a positive flow-on effect on the consumer population.

This initiative has also created another career pathway for mental health nurses who are committed to their clinical work, but who no longer wish to work in the hospital-based sectors. As the mental health workforce is shrinking and the population is ageing, many have now received an incentive to remain in the workforce. The credentialing process ensures that mental health nurses working in the field of general practice have attained an adequate standard of clinical practice. Feedback from the consumers, the clinics and the clinicians is overwhelmingly positive. It is hoped that this service will continue to grow.

DISCUSSION QUESTIONS

1   What is the importance of including mental health nurses as members of the primary health-care team?

2   If you were to take up such a role, what do you consider are the skills and level of knowledge required of an effective nurse practitioner in primary health care?

3   'Clinical supervision, peer support and debriefing are important aspects of professional practice.' Discuss.

TEST YOURSELF

1   Primary health care is defined as:
   a   health care that emphasises first contact and assumes responsibility for both treatment and health maintenance
   b   an incomplete state of physical, mental and social well-being and not merely the absence of disease or infirmity
   c   providing partial care by a multidisciplinary team
   d   health care provided by a GP alone

2   The breadth of primary health care encompasses:
   a   prevention, detection of illness and early diagnosis
   b   management of illness, complications and terminal care
   c   rehabilitation and counselling
   d   all of the above

3   The primary role of the mental health nurse in primary care is to:
   a   assess and treat people with mental and physical illness within a general practice
   b   focus on mental health issues solely
   c   assist people to adopt and maintain healthy practices and lifestyles
   d   communicate information about resources

4   The mental health nurse incentive program (MHNIP):
   a   focused on providing care to people with private health insurance
   b   was provided by credentialed mental health nurses
   c   provided mental health care to those who are ineligible for other services
   d   relied on GPs to credential mental health nurses

USEFUL WEBSITES

Australian College of Mental Health Nurses: www.acmhn.org/

Australian Government—Primary Health Networks (PHNs): www.health.gov.au/internet/main/publishing.nsf/content/primary_health_networks

Department of Health—Primary mental health care services for people with severe mental illness: www.health.gov.au/internet/main/publishing.nsf/Content/2126B045A8DA90FDCA257F6500018260/$File/4PHN%20Guidance%20-%20Severe%20mental%20illness.PDF

New Zealand Ministry of Health—Mental health: www.health.govt.nz/our-work/mental-health-and-addictions/mental-health

Nursing and Midwifery Board of Australia—Professional Standards: www.nursingmidwiferyboard.gov.au/Codes-Guidelines-Statements/Professional-standards.aspx

Primary Health Care Research and Information Service: www.phcris.org.au

REFERENCES

American Psychiatric Association (2013). *Diagnostic and statistical manual of mental disorders* (5th ed.). Arlington: American Psychiatric Association.

Australian Bureau of Statistics (1999). *National survey of mental health and well-being.* Canberra: Australian Government Printing Service.

Australian Bureau of Statistics (2007). *National survey of mental health and wellbeing: Summary of results.* Cat. No 4326.0. Canberra: ABS.

Australian Bureau of Statistics (2009). *Mental health: Australian social trends.* Cat. No 4102.0. Canberra: ABS.

Australian Government Department of Health (2016a). *PHN Background.* Retrieved from www.health.gov.au/internet/main/publishing.nsf/Content/PHN-Background.

Australian Government Department of Health (2016b). *Stepped Care.* Retrieved from www.health.gov.au/internet/main/publishing.nsf/Content/2126B045A8DA90FDCA257F6500018260/$File/1PHN%20Guidance%20-%20Stepped%20Care.PDF.

Australian Human Rights Commission (1993). *Report of the national inquiry into the human rights of people with mental illness.* Canberra: Australian Government Publishing Service.

Australian Medical Association (2006). *Primary health care: Position statement.* Canberra: Royal Australian College of General Practitioners.

Britt, H., Miller, G. C., Henderson, J., Bayram, C., Harrison, C., Valenti, L., Charles, J. (2015). General Practice activity in Australia 2014–15. *General Practice series, 38.*

Community Mental Health Australia (2012). *Taking our place—Community Mental Health Australia: Working together to improve mental health in the community.* Sydney: CMHA.

Dawson, D., & MacMillan, H. L. (1993). *Relationship management of the borderline patient.* New York: Brunner/Mazeil.

Department of Health and Aged Care (2000). *National action plan for promotion, prevention and early intervention for mental health.* Canberra: Mental Health and Special Programs Branch, Department of Health and Aged Care.

Elder, R., Evans, K., & Nizette, D. (2009). *Psychiatric and mental health nursing* (2nd ed.). Sydney: Mosby Elsevier.

Happell, B., Palmer, C., & Tennent, R. (2010). Mental Health Nurse Incentive Program: contributing to positive consumer outcomes. *International Journal of Mental Health Nursing, 19*(5), 331–339.

Harris, M., & Harris, E. (2006). Facing the challenges: General practice in 2020. *Medical Journal of Australia, 185*(2), 122–124.

Lakeman, R. (2013). Mental health nurses in primary care: Qualitative outcomes of the Mental Health Nurse Incentive Program. *International Journal of Mental Health Nursing, 22*(5), 391–398.

Lakeman, R., & Bradbury, J. (2014). Mental health nurses in primary care: Quantitative outcomes of the Mental Health Nurse Incentive Program. *Journal of Psychiatric & Mental Health Nursing, 21*(4), 327–335.

Lunnay, B., McIntyre, E., & Oliver-Baxter, J. (2014). *Fact sheet: Primary health care matters* (2nd ed.). Adelaide: Primary Health Care Research and Information Service.

MacLochlainn, A., Ryan, M., & O'Mara, R. (1994). *Information for debriefers.* Sydney: Mental Health Liaison, St Vincent's Hospital.

Martin, C. (2009). A long way to go. *Australian Nursing Journal Mental Health, 17*(2).

Meehan, T., & Robertson, S. (2013). The Mental Health Nurse Incentive Program: Reactions of general practitioners and their patients. *Australian Health Review, 37*(3), 337.

NICE (2014). Psychosis and schizophrenia in adults: Prevention and management. *Clinical guideline [CG178].* Retrieved from www.nice.org.uk/guidance/cg178/chapter/1-recommendations?unlid=7841963720162313751#promoting-recovery-and-possible-future-care-2.

Oades, L., Deane, F., Crowe, T., Lambert, W.G., Kavanagh, D., & Lloyd C. (2005). Collaborative recovery: An integrative model for working with individuals who experience chronic and recurring mental illness. *Australasian Psychiatry. 13*(3), 279–284.

Peplau, H. E. (1952). *Interpersonal relations in nursing.* New York: G. P. Putnam & Sons.

RANZCP (2016). Royal Australian and New Zealand College of Psychiatrists clinical practice guidelines for the management of schizophrenia and related disorders. *Australian and New Zealand Journal of Psychiatry, 50*(5), 1–117.

Stein-Parbury, J. (2005). *Patient and person* (3rd ed.). Marrickville: Elsevier.

Theophilos, T., Green, R., & Cashin, A. (2015). Nurse practitioner mental health care in the primary care context: A Californian case study. *Healthcare, 3*, 162–171.

Whiteford, H., Ferrari, A., & Degenhardt, L. (2016). Global burden of disease studies: Implications for mental and substance use disorders. *Health Affairs, 35*(6), 1114–1120.

WONCA (2008). *Integrating mental health into primary care: A global perspective.* WHO & World Organization of National Colleges, Academies and Academic Associations of General Practitioners/Family Physicians.

World Health Organization (2008). *The world health report 2008: Primary health care now more than ever.* Geneva: WHO.

World Health Organization (2016a). *Global Health Estimates 2014 Summary Tables.* Health statistics and Information systems. Retrieved from www.who.int/healthinfo/global_burden_disease/estimates/en/index2.html.

World Health Organization (2016b). *Depression: Fact sheet.* Retrieved from www.who.int/mediacentre/factsheets/fs369/en/.

CHAPTER 6

Resilience, Recovery and Reconnection

KAREN-LEIGH EDWARD,
ANTHONY WELCH AND
LOUISE BYRNE

KEY TERMS

- reconnection
- recovery
- resilience

Acknowledgment

The authors would like to acknowledge the contribution of Stephen Elsom who co-wrote this chapter in the second edition.

KEY OUTCOMES

AFTER READING THIS CHAPTER, YOU SHOULD BE ABLE TO:

- describe what is meant by the terms 'resilience', 'recovery' and 'reconnection'
- describe the applicability of resilience, recovery and reconnection to the clinical practice setting
- identify the types of skills and attitudes that you will require in facilitating resilience, recovery and reconnection with consumers in your care.

Introduction

This chapter introduces you to the notions of resilience and recovery in providing best health-care interventions for individuals and groups in the mental health setting. The chapter begins by providing a foundation from which to explore what resilience means in the mental health context and how to foster resilience in others as a therapeutic approach. The chapter then explores what recovery is, and how this can be understood from the perspective of consumers of mental health services.

Resilience

Resilience is used to explain the ability of people to roll with the punches and cope with life events, both negative and positive (Edward, 2013); to transcend such events and grow from the experience in most cases. A resilient individual can bend, yet subsequently recover. Resilient people allow themselves to feel grief, anger, loss and confusion when hurt and distressed, but they do not let it become a permanent feeling state. Being resilient can develop by allowing healing in the initial stages of mental illness (such as depression); by using active problem-solving and developing skills to address the situation, the person can then move towards more resilient behaviour patterns and adaptation or adjustment, and then incorporate these changed behavioural patterns into their everyday lives (Edward, 2005a, 2007, 2013; Hernandez, Gangsei & Engstrom, 2007; Landau, 2007; Lee et al., 2013). Studies related to resilience and mental illness support that personality type, and resilient behaviours provide protection from the experience of being stressed—enhancing the capacity to 'live with an illness or a disorder' rather than allowing

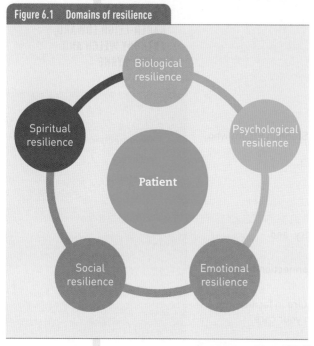

Figure 6.1   Domains of resilience

Edward (2013)

the illness to consume the sufferer (Earvolino-Ramirez, 2007; Edward, Welch & Chater, 2009; Garcia-Dia et al., 2013). Previous research on the effects of severe psychological stress and coping towards recovery has focused on stress-related psychopathology (Badal, 2003; Cassano & Fava, 2002; Charney, 2004; Edward, 2005a, 2005b, 2007; Edward & Warelow, 2005; Edward, Welch & Chater, 2009). Charney (2004) developed a psychobiological model of resilience to counteract extreme stress. He proposed an integrative model that included the notions of resilience and vulnerability, and that encompassed the neurochemical response patterns to acute stress and the neural mechanisms mediating reward, fear conditioning, extinction and social behaviour. The neural mechanisms of reward and motivation (hedonic, hopefulness and learned helpfulness), fear responsiveness (effective behaviours despite intense emotion) and adaptive social behaviour were found to be relevant to resilient traits. An opportunity exists to advance our understanding of resilience and the neurobiological basis of behaviour to facilitate the discoveries needed to predict, prevent and treat stress-related psychopathology. Three constitutional factors that enhanced feelings of resilience are robust measures of self-efficacy, well-defined faith lives and the ability to reframe perceived obstacles to daily living. In conjunction with these emotional and cognitive factors, relational/psychosocial factors also play a significant role in enhancing the experience of resilience for individuals. An important psychosocial factor that mediated resilience is close and positive relationships, and such relationships served as sources of support within and outside the family at various developmental moments. In this context, resilience can be conceptualised as a biopsychosocial-emotional-spiritual phenomenon and is conducive to the practice of nursing, which is holistic and based in the biopsychosocial-emotional-spiritual domains (see Figure 6.1).

CRITICAL THINKING OPPORTUNITY

1   What is your understanding of the concept of resilience? How does your understanding compare to the latest research to this concept?

2   What skills do you need to develop to enhance your ability to engage consumers in developing a therapeutic alliance to improve resilience?

How can you enhance resilience and resiliency?

Mental health consumers and clinicians work together in a therapeutic alliance to assist the person in the process of recovery from mental illness by identifying the abilities acquired through the experience of the episode or relapse. This therapeutic alliance works towards offering alternatives beyond symptoms and deficits for individuals and their carers, challenging the realities of social exclusion that relate to stigma attached to mental illness, and working collaboratively in the direction of changing the balance of power (Murphy & Dillon, 2003). Nursing care interventions such as talking, crying, laughing and relating to consumers are all forms of caring, and all shape part of the therapeutic relationship. These types of care interventions provide support for healthy development and living, and foster resilience in terms of allowing healing to take place while engaging consumers in the therapeutic relationship whereby counselling and other therapeutic interventions related to resilience can occur. Resilience-therapeutic interventions such as these are aimed at building consumers' abilities in avoiding giving in to negative experiences such as feeling fear, anger, anxiety, distress, helplessness and hopelessness, which decrease an individual's ability to problem-solve, thus weakening their resiliency.

> Because I've had to deal with the worst of the worst to see how good it is on the other side, it helps to push you along without even thinking. When I look back on the bad it was I think: 'How did I get through that?' You know … you don't even know you're doing it. I found strength in the day to day … my family matter to me, my home matters to me and the love I had with my grandparents mattered to me. These are the things that got me through the depression.

As a nurse in the care of this person, what are the elements of resilience that you can work on with this consumer in the therapeutic alliance?

Recovery

Background to the recovery movement

The concept of recovery has its origins in the writings of John Perceval, the son of one of England's prime ministers, in which he describes his experience of recovering from psychosis between the years 1830 and 1832. His journey of recovery is chronicled in his book *Perceval's Experience*. Throughout the 1980s, consumer-survivors, many of whom were mental health professionals, began to speak out about their experiences of mental illness and their personal journey of recovery (Deegan, 1988; Hougton, 1982; Leete, 1989), which gave birth to the *consumer-recovery movement* (Carpenter, 2002) bringing the concept of recovery into mainstream mental health care. This movement gained strength through the support of William Anthony, a respected American authority on mental health rehabilitation, who challenged the American mental health-care system, which, at that time, was working from the assumption that mental illness was essentially a 'chronic' condition with little, if any, chance of the person achieving a return to health. Symptom relief rather than a focus on recovery was the central goal of mental health services (Anthony, 1993, 2007; Carpenter, 2002). Since that time, the recovery movement, supported by mental health services research, has been instrumental in influencing a change in government mental health policy in a number of countries, including Canada, the UK, Ireland, New Zealand and Australia. Each of these countries has developed its own perspectives on what constitutes recovery. Since the 1980s, recovery has been part of the language of people with lived experience, carers, advocates, health services management and health-care practitioners of mental health-care services.

Recovery defined

Since the beginning of the recovery movement and its subsequent development, there have been many attempts to define what actually constitutes the act or process of recovery. A variety of views has been put forward, but without any general agreement. America and Canada view recovery as the consumer's unique self-determined personal journey supported by mental health services. The UK and Ireland, through the National Institute for Mental Health in England (NIMHE) and the Mental Health Commission of Ireland, endorsed a recovery model as the guiding principle of mental health service and community education, placing the consumer at the centre of mental health care. Both New Zealand and Australia adopted a more inclusive model of recovery.

The nature of recovery and the apparent lack of consensus or a globally accepted definition only serves to highlight the complexity of individual experiences of mental health challenges and the different ways by which individuals and their families construct their own path to wellness and well-being at different points of their illness experience (Lester & Gask, 2006). Green's definition of recovery from mental illness captures the dynamic nature of the recovery process:

> Recovery [is] the active process of moving toward achieving well-being and a satisfying life, or the process of maintaining a stable level of well-being, mindful that these processes and states include a range of well-being statuses, life satisfaction, or progress towards those ends, just as is true among individuals who do not have mental health problems (Green, 2004, p. 296).

Patricia Deegan, a notable consumer/survivor, and a strong advocate of the recovery movement, shares her personal experiences of mental illness and what recovery means to her:

> The concept of recovery is rooted in the simple yet profound realization that people who have been diagnosed with mental illness are human beings ... Those of us who have been diagnosed are not objects to be acted upon. We are fully human subjects who can act and in acting, change our situation. We have a voice and can learn to use it. We have the right to be heard and listened to. We can take a stand toward what is distressing to us and need not be passive victims of an illness. We can become experts in our own journey of recovery (Deegan, 1996, p. 92).

The two descriptions provided by Green (2004) and Deegan (1996) suggest that recovery is a highly individual process. It is not about being normal in the eyes of health-care professionals and society, but a personal search for who one is amid the challenges of rebuilding a meaningful life—a life worth living—irrespective of whether the person is free from or continues to live with mental health challenges (Carpenter, 2002).

Green (2004) and Deegan (1996) highlight that there is no singular, definable pathway, but multiple paths based on each person's needs, values, aspirations or goals, and ability to take back control of her life. Emphasis is placed on the person as the arbitrator and decision-maker of what constitutes quality of life. At the core of the recovery movement are a number of key values:

- accepting the reality of the illness
- recognising that one is still a whole person despite the illness experience
- understanding that recovery is about the whole self and not just the illness
- being self-determining or self-choosing
- accepting one's limitations while acknowledging one's strengths
- recognising that recovery is unique to each person
  having hope for the future and that recovery is possible
- being open to new possibilities
- taking an active role in regaining control over one's life (Alves & Cleveland, 1999; Deegan, 1996; Parker, 2014).

These values underpin the concept of resilience, which is concerned with drawing on the person's strengths and experiences in confronting and overcoming the daily challenges of mental illness (Edward, Welch & Chater, 2009; Hong & Welch, 2013).

Recovery from New Zealand and Australian perspectives

Since 1998, mental health services in New Zealand have been required by government policy to adopt a recovery approach to consumer care and management (O'Hagan, 2004). Although there was growing interest in the use of a recovery model within the health-care sector, it was not until the release of the Mental Health Commission's (1998) *Blueprint for Mental Health Services in New Zealand* that recovery as a model of mental health service provision became a reality. The approach taken by New Zealand differed from the North American model in that recovery is seen as a social-economic-political process, with consumers having ownership of their recovery process (O'Hagan, 2004). In developing a model of recovery that reflected the New Zealand context, emphasis has been placed on citizenship, the breaking down of stigma and discrimination, diversity of ways of responding to mental health concerns, human rights, advocacy, and bicultural partnership between Māori and people of European descent (Mental Health Commission, 1998).

Although New Zealand in many respects has led the way in the recovery movement, Australia has made significant moves in recent years to embed recovery as a core value in mental health-care delivery, placing recovery clearly on the national agenda. The *Fourth National Mental Health Plan* (Commonwealth of Australia, 2009), which covered the period 2009–2014, identified social inclusion and recovery as the number-one priority. An implementation strategy was agreed by the Australian Health Ministers' Conference in December 2010. The Australian Action Plan 2011–2012 and the Roadmap for National Mental Health Reform 2012–2020 placed recovery at the centre of mental health-care delivery.

Despite significant inroads to the adoption of a national recovery model of mental health service, considerable work remains. One of the major barriers to the implementation of a recovery model of mental health service is the lack of consensus about what actually constitutes recovery (see Box 6.1).

BOX 6.1 DEFINITIONS OF RECOVERY

Recovery has been defined in various ways, depending on the source (policy makers and peak bodies), including:

- a process of returning to a 'pre-morbid' level of functioning; a situation in which personal growth and development has occurred
- a point at which the use of mental health resources and services is no longer required by the individual and family

- the ability to fulfil role expectations and obligations irrespective of functional limitations imposed on the individual as a result of his illness experience
- symptom remission
- a state of well-being and satisfaction with one's life.

Beginning the journey of recovery

The process of recovery from mental illness is not something that just happens to an individual. More often than not, it begins in the depths of numb apathy, confusion and uncertainty. Deegan (1996) describes her journey of recovery in the case study, 'Patricia's story'.

ABOUT THE CONSUMER   Patricia's story

Patricia engages with you in relaying her experience of recovery:

> Prior to becoming active participants in our own recovery process, many of us find ourselves in a time of great apathy and indifference. It is a time of having a hardened heart—of not caring anymore. It is a time when we feel ourselves to be among the living dead: alone, abandoned and adrift on a dead and silent sea without course or bearing. If I turn my gaze back I can see myself at 17 years old, diagnosed with chronic schizophrenia, drugged on Haldol and sitting in a chair. As I conjure the image the first thing I can see are the girl's yellow, nicotine-stained fingers. My fingers. I can see her shuffled, stiff, drugged walk. Her eyes do not dance. The dancer has collapsed and her eyes are dark and they stare endlessly into nowhere.

In the unit, people come and people go. People urge her to do things to help herself, but her heart is hard and she cares about nothing except sleeping, sitting and smoking cigarettes. Her day consists of this: at eight in the morning she forces herself out of bed. In a drugged haze she sits in a chair, the same chair every day. She begins smoking cigarettes. Cigarette after cigarette. Cigarettes mark the passing of time. Cigarettes are proof that time is passing and that fact, at least, is a relief. From 9 a.m. to noon she sits and smokes and stares. Then she has lunch. At 1 p.m. she goes back to bed to sleep until 3 p.m. At that time she returns to the chair and sits and smokes and stares. Then she has dinner. Then she returns to the chair at 6 p.m. Finally it is 8 o'clock in the evening, the long-awaited hour—the time to go back to bed and to collapse into a drugged and dreamless sleep.

Patricia tells you that this scenario unfolds the next day and the next and then the next, until the months pass by in numbing succession, marked only by the next cigarette and the next …

> During this time people would try to motivate me. I remember people trying to make me participate in food shopping on Wednesday or to help bake bread or to go on a boat trip. But nothing anyone did touched me or moved me or mattered to me. I had given up. Giving up was a solution for me. The fact that I was unmotivated was seen as a problem by the people who worked with me. But for me, giving up was not a problem, it was a solution. It was a solution because it protected me from wanting anything. If I didn't want anything, then it couldn't be taken away. If I didn't try, then I wouldn't have to undergo another failure. If I didn't care, then nothing could hurt me again. My heart became hardened. The spring came and went and I didn't care. Holidays came and went and I didn't care. My friends went off to college and started new lives and I didn't care. A friend whom I had once loved very much came over to visit me and I didn't care. I remember sitting and smoking and saying almost nothing. And as soon as the clock struck 8, I remember interrupting my friend in mid sentence and telling her to go home because I was going to bed. Without even saying goodbye I headed for my bed. My heart was hard. I didn't care about anything.
>
> I cannot remember the specific moment when I turned the corner from surviving to becoming an active participant in my own recovery process. My efforts to protect my breaking heart by becoming hard of heart and not caring about anything lasted a long time. One thing I can recall is that people around me did not give up on me. They kept inviting me to do things. I remember, one day, for no particular reason, saying yes to helping with food shopping. All I would do was push the

shopping trolley. But it was a beginning. And truly, it was through small steps like these that I slowly began to discover that I could take a stand towards what was distressing to me.

Patricia's mood lifts as she talks of her recovery journey:

My journey of recovery is still ongoing. I still struggle with symptoms, grieve the losses that I have sustained, and have had to get involved in treatment for the sequaela child abuse. I am also involved in self-help and mutual support, and I still use professional services including medications, psychotherapy and hospitals. However, now I do not just take medication or go to the hospital. I have learned to use medications and to use the hospital. This is the active stance that is the hallmark of the recovery process.

REFLECTION QUESTIONS

1   In your view, is the recovery process an ongoing dynamic experience, or does recovery have an endpoint? How does your position on this matter compare to the latest research on recovery?

2   Referring to the contemporary literature, identify the most recent movements towards destigmatisation and re-engagement with community for those who experience mental illness in your part of the world. What do you think are the skills you will require to enable you to work effectively with those who are embarking on their own recovery process?

Facilitating recovery: qualities of mental health services and mental health-care providers

Recovery from mental illness is not achieved in isolation but in partnership with mental health services and mental health-care providers. In order to facilitate a recovery process for any consumer, both the mental health service and mental health-care providers require a paradigm shift away from traditionally accepted models of delivery, with their emphasis on pathology and disability, to one of wellness and well-being. Such a shift in focus is underpinned by a number of basic assumptions and key elements, as discussed in Box 6.2.

BOX 6.2   BASIC ASSUMPTIONS AND KEY ELEMENTS OF A RECOVERY-FOCUSED MENTAL HEALTH SYSTEM

Basic assumptions

Anthony (1993, pp. 530–5) identified eight basic assumptions that underpin a recovery-focused system of mental health:

1   Recovery can occur without professional intervention: the key to recovery is held by the consumer, not health-care professionals who facilitate recovery.

2   A common denominator of recovery is the presence of people who believe in and stand by the person in need of recovery; central to an individual's recovery is having someone in whom one can trust to 'be there' in times of need.

3   A recovery vision is not a function of one's theory about the causes of mental illness: recovery may occur irrespective of an individual's view of causation.

4   Recovery can occur even though symptoms recur: the episodic recurrence of mental illness may impede but does not prevent recovery.

KAREN-LEIGH EDWARD, ANTHONY WELCH AND LOUISE BYRNE

5 Recovery changes the frequency and duration of symptoms: the recurrence of symptoms may be intense as previous episodes, but the frequency and duration seem to lessen.

6 Recovery does not feel like a linear process: recovery is a gradual process characterised by periods of personal growth, rapid or slow change and setbacks.

7 Recovery from the consequences of the illness is sometimes more difficult than recovering from the illness itself: disability, marginalisation, discrimination, disempowerment and inequality are often more difficult to deal with than the illness itself.

8 Recovery from mental illness does not mean that one was not mentally ill: accepting that one has been mentally ill and working towards recovery is an important source of knowledge about the recovery process.

Key elements

Parkham (2007) described the key elements of a recovery-focused health-care system:

- the development of mental health policy that focuses on health promotion, embracing a social view of health and articulating the social, political and economic determinants influencing mental health and well-being
- a convergence of and collaboration with various workforce sectors and systems: mental health and public health
- a collaboration between levels of government in establishing health-care priorities
- a convergence of sectors, such as mental health, general health, education, media, workplaces and community groups and organisations
- systemic or structural change: a convergence of individual and systemic change directed towards health promotion, enhancing resilience and illness prevention.

Principles of recovery-oriented mental health practice

The purpose of developing and implementing principles of recovery-oriented mental health practice is to provide a framework in which mental health care is delivered in a manner that values and supports the recovery of mental health consumers (Commonwealth of Australia, 2010). The recovery principles adopted by the Australian Government have been adapted from the Hertfordshire Partnership NHS Foundation Trust Recovery Principles in the UK.

Uniqueness of the individual

Recovery-oriented mental health practice:

- recognises that recovery is not necessarily about cure but is about having opportunities for choices and living a meaningful, satisfying and purposeful life, and being a valued member of the community
- accepts that recovery outcomes are personal and unique for each individual and go beyond an exclusive health focus to include an emphasis on social inclusion and quality of life
- empowers individuals so they recognise that they are at the centre of the care they receive.

Real choices

Recovery-oriented mental health practice:

- supports and empowers individuals to make their own choices about how they want to lead their lives and acknowledges choices need to be meaningful and creatively explored

- supports individuals to build on their strengths and take as much responsibility for their lives as they can at any given time
- ensures that there is a balance between duty of care and support for individuals to take positive risks and make the most of new opportunities.

Attitudes and rights

Recovery-oriented mental health practice:

- involves listening to, learning from and acting upon communications from the individual and their carers about what is important to each individual
- promotes and protects each individual's legal, citizenship and human rights
- supports each individual to maintain and develop social, recreational, occupational and vocational activities that are meaningful to the individual
- instils hope in an individual's future and ability to live a meaningful life.

Dignity and respect

Recovery-oriented mental health practice:

- consists of being courteous, respectful and honest in all interactions
- involves sensitivity and respect for each individual, particularly for their values, beliefs and culture
- challenges discrimination and stigma wherever it exists within our own services or the broader community.

Partnership and communication

Recovery-oriented mental health practice:

- acknowledges each individual is an expert on their own life and that recovery involves working in partnership with individuals and their carers to provide support in a way that makes sense to them
- values the importance of sharing relevant information and the need to communicate clearly to enable effective engagement
- involves working in positive and realistic ways with individuals and their carers to help them realise their own hopes, goals and aspirations.

Evaluating recovery

Recovery-oriented mental health practice:

- ensures and enables continuous evaluation of recovery-based practice at several levels
- allows individuals and their carers to track their own progress
- uses the individual's experiences of care to inform quality improvement activities within the mental health practice service.

Consumer perspective on recovery

Recovery at its core is about attitude and making the choice to 'be with' someone in their journey, to be respectful and to find ways to empower their control of their own experience. When consumers are acutely unwell, particularly when they have been involuntarily admitted, there can be a temptation to assume that no level of autonomy is possible. However, there will always be ways to ensure the consumer can make choices. Small things like a choice of drink or where to sit might not seem important, but to someone who has lost control over their emotions and ultimately their liberty, any small ability to choose can be significant.

A common mistake people make in trying to come from a recovery perspective is forgetting that it is the consumer's journey; that their healing and each step of the journey will happen when they are ready, not when the clinician might wish it for them.

The most important thing to remember is that everyone can potentially experience recovery. It is not for anyone else to decide whether a consumer will engage with their recovery journey. In the meantime, all others can do is hold onto hope for them—and it is imperative that they do so (Meehan & Glover, 2007).

The role of consumers in recovery is intrinsic and historic, but often not influential enough. This is true for individuals in their healing journey and consumer workers employed within the sector to assist with ongoing recovery implementation, discussed in Box 6.3.

BOX 6.3 CONSUMER WORKERS

What is a consumer worker?

- A consumer worker has previously experienced mental health challenges in a way that has significantly and unexpectedly altered the course of their life. Most have accessed mental health services and received a diagnosis. As part of their mental health challenge, consumer workers have frequently experienced loss of status: socially or within employment. Many have faced discrimination and a loss of personal identity (Mead & MacNeil, 2006).

- Along with the crucial qualification of having experienced recovery, consumer workers can truly understand what current consumers are facing, socially and emotionally.

- An important role of consumer workers is to advocate for current consumers. This occurs at individual and systemic levels.

- The consumer workforce is rapidly growing in Australia and other recovery-oriented countries. The value of consumer workers is recognised by government policy (Australian Government, 2012) and a growing body of research.

The existing and potential role of consumers in a recovery-oriented system

While contention does exist about what constitutes recovery from the perspective of clinicians, managers and policy writers, consumers and consumer workers have a deep, internal understanding of not only what recovery is, but also what it feels like (Ostrow & Adams, 2012).

Consumer participation is acknowledged as crucial to the meaningful implementation of recovery (Byrne et al., 2013; Department of Health and Ageing, 2013; Gordon & Ellis, 2013). However, progress has been spasmodic and has not yet realised the earlier articulated goals of the consumer movement or government policy (Ning, 2010).

A growing body of evidence suggests both the ongoing confusion surrounding recovery concepts, and the still emergent prevalence of recovery within mental health services, would be significantly assisted by allowing more meaningful leadership of recovery education and implementation by consumer workers (Byrne, Happell & Reid-Searl, 2015).

It is anticipated the ongoing development of more senior roles for consumers, both within mental health services and the wider sector, will allow consumer-led recovery concepts to be more impactful and effective (Slade, Adams & O'Hagan, 2012).

Models of recovery

With the move away from the long-held view of mental illness as a chronic unremitting disorder and towards a position of optimism and the potential for recovery, a number of models focusing on the concept of recovery have been developed. Two examples of these models are the tidal model of recovery and the recovery alliance theory of mental health recovery model.

Tidal model of recovery

The tidal model (Barker, 2001; Barker & Buchanan-Barker, 2010) was developed from a five-year study at Newcastle University, England, of 'the need for nursing'. The Need for Nursing Study sought to clarify the discrete activities or roles of nursing within a multidisciplinary care and treatment process (Barker, 2001). The model focuses on the fundamental (radical) care processes across a 'care continuum' that represents the hospital–community divide. Emphasis is placed on care rather than the setting in which the care is provided.

Three discrete forms of care are identified—critical, transitional and developmental—representing what Barker (2003, p. 99) terms 'the different, hypothetical stages of the care process'. These three forms of nursing care are considered to be complementary to the care and treatment provided by other health-care disciplines operating as part of the multidisciplinary health-care team, with its primary emphasis on the lived experience of the person-in-care and his need for nursing. The term 'tidal' (tides) is a metaphor for a person's lived experiences, and is captured by the following quote (Brookes, Murata & Tansey, 2008, p. 24): 'Tides ebb and flow; they are constantly changing and full of possibilities. Our lives are like sea voyages. At times we sail smoothly, at other times we may be cast adrift or driven off course; we may even be shipwrecked and in need of a safe haven' (Barker, 2003; Barker & Buchanan-Barker, 2005, 2010). Nurses are the lifesavers: they recognise that someone is in distress and provide assistance—at the same time never risking their own lives. Nurses, like lifeguards, are vigilant—constantly scanning the environment and the people in it—and ready, when needed, to go to the rescue.

The model provides a flexible and creative approach to responding to a person's health-care needs that emerge as part of living (see Box 6.4). The use of narrative is central to the model, providing the person with opportunities to explore the construction of her experiences through the nurse–consumer therapeutic alliance. This model has been described by Keen (2005, p. 213) as 'research based, collaborative, person centred, solution focused, narrative systematic and, above all, pragmatic'.

BOX 6.4 THE TEN COMMITMENTS OF THE TIDAL MODEL

Buchanan-Barker (2004) and Buchanan-Barker and Barker (2008) stipulated ten commitments (essential values) of the tidal model:

1 *Value the voice*—the person's story is the beginning and endpoint of the whole helping encounter. The person's story embraces not only the account of the person's distress but also the hope for its resolution. This is the voice of experience.

2 *Respect the language*—the person has developed a unique way of expressing the life story, of representing to others that which

KAREN-LEIGH EDWARD, ANTHONY WELCH AND LOUISE BYRNE

the person alone can know. The language of the story—complete with its unusual grammar and personal metaphors—is the ideal medium for lighting the way.

3 *Develop genuine curiosity*—the person is writing a life story but is not an 'open book'. We need to develop ways of expressing genuine interest in the story so that we can better understand the storyteller.

4 *Become an apprentice*—the person is the world expert on the life story. We can begin to learn something of the power of that story, but only if we apply ourselves diligently and respectfully to the task by becoming the apprentice.

5 *Reveal personal wisdom*—the person has developed a powerful storehouse of wisdom in the writing of the life story. One of the key tasks for the helper is to assist in revealing that wisdom, which will be used to sustain the person and to guide the journey of reclamation.

6 *Be transparent*—the person and the professional helper become a team. If this relationship is to prosper, both must be willing to let the other into their confidence. The professional helper is in a privileged position, and should model this confidence building by being transparent at all

times, helping the person to understand exactly what is being done and why.

7 *Use the available toolkits*—the person's story contains numerous examples of 'what has worked' or 'what might work' for this person. These represent the main tools that need to be used to unlock or build the story of recovery.

8 *Craft the step beyond*—the helper and the person work together to construct an appreciation of what needs to be done now. The first step is the crucial step, revealing the power of change and pointing towards the ultimate goal of recovery.

9 *Give the gift of time*—there is nothing more valuable than the time the helper and the person spend together. Time is the midwife of change.

10 *Know that change is constant*—the tidal model assumes that change is inevitable, for change is constant. This is the common story for all people. The task of the professional helper is to develop awareness of how that change is happening and how that knowledge might be used to steer the person out of danger and distress back on to the course of reclamation and recovery.

Brookes, Murata & Tansey (2008, p. 24)

Recovery alliance theory of mental health recovery model

Apart from a number of models of recovery developed in recent years, theories of the recovery process have also been put forward. One such theory is the recovery alliance theory of mental health (RAT) developed by Shanley and Jubb-Shanley (2007), which has been developed as an alternative to the traditional medical model that dominated mental health. The theory was constructed in response to social changes and changes in the mental health field, including liberalisation of legislation, decentralisation of decision-making, growing support for a more consumer-centred service and a move to a recovery-focused approach to treatment and management of people with a mental illness (Shanley & Jubb-Shanley, 2007). In the development of the theory, consideration was given to cultural and geographical diversity across mental health settings: metropolitan, rural and remote areas of Australia.

The theory brings together the philosophical underpinnings of the recovery-oriented approach (Anthony, 1993) and Bordin's (1994) conception of the working alliance model. The recovery alliance theory consists of three concepts: coping, working alliance, and self-responsibility and control. The theory also includes four concepts that form the meta-paradigm of mental health nursing—person, mental health, mental health nursing and environment—and six outer constructs: humanistic philosophy, recovery, partnership, strengths focus, empowerment and common humanity. Characteristics of the philosophy underpinning the recovery alliance theory are as follows:

- Individuals are social animals and share a common humanity.
- Individuals have the potential for growth through awareness of and interaction with self and others.
- The individual's growth is enhanced by a respectful approach in validating the person's ability to deal competently with his or her own life experiences.
- Individuals have the ability to make choices and to exercise control in decisions affecting their lives.
- Individuals cannot be categorised in that they are composed of many different facets, of which none stands alone (Shanley & Jubb-Shanley, 2007, p. 737).

The recovery alliance theory of mental health provides a comprehensive framework for the practice of mental health nursing across the spectrum of mental health settings. The constructs and philosophical underpinnings are consistent with the emerging global patterns of mental health care and management.

CRITICAL THINKING OPPORTUNITY

1 In your review of the current mental health-care system, what is your assessment of whether a recovery-focused model of care is evident?

2 What are your beliefs and attitudes about a person who has experienced a mental illness?

3 Do you believe that a person can recover from a mental illness?

4 What do you think are the personal qualities or strengths an individual needs to recover from a mental illness?

5 What is needed for the effective implementation of a recovery-focused model of mental health care?

ABOUT THE CONSUMER   Suassan's story

An 18-year-old female by the name of Suassan has been admitted to your unit after being found wandering alone in the early hours of the morning. On admission, Suassan presented as dishevelled in appearance, confused, withdrawn and guarded in her response to being questioned. During the course of the admission interview, Suassan briefly talked about her life in Somalia prior to migrating to Australia two years ago. She talked of the family's life of poverty and daily violence as a consequence of war and civil unrest. Although only 16 years old at the time, Suassan was the one person who was able to hold the family together. Her abilities to forage for food, to instil a sense of hope for a better future and to assist her mother to care for the family were evident in her stories. However, since her arrival she has found it difficult to make friends and complete her high-school education. Her family, which consists of her parents, two brothers aged 10 and 12 and one sister aged 6, live in a small inner-city apartment sponsored by the Ministry of Housing. The initial assessment indicates that Suassan is depressed and requires a period of hospitalisation for symptom management. You have been asked by the unit manager to develop an initial nursing care plan for Suassan.

How would you work with Suassan to develop personal resilience in moving towards recovery?

REFLECTION QUESTION

KAREN-LEIGH EDWARD, ANTHONY WELCH AND LOUISE BYRNE

Reconnection

A central component of the recovery process is the ability of the person who has experienced mental illness or disability to reconnect with the everyday world in meaningful and self-affirming ways. The manner in which each person re-engages with life is one of personal preference based on her or his values, needs and aspirations for the future. Key elements in achieving a sense of reconnection involve regaining a sense of independence, control and self-worth, and being willing to gradually move from the support of health-care professionals to the natural everyday supports of family, friends and the local community (Kartalova-O'Doherty & Tedstone Doherty, 2010). Essentially, reconnecting is about improving one's quality of life.

Reconnection is also considered a socially adaptive response for those at risk of being socially excluded (Derfler-Rozin, Pillutla & Thau, 2010). For those who experience mental illness, the potential for social exclusion is relatively high. Social exclusion can be generated by oneself (because of feelings of low self-esteem or as a consequence of symptoms of mental illness such as depression) or can result from stigma attached to mental illness or life circumstances, such as poverty and deprivation. Social exclusion, irrespective of the reason (which can be manifold), results in people being marginalised. An individual can be the recipient of social exclusion practices if 'he or she is unable for reasons beyond his or her control to participate in social events or community activities over a period of time despite wishing to be involved' (Burchardt, 2000).

Other authors suggest that social exclusion has key elements, including a lack of personal and community resources (a multidimensional element); exclusion at a particular point in time within a particular group (a relative element); exclusion because of the current situation and having little prospect for the future (a dynamic element); and a disconnection between the individual and the rest of society (a relational element) (Atkinson, 1998; Chakravarty & D'Ambrosio, 2006; Sen, 2000).

Hope and self-efficacy

Hope and self-efficacy are central components to resilience, recovery and reconnection.

The concept of hope

The concept of hope has been described as a life-sustaining force essential to life (Fromm, 1968; Frankl, 1962; Marcel, 1951) and valued by thinkers of all ages—whether scientist, religious, spiritually minded, atheist or agnostic—as contributing to a person's quality of life and well-being. For Eric Fromm (1968), one of the founding fathers of psychoanalysis as well as a sociologist, hope is a fundamental requirement essential for personal transformation. From the perspective of Gabriel Marcel (1951), a French philosopher of the twentieth century, hope is paradoxical in nature in that it surfaces in situations that seem hopeless. Victor Frankl, an existentialist psychiatrist, was imprisoned in Auschwitz concentration camp during the Second World War, and witnessed many atrocities. As a result, he came to view hope as essential for survival. In his writings, an underlying theme was not to give up hope, which he called *meaning to live*. For Frankl, one constructs meaning in life by rising above what is perceived to be hopeless situations. Since these seminal works there has been considerable research into the place of hope in human existence (Bernardo, 2010; Snyder, 2002; Venning et al., 2011).

Although there have been many definitions of hope generated over time, two definitions have been chosen that embody the essential nature of hope. Groopman (2004) offers a succinct and useful definition that can be applied to everyday life situations. Hope is 'the elevating feeling we experience when we see—in the mind's eye—a path to a better future [with realistic expectations that the future may present with] significant obstacles and deep pitfalls along that path' (p. xiv). Miller (2000) defined hope as 'a state of being characterized by an anticipation of a continued good state, an improved state or a release from perceived entrapment … [it] is an anticipation of a future that is good and is based upon: mutuality, psychological well-being, purpose and meaning in life as well as a sense of the possible' (pp. 523–4). Both of these definitions provide a comprehensive conceptualisation of what constitutes hope.

Hope as a construct is not linear in nature or an uninterrupted feeling of realistic optimism, but can be momentarily diminished by life experiences that surface moments of doubt and uncertainty. It is also a multidimensional concept encompassing affective, cognitive and behavioural aspects of a person to manage stress and crises (Snyder, Rand & Sigmon, 2002). A person's spirituality has also been found to be an important source in fostering hope (Duggleby & Wright, 2007). Spirituality is the essence of the person, the core of an individual's being. It is the process of searching for meaning and purpose in life and underpins everyday activities in which one engages (Bassett, Lloyd & Tse, 2008). Spirituality has the potential to boost a person's self-esteem and sustain hope (Longo & Paterson, 2002).

One of the major contributions to psychological theories of hope in the past two decades has been Snyder's hope theory (2002), which has three major components of hope: goals, agency and pathways. The cornerstone of the theory is approaching life in a goal-oriented way—clearly conceptualising goals. The second component is pathways—conceptualisation or identification of different ways to achieve your goals rather than relying on one pathway that may or may not work. The third component is the notion of agency—believing that you can instigate change and achieve established goals. According to Snyder's hope theory, a goal can be anything an individual desires to experience, become or create. The goal may be a lifelong pursuit or something brief such as getting to work. Pathways represent a person's perceived capacity to set in place realistic and workable ways by which the established goals can be achieved. Agency involves the person engaging in what Snyder terms 'internal speech', which involves the person engaging in self-talk; for example, 'I believe I can do this' or ' I am not going to fail'. However, agency is not limited to the individual taking action by themselves (direct agency) but can also involve others acting on behalf of the person (proxy agency) or through group action (collective agency). What becomes important is how the individual assesses the situation, clearly identifies goals that are realistic and achievable, identifies pathways or ways by which the goals can be achieved, and identifies what type of agency would be appropriate in moving to a successful outcome.

Hope in and of itself is not sufficient for being resilient, transcending difficult times in one's life, and recovering from mental health challenges. A personal belief in one's own ability and self-worth—self-efficacy—is also required.

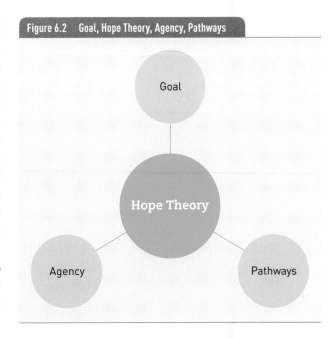

Figure 6.2 Goal, Hope Theory, Agency, Pathways

Goal

Hope Theory

Agency

Pathways

KAREN-LEIGH EDWARD, ANTHONY WELCH AND LOUISE BYRNE

1 In a review of Snyder's hope theory (2002), what do you understand about the concepts—goal setting, agency and pathways—in working with consumers experiencing mental health challenges and their families?

2 What are your beliefs and attitudes about the importance of hope within the therapeutic relationship from both the perspectives of the consumer and the health-care professional?

Self-efficacy

Self-efficacy can be defined as the perception or belief that 'one posses[es] specific skills to make changes given a specific situation' (Hartley & Vance, 2008, p. 522). Self-efficacy is a key personal factor in Albert Bandura's social cognitive theory (1986) and has a specific meaning that is different from such concepts as self-confidence, self-worth, self-esteem and outcome expectations. Self-confidence is concerned with a general capability self-belief, while self-worth purports a view of self-concept in which beliefs in one's competence are central to the self-system and the need to perceive oneself as competent. Self-esteem is an overall evaluation of oneself through the process of self-judgment (Schunk & Pajares, 2005). Outcome expectations focuses on beliefs about anticipated outcomes of actions (Bandura, 1997).

Bandura (1997) further suggested that self-efficacy is concerned with human functioning. For Bandura, 'human functioning results from a dynamic interplay among personal, behavioural, and environmental influences'(p. 36), which he termed 'reciprocal determinism'. The interplay between these three concepts 'create interactions that result in a triadic reciprocity'(Bandura, 1977, p. 35). The reciprocal nature of these three determinants of human functioning provide opportunities for self-reflection, the development of self-knowledge and the assessment of one's abilities to successfully problem-solve challenging situations. People with high self-efficacy are able to set challenging goals and have a strong commitment to achieving their goals, even in the face of setbacks or failure. On the other hand, individuals with low self-efficacy tend to view the task at hand as more difficult than it actually is, which acts as a deterrent in reaching one's goals.

Both hope and self-efficacy are inextricably intertwined with the concepts of resilience and recovery. As mentioned at the beginning of this chapter, the resilient person is not only able to bend with the pressures, disappointments and struggles of daily life—buoyed by a belief in their ability to problem-solve their way out of situations—but is also able to look to the future with hope, realistic optimism and agency. In other words, hope and self-efficacy provide the soil for the development of personal resilience in meeting the challenges of daily life with a sense of self-determination.

In terms of recovery, which has previously been defined as 'an active process of moving towards achieving a personal sense of well-being and a satisfying life'(Green, 2004, p. 296), self-efficacy, self-worth and having hope are central concepts. In other words, the process of recovery from mental illness is grounded in the notions of resilience, self-efficacy and hope.

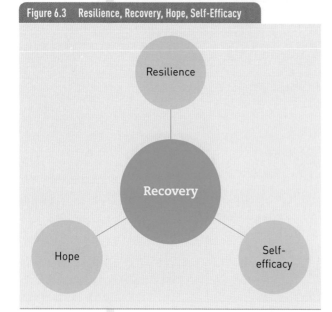

Figure 6.3 Resilience, Recovery, Hope, Self-Efficacy

1 What are your beliefs and attitudes about the place of agency or self-efficacy in working with consumers experiencing mental illness?

2 What is needed for the effective implementation of care in which the consumers' sense of agency or self-efficacy is promoted?

CRITICAL THINKING OPPORTUNITY

Implications for health-care professionals

From the perspective of a recovery approach to care, mental health professionals play an important role in supporting mental health consumers to reconnect to the everyday world after experiencing mental illness. Apart from having to cope with the experience of mental illness or disability, the mental health consumer is also faced with challenges of dealing with internalised stigma, social stigma, low self-esteem, feeling devalued and struggling to make sense of their fractured world. Health professionals therefore require particular skill in working with the consumer and their family in developing personal resilience, meeting the challenges of mental illness as part of the recovery process, and looking to the future with hope and a sense of self-efficacy.

Having a commitment to working with the consumer and acknowledging them as the driver of their care is an essential starting point for the development of the recovery alliance relationship. Valuing the importance of the need for the consumer to regain a sense of independence, control and self-worth is necessary for the consumer to begin coming to terms with their illness experience and then move forward in life. Feeling genuinely supported by health-care professionals is pivotal to the consumer being successful in making this transition from illness to wellness and well-being, despite continuing to experience symptoms of mental illness (Levine et al., 2013). Genuine support from health-care professionals involves being hope carriers (Bland & Darlington, 2002); that is, having hope and belief in the consumer's ability to engage in decision-making in setting realistic and achievable goals and having a commitment to work in partnership with the consumer in exploring future options for living quality of life as determined by the consumer.

Nurses are well placed in working with consumers and their family to assist them to reconnect with life after mental illness, using strategies that are resilience-focused, person-centred, recovery-oriented and underpinned by a realistic sense hope for the future; and a commitment to enhancing the consumers' sense of agency or self-efficacy in making personal choices about their future.

In what ways can you embed the concepts of resilience, recovery, hope and self-efficacy into your professional practice in a therapeutical and meaning way for both yourself and the consumer?

CRITICAL THINKING OPPORTUNITY

Care planning

The following is an example care plan for Suassan with a recovery focus. The areas of daily living that are considered include biopsychosocial factors. The plan is mapped out using the nursing process (assessment, planning, implementation and evaluation). Remember, the success is in the detail, so be specific about who, when and what in the collaborative plan; and never include someone in the plan if they were not consulted in the planning process.

KAREN-LEIGH EDWARD, ANTHONY WELCH AND LOUISE BYRNE

Care Plan 1

Date: [Today's date]						
Consumer: Suassan Case Manager: Dave						
Areas of daily living address	**Assessment of current situation**	**Goal**	**Plan (undertaken with consumer)**	**Implementation**	**Who is responsible (including only those who have been consulted in the planning process)**	**Evaluation/ review date**
Mental health	Depressed mood Guarded, confused and withdrawn	Manage depressed mood Maximise communication	Present treatment options for managing depression. Provide opportunities for consumer input to decision-making about treatment options. Work towards establishing a therapeutic partnership. Provide opportunities to explore achievable and meaningful goals.	Schedule a meeting with consumer to discuss treatment options. Identify outcomes of treatment choices. Engage in open and transparent communication with consumer. Set timelines for achieving identified goals.	Dave and Suassan	Review monthly
Social	Social isolation	Identify reasons and solutions for social isolation	Utilise face-to-face time with consumer to explore her feelings of social isolation. Work with consumer to identify ways to successfully manage her social situation.	Negotiate regular meeting times to meet with consumer. Set agenda for discussion that has been mutually agreed on. Identify strategies for overcoming social isolation that are meaningful to the consumer.	Dave and Suassan	Review monthly

Date: [Today's date]						
Substance using behaviours	Nil					
Risk behaviours	Potential for self-harm	Harm minimisation	Work with consumer to identify level of risk of self-harm and strategies for harm minimisation. Empower consumer to accept responsibility for own behaviour.	Negotiate mutually agreed contract to reduce risk of self-harm. Support to consumer to take control (where appropriate) of their actions.	Dave and Suassan	Review monthly

SUMMARY

This chapter has provided you with contemporary evidence-based knowledge of resilience, recovery, reconnection, hope and self-efficacy within the context of a therapeutic relationship. You will now have a nascent understanding of what is meant by these terms, and an enhanced ability in conceptualising the applicability of this information to your practice. There are key characteristics and skills highlighted throughout this chapter that you will need to develop throughout your career in order to facilitate resilience through adopting a recovery-focused approach when working with consumers and their families to promote a sense of wellness and personal well-being while reconnecting with life.

DISCUSSION QUESTIONS

1   What is resilience, and how might you foster resilience in your care practices?
2   What are the various definitions of recovery? How do the various definitions of recovery impact the type of nursing care you provide?
3   What is the importance of hope within the therapeutic relationship when working with individuals who are recovering from mental health challenges?
4   In what ways can you as a mental health professional promote a sense of agency or self-efficacy in your care practices?

KAREN-LEIGH EDWARD, ANTHONY WELCH AND LOUISE BYRNE

TEST YOURSELF

1 The term resilience is:

   a used to explain the ability of people to roll with the punches and cope with life events, both negative and positive

   b used to explain the inability of people to roll with the punches and cope with life events, both negative and positive

   c used to explain the ability of people to roll with the punches and cope with life events that are negative

   d used to explain the inability of people to cope with life events, both negative and positive

2 Recovery is:

   a the same for all people

   b not achievable for most people

   c a highly individual process

   d a roller-coaster ride for most people

3 According to Anthony (1993), recovery:

   a is when all the symptoms are absent

   b can occur even though symptoms recur

   c cannot occur when the person has episodic mental illness

   d is not possible for consumers with mental illness

4 Snyder's hope theory (2002) has three major components:

   a goals, assertiveness and pathways

   b goals, attentiveness and perseverance

   c gratitude, agency and pathways

   d goals, agency and pathways

USEFUL WEBSITES

Department of Health—Principles of recovery oriented mental health practice: www.health.gov.au/internet/publications/publishing.nsf/Content/mental-pubs-i-nongov-toc~mental-pubs-i-nongov-pri

Mental Health Foundation of New Zealand—Destination: Recovery: https://www.mentalhealth.org.nz/assets/Our-Work/Destination-Recovery-FINAL-low-res.pdf

Tidal Model: www.tidal-model.com

World Health Organization—Mental health, resilience and inequalities: http://www.euro.who.int/__data/assets/pdf_file/0012/100821/E92227.pdf?ua=1

REFERENCES

Alves, D., & Cleveland, P. (1999). *The Maori and the crown: An indigenous people's struggle for self-determination*. Auckland: Greenwood Publishing Group.

Anthony, W. (1993). Recovery from mental illness: The guiding vision of the Mental Health Service in the 1990s. *Psychosocial Rehabilitation Journal, 16*(4), 11–23.

Anthony, W. (2007). *Toward a vision of recovery for mental health and psychiatric rehabilitation services*. Boston: Centre for Psychiatric Rehabilitation, Boston University.

Atkinson, A. (1998). Social exclusion, poverty and unemployment. In A. Atkinson & J. Hills (Eds.), *Exclusion, employment and opportunity*.

London: Centre for the Analysis of Social Exclusion, London School of Economics.

Australian Government (2012). *National mental health commission paid participation policy: For people with a lived experience of mental health difficulties, their families and support people*. Canberra: National Mental Health Commission.

Badal, D. W. (2003). *Treating chronic depression: Psychotherapy and medication.* Northvale: Jason Aronson.

Bandura, A. (1977). Self-efficacy: Toward a unifying theory of behavioral change. *Psychological Review, 84*(2), 191–215.

Bandura, A. (1997). *Self-efficacy: The exercise of control.* New York: Freeman.

Barker, P. (2001). The tidal model: Developing an empowering, person-centred approach to recovery within psychiatric and mental health nursing. *Journal of Psychiatric and Mental Health Nursing, 8*(3), 233–240.

Barker, P. (2003). The tidal model: Psychiatric colonization, recovery and the paradigm shift in mental health care. *International Journal of Mental Health Nursing, 12*(2), 96–102.

Barker, P., & Buchanan-Barker, P., (2005). The tidal model: A guide for mental health professionals. London and New York: Brunner-Routledge.

Barker, P., & Buchanan-Barker, P. (2010). The tidal model of mental health recovery and reclamation: Application in acute care settings. *Issues in Mental Health Nursing, 31*(3), 171–180.

Bassett, H., Lloyd, C., & Tse, S. (2008). Approaching in the spirit: Spirituality and hope in recovery from mental health problems. *International Journal of Therapy and Rehabilitation, 15*(6), 254–261.

Bernardo, A. B. I. (2010). Extending hope theory: Internal and external locus of trait hope. *Personality and Individual Differences, 49*, 944–949.

Bland, R., & Darlington, Y. (2002). The nature and sources of hope: Perspectives of family caregivers of people with serious mental illness. *Perspectives in Psychiatric Care, 38*(2), 61–68.

Bordin, E. S. (1994). Theory and research on the therapeutic working alliance: New directions. In A. O. Harvath & L. S. Greenberg (Eds.), *The working alliance: Theory, research and practice* (pp. 13–17). New York: John Wiley.

Brookes, N., Murata, L., & Tansey, M. (2008). Tidal waves: Implementing a new model of mental health recovery and reclamation. *Canadian Nurse, 104*(8), 22–27.

Buchanan-Barker, P. (2004). *Uncommon sense: The value base of the tidal model.* Retrieved from www. tidal-model.com/New%20Uncommon%20sense. htm.

Buchanan-Barker, P., & Barker, P. (2008). The tidal commitments: Extending the value base of mental health recovery. *Journal of Psychiatric and Mental Health Nursing, 15*(2), 93–100. doi: 10.1111/j.1365–2850.2007.01209.x.

Burchardt, T. (2000). Social exclusion: Concepts and evidence. In D. Gordon & P. Townsend (Eds.), *Breadline Europe: The measurement of poverty.* Bristol: Policy Press.

Byrne, L., Happell, B., Welch, A., & Moxham, L. (2013). Reflecting on holistic nursing: The contribution of an academic with lived experience of mental health service use. *Issues in Mental Health Nursing, 34*(4), 265–272.

Byrne, L., B. Happell, & K. Reid-Searl (2015). Recovery as a lived experience discipline: A grounded theory study. *Issues in Mental Health Nursing, 36*(12), 935–943.

Carpenter, J. (2002). Mental health recovery paradigm: Implications for social work. *Health and Social Work, 27*(2), 1–13.

Cassano, P., & Fava, M. (2002). Depression and public health: An overview. *Journal of Psychosomatic Research, 53*(4), 849–857.

Chakravarty, S. R., & D'Ambrosio, C. (2006). The measurement of social exclusion. *Review of Income and Wealth, 52*(3), 377–398.

Charney, D. S. (2004). Psychobiological mechanisms of resilience and vulnerability: Implications for successful adaptation to extreme stress. *American Journal of Psychiatry, 161*(2), 195–216.

Commonwealth of Australia (2009). *Fourth national mental health plan: An agenda for collaborative government action in mental health 2009–2014.* Barton.

Commonwealth of Australia (2010). *National standards for mental health services.* Barton, ACT.

Deegan, P. (1988). Recovery: The lived experience of rehabilitation. *Psychosocial Rehabilitation Journal, 11*(4), 11–19.

Deegan, P. (1996). Recovery as a journal of the heart: Mentally ill: Rehabilitation. *Psychiatric Rehabilitation Journal, 19*(3), 91–100.

Department of Health and Ageing (2013). *A national framework for recovery-oriented mental health services: Policy and theory.* Canberra: Commonwealth of Australia.

Derfler-Rozin, R., Pillutla, M., & Thau, S. (2010). Social reconnection revisited: The effects of social exclusion risk on reciprocity, trust, and general risk-taking. *Organizational Behavior and Human Decision Processes, 112*(2), 140–150.

Duggleby, W., & Wright, K. (2007). The hope of professional caregivers caring for persons at the end of life. *Journal of Hospice and Palliative Nursing, 9*(1), 42–49.

Earvolino-Ramirez, M. (2007). Resilience: A concept analysis. *Nursing Forum, 42*(2), 73–82. doi: 10.1111/j.1744–6198.2007.00070.x.

Edward, K. (2005a). The phenomenon of resilience in crisis care mental health clinicians. *International Journal of Mental Health Nursing, 14*(2), 142–148.

Edward, K. (2005b). Resilience: A protector from depression. *Journal of the American Psychiatric Nurses Association, 11*(4), 241–243.

Edward, K. (2007). The phenomenon of resilience as described by people who have experienced mental illness. PhD thesis. Melbourne: RMIT University.

Edward, K. L. (2013). Chronic illness and wellbeing: Using nursing practice to foster resilience as resistance. *British Journal of Nursing, 22*(13), 741–746.

Edward, K., & Warelow, P. (2005). Resilience: When coping is emotionally intelligent. *Journal of the American Psychiatric Nurses Association, 11*(2), 101–102.

Edward, K., Welch, A., & Chater, K. (2009). The phenomenon of resilience as described by adults who have experienced mental illness. *Journal of Advanced Nursing, 65*(3), 587–595.

Frankl, V. E. (1962). *Man's search for meaning* (3rd ed.). New York: Simon & Schuster.

Fromm, E. (1968). *The revolution of hope.* New York: Harper & Row.

Garcia-Dia, M. J., DiNapoli, J. M., Garcia-Ona, L., Jakubowski, R., & O'Flaherty, D. (2013). Concept analysis: Resilience. *Archives of Psychiatric Nursing, 27*(6), 264–270.

Gordon, S. E., & Ellis, P. M. (2013). Recovery of evidence-based practice. *International Journal of Mental Health Nursing, 22*(1), 3–14.

Green, C. (2004). Fostering recovery from life-transforming mental health disorders: A synthesis and model. *Social Theory and Health, 2*(4), 293–314.

Groopman, J. (2004). *The anatomy of hope: How people prevail in the face of illness.* New York: Random House.

Hartley, M., & Vance, D. E. (2008). Hope, self-efficacy, and functional recovery after knee and hip replacement surgery. *Rehabilitation Psychology, 53*(4), 521–529.

Hernandez, P., Gangsei, D., & Engstrom, D. (2007). Vicarious resilience: A new concept in work with those who survive trauma. *Family Process, 46*(2), 229–241. doi: doi:10.1111/j.1545–5300.2007.00206.x.

Hong, R. R., & Welch, A. (2013). The lived experiences of single Taiwanese mothers being resilient after divorce. *Journal of Transcultural Nursing, 24*(1), 51–59.

Houghton, J. F. (1982). First person account: Maintaining mental health in a turbulent world. *Schizophrenia Bulletin, 8*(3), 548–552.

Kartalova-O'Doherty, Y., & Tedstone Doherty, D. (2010). *Reconnecting with life: Personal experiences of recovering from mental health problems in Ireland.* Dublin: Health Research Board.

Keen, T. (2005). In P. J. Barker & P. Buchanan-Barker, *The tidal model: A guide for mental health professionals.* London: Brunner-Routledge.

Landau, J. (2007). Enhancing resilience: Families and communities as agents for change. *Family Process, 46*(3), 351–365. doi: 10.1111/j.1545–5300.2007.00216.x.

Levine, S. Z., Rabinowitz, J., Ascher-Svanum, H., Faries, D. E, & Lawson, A. H. (2013). Comparing symptom response among antipsychotic medications in CATIE. *Journal of Clinical Psychopharmacology,* 33(1), 123–126.

Lee, J. H., Nam, S. K., Kim, A., Kim, B., Lee, M. Y., & Lee, S. M. (2013). Resilience: A meta-analytic approach. *Journal of Counseling & Development, 91*(3), 269–279.

Leete, E. (1989). How I perceive and manage my illness. *Schizophrenia Bulletin, 15*(2), 197–200.

Lester, H., & Gask, L. (2006). Delivering medical care for patients with serious mental illness or promoting a collaborative model of recovery? *British Journal of Psychiatry, 188*(5), 401–402.

Longo, D., & Paterson, S. (2002). The role of spirituality in psycho-social rehabilitation. *Psychiatric Rehabilitation Journal, 25,* 333–340.

Marcel, G. (1951). *Homo viator* (E. Craufurd, Trans.). Chicago: Henry Regnery Co.

Mead, S., & MacNeil, C. (2006). Peer support: What makes it unique? *International Journal of Psychosocial Rehabilitation, 10*(2), 29–37.

Meehan, T., & Glover, H. (2007). Telling our story: Consumer perceptions of their role in mental health education. *Psychiatric Rehabilitation Journal, 31*(2), 152–154.

Mental Health Commission (1998). *Blueprint for mental health services in New Zealand.* Wellington: MHC.

Miller, J. F. (2000). *Coping with chronic illness: Overcoming powerlessness.* Philadelphia: F. A. Davis.

Murphy, B., & Dillon, C. (2003). *Interviewing in action: Relationship, process and change* (2nd ed.). Toronto: Brooks/Cole.

Ning, L. (2010). Building a 'user-driven' mental health system. *Advances in Mental Health, 9*(2), 112–115.

O'Hagan, M. (2004). Recovery in New Zealand: Lessons for Australia? *Australian e-Journal for the Advancement of Mental Health, 3*(1). Retrieved from www.auseinet.com/vil3iss1/ohaganeditorial.pdf.

Ostrow, L., & Adams, N. (2012). Recovery in the USA: From politics to peer support. *International Review of Psychiatry, 24*(1), 70–78.

Parker, J. (2014). Recovery in mental health. *South African Medical Journal, 104*(1), 77. Retrieved February 6 2017 from www.scielo.org.za/scielo.php?script=sci_arttext&pid=S0256–95742014000100033&lng=en&tlng=en.

Parkham, J. (2007). Shifting mental health policy to embrace a positive view of health: A convergence of paradigms. *Health Promotion Journal of Australia, 18*(3), 173–175.

Schunk, D. H., & Pajares, F. (2005). Competence beliefs in academic functioning. In A. J. Elliot & C. Dweck (Eds.), *Handbook of competence and motivation* (pp. 85–104). New York: Guildford Press.

Sen, A. (2000). *Social Exclusion: Concept, Application, And Scrutiny.* Phillipines: Asian Development Bank.

Shanley, E., & Jubb-Shanley, M. (2007). The recovery alliance theory of mental health nursing. *Journal of Psychiatric and Mental Health Nursing, 14*(8), 734–743.

Slade, M., Adams, N., & O'Hagan, M. (2012). Recovery: Past progress and future challenges. *International Review of Psychiatry, 24*(1), 1–4.

Snyder, C. R. (2002). Hope theory: Rainbows in the mind. *Psychological Inquiry, 13,* 249–275.

Snyder, C. R., Rand, K. L., & Sigmon, D. R. (2002). Hope theory: A member of the positive psychology family. In C. R. Snyder & S. J. Lopez (Eds.), *Handbook of positive psychology* (pp. 257–276). Oxford: Oxford University Press.

Venning, G., Kettler, L., Zajac, J., Wilson. A., & Eliott, J. (2011). Is hope or mental illness a stronger predictor of mental health? *International Journal of Mental Health Promotion, 13*(2), 32–39.

CHAPTER 7

Nurses' Health and Self-care

GLENN TAYLOR,
DANIEL NICHOLLS AND
WENDY CROSS

KEY OUTCOMES

AFTER READING THIS CHAPTER, YOU SHOULD BE ABLE TO:

- understand the possible personal effects of working in mental health
- see how these effects may have an impact upon your clinical relationships
- have strategies to employ in meeting the emotional demands of mental health nursing
- recognise the importance of reflection and practice development in both accountable practice and self-care.

KEY TERMS

- self-care
- clinical supervision
- counter-transference
- compassion fatigue
- facilitation
- reciprocity
- reflection
- stress
- transference

Introduction

This chapter is divided into three sections. The first discusses the essential elements of self-care, the second describes the self-care of clinical supervision, and the last section examines the crucial element of self-care that is practice development.

SECTION 1 THE ESSENTIAL ELEMENTS OF SELF-CARE

GLENN TAYLOR

Self-care defined

According to Bunn (2010), self-care begins with understanding that the body possesses its own in-built intelligence. Living in harmony with the 'natural laws' of life supports our body's inner intelligence. This allows us to heal and nourish the body from within so we need fewer 'things' outside of ourselves to prop us up. Those from traditional cultures have practised the principles described by Bunn for thousands of years with favourable results: 'If we were to isolate one factor common to the world's healthiest and longest living populations, it would be that they have predominantly lived in harmony with the natural laws of life' (Bunn, 2010, p. 22).

Fundamental to the success of any nurse–consumer therapeutic relationship is the presence of a 'healthy' mental health nurse. Effective self-care practices on the part of the mental health nurse are as important to the therapeutic relationship as any nursing practice or intervention. Without this, the care provided will not be as effective, therapeutic or successful. In fact, it could be unhelpful or even harmful. Personal insight and emotional maturity are essential characteristics of the mental health nurse and provide the platform from which we launch our practice. Keeping these at healthy levels requires diligence and discipline on the part of the individual.

Self-care is reliant on self-awareness, reflection, insight, self-regulation, planning, commitment, action and evaluation. Interestingly, these are the very qualities required of an effective, practising mental health nurse. Optimum self-care involves balance in all aspects of life: physical, psychological and spiritual. Achieving life balance not only benefits the well-being of the mental health nurse but also provides the public with a healthy treatment agent in the delivery of nursing care; that is, the mental health nurse.

Diligence with self-care practices positively influences everyone in the therapeutic environment as the nurse acts as both a role model and a teacher. Those influenced include the consumer's family and significant others. We can also act as role models to our colleagues, associates, family and friends who will come to appreciate the benefits of self-care as they see for themselves our increased ability to deal with the stressors in our lives.

The role of the mental health nurse

What motivates someone to become a mental health nurse? Is it an inherent or instinctive desire to help another? Is it based on the individual's values or philosophical beliefs of providing care to the disadvantaged in our society? Is it motivated by a desire to learn more about the human condition? These questions allow us to look at our own motivations in our career choice and are directly relevant to how we view self-care.

Individuals are best placed to achieve a therapeutic partnership when they possess the personal characteristics and skill set that assist them to undertake the role. Using one's self as the therapeutic agent provides the foundation for providing the care that is required by the consumer and their significant others. Use of self requires an ability to show empathy without emotional attachment, to withhold judgment of the consumer throughout the relationship, and to remain in control and focused while caring for and nurturing an individual who may be experiencing significant distress related to their condition.

Innovation, creativity and ingenuity are important and commonly displayed characteristics in mental health nurses. These attributes assist us when confronted by challenges and potential barriers to effective communication with the consumer. Honing these attributes requires resilience and determination on the part of the mental health nurse and the ability to pause and question our methods before finding something from within that we can activate to provide an alternative approach.

Of the many tasks of the mental health nurse, there are few more important than the ability to listen, reflect and initiate an empathic, therapeutic response. This is a function that can be underestimated and requires great skill and finesse. Demonstrating to the consumer that we care for them and displaying an understanding of the context of their presentation can be powerful and reassuring.

Being confronted by uncontrollable events is a common occurrence for the mental health nurse. Managing these events for the best possible outcome requires versatility and adaptability. The roles we undertake (carer, helper, advocate, counsellor and administrator) make demands on us every time we step into the role. And just as we manage these events we manage ourselves—this is self-care.

How health is challenged for the mental health nurse

Mental health nurses are trained to give of themselves professionally. However, we are prone to giving too much of ourselves at times. Mental health nurses often put themselves later or last and do not replenish their stocks in a timely manner. Continuing to practise in a depleted state is ill-advised as it places us at risk of illness, which, in turn, risks the safety of the consumer.

It is useful to remind ourselves that mental health nurses are people first. A qualification in nursing doesn't protect mental health nurses from the challenges presented by our work. We are human, complete with fears, anxieties, faults, flaws and failings. For the most part we manage our life insecurities satisfactorily. However, in times of stress or trauma unexpected thoughts and feelings may surface, casting doubt over the individual nurse's ability to succeed in our profession.

We as mental health nurses are influenced by our experiences in life. This is also known colloquially as our 'baggage'. Our life 'baggage' can shape the way we view the world. Our family of origin, childhood and upbringing, environment and social influences all shape us. Of course, not all circumstances and experiences are as negative as the term 'baggage' might imply, so we need to have a balanced view of what we bring to nursing. This balanced view can also be transferred to consumers and their families who sometimes see their current situation in highly negative terms.

Our personal circumstances and experiences influence the way nurses support those for whom we care. Mental illness and other challenging life events are likely to expose and accentuate the fears, anxieties, faults, flaws and failings of our consumers. Witnessing these in those we care for can prove challenging and detrimental to our own health as our values and beliefs are regularly challenged, leaving us with sometimes unanswerable questions. Why do people experience mental illness? Why do some of our consumers remain unwell? These questions can challenge our own beliefs about ourselves and our worldviews.

It is important to remember that external factors that exist to challenge our health as a mental health nurse are numerous, and most are out of our control. The more obvious contributing factors are those tangible in form, such as crude violence, threats of homicide and suicide, and antisocial behaviours. Dealing with people in acute distress and in acutely distressing situations is confronting and unsettling, and can result in poor physical and psychological health for the mental health nurse if not identified and managed early.

Arguably less confronting, though just as detrimental to the health of the mental health nurse, are the feelings raised when working in inadequately staffed departments, areas of high demand for service and unrelenting workloads: 'Compounding these feelings is the loss of control they [mental health nurses] experience in their work environments' and a 'lack of support and understanding from organisational management' (Currid, 2008, p. 3).

Then there are the practical components that can negatively impact upon our ability to live the healthiest possible life. The range of side effects experienced by mental health nurses who work a rotating roster or shiftwork can be extensive. These may include disturbed sleep patterns, poor diet, limited exercise due to tiredness, and poor exposure to sunlight. Maintaining healthy personal relationships with our family and friends can also prove challenging due to the often antisocial hours we work.

Less obvious and potentially no less damaging are those events or occurrences that trigger our fears and insecurities, causing us to question our reality and potentially leading to a breakdown in our self-confidence, self-esteem and self-worth. These are often subtle in execution and may include manipulative,

GLENN TAYLOR, DANIEL NICHOLLS AND WENDY CROSS

intimidating or bullying behaviours. These behaviours may come from colleagues, employers or those senior to us. This may also emanate from the consumer or others involved in their care.

Blurred and inconsistent nurse–consumer boundaries include the notion of transference (where someone receiving care attaches to their caregiver feelings formerly held towards other significant people) and counter-transference (where a therapist forms an emotional attachment towards a consumer based on a perceived connection to the consumer). Within the therapeutic relationship, self-sacrificing attitudes and unrelenting standards held by the mental health nurse can all present challenges to the health of the individual.

Burnout is a recognised professional risk to mental health nurses. Billeter-Koponen and Freden (2005, p. 21) defines burnout as 'a long-lasting, work related mental condition, which is characterised by exhaustion, dissatisfaction and low capacity'. Continued exposure to these factors will eventually result in a breakdown of the health of the mental health nurse.

CRITICAL THINKING OPPORTUNITY

1   What life experiences do you think could challenge you as a mental health nurse?

2   How will you recognise your positive growth and development as a mental health nurse?

Recognising if your health is being affected

Assessing one's own health can be difficult. This is particularly true when one is in a heightened state of arousal, is experiencing increased levels of distress and anxiety, or is in a state of impaired health. As a proactive measure it is advisable to undergo a health assessment with a trained professional who is equipped with the appropriate skills, such as your GP, a mental health specialist, a counsellor or a specialised industry support service.

Examining alterations in physical, psychological and spiritual health will help to identify health deficits and open discussions for remedial action. Physical alterations might include:

- sleep disturbance
- loss of appetite
- lowered energy levels
- becoming easily fatigued
- fluctuations in weight
- persistent or unexplained somatic complaints.

Psychological alterations can include:

- loss of spark, enthusiasm and zest for life
- atypical fluctuations in mood, including displays of anger and frustration
- preoccupation with work when rostered off
- feeling burdened or overwhelmed by professional responsibilities
- being easily distracted or struggling to concentrate
- experiencing a sense of dread or despair
- feeling a heightened self-criticism and negativity
- feeling disconnected from relationships with others of significance
- practising avoidance strategies such as an increase in substance use.

Spiritual alterations might include:

- questioning one's core values and beliefs
- a loss of interest in regular spiritual processes
- feeling lost or lacking direction
- questioning the purpose or the value of the contribution you make to the world
- experiencing a sense of imbalance with life.

Staying healthy

The World Health Organization (1948, p. 100) defines health as 'a state of dynamic harmony between the body, mind and spirit of a person and the social and cultural influences which make up his or her environment'. It views our health holistically and considers the individual as a multidimensional and complex system. In order to achieve and maintain 'harmony of health' as a mental health nurse, it is important to identify our fundamental values—the things that define who we are and how we live our lives. Harris (2007, p. 198) defines values as 'our heart's deepest desires: how we want to be, what we want to stand for and how we want to relate to the world around us'. Identifying our values and committing to them provides us guidance and a template for life. It provides a road map that helps us better manage life challenges when they present. Such examples of an individual's values include integrity, compassion and honesty.

It may be beneficial for the mental health nurse to undertake the 'Clarifying your values' exercise developed by Tobias Lundgren (see 'Useful websites' at the end of this chapter) or a tool of similar design.

Linked to an individual's values is the sense of purpose or meaning they obtain from their life—their spirituality. Hassed (2008, p. 82) believes 'spirituality relates to how we find meaning and purpose, how we connect with others in society, and how we understand our place on the planet and within the universe'. As mental health nurses it is beneficial to have an insight into our belief system. It is something that will be challenged regularly in our practice. It helps us better understand, empathise and provide support to those we care for. It is the moral and ethical compass we use in our decision-making process as health professionals. Our spiritual health is fundamental in our work, and good spiritual health underpins good mental health.

Striking a spiritual balance starts with understanding self. Personal insights are challenged and processed through supervision. This provides us opportunities to test our belief systems, and question and challenge our behaviours and the way we operate as mental health nurses.

As mental health nurses we are confronted by the illness and suffering experienced by our fellow human beings. This can be challenging and disturbing. It can cause us to be disillusioned and lead us to question whether things are fair and just in the universe. In other words, it may prompt a search for meaning. According to Hassed (2008, p. 83), ways we look for meaning in life include:

- meaningful relationships and how we respect others around us
- making a contribution to the world through our work
- a sense of connectedness and transcending individuality
- experiencing science and nature
- a respect for social justice, morality and rights
- a connection with one's natural environment
- religion.

Good general health

Bunn (2010, pp. 21–2) believes 'health is our natural state' and that 'there is an order and innate harmony underlying everything in nature'. We can maintain good general health and thrive 'if given the right basic ingredients to support the body's natural self-healing mechanisms'.

The basic ingredients to general good health include:

- A balanced diet—consume nourishing whole foods, including fruits, vegetables, nuts, seeds and grains. Plan your meal times and eat larger amounts during the day and less in the evening to reduce stress on the digestive system and aid sleep and regeneration.
- Healthy sleep patterns—reduce physical and mental activity before bed to promote good sleep. Prioritising sleep between shifts and developing healthy patterns of sleep in conjunction with your roster demands will assist energy levels.
- Regular exercise—plan and prioritise physical activity in your week.
- Relaxation—choose an activity that you enjoy and that will complement your lifestyle. Taking planned time away from the workplace is designed to give us the opportunity to unwind and recharge.
- Exposure to sunlight—shift workers are susceptible to vitamin D deficiency. Plan to get outdoors and incorporate regular sun exposure into your routine.
- Keeping hydrated—keep water at hand. Make it easy to access, particularly at work where it can be easy to lose track of time and not prioritise your hydration.
- Getting fresh air—in your break find the time to get outdoors and take in some fresh air. This is particularly relevant to those working in enclosed and air-conditioned environments.
- Scheduled health checks—take responsibility for your own health. Your role as a mental health nurse will challenge your health and like the rest of society you are susceptible to illness. Be proactive and schedule regular appointments with your GP. It is good role modelling for others in your life.

The demands of the mental health nursing role challenge our body's 'natural' harmony; committing to a life that balances our physical, psychological and spiritual needs will better position us to be effective contributors in our professional and personal lives.

ABOUT THE CONSUMER   Ashley's story

Ashley is a 23-year-old mental health nurse. She is half way through her 12-month graduate nurse program in a busy, metropolitan health service. It was not her first-choice employment option. She works full-time and is regularly exhausted when she gets home from work. Ashley excelled at university, but she lacks self-confidence. She has ambitions to work in the community sector in the near future.

She is the eldest of three children and lives at home with her parents and siblings. She has a partner who is 10 years her senior. He has a 5-year-old child from a previous relationship. Ashley's youngest sister has been diagnosed with bulimia nervosa, and her mother relies on Ashley for emotional support. Ashley is very popular in her peer group and has a large circle of friends, but between working, supporting her sister and mother, and spending time with her partner, she finds few opportunities to see them. She also struggles to find the time to go shopping, exercise or just relax with a book. Ashley has expressed an interest in reigniting her passion for cycling, which she has neglected in recent years.

REFLECTION QUESTIONS

1   Do you think Ashley is exercising sufficient self-care?

2   What values and beliefs do you think Ashley would hold as most important?

3   What strategies do you think Ashley could implement to meet her personal needs without neglecting her other responsibilities?

4   What external supports do you think Ashley could use to help her achieve this?

5   What are three outcomes Ashley could expect to achieve from the process?

6   How will Ashley know if she has successfully achieved these?

SECTION 2   CLINICAL SUPERVISION AS SELF-CARE

DANIEL NICHOLLS

> *Yet isn't it clear to everyone that the world is not, and has never been, what it ought to be? And who knows, or has ever known, what this 'ought' should be? The 'ought' is utopian; it has no proper topos or place in the world.*
>
> Hannah Arendt, *The Life of the Mind* (1978, p. 196)

You might be asking the question: what has supervision got to do with self-care? This is an important question—a question we should let stand for a while to see where it will take us (Le Dœuff, 1991; Nicholls, 2007; Nicholls & Mitchell-Dawson, 2002). One way to let a question stand is to constantly engage with it—to speak to it in different ways. We can constantly address a question in the same way that we constantly check ourselves in our motivations and actions. That is the very nature of clinical supervision, after all, to examine ourselves in our clinical interactions.

This section of the chapter is presented as a dialogue between two people. First, it is more interesting to read a discussion rather than a slab of writing that can have the appearance of a monologue. Second, when we examine ourselves we do so in the form of a dialogue: we put a point forward and then challenge it. For example, if you are trying to decide where to go for your next holiday, you may have several possible choices and you gradually rule out all but one by considering the positive and negative aspects of each possibility: cost, distance, theme, etc. It is as if you have an imaginary friend who asks relevant questions concerning your choice.

Finally, the dialogue is an ancient device or method employed to get a point across. Plato used it for the Socratic dialogues of the fourth century BCE (for example, Plato, 1956), Bishop Berkeley used it in the 1700s (Berkeley, 1965) and Martin Heidegger used it in the twentieth century (Heidegger, 1966).

Use of the dialogue would certainly have assisted these writers in presenting their arguments and counter-arguments. However, this did not mean that they were then immediately understood—it takes some work to see what they are up to at each stage of the argument. The dialogue allows or compels this work, which makes it the ideal vehicle for clinical supervision, which is all about being alert to the things we are telling ourselves—our internal dialogue, which includes our thinking and emotions (for insights to emotions in clinical supervision see McLaren, Stenhouse & Ritchie, 2016). You can go more slowly with a dialogue, examining each point as it arises—just like in clinical supervision.

The two characters of this dialogue are Lucy and Ben. Ben is someone who is considering asking Lucy to be his supervisor, but wants to talk to her about it first. We already see here an important element of clinical supervision—the supervisee choosing their own supervisor. Another important element is that we discuss our intention with the potential supervisor. There may be reasons that we cannot have that person as a supervisor. Some of those reasons may emerge in this dialogue.

We will also have a third person contributing to the dialogue. That person is you, the reader. For you are not passive in this reading. You have an opinion and questions that are important for you. Write down your own responses to Ben and Lucy and consider them with regard to your own supervisory relationship.

BOX 7.1   BEN AND LUCY'S DIALOGUE

Ben

I'm wondering about the appropriateness of you being my supervisor. I'm thinking of a couple of things: we work together on the ward and you are not that much more experienced than I am.

Lucy

It's a good question, Ben. But the way I see it there is no problem with us working together. The supervision will be confidential, which means I can't discuss anything we talk about with anyone else. If you ever think that it impacts on our working relationship on the ward, then I think we can contract that you will discuss that with me. As to the question of experience, I don't see supervision being about one person knowing more than another. I see it rather as me being able to reflect back to you the issues you present. That means I need to know how to listen to you. And because we have more or less the same level of experience, that might be a good thing. What do you think?

REFLECTION QUESTIONS

1 If you were Ben, do you think confidentiality would be an issue if Lucy were your supervisor?
2 What do you see as Lucy's potential role?
3 How could Lucy assist Ben with reflection?

Ben

Yes, that sounds reasonable. However, what if I come up with a problem that's bigger than both of us?

Lucy

My answer to that is that clinical supervision, as I see it, is not about problem-solving, but rather about strengthening our ability to problem-solve; both your ability and my ability. That's why I like to see it as a supervisory relationship—we both benefit.

REFLECTION QUESTIONS

1   What do you think Lucy means when she says that clinical supervision is not about problem-solving?
2   How do you think Lucy might benefit from the relationship?

Ben

OK then, so what you are saying is that I must solve my own problems and that clinical supervision will help me to be able to do this. How does this help with my self-care if I am struggling to solve a problem? Won't it mean that I will be left to struggle alone?

Lucy

Well, you won't be alone, will you, when you know I'm listening to you and following on with your reasoning around your problems. I'll be reflecting back to you what you say to me so that you can better hear what you are saying to yourself. And as to the question of being alone, aren't we always alone, in some senses, when we are with a consumer? Of course, the consumer is there, but the she or he doesn't have our perspective on things, no matter how knowledgeable and insightful they might be, just as we don't have the perspective of the consumer.

That is the very nature of the clinical divide, something that might be worth considering at some stage. The other point, of course, is that often there is no other clinician there but ourselves. This makes clinical supervision doubly important because that means I can be a third person for your interaction with the consumer. With practice, you can even imagine what I might say to you while you are there with the consumer—just as I will imagine the consumer and the interaction from what you choose to bring to supervision. An aspect of this is called the parallel process, whereby the way we act together in supervision reflects the way you act with the consumer. It's quite complex and worth thinking about, and also a bit of a paradox: on the one hand we are always alone, on the other hand it is not possible to be alone as an interactive person. [See Crowe and colleagues (2011) for a discussion of parallel process.]

REFLECTION QUESTIONS

1   What do you understand by the term 'parallel process'?
2   How might clinical supervision assit you when you are alone with a consumer?

Ben

How am I going to be able to come to decisions if I am constantly presented with paradoxes? I want results, not unanswerable questions.

Lucy

Surely you don't mean that you want me to answer your questions for you!

REFLECTION QUESTIONS

1   What do you understand by the word 'paradox'?
2   How would you answer Ben's question?

Ben

No. But I'd like to think that there is an answer.

Lucy

Whose answer, Ben? Yours or mine? Now I'm not trying to be cryptic here, but we all know that there may be several possible answers to a question. The real answer, if there is one, will depend on us knowing every possible facet of the situation. That is why I can't make decisions for consumers. I don't live in their skin. I can be there for them, be available and attentive, and provide them information. But I can't make their decisions.

GLENN TAYLOR, DANIEL NICHOLLS AND WENDY CROSS

REFLECTION QUESTIONS

1 Is it possible to know everything about a situation?
2 What do you think Ben needs from Lucy right now?

Ben

So what you're saying is that clinical supervision reflects or parallels the process whereby I try to assist consumers with getting on with their lives—being with them as they make mistakes and learn from them. Fair enough! However,

I can't afford to make a mistake as it may have a disastrous impact on the consumer's life and well-being.

Lucy

Does that mean you never make a clinical error?

REFLECTION QUESTIONS

1 Is it reasonable to expect that we never make clinical errors?
2 What do you think should we do if we make a clinical error?

Ben

Yes, I guess I do make errors. And I guess you're going to tell me that while the error might be grave, it will be graver still if I don't stop to reflect on it and learn from it—for I might continue to make the same error. I guess you're also going to tell me that I need to reflect also on what I see to be the positive aspects of an interaction, both in order to see clearly what I do well but also

to be fairly certain that I haven't made an error (even though I think I haven't).

Lucy

Well, Ben, I can see you are your own best critic. That means you won't see clinical supervision as positive or negative criticism. It's rather a constant re-evaluation. And not by me, but by you yourself.

REFLECTION QUESTIONS

1 How has Ben achieved greater understanding?
2 How is re-evaluation different from criticism?

Ben

I see. I have come to the position where I can now have an answer, of sorts, about the self-care aspect of clinical supervision. Reflecting on myself, in my interactions, means taking responsibility for myself; being accountable. This means I will become more confident

and competent. I will have a more complete professional persona.

Lucy

Yes. It might also mean that you and I will become more assertive in our interdisciplinary interactions as we will have pretty thoroughly examined our own interactive processes.

REFLECTION QUESTIONS

1 Do you agree that clinical supervision can increase assertiveness?
2 What do you think are the key components of assertiveness?

Ben

Thank you, Lucy, for helping me get to this point. I don't feel at all that you are placing yourself in a position of power over me. You are someone who will be there with me in my own reflections on practice.

Lucy

Thank you, Ben, for doing me the honour of trusting me with your thoughts and feelings. You have given me a lot to think about; for example, around the question of paradoxes. Here's another, then: in giving me something to think about, have you become my supervisor? Naturally, neither of us has to answer this—I merely flag it for further reflection.

1 Who do you think is the 'actual' supervisor here?

2 Do we still need clinical supervision when we become proficient at reflecting on our practice?

3 Who do you think has power in a supervisory relationship?

4 Do you think there is an emotional element to clinical supervision? See if you can find instances of this in the interaction between Lucy and Ben.

SECTION 3 SELF-CARE THROUGH PRACTICE DEVELOPMENT

WENDY CROSS

Defining practice development is not easy as there a a number of diverse thoughts on the subject (Sanders, Odell & Webster, 2013). However, this definition by Manley, McCormack and Wilson (2008, p. 9) sums it up and includes the main dimensions:

> [Practice development is] a continuous process of developing person-centred cultures. It is enabled by facilitators who authentically engage with individuals and teams to blend personal qualities and creative imagination with practice skills and practice wisdom. The learning that occurs brings about transformations of individual and team practices. This is sustained by embedding both processes and outcomes in corporate strategy.

The key terms in this definition are 'person-centredness', 'facilitation', 'authentic engagement' and 'learning'.

Person-centredness

According to McCance, McCormack and Dewing (2011) the term 'person-centredness' is becoming more familiar within health and social care across the world to describe standards of care that ensure that the consumer is the focus of care delivery. Person-centredness has its roots in the work of Carl Rogers and John Heron (McCance, McCormack & Dewing, 2011).

McCormack, McCance and Maben (2013, p. 193) suggest five key principles that need to be in place for a health service to be considered person-centred:

1 the meeting of needs through caring processes
2 the existence of nurturing relationships
3 the promotion of social belonging
4 the creation of meaningful spaces and places
5 the promotion of human flourishing.

Person-centredness relates to the status that is given to others in the context of their relationship and social being. It inherently reflects recognition, respect and trust. McCormack (2004) states that person-centredness focuses on four ways of being: being in relation, being in a social world, being in place and being with self. These ways of being mean that people exist in relation to each other: they are social, they are contextualised and they develop a sense of self through the recognition, respect and trust of others. It is the concept of being with self that we address in this chapter.

Manley (2004) states that self-knowledge is essential for the enabling of others towards empowerment, and the intentional use of self is crucial for the critical companion. Two main attributes are knowing our own beliefs and values, and being authentic (Shaw et al., 2008). When we recognise our own attitudes, ways of thinking and principles, we are able to comprehend how they relate to our decisions and behaviours. We can then develop the ability to analyse these decisions and behaviours with a view to modifying them to suit the context and the particular situations in which they occur. Nurses who are self-aware are in a better position to use self with the intention of facilitating change in others.

Being authentic involves consistency, integrity and transparency. In their literature review about the characteristics, qualities and skills of practice developers, McCormack and Garbutt (2003b) note that practice developers embody a range of authentic attributes and that these attributes cluster around support and mentoring, empathy, the innate valuing of others and transformational leading. All practice development work involves facilitation of some sort.

Facilitation

A technique by which one person makes things easier for others.

Kitson, Harvey and McCormack (1998, p. 152)

Facilitation includes a broad assortment of functions from providing help to achieve specific tasks to using techniques that encourage individuals and teams to review their attitudes, habits, skills and ways of thinking and working (Larsen et al., 2005). Kitson and colleagues (1998) proposed that facilitators have key roles in helping individuals and teams to change in terms of understanding why and how. Facilitators use a range of interpersonal skills and attributes to effect change. The terms 'change agent' and 'change management' are linked to facilitation, which is derived from counselling, student-centred learning and humanistic psychology. Facilitation refers to the processes of enabling individuals and groups to understand the processes they must go through to effect change in themselves, their work or others. The focus is on experiential learning through critical reflection, challenging cultures and customs, and coping with psychological barriers.

Facilitation has been linked with:

- problem-based learning (Barrows & Tamblyn, 1980)
- active learning (Dewing, 2010)
- quality management, prevention and audits (Loftus-Hill & Harvey, 2000)
- reflective practice and clinical supervision (Mills, Francis & Bonner, 2005)
- practice development and action research (McCormack & Garbutt, 2003a)
- critical companionship (Titchen, 2003)
- evidence translation (Crisp & Wilson, 2011).

Most descriptions of facilitation include 'amalgam' models, where there is a balance between goal attainment and the development of individuals and group processes: 'Overall … the purpose of facilitation can vary from providing help and support to achieve a specific goal to enabling individuals and teams to analyze, reflect and change their own attitudes, behaviour and ways of working' (Harvey et al., 2002, p. 580).

The role of the facilitator

According to Harvey and colleagues (2002) in their concept analysis, there are many interpretations of the facilitation role. They state that facilitation can focus on the 'practical hands on' approach or more sophisticated and complicated roles. They divide these roles into two broad groups: doing for others and enabling others (see Table 7.1). Most roles, however, contain elements of both.

TABLE 7.1 FACILITATION ROLES

Facilitation roles	
Doing for others	**Enabling others**
Practical-task driven, with a focus on administration, support and undertaking specific tasks: ■ episodic contact ■ practical and technical help ■ didactic teaching ■ external agent ■ low intensity with wide coverage.	Developing others, exploring and releasing the potential of others: ■ sustained partnership ■ developmental ■ adult leaning ■ internal or external agent ■ high intensity with narrow coverage.

Heron's (1989) model of facilitation reflects both dimensions. Heron addresses issues of emotion, resistance and meaning, as well as facilitation's role in managing the completion of the task. Heron notes that facilitators act in different ways at different times depending on the individual's or group's need at the time and the stage of development. So a facilitator may be directive or non-directive as the situation demands. This, of course, implies purpose: facilitation is purposeful.

Heron studied interventions utilised during counselling (though they are useful for clinical supervision as well), advising the use of a taxonomy for the analysis and categorisation of such interventions. He suggested six primary categories—prescriptive, informative, confrontative, cathartic, catalytic and supportive—and proposed that all interventions could be subsumed under one of the categories. He further sorted the six styles into two basic categories: authoritative and facilitative (see Table 7.2).

TABLE 7.2 INTERVENTIONS

Authoritative interventions	**Facilitative interventions**
Prescriptive: the facilitator explicitly gives direction by giving advice or direction.	**Cathartic:** the facilitator attempts to help the individual move on through the expression of thoughts or emotions previously unacknowledged or unexpressed.
Informative: the facilitator intends to provide information or instruction.	**Catalytic:** interventions are focused on helping the individual become increasingly self-directed and reflective. They aim to raise the developmental level of the individual as a professional.
Confrontative: the facilitator challenges beliefs or behaviours. Such confrontation does not imply aggression, but rather invites consideration of some aspect of individual's work or themselves that was perhaps previously taken for granted.	**Supportive:** the facilitator attempts to reinforce confidence through focusing on areas of competence, and attending to what individuals do well.

Critical companionship

> Critical companionship is a helping relationship, in which an experienced facilitator accompanies another on an experiential learning journey, using methods of 'high challenge' and 'high support' in a trusting relationship. It is a metaphor and framework for learning.
>
> Titchen (2003, p. 33)

The overall purpose of critical companionship is to enable others to practise in ways that are person-centred and evidence-based. This can be employed on a one-to-one basis or within a number of learning contexts. It is anticipated that critical companionship will support and develop high-level critical reflection and metacognitive skills, and would enable individuals to interrogate their own practice and continually develop their learning.

Critical companionship has been informed by the theoretical perspectives of Mezirow (1990), Rogers (1983) and Schön (1987), and combines critical social science, humanism, phenomenology, spirituality and reflective practice. It is an example of holistic facilitation (Harvey et al., 2002).

Features of the critical companionship relationship

According to Titchen (2003), critical companionship occurs across a number of domains within a framework. The domains interconnect and overlap, and reflect different kinds of knowledge. The domains include relationship, rationality–intuitive and facilitation, and are examined in detail below. Titchen's model is reproduced in Figure 7.1.

Relationship domain

- Particularity—knowing practitioners or learners as unique beings in the context of specific situations through listening to their stories and self-reflections and attending to cues.
- Reciprocity—the exchange of knowledge, thoughts, ideas and actions; and acknowledgment of the gifts of care, concern, satisfaction and wisdom.
- Mutuality—working in partnership and equality; sharing responsibility for the relationship.
- Graceful care—being with the practitioner through presence, touch and body language. This involves genuineness, generosity (with self, knowledge and time), kind intention, undivided attention, reassurance in times of stress and disappointment, appropriate balance, self-management, the use of humour and valuing the practitioner in their uniqueness.

Rationality–intuitive domain

- Saliency—knowing what is important (from both perspectives) and attending to it.
- Temporality—relates to time (past, present and future), timing (making focused time and acting at the right time) and pacing oneself (regulation of interaction).
- Intentionality—acting deliberately, consciously and thoughtfully, using all the strategies.

Facilitation domain

- Consciousness-raising—bringing to consciousness actions, thoughts and behaviours for greater understanding.
- Problematisation—raising awareness of issues that might not be perceived as problems or helping to find the solution to problems posed by the practitioner.

Figure 7.1 Critical companionship framework

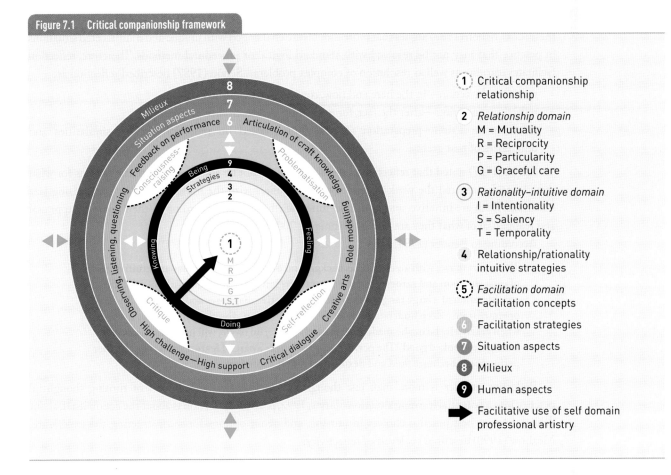

1 Critical companionship relationship

2 *Relationship domain*
M = Mutuality
R = Reciprocity
P = Particularity
G = Graceful care

3 *Rationality–intuitive domain*
I = Intentionality
S = Saliency
T = Temporality

4 Relationship/rationality intuitive strategies

5 *Facilitation domain*
Facilitation concepts

6 Facilitation strategies

7 Situation aspects

8 Milieux

9 Human aspects

➤ Facilitative use of self domain professional artistry

- Self-reflection—reflecting on and evaluating experiences, actions, behaviours, thoughts and feelings, with a focus on those that are inhibiting growth.
- Critique—collaborative critical reflection of the event and the context it occurred in, through articulating craft knowledge, active attending, feedback, high challenge and high support, critical dialogue and role modelling using creativity (Titchen, 2003).

The place of reflection in caring for self

> [Reflection is a] window through which the practitioner can view and focus self within the context of her own lived experience in ways that enable her to confront, understand and work towards resolving the contradictions within her practice between what is desirable and actual practice.
>
> Johns (2000, p. 34)

Dewey (1933) introduced the notion of reflection in relation to critical thinking, whereby a person may give solemn contemplation to a certain issue. It involves rational and intellectual thinking that is holistic and includes emotions. A reflective person is unprejudiced, unconditional and accountable. Furthering these ideas, Schön (1987) argues that professionals are challenged with unique and multifaceted situations in practice that may not be resolved with standard logical or procedural methods. Therefore, reflection facilitates learning as well as resolution of complex problems. Schön (1987) described reflection as:

- reflection-in-action—in the here and now, conscious, spontaneous
- reflection-on-action—after the fact, for evaluating the experience or event
- reflection-for-action—preparation for the future, based on reflection on the similarities and differences of past events.

Schön (1987) noted that reflective professionals might not be able to articulate the reasons for what they do, and compared the work of reflective practitioners with the music created by improvising jazz musicians. Both are intuitive, and both fine-tune their behaviours according to their constant appraisal and reappraisal of what they are doing (Hannigan, 2001).

According to Benner (1984, p. 34):

> The expert nurse, with an enormous background of experience, now has an intuitive grasp of each situation and zeroes in on the accurate region of the problem without wasteful consideration of a large range of unfruitful, alternative diagnoses and solutions. The expert operates from a deep understanding of the total situation. The chess master, for instance, when asked why he or she made a particularly masterful move, will just say: 'Because it felt right; it looked good.' The performer is no longer aware of features and rules; his/her performance becomes fluid and flexible and highly proficient.

Reflective practice is more than just thoughtful practice; it is the process of turning thoughtful practice into a potential learning situation (Jarvis, 1992, p. 180). Reflection is about the action itself, about deliberation on best practice choices in nursing, and about options for reconstructing the experience. Mezirow (1990) describes six levels of reflectivity:

1 reflectivity—being generally aware of self and others
2 affective reflectivity—awareness of feelings
3 discriminant reflectivity—awareness of how we make decisions and their impact
4 judgmental reflectivity—awareness of values and assumptions
5 conceptual reflectivity—awareness of the concepts underpinning our decisions and the critical analysis of the need for further learning
6 theoretical reflectivity—understanding self in context and the ability to alter assumptions based on new knowledge.

Reflection enables us to use our knowledge, skills and attitudes to gain a deeper understanding of self, and how that affects the ways in which we work as nurses and the impact the nursing work has on our own well-being. Reflection and self-awareness are essential for self-care.

BOX 7.2 THE TEN CS OF REFLECTION

1 Commitment—self and nursing matter, being responsible for self, and being open, curious and willing to change customary ways of responding.

2 Contradiction—exposing the contradictions between real and ideal aspects of practice.

3 Conflict—using the power within inconsistencies of practice to take action.

4 Challenge and support—non-threatening confrontation of attitudes, beliefs and behaviour.

5 Catharsis—dealing with and letting go of unhelpful feelings.

6 Creation—seeing new ways of regarding and responding to practice.

7 Connection—applying new understandings to the real world of practice.

8 Caring—taking advantageous practices into everyday living.

9 Congruence—reflection and acting in concert.

10 Constructing personal knowledge in practice—joining personal knowledge with other ways of knowing to create practice knowledge.

Johns (2000)

Reflective techniques and triggers

There are several techniques that can be used to facilitate reflection. It can be structured or freeflowing, or in combinations that meet your individual needs. Self-reflection is undertaken alone, and can be facilitated through the use of a diary. Situations can be viewed in person-centred ways using a reflective framework. Some triggers you might use appear below. Eventually they will become inherent in the way you think about all situations, whether at work or elsewhere.

- What happened in that situation?
- Who was involved?
- How did the person behave? How did I behave?
- What was the impact of everyone's behaviour?
- How do I feel about this person?
- What assumptions have I made regarding this person and/or their care?
- What are their beliefs about the situation?
- What can I do to help this person?
- How can I work with this person?
- What would I do differently?
- What can I change?

In a facilitated discussion, a more structured approach is taken. Manley and McCormack (2003) suggest the following triggers to aid reflection:

- Describe the situation.
- What are the essential contributing factors?
- What were you trying to achieve?
- What are the consequences of your actions? For you? For others?
- What were you feeling?
- What were others feeling? How do you know this?
- What influenced your actions? (Knowledge? Assumptions?)
- Were there other choices available?
- If another choice were made, what would be the consequences? How do you know this?
- Could you have dealt better with this situation?
- How are you feeling now?
- What have you learnt from the experience?

Johns (2000) states that structured reflection focuses on looking in at oneself and looking out at the situation itself. Reflection should focus on your own significant thoughts and emotions and at the same time explore the experience, with particular attention to significant factors; critical understanding; values, assumptions and ethics; and empirics and the relationship of this experience with your learning from previous experiences. You should come away with a sense of deeper understanding of self and new ways of practising. Whatever you decide fits best with your philosophical outlook, the importance of learning about self underpins self-care and the idea that self-awareness can be achieved through clinical supervision, critical companionship and structured facilitation.

CRITICAL THINKING OPPORTUNITY

1 How would you rate your level of person-centredness?

2 How do you demonstrate your authenticity?

3 What do you need to do to develop your facilitation skills?

4 Do you have a critical companion? What will you do to obtain one?

5 Contemplate reflecting about yourself. Identify three important aspects for your development.

SUMMARY

To care for ourselves we must address the concept on many levels: physical, personal, professional, psychological and practical. As mental health nurses, we need to be able to recognise when our health is being challenged and adopt a range of strategies to look after ourselves, in order to provide the possible care for consumers. Open reflective dialogue within clinical supervision is critical, as are the thoughtful consideration of person-centredness, facilitation, critical companionship and reflection. We hope that the essential ingredients of self-care will be incorporated into your life forever.

DISCUSSION QUESTIONS

1 What do you think a good anti-stress plan for a mental health nurse should include?

2 Consider substance misuse in nursing. What are the key considerations?

3 Discuss with another student how you think clinical supervision could be significant in your future nursing activities.

4 Discuss the concepts of person-centredness, facilitation, authentic engagement and learning. How can each of these concepts contribute to your self-awareness and practice development?

TEST YOURSELF

1   The role of the mental health nurse is:

   a   To show empathy without emotional attachment

   b   Withhold judgement of the consumer throughout the relationship

   c   Remain in control and focused

   d   Caring for and nurturing the consumer through their illness experience

   e   A and C

   f   All of the above

2   Ways we as individuals look for meaning in life include the following except:

   a   Making meaningful relationships and respecting others around us

   b   Having a sense of connectedness and transcending individuality

   c   Having respect for social justice, morality and rights

   d   Not needing to appreciate one's natural environment

3   Which of the following are needed for a health care service to be considered person-centred:

   a   The meeting of needs through caring processes

   b   The existence of nursing relationships

   c   The promotion of social belonging

   d   The promotion of human flourishing

   e   None of the above

   f   All of the above

4   Which of the following statements is incorrect in relation to reflective practice:

   a   Reflectivity is being generally aware of self and others

   b   Affective reflectivity is being aware of feelings of self and others

   c   Judgemental reflectivity is being aware of values and assumptions

   d   Conceptual reflectivity is understanding self and the ability to alter assumptions based on new knowledge

USEFUL WEBSITES

Australian Clinical Supervision Association: http://clinicalsupervision.org.au

Clarifying your values: http://thehappinesstrap.com/wp-content/uploads/2017/06/ACT_Made_Simple_-_Client_Handouts_and_Worksheets.pdf

REFERENCES

Arendt, H. (1978). *The life of the mind.* New York: Harcourt Brace Jovanovich.

Barrows, H. S., & Tamblyn, R. M. (1980). *Problem-based learning: An approach to medical education.* New York: Springer.

Benner, P. (1984). *From novice to expert: Excellence and power in clinical nursing practice.* Reading: Addison-Wesley.

Berkeley, G. (1965). Three dialogues between Hylas and Philonous. In D. Armstrong (Ed.), *Berkeley's philosophical writings.* New York: Macmillan.

Billeter-Koponen, S., & Freden, L. (2005). Long-term stress, burnout and patient-nurse relations: Qualitative interview study about nurses' experiences. *Nordic College of Caring Sciences, 19,* 20–27.

Bunn, M. (2010). *Ancient wisdom for modern health: Rediscover the simple, timeless secrets of health and happiness.* NSW: Enlightened Health Publishing.

Crisp, J., & Wilson, V. (2011). How do facilitators of practice development gain the expertise required to support vital transformation of practice and workplace cultures? *Nurse Education in Practice,* *11*(3), 173–178.

Crowe, T. P., Oades, L. G., Deane, F. P., Ciarrochi, J., & Williams, V. C. (2011). Parallel process in clinical supervision: Implications for coaching mental health practitioners. *International Journal of Evidence Based Coaching and Mentoring,* *9*(2), 56–66.

Currid, T. (2008). Experience of stress in acute mental health nurses. *Nursing Times,* *104*(2), 39–40.

Dewey, J. (1933). *How we think.* Boston: Heath.

Dewing, J. (2010). Moments in movement. *Nurse Education in Practice,* *10*(1), 22–26.

Hannigan, B. (2001). A discussion of the strengths and weaknesses of 'reflection' in nursing. *Journal of Clinical Nursing,* *10*(2), 278–283.

Harris, R. (2007). *The happiness trap: Stop struggling, start living.* Wollombi: Exisle Publishing.

Harvey, G., Loftus-Hills, A., Rycroft-Malone, J., Titchen, A., Kitson, A., McCormack, B., & Seers, K. (2002). Getting evidence into practice: The role of facilitation. *Journal of Advanced Nursing,* *37*(6), 577–588.

Hassed, C. (2008). *The essence of health: The seven pillars of wellbeing.* North Sydney: Ebury Press.

Heidegger, M. (1966). Conversation on a country path about thinking. In M. Heidegger, *Discourse on thinking* (J. M. Anderson & E. H. Freund, Trans.). New York: Harper and Row.

Heron, J. (1989). *The facilitator's handbook.* London: Kogan Page.

Jarvis, P. (1992). Reflective practice in nursing. *Nurse Education Today,* *12*(3), 174–181.

Johns, C. (2000). Working with Alice: A reflection. *Complementary Therapies in Nursing and Midwifery,* *6*(4), 199–203.

Kitson, A., Harvey, G., & McCormack, B. (1998). Enabling the implementation of evidence-based practice: A conceptual framework. *Quality in Health Care,* *7*(3), 149–158.

Larsen, J., Maundrill, R., Malone, J., & Mouland, L. (2005). Practice development facilitation: An integrated strategic and clinical

approach. *Practice Development in Healthcare,* *4*(3), 142–149.

Le Dœuff, M. (1991). *Hipparchia's choice: An essay concerning women, philosophy, etc.* Oxford: Blackwell.

Loftus-Hill, A., & Harvey, G. (2000). *A review of the role of facilitators in changing professional health care practice.* Oxford: RCN Institute.

Manley, K. (2004). Transformational culture: A culture of effectiveness. In B. McCormack, K. Manley & R. Garbutt (Eds.), *Practice development in nursing* (pp. 33–50). Oxford: Blackwell.

Manley, K., & McCormack, B. (2008). Practice development: Purpose, methodology, facilitation and evaluation. *Nursing in Critical Care,* *8*(1), 22–29.

Manley, K., McCormack, B., & Wilson, V. (2008). *International practice development in nursing and healthcare.* Chichester: Wiley-Blackwell.

McCance, T., McCormack, B., & Dewing, J. (2011). An exploration of person-centredness in practice. *Online Journal of Issues in Nursing,* *16*(2), 1.

McCormack, B. (2004). Person-centredness in gerontological nursing: An overview of the literature. *International Journal of Older People Nursing,* *13*(3a), 31–38.

McCormack, B., & Garbutt, R. (2003a). *A concept analysis of practice development.* Oxford: RCN Institute.

McCormack, B., & Garbutt, R. (2003b). The characteristics, qualities and skills of practice developers. *Journal of Clinical Nursing,* *12*(3), 317–325.

McCormack, B., McCance T., & Maben, J. (2013). Outcome evaluation in the development of person-centred practice. In McCormack, B., Manley K., & Titchen A. (Eds.), *Practice development in nursing and healthcare* (2nd ed.). Chichester: Wiley-Blackwell.

McLaren, Stenhouse & Ritchie, (2016). *Mental health nurses' experiences of managing work-related emotions through supervision.* Journal of Advanced Nursing, 72(10), 2423–2434. DOI: 10.1111/jan.12995.

Mezirow, J. (1990). A critical theory of adult learning and education. *Adult Education,* *32*(1), 3–24.

Mills, J., Francis, K., & Bonner, A. (2005). Mentoring, clinical supervision and preceptoring: Clarifying the conceptual definitions for Australian rural nurses. A rev of the literature. *Rural and Remote Health,* *5*(3), 410.

Nicholls, D. (2007). Essential skills for a succes supervisory partnership to flourish. In J. Dri (Ed.), *Practising clinical supervision for health professionals: A reflective approach* (2nd ed.). London: Baillière Tindall and Royal Colleg Nursing.

Nicholls, D., & Mitchell-Dawson, B. (2002). Promoting mental health in nurses through clinical supervision. In L. Morrow, I. Verins E. Willis (Eds.), *Mental health and work: Iss and perspectives.* Adelaide: Commonwealth o Australia.

Plato (1956). *Protagoras and meno* (W. K. C. Guthrie, Trans.). London: Penguin.

Rogers, C. (1983). *Freedom to learn for the 80s.* London: Charles E Merrill.

Sanders, K., Odell, J., & Webster, J. (2013). Lea to be a practice developer. In B. McCormack K. Manley & A. Titchen (Eds.), *Practice development in nursing and healthcare* (2nd E Chichester: Wiley-Blackwell.

Schön, D. A. (1987). *The reflective practitioner: I professionals think in action.* Aldershot: Avebu

Shaw, T., Dewing, J., Young, R., Devlin, M., Boomer, C., & Legius, M. (2008). Enabling practice development: Delving into the conc of facilitation from a practitioner perspective K. Manley, B. McCormack & V. Wilson (E *International practice development in nursing a healthcare.* Chichester: Wiley-Blackwell.

Titchen, A. (2003). Critical companionship: Pa *Nursing Standard,* *18*(9), 33–40.

World Health Organization (1948). Preamble t Constitution. *Official Records of the World Hea Organization,* *2*. Geneva: WHO. Test yourse

CHAPTER 8

Law and Ethics

SCOTT TRUEMAN

Acknowledgment

The author would like to acknowledge the contribution of Beth Bennett and Anna Bennett who wrote this chapter in the second edition.

LEARNING OBJECTIVES

AFTER READING THIS CHAPTER, YOU SHOULD BE ABLE TO:

- identify what ethics is, and what it is not
- recognise key areas in mental health practice requiring ethical and legal analysis
- demonstrate an understanding of the legal context in which all mental health practice occurs
- discuss key components of mental health and guardianship legislation in your jurisdiction and recognise how these apply to your practice
- apply ethical reasoning to decision making in mental health practice.

KEY TERMS

- autonomy
- beneficence
- capacity
- consent
- deontology
- duty of care
- justice
- negligence
- non-maleficence
- teleology
- utilitarianism
- virtue ethics

Introduction

This chapter discusses the practice of mental health nursing both ethically and legally and as required professionally by the national registration authority (Australian Health Practitioner Regulation Agency; AHPRA). The regulative framework for mental health nurses is complex and extensive.

The first section of this chapter discusses ethical theories, principles and values and how they relate to mental health nursing. It is very important to understand that ethics is not the law and the law is not ethics. They are distinct but related. The second section of the chapter covers the interface of the law and professional regulation of mental health nursing. The last section canvasses some specific mental health nursing issues (such as privacy, confidentiality and professional boundaries), and discusses them with reference to the law and ethics.

What ethics is, and what it is not

A definitive definition of what is ethics is illusive. Ethics is the branch of study dealing with what is the proper course of human action. It answers the question, 'What do I do that is just and right?' by studying what is right and wrong in human endeavours. At a more fundamental level, it is the method by which we categorise our values and pursue them.

What ethics is *not*:

- the law—law and ethics intertwine, they are distinctly different; the law is a system of rules that a society or community recognises as regulating the actions of its members
- acting in accordance with one's feelings
- acting pursuant to religious beliefs
- doing 'whatever society accepts' or acting in accordance with public opinion
- complying with a health services or institutional policies or procedures
- acting pursuant to an ideology—it is not a means to advocate or justify strong personal views or beliefs without credible evidence (Johnstone, 2013).

Ethical frameworks and principles

A variety of ethical theories and principles exist. Those that relate to health care are discussed in this section and have been identified by Beauchamp and Childress (2013).

Deontology (or intrinsiticalist theories)

The word deontology derives from the Greek words for duty (*deon*) and science (or study) of (*logos*). The theory of deontology asserts that persons are morally obliged (have a duty) to act in accordance with universal principles and rules that are intrinsically right and must be always followed. It was formulated by Immanuel Kant (1724–1804) on the basis that humans (unlike other animals) have a capacity for reason. This makes them moral free agents to act in accordance with, and for the sake of, a moral law or duty—not influenced by the willing of an outcome or result. Hence, if telling the truth is inherently 'good' (as opposed to lying), then telling the truth must universally be adhered to, despite the circumstances. Therefore, the nurse tells the truth even if it offends or enrages the consumer.

Criticisms of deontology are first that deontological moral systems provide no clear way to resolve conflicts between competing moral duties. A second criticism is that deontological theories do not readily allow for 'grey' areas where the morality of an action is questionable. Rather, they are systems that are based upon absolutes—absolute principles and absolute conclusions. In reality, moral questions often involve 'grey areas' rather than absolute 'black and white' choices. Third is the question of just which duties qualify as those that we should all follow, regardless of the consequences. Duties that might have been valid in the eighteenth century are not necessarily valid now; for example, deinstitutionalisation versus the use of asylums.

Teleology

The word teleology derives from the Greek *telos*, meaning 'end' and *logos* meaning 'reasoned discourse'. Some writers also refer to it as consequentalism (results-based ethics). It is a general term denoting theories concerned with evaluating the 'value' of determining the consequential outcome of one's actions. The right act(ion) is one that results in or produces (maximises) the greatest degree or level of happiness and 'good'. It therefore rejects the assertions made by deontological ethics. A utilitarian examines and weighs up the beneficial and harmful outcomes of alternative actions, and decides upon the action with the greatest benefit (utlitity) and least harm as being the right action (Bentham, 1962/1789; Mill, 1962/1861).

While there exist a number of criticisms of consequentialism, the two major criticisms are:

- *Impracticability*—one cannot calculate in advance all the effects, on all of those affected.
- *Insufficiency (of scope)*—how do you measure the universal basis of what is a good or harmful result for everyone in every situation?

There is a proposal for a trial of a new drug to treat psychosis.

1 How would a utilitarian decide whether the trial should go ahead?

2 How would a deontologist decide whether the trial should proceed?

Virtue ethics

Although virtue ethics is an ancient theory associated with the Greek philosopher Aristotle (384–322 BCE), it continues to be examined as a theory for professional practice (Begley, 2005; Crowden, 2004; Oakley & Hocking, 2001) and nursing practice (Armstrong, 2006; Hodkinson, 2008; Newham, 2015), including mental health nursing (Lutzen & da Silva, 1996; Mckie & Swinton, 2001). It identifies and emphasises the virtues, or moral character, of the person (nurse) in contrast to deontology that emphasises duties or rules, or teleology that emphasises the consequences of actions. Of all the virtuous traits a nurse can possess, Beauchamp and Childress (2013) identify five 'focal' virtues when providing health care:

- *compassion*—having active regard for a consumer's well-being while being emotionally responsive; for example, sympathy and tenderness (Blum, 1980)
- *discernment*—being insightful, understanding and astute in judgment
- *trustworthiness*—having 'a confident belief in and reliance on the moral character and competence of another person' (Beauchamp & Childress, 2013, p. 39)
- *integrity*—having honesty, uprightness, probity, rectitude and honour as part of a strong personal moral character
- *conscientiousness*—when a nurse 'is motivated to do what is right because it is [the] right' course of action (Beauchamp & Childress, 2013, p. 42).

See also the seven virtuous traits identified by Pellegrino (1995) to be a 'good' clinician (pp. 268–270).

Being a virtuous nurse is not enough in and of itself; it also requires practical wisdom in its execution. Knowing when and how to be virtuous in the circumstances is fundamental. A nurse needs practice and experience to gain wisdom of how to act virtuously.

1 What moral virtues or character traits should a mental health nurse posses?

2 Are those moral virtues or character traits different from non-mental health nurses? If so what are these differences and why do they occur?

3 If not moral virtues, what do you think makes people act ethically?

Ethical principles

Ethical principlism is the delivery of health care based on sound moral principles. The moral principles are mutually recognised as providing correct moral reasons for taking moral actions (Johnstone, 2016). Benjamin (2001) and Little (2001) assert that ethical principlism for ethical decision making and problem solving within health care is becoming more acceptable. With reference to Beauchamp and Childress (2013), this chapter identifies four principles—autonomy, beneficence, non-maleficence and justice—derived from common morality, or 'the set of norms shared by all persons committed to morality' (Beauchamp & Childress, 2013, p. 3).

Autonomy

The word *autonomy* derives from the Greek *autos-nomos* meaning 'self-rule' or 'self-determination'. Accordingly, an autonomous decision is described as one that is made freely and without undue influence, by a competent person (consumer), in full knowledge and understanding of the relevant information necessary to make such a decision. For John Stuart Mill (1962), the concept of respect for autonomy involves the capacity to think, decide and act on the basis of such thought and decision freely and independently. Mill advocated for the principle of autonomy ('the principle of liberty') provided it did not cause harm to others.

Upholding and respecting the principle of autonomy presents certain challenges for mental health nurses and consumers. Autonomy encompasses a level of cognitive ability or functioning to understand, choose and make judgments. In some circumstances the consumer may be ill to a degree that they are unable to judge. In these circumstances the consumer has lost the 'capacity' to make decisions in their best interests and well-being. Accordingly, there exists legislative authorisation for compulsory treatment and care, even in the absence of consent (Arya, 2012; Callaghan & Ryan, 2012).

A recent development in relation to autonomy is the preparation of psychiatric advance directives (PADs) by competent consumers for use should they lose decision-making capacity during acute episodes of mental illness (Nicaise, Lorant & Dubois 2013; Swanson et al., 2008; Weller, 2008, 2012; Wilder et al., 2010). The PAD may address areas such as:

- appointment of an agent to represent the appointee's interests (Srebnik, 2005)
- instructions about treatment, including medications, restraint and seclusion
- who should be notified in the event of admission to hospital
- who may visit the person while in hospital.

PADs are recognised in New Zealand (Health Services Commissioner, 2009) and explicitly in some states of Australia; for example, *Mental Health Act 2015* (ACT), ss 24–32 and *Mental Health Act 2014* (Vic), ss 19–22). Other states and territories rely on other Acts—for example, *Advanced Personal Planning Act 2013* (NT), *Powers of Attorney Act 1998* (Qld) and *Guardianship and Administration Act 1990* (WA)—while others are silent (NSW, South Australia and Tasmania). PADs, where legally recognised, are one way that the law protects and upholds a consumer's autonomy (Nicaise, Lorant & Dubois, 2013; Berghmans & van der Zanden, 2012). When nurses override a consumer's autonomy and act paternalistically, it is typically justified using arguments about the consumer's best interests, based on the principles of beneficence and non-maleficence. In jurisdictions where PADs are legislatively recognised, they may still be overridden if their contents are inconsistent with what is in the consumer's best interests.

Beneficence

Beneficence originates from the Latin word *benefactum*, meaning 'good deed'. The principle of beneficence prescribes 'above all, do good'. It therefore places on a nurse a positive obligation to act for the benefit of others (consumers) (Beauchamp & Childress, 2013). It is important to note that the principle does not involve a secondary type of beneficence, namely 'ideal beneficence', which comprises extreme acts of generosity or attempts to benefit others on all possible occasions (Johnstone, 2016). Acts of beneficence made by nurses towards or for consumers include compassion, empathy, kindness, sympathy, mercy, friendship and altruism. Examples of beneficence are nurses advocating on behalf of consumers, counselling a non-compliant consumer to take their medications and arranging accommodation for a homeless consumer.

Non-maleficence

Non-maleficence is based on the Latin maxim *primum non nocere* or 'First, do no harm'. It is a positive obligation on nurses to avoid the infliction of harm on consumers. (Beauchamp & Childress, 2013). Harm is the 'invasion, violation, thwarting, or the "setting back" of a person's significant interests' (Johnstone, 2016, p. 38) to the detriment of their welfare (Beauchamp & Childress, 2013; Feinberg, 1984).

As a generality, obligations of non-maleficence are given paramountcy over those of beneficence, particularly when beneficent acts are not morally justifiable (Beauchamp & Childress, 2013). This is not always true though. To cause momentary pain by giving an antipsychotic injection has paramouncy over not causing the pain, whereby the consumer becomes floridly psychotic and involuntarily hospitalised.

However, depending on the values a person [nurse] holds, 'what constitutes benefit for one person, may be harm for another' (Gillon, 1995, p. 25). This invokes the notion of moral relativism: that moral judgments are true or false only relative to some particular standpoint and that no standpoint is uniquely privileged over all others. Not only does this raise questions about how we are to decide what is good and bad (or beneficial and harmful), but also whether paternalism can be defended on moral grounds.

In mental health care, resort to paternalism may arguably be justifiable on the basis of protecting the consumer's long-term autonomy by acting in their 'best interests' while mentally ill. For example, involuntarily detaining a depressed consumer may be welcomed by the consumer when they are no longer depressed. This is essentially Young's (1986) approach, when he points out that it is our *dispositional autonomy* (that is, our dominant concerns over time) rather than *current autonomy* (our immediate interests) that are central to our views of our lives; that is, the consumer's illness deprives the capacity to make decisions about their life consistent with their dispositional autonomy (Robertson & Walters, 2014).

A further means to examine paternalism is to distinguish between soft and hard (or weak and strong) paternalism. Soft paternalism means making decisions on behalf of consumers whose agency is limited (for example, if their ability to act in a voluntary way is affected by cognitive impairment, addiction or severe depression). Situations where interference is justified only where the consumer's conduct is 'substantially non-voluntary or when temporary intervention is necessary' (Feinberg, 1971, pp. 113, 116); for example, a short period of psychogenic distress. Hard paternalism means overriding informed, voluntary and autonomous choices (Beauchamp & Childress, 2013, pp. 216–19), justified as 'it is proper to protect or benefit the [consumer] even when [their] contrary choices are informed and voluntary' (Beauchamp, 1978, p. 1197). An example is when a consumer with capacity is strongly advised against discharge to situations of almost certain domestic violence.

To justify any act of hard paternalism, Beauchamp and Childress (2013, p. 222) propose the following conditions need to be met:

- A consumer is at risk of significant preventable harm.
- The paternalistic action will probably prevent the harm.
- The benefits of the paternalistic action outweigh the risks.
- There is no reasonable alternative.

- It is the least autonomy-restrictive alternative, and will achieve the benefits and reduce the risks.
- In almost all circumstances, the paternalistic action does not substantially restrict autonomy.

Johnston (2016, pp. 178–9) identifies three possible stances to justify resort to paternalism:

- *pro-paternalism*—paternalism is *always justified* 'to protect consumers against themselves' (Hart, 1963, p. 31)
- *anti-paternalism*—it is *never justified* (Childress, 1982)
- *prima facie paternalism*—is *sometimes justified* depending on the circumstances. Two conditions are required:
  - the evils prevented from occurring to the [consumer] are greater than the wrongs (if any) caused by the violation of the moral rule
  - it can be universally justified under relative similar circumstances (Silber, 1989, p. 453).

CRITICAL THINKING OPPORTUNITY

A floridly psychotic consumer refuses oral medication, so security officers are called. Four large men hold the consumer down and the nurse administers the medication intramuscularly.

1   In what, if any circumstances, could this be justified paternalism?

2   In what circumstances would this be soft paternalism?

3   In what circumstances would the action breach obligations to act non-maleficently?

Justice

A universally agreed definition of justice does not exist (Nussbaum, 2006; Powers & Faddern, 2006; Sen, 2009). The principle of justice originates from the writings of Aristotle more than two thousand years ago—that 'equals should be treated equally and unequals unequally'. Justice in terms of fairness is referred to by Beauchamp and Childress (2013) as 'what is owed and due' (Johnston, 2013, p. 250).

One means to ensure fair and equitable distribution of scarce resources (according to distributive justice) is posited by Rawls (1971). According to Rawls (p. 302) social and economic inequalities are to be arranged so that;

- they are to be of the greatest benefit to the least-advantaged members of society, consistent with the just savings principle (*the difference principle*)
- offices and positions must be open to everyone under conditions of *fair equality of opportunity*.

Justice concerning mental health consumers requires society and nurses to consider whether their actions and attitudes help to redress the discrimination and burden of disability experienced by mental health consumers.

Our society uses a variety of criteria for distributive justice, including the following:

1   to each person an equal share
2   to each person according to need
3   to each person according to effort
4   to each person according to contribution
5   to each person according to merit
6   to each person according to free-market exchanges

Beauchamp & Childress, 2013, p. 253

Irrespective of the criteria utilised, as Rawls states, consumers are part of the 'least-advantaged members of society'. Ultimately, the actual application of 'doing' justice is a matter of the circumstances of each individual case (Buchanan, 2009).

Ethics of care

The notion of an 'ethics of care' differs from other ethical theories in that it does not focus on the autonomy or rationality of the individual (nurse), but rather focuses on the interdependence we as human beings have for each other (Ozolins & Grainger, 2015). It emphasises caring in the sense of 'care[ing] for, and taking care of others' (Beauchamp & Childress, 2013, p. 34; Little, 1998; McCarthy, 2006). The emphasis is on traits such as empathy, compassion and sensitivity to others, ultimately linking ethics of care to virtue ethics. Hence, because of these traits, ethics of care is central and fundamental to nurses delivering mental health care (Bowden, 1995; Cooper, 1991; Finfgeld-Connett, 2008; Gaut, 1992; Volker, 2003).

Ethics of care is not without its critics. Gilligan (1982) argues such an ethic is 'hopelessly vague', Allmark (1995) that it is 'obscuring more than it promotes' (p. 20; Johnston, 2016) and Curzer (1993) rejects the notion of such an ethic even existing. Further criticisms include the conceptual ambiguity of the notion of care and caring.

CRITICAL THINKING OPPORTUNITY

1   Does an ethics of care link to other theoretical approaches to mental health nursing?

2   Is caring the central value of nursing?

3   Are there any problems with the claim, 'Caring is the core value of nursing'?

By contrast, rights-based theory draws attention to needs that are considered to be universal and impartially determined.

Moral rights-based theory

Moral rights-based ethics is central to the idea that people (consumers) possess certain rights merely by virtue of being born human (Martin & Nickel, 1980). Johnston (2013) identifies three types of 'rights';

- *inalienable rights*—which are unable to be transferred under any circumstances; for example, the right to life
- *absolute rights*—which are unable to be overridden under any circumstances; for example, if the right to life is absolute then it cannot be overridden in any circumstances such as war, abortion or self-defence
- *prima-facie rights*—which can be overridden by stronger moral claims; for example, the right to life is overridden in situations of war or self-defence.

Johnstone (2009b) states that 'moral rights … generally entail claims about some special entitlement or interest which ought, for moral reasons, to be protected', and these interests include 'life, freedom, happiness, privacy of information, self-determination, fair treatment and bodily integrity' (p. 49). Johnstone recognises the increased use of 'rights language' in organisational, national and international documents (and the Australian Nursing and Midwifery Council [2008a] *Code of Ethics* illustrates her point). But while claims about rights may be a mechanism for improving the well-being of people who are disadvantaged, including people with mental illness, the moral basis for such rights is diverse.

SCOTT TRUEMAN

The bases for rights include: natural law and divine command; common humanity; rationality; interests or preferences; and human experience of grievous wrongs, whereby injustice is redressed and prevented (Johnstone, 2013). Measures to address and prevent wrongs have led to the *Universal Declaration of Human Rights* (Dershowitz, 2005, cited in Johnstone, 2009b), as well as international agreements about research involving human beings in the *Nuremberg Code* in 1949 and the subsequent *Declaration of Helsinki* (World Medical Association, 2008).

Codification of such rights into law arguably serve to protect human and moral rights, and assist to redress mental health discrimination (Beauchamp & Childress, 2013; Callaghan & Ryan, 2012). This can be significant for people with mental illness: the codification of rights in statutory law may provide a redress for discrimination. There is some evidence of this in Victoria since the passage of the *Charter of Human Rights and Responsibilities Act 2006* (for example, *Kracke v Mental Health Review Board & Ors* 2009 and *PJB v Melbourne Health & Anor* 2011). Note that the ACT is the only other Australian jurisdiction with a Human Rights Act. New Zealand has had a Bill of Rights Act since 1990.

CRITICAL THINKING OPPORTUNITY

1 Is there such a thing as rights?

2 How do you justify your answer?

Moral 'problems'

Mental health nurses frequently encounter moral problems and dilemmas. Only moral problems and dilemmas require a moral solution. A non-moral problem or dilemma does not. For example, whether to elevate a consumer's bed to accommodate a second nurse's height is a practical issue and issues of morality do not arise. By contrast, a decision to involuntarily seclude a consumer necessarily involves issues breaching the consumer's autonomy and acting beneficently.

Johnstone (2016) identifies nine different types of moral problems encountered by [mental] health practitioners (presented in Table 8.1).

TABLE 8.1 TYPES OF MORAL PROBLEMS

Moral problem	Definition	Example
Moral unpreparedness and incompetence	The nurse enters a clinical situation without the necessary moral skills, knowledge, experiences and competencies	Witnessing a more senior colleague excessively restrain a psychotic consumer and not reporting or intervening to stop the abuse
Moral unpreparedness and incompetence	Where a nurse is confronted by a moral problem but does not recognise it exists	Not recognising that the excessive force used is not morally unjustified
Moral indifference and blindness	Uninterest and no concern by the nurse to the moral problem; that is, accepting a situation is an institutional norm (Aroskar, 1986)	Indifference to the disproportionate degree of force used in the circumstances

Moral problem	Definition	Example
Amoralism	Indifference, rejection or absence of concern for morality in the circumstance	Accepting that psychotic consumers need to be restrained and hence 'whatever it takes' to achieve their seclusion is acceptable
Immoralism	A deliberate violation or breach of accepted ethical behaviour by a nurse	Knowing that excessive force is being used to seclude a consumer without justifiable circumstances, but irrespective agrees to the same
Moral complacency	A fixed or wedded position to the primacy of a nurse's own moral position (Unwin, 1985)	Irrespective of the 'harm' or 'seclusion reduction policies', the nurse supports that seclusion is legitimate and necessary
Moral fanaticism	A fixed or wedded position by the nurse, defended by a lack of critical self-reflectiion (Hare, 1981)	Irrespective of the 'harm' or 'seclusion reduction policies', the nurse supports that seclusion is legitimate and necessary, and will not reflect on their own beliefs/position
Moral dilemmas	Situation requiring a choice by the nurse between two desirable or undesirable alternatives	Deciding between physically or chemically restraining an aggressive consumer
Moral distress	Where a nurse feels constrained in acting in accordance with a personal moral stance and either does nothing or believes what has been done is wrong (Jametone, 1993)	Assisting in physically restraining a consumer when feeling it was unnecessary in the circumstances

International obligations underpinning Australian mental health laws

People with a mental health illness or disorder are usually viewed by society as being vulnerable, requiring their interests to be protected. Violation of their human rights may be due either to abuse or neglect. The recognition of this protection is reflected in the ratification of various codified international declarations and conventions that aim to protect and promote the interests of mental health consumers (McSherry, 2008).

Internationally Australia has ratified:

- *The Convention Against Torture*
- *The Convention on the Elimination of All Forms of Discrimination against Women*
- *The Convention on the Elimination of All Forms of Racial Discrimination*
- *The Convention on the Rights of Persons with Disabilities*
- *The Convention on the Rights of the Child*
- *The International Covenant on Civil and Political Rights*
- *The International Covenant on Economic, Social and Cultural Rights.*

SCOTT TRUEMAN

Additionally, in 1991 Australia recognised the United Nation's *Principles for the Protection of Persons with Mental Illness and the Improvement of Mental Healthcare. Mental Health: New Understanding, New Hope.* These can be summarised as follows:

- A mentally ill person is to have all the rights of any other person, and is to be free from discrimination.
- The determination that a person has a mental illness shall be made in accordance with internationally accepted principles.
- A person is to be able to live and work within the community to the extent of his or her capabilities.
- Treatment is to be based on the principle of the 'least restrictive alternative', and is to be individualised, discussed with the consumer and reviewed regularly.
- Consumers are to be protected from exploitation, abuse and degrading treatment.
- A person is not to be detained involuntarily unless it is necessary for the safety of the person or others, or to prevent serious deterioration in the person's condition.
- Where detention is necessary, it may be for a short period pending review and should involve the least restrictive measures for the least necessary time, and follow legislatively established procedures.

Subsequently in 2008, Australia adopted the United Nations *Convention on the Rights of Persons with Disabilities* (CRPD). The CRPD expressly refers to people with a mental health illness or disorder (and encompasses health generally) but in so doing invests in mental health consumers four overarching 'rights of protection';

- the right to liberty and security of the person (Article 14.1)
- the right to equal recognition before the law (Article 12)
- the right to enjoy the highest attainable standard of health (Article 25)
- the right to respect for physical and mental integrity (Article 17).

Law and nursing practice

In Australia, nursing and other health practitioners, including students, are registered with and regulated by, the Australian Health Practitioner Regulation Agency (AHPRA) and through boards such as the Nursing and Midwifery Board of Australia (NMBA). AHPRA and the NMBA operate under what is known as statutory law; that is, an Act of Parliament. In Australia there is uniform regulation of nurses, as the parliaments of all Australian states and territories passed the *Health Practitioner Regulation National Law Act*, also known as the National Law. This mandates registration of health practitioners annually, certification, and reporting of any adverse relevant events (for example, a charge or finding of guilt relating to serious criminal offences).

New Zealand nurses' practice is governed by Nursing Council of New Zealand (Te Kaunihera Tapuhi o Aotearoa). This is a statutory body authorised under the *Health Practitioners Competence Assurance Act 2003*. Both the New Zealand and Australian Acts are primarily concerned with protecting the safety of the public. The nursing regulatory boards are therefore authorised to make judgments about individual nurses' eligibility to register and practise. Decisions made by regulatory boards are subject to court rulings on appeal.

The National Law (Australia) defines professional misconduct, unprofessional conduct and notifiable conduct (ss. 5, 140); and the relevant board (for example, the NMBA) may investigate nurses whose practice or conduct is or may be unsatisfactory. For example, the board may assess a nurse's knowledge, skill, judgment or care, and evaluate this in relation to the standard reasonably expected of a nurse of an equivalent level of training or experience. Additionally, the Act authorises boards to intervene if nurses or students have an impairment (such as a physical or mental health impairment) that affects consumer' safety. Furthermore, there is a mandatory requirement for nurses, employers and (in the case of students) educators to report such an impairment (ss. 140, 143); that is, impairment is one ground for 'notifiable conduct'. The other grounds for notifiable conduct (and hence mandatory reporting) are when a nurse:

- provides care while affected by alcohol or drugs
- engages in sexual misconduct in connection with practice
- places consumers at risk of harm by significantly departing from professional standards (s. 140).

The NMBA has adopted the former Australian Nursing and Midwifery Council's competency standards (ANMC, 2006) and codes (ANMC, 2008a, 2008b) to articulate minimum standards—including compliance with relevant law—and the values that should inform practice. Similarly, the Nursing Council of New Zealand (2012a) refers to Acts that impose legal obligations on New Zealand nurses, as well as the council's expectations about the values nurses are expected to demonstrate. Failure by nurses to practise according to the standards of conduct and values could lead to disciplinary proceedings (ANMC, 2008a, 2008b; Nursing Council of New Zealand, 2012a), with the form of investigation, hearing and outcome outlined in the regulatory legislation regimes.

CRITICAL THINKING OPPORTUNITY

1   Review nurse regulatory authority websites (AHPRA or NZNC) and legal websites. What are the outcomes of some disciplinary hearings?

2   What degree or level of information or evidence do nurses need for mandatory reporting of a health practitioner colleague to AHPRA or NZNC? Are such notifications confined to nurses and midwifes?

Mental health law

Arising from the very nature of having a mental illness, consumers are vulnerable to abuse, neglect and ill treatment. This primarily occurs because their autonomy is breached due to an assessed lack of legal capacity to make decisions for themselves in their best interests. Detention, treatment and care can be undertaken without consent and even against the expressed wishes of the consumer; in such circumstances the law must protect the consumer's civil, human rights and interests from unnecessary, arbitrary and unreasonable encroachment.

Mental health legislation

New Zealand and each Australian state and territory have legislation regarding mental health consumers (see Table 8.2). The relevant Acts outline the obligations of government in the provision of care; criteria protecting people subject (or not) to the Act; and requirements for the provision of involuntary, community and other treatments. These legislative frameworks interplay with the work of nurses, including the initial assessment phase, transportation of the person exhibiting a mental illness/mental disorder, subsequent medical review and possible hospitalisation, as well as the provision and review of treatment.

TABLE 8.2 AUSTRALIAN AND NEW ZEALAND MENTAL HEALTH LEGISLATION	
Jurisdiction	**Act**
Australian Capital Territory	*Mental Health Act 2015*
New South Wales	*Mental Health Act 2007*
Northern Territory	*Mental Health and Related Services Act 1998*
Queensland	*Mental Health Act 2016*
South Australia	*Mental Health Act 2009*
Tasmania	*Mental Health Act 2013*
Victoria	*Mental Health Act 2014*
Western Australia	*Mental Health Act 2014*
New Zealand	*Mental Health (Compulsory Assessment and Treatment) Act 1992*

The various Acts outline the 'Objects' of each Act and important sections by canvassing the following:

- definitions of mental illness and mental disorder (see below)
- voluntary admissions
- involuntary admissions
- review, discharge, leave and treatment (including community)
- mental health review tribunals
- contentious treatments (electro-convulsive therapy and psychosurgery)
- forensic mental health.

Legal definitions of mental illness

Given the importance of identifying who is lawfully subject to the legislation, the definitions of mental illness in the Acts are significant (see Table 8.3). There is abundant commonality in the Acts concerning the definition of 'mental illness' and 'mental disorder' (for example, *Z v Mental Health Review Tribunal* 2015).

Most, but not all Acts list a number of behaviours and personal characteristics that are *not* indicative of mental illness:

- a person holds or is a member of a particular religious, cultural, political organisation or holds a philosophical belief, opinion and/or activity
- a person has a particular sexual preference or orientation or is sexually promiscuous
- a person engages in indecent, immoral or illegal conduct
- a person has an intellectual disability
- a person uses alcohol or other drugs
- a person is involved in, or has been involved in, personal or professional conflict
- a person engages in antisocial behaviour.

CRITICAL THINKING OPPORTUNITY

1   In your jurisdiction, what is defined as mental illness or a mental disorder, and what behaviours and/or beliefs are not?

2   How do these differ from definitions and exclusions in other jurisdictions?

3   What are some possible reasons for the differences?

TABLE 8.3 LEGISLATIVE DEFINITIONS OF MENTAL ILLNESS

Jurisdiction and Act	Part of Act	Notes
Australian Capital Territory: *Mental Health Act 2015*	Dictionary	Mental dysfunction: a disturbance or defect, to a substantially disabling degree, of perceptual interpretation, comprehension, reasoning, learning, judgment, memory, motivation or emotion. Mental illness: a condition that seriously impairs (either temporarily or permanently) the mental functioning of a person and is characterised by the presence in the person of any of the following symptoms: (a) delusions; (b) hallucinations; (c) serious disorder of thought form; (d) a severe disturbance of mood; (e) sustained or repeated irrational behaviour indicating the presence of the symptoms referred to in paragraph (a), (b), (c) or (d).

New South Wales: *Mental Health Act 2007*	s. 4(1)	Mental illness means a condition which seriously impairs, either temporarily or permanently, the mental functioning of a person and is characterised by the presence in the person of any one or more of the following symptoms:
		a) delusions,
		b) hallucinations,
		c) serious disorder of thought form,
		d) a severe disturbance of mood,
		e) sustained or repeated irrational behaviour indicating the presence of any one or more of the symptoms referred to in paragraphs (a)–(d).
		
		A mentally ill person:
		1) A person is a mentally ill person if the person is suffering from mental illness and, owing to that illness, there are reasonable grounds for believing that care, treatment or control of the person is necessary:
		    a) for the person's own protection from serious harm, or
		    b) for the protection of others from serious harm.
		2) In considering whether a person is a mentally ill person, the continuing condition of the person, including any likely deterioration in the person's condition and the likely effects of any such deterioration, are to be taken into account.

Northern Territory: *Mental Health and Related Services Act 1998*	s. 6	When person has a mental illness:
		(1) A person has a mental illness if the person has a condition that:
		    (a) is characterised by a disturbance of thought, mood, volition, perception, orientation or memory; and
		    (b) significantly impairs (temporarily or permanently) the person's judgment or behaviour

Queensland: *Mental Health Act 2016*	s. 10	Meaning of mental illness; (1) Mental illness is a condition characterised by a clinically significant disturbance of thought, mood, perception or memory.
South Australia: *Mental Health Act 2016*	s. 3	Mental illness means any illness or disorder of the mind

Jurisdiction and Act	Part of Act	Notes

Tasmania: *Mental Health Act* 2013	s. 4	Meaning of mental illness;
		(1) (a) a person is taken to have a mental illness if he or she experiences, temporarily, repeatedly or continually –
		  (i) a serious impairment of thought (which may include delusions); or
		  (ii) a serious impairment of mood, volition, perception or cognition

Victoria: *Mental Health Act* 2014	s. 4	Mental illness is a medical condition that is characterised by a significant disturbance of thought, mood, perception or memory.

Western Australia: *Mental Health Act* 2014	s. 6	Person has a mental illness:
		(1) A person has a mental illness if the person has a condition that —
		  (a) is characterised by a disturbance of thought, mood, volition, perception, orientation or memory; and
		  (b) significantly impairs (temporarily or permanently) the person's judgment or behaviour.

New Zealand: *Mental Health (Compulsory Assessment and Treatment) Act* 1992	ss. 2, 7A(2)	Mental disorder in relation to any person, means an abnormal state of mind (whether of a continuous or an intermittent nature), characterised by delusions, or by disorders of mood or perception or volition or cognition, of such a degree that it: (a) poses a serious danger to the health or safety of that person or of others; or (b) seriously diminishes the capacity of that person to take care of himself or herself A practitioner must consult the family or whanau of the proposed consumer.

BOX 8.1 BURNETT V MENTAL HEALTH TRIBUNAL (1997)

This case involved a challenge to a decision of the ACT Mental Health Tribunal. The ACT Supreme Court set aside an order to detain and administer psychiatric treatment to Geraldine Burnett, a 38-year-old woman who suffered from a mild psychotic disorder.

Burnett had at various times been taken into custody after aggressive behaviour towards her neighbours. She had been admitted five times to the psychiatric unit at Canberra Hospital prior to her admission on 11 October 1997, when she allegedly physically abused her neighbour.

The Mental Health Tribunal ordered Burnett to be involuntary detained for 28 days and to receive psychiatric treatment. Burnett appealed to the ACT Supreme Court seeking judicial review, as natural justice had not be afforded to her.

Sections 23 to 29 of the *Mental Health (Treatment and Care) Act* 1994 (ACT) (now repealed) outlined the conditions that needed to be met before a consumer could be detained or involuntarily treated. These included *inter alia* that a consumer must be suffering from a 'psychiatric illness' before the tribunal could make an order for psychiatric treatment, and that an involuntary commitment order could only be made if it was necessary for the person's own protection or the protection of others.

The court held that it was unlawful to detain and administer treatment involuntarily to Burnett. The court was not satisfied that Burnett's mental illness was severe enough to meet the definition of psychiatric illness under the Act. It found that the evidence of her condition was insufficient to justify the involuntary treatment.

The court found that it was not necessary to detain Burnett for her own protection. The court held that it would be necessary to detain someone in order to protect them from suicide, self-mutilation or some other physical harm. However, it found that the Tribunal had not established satisfactory evidence that this was the case.

REFLECTION QUESTIONS

1   How does this case show that definitions of mental illness in the Acts are significant?

2   When a person challenges their detention in a mental health facility, what is the appeal process in your jurisdiction?

A more recent case, *Re J (No2)* (2011), related to the nature of harm. The 'harm' contemplated in *Re J (No2)* was unusual as it related not to physical but to financial harm. Mr J was involuntarily detained under the *Mental Health Act 2007* (NSW) when he exhibited signs of mania. Shortly before detention, he had received a large life insurance payout because he was terminally ill, and was liberally spending the $700,000 payout.

On appeal there were two issues. First, whether continued involuntary detention could be justified on the ground that Mr J might suffer financial harm when he was not capable of making a proper judgment about the wisdom of the expenditure *due to* his mental illness. Second, was the *least* restrictive means being taken to treat the mental illness?

Mr J successfully appealed to the Supreme Court after his application for discharge was refused by the Mental Health Review Tribunal. The court interpreted the Act meaning that involuntary detention is to be a measure of *last resort* to protect against harm. In the present case, that protection could have been provided by a financial management order if the tribunal or the court was satisfied that Mr J was not capable of managing his affairs. Such an order would prevent the continued involuntary detention of Mr J and prevent any financial 'harm'.

Involuntary treatments

The various Mental Health Acts authorise detention and treatment of consumers where it can be shown that they satisfy specified criteria. The Acts also specify time periods for assessment, examination and review of treatment orders, whether these are in the form of detention or community treatment orders.

XX v WW and Middle South Area Mental Health Service (2014) demonstrates that Involuntary Treatment Orders (ITO) are not to made so as to circumvent the authority of a Mental Health Tribunal. Three hours after an ITO had been discharged by a tribunal, a mental health nurse made the decision to recommend the consumer be subject to a further ITO before being physically discharged. The Supreme Court ruled that nurses cannot order people to be detained for involuntary treatment simply because they disagree with a decision of a tribunal.

The use of prescribed treatments such as electroconvulsive therapy, psycho-surgery and seclusion and restraint are regulated in Mental Health Acts and Regulations (see Table 8.4). The use of seclusion and restraint remains controversial.

Generally, medical authorisation is required to confine or restrain consumers. However, in an emergency, a senior nurse may be authorised to do so, with a requirement for subsequent medical review and authorisation within a specified time. The Acts and, in some jurisdictions, Regulations (or

TABLE 8.4 SECLUSION AND RESTRAINT: DEFINITIONS		
Seclusion		The confinement of a consumer at any time alone in a room or area from which free exit is prevented.
Restraint	Physical restraint	The restriction of an consumer's freedom of movement by physical or mechanical means (for example, handcuffs, harnesses or straps)
	Chemical restraint	When medication that is sedative in effect is prescribed and dispensed to control a consumer's behaviour
	Emotional restraint	Where a consumer is 'conditioned' to an extent that there is a loss of confidence in being able to express their views openly and honestly to staff for fear of consequences that are, for example, coercive and threatening in nature (for example, a consumer being told if they will not calm down they will be secluded)

TABLE 8.5 REGULATION OF SECLUSION AND RESTRAINT IN AUSTRALIA AND NEW ZEALAND		
Jurisdiction	**Act**	**Provisions**
Australian Capital Territory	*Mental Health Act 2015*	s. 88
New South Wales	*Mental Health Act 2007*	'Seclusion' not mentioned per se but see s. 68(f)
Northern Territory	*Mental Health and Related Services Act 1998*	s. 62
Queensland	*Mental Health Act 2016*	Specifically s. 284 but generally concerning 'seclusion' in Parts 3–5
South Australia	*Mental Health Act 2016*	
Tasmania	*Mental Health Act 2013*	s. 56
Victoria	*Mental Health Act 2014*	ss. 105–116
Western Australia	*Mental Health Act 2014*	ss. 211–225
New Zealand	*Mental Health (Compulsory Assessment and Treatment) Act 1992*	s. 71

subordinate legislation) provide details about the maximum duration of seclusion and requirements such as frequency of observation; provision of food, water, bedding, toilet needs and maintenance of a register concerning the use of restraint and seclusion. Table 8.5 highlights these parts of the various Acts referring to seclusion and restraint.

While this chapter does not review the jurisdiction of coroners in Australia and New Zealand, it is noted that the death of a person who is an involuntary consumer (whether in seclusion or not, at the time of death), and any unexpected death, would be reportable to the coroner

Community treatment orders

The move from institutional to least restrictive care of people with mental illness has led to community-based treatment being authorised under the various mental health Acts (see *Antunovic v Dawson* (2010)). Community treatment orders (CTOs) permit consumers to reside in non-institutional settings, but usually require the consumer to comply with treatment, such as taking prescribed medication and attending counselling and regular mental health service appointments (see *M v Mental Health Review Tribunal & Ors* (2015)). CTOs may require the consumer to live in a specified facility and not engage in certain activities or associate with certain people. A breach of a CTO can authorise involuntary hospitalisation.

The prescriptive nature of CTOs has led to debate about the coercive nature of this legislative development. This debate helps to show the interface between ethics and the law in mental health practice (Burns & Dawson, 2009; Everett, 2001; Kisely, Campbell & Preston, 2005; Light et al., 2012a, 2012b; McSherry & Freckelton, 2013; O'Reilly, 2004); namely, on what basis is it just to lawfully deprive a person of freedom(s)?

CRITICAL THINKING OPPORTUNITY

Locate the code of ethics and code of conduct used by your nurse regulatory authority (for example, see www. nmba.org.au and www.nursingcouncil.org.nz).

1   If ethics should not be codified, what does your nurses' code say about its purpose?

2   Is the code of ethics distinguished from a code of conduct? If so, how is it distinguished?

Legal and ethical issues in mental health

While there are myriad legal and ethical issues, here we discuss four: consent, guardianship, negligence, and duty of care and standard of care.

Consent

Fundamental to the ethical principle of autonomy is that any consumer (with capacity) has the right to refuse treatment, even if it is contrary to the best medical evidence and advice. Ultimately, the consent of a consumer is required for treatment and care to be provided. The courts (see, for example, *Rylan v Fletcher (1992)*) jealously guard this human right, pronouncing that the consumer's consent is paramount and without it a health practitioner may be potentially liable to prosecution for assault, battery or false imprisonment (depending on the clinical circumstances). Definitions of these terms appear in Table 8.6.

TABLE 8.6   ASSAULT, BATTERY AND FALSE IMPRISONMENT: DEFINITIONS

Offence	Definition	Example
Assault	An act intended to cause an imminent apprehension of harmful or offensive contact in the victim (consumer)	Threatening to forcefully restrain and seclude a consumer; see *Logdon v DPP* (1976)
Battery	An act of deliberate physical contact with another (consumer) intended to be harmful or offensive	Giving a medication injection without the consent or against the wishes of a consumer; see *Carter v Walker* (2010)
False Imprisonment	The illegal confinement of another (consumer) against their will by a second person in such a manner as to violate the confined individual's (consumer's) right to be free from restraint of movement	Locking a voluntarily admitted consumer in their hospital room or in a locked ward against their wishes; see *Watson v Marshall & Cade* (1971)

Three types of consent can be provided:

1 *implied*—arises from the actions or conduct of the consumer; for example, rolling up a sleeve while an injection is being prepared
2 *express*—the consumer verbalises to the nurse their consent
3 *written*—for example, the consumer signs a consent form.

Even so, to be a legal 'consent' the consumer needs to additionally satisfy the following criteria. Consent must be:

■ *voluntary* and *freely given*—with the understanding that it can be withdrawn at any time; consent obtained through threat or coercion would not meet this condition
■ *specific*—only the act to which the consumer has consented can be carried out
■ given by a *competent person*—with some exceptions this means an adult (a person 18 years or older), who is able to understand the nature and effect of the proposed care, and who makes a choice in relation to that care.

Without a consumer's consent there must be a lawfully justifiable reason; see *Schloendorff v Society of New York Hospitals* (1914) per Justice Cardozo. Such a reason may emanate from either the common law or mental health legislation. In both instances, the central issue is that the consumer does not, due to their mental health illness, have 'legal' capacity.

BOX 8.2 HART V HERRON (1984)

Mr Hart attended the admission clinic of a psychiatric hospital seeking information about a procedure he was to undergo. He was agitated, and was offered medication for this, then given deep sleep treatment and electro-convulsive therapy without his consent. The court rejected the argument that attendance at the hospital amounted to implied consent to subsequent treatment. The treating medical practitioner was found liable in battery, while the hospital was liable for false imprisonment.

REFLECTION QUESTIONS

1 What would be required for Mr Hart's medical interventions to be lawful?
2 What could a nurse have done to ensure that Mr Hart's legal rights were protected?

Guardianship

Issues of guardianship arise when an adult lacks legal capacity or competency and therefore is deemed unable to provide a valid consent. *Re C (Adult: Refusal of Treatment)* (1994) concerned whether a man who suffered from a mental illness was capable of refusing treatment to amputate a limb that was gangrenous. Judge Thorpe stated in relation to assessing whether a person has capacity is to enquire whether the person has a sufficient understanding of 'the nature, purpose and effects of the proffered treatment' (p. 295).

In *White v The Local Health Authority & Anor* (2015), the consumer had been an involuntary admission in the hospital, but at the time of the application she had 'voluntary' status due to an order for release from a Mental Health Tribunal. The consumer sought a court order for release. This was opposed by consumer's guardian and the hospital formed the view that the *Mental Health Act 2007* (NSW) and *Guardianship Act 1987* (NSW) both authorised her continued detention. The court found that the guardianship order was sufficient to displace the consumer's wishes and operated to authorise the 'voluntary' admission despite her wishes to the contrary. However, once the tribunal had made a decision authorising the consumer's discharge, the guardian was constrained by the *Guardianship Act* from acting or making a decision contrary to the tribunal's decision. As a result, the court ordered the consumer be discharged from the facility.

Parents are able to provide consent to treatment for their children under 18 years, and in some jurisdictions the consent of younger people is lawful between 12 and 18 years of age (*Gillick v West Norfolk & Wisbech Area Health Authority* (1985)) in certain circumstances. When an adult, because of a mental impairment, is unable to consent to treatment, there is legal provision for substitute decision-makers. Kerridge et al. (2013) list these as:

- the Supreme Courts of each Australian jurisdiction (states and territories)
- guardianship authorities, and the guardians they appoint
- agents appointed by consumers to act for them if they become incapacitated
- the 'person responsible' as identified in guardianship legislation.

Note that in New Zealand the High Court is equivalent in the court hierarchy to Australia's Supreme Courts.

Each jurisdiction has guardianship legislation (see Table 8.7) that facilitates consent for treatment on behalf of adults who do not have the capacity to make decisions; and in Australian jurisdictions (with the exception of the Australian Capital Territory and the Northern Territory), the consent of a relative or carer may be lawful where no other legal guardian has precedence (Kerridge et al., 2009). For example, the *Guardianship and Administration Act 1986* (Vic) includes a hierarchy whereby a person appointed by the Victorian Civil and Administrative Tribunal (VCAT), under a guardianship order, and by the consumer as an enduring guardian all precede the consumer's spouse or domestic partner and primary carer; and all the former precede the further hierarchy of nearest relative (ss. 3, 37).

Depending on the circumstances of the consumer for whom an order is made, the authority of the guardian may be full or limited (for example, in decision-making scope and/or period of authorisation).

TABLE 8.7 GUARDIANSHIP LEGISLATION AND AUTHORITIES IN AUSTRALIA AND NEW ZEALAND

Jurisdiction	Act	Authority
Australian Capital Territory	*Guardianship and Management of Property Act 1991*	Guardianship and Management of Property Tribunal
New South Wales	*Guardianship Act 1987*	Guardianship Tribunal
Northern Territory	*Adult Guardianship Act 1988*	Guardianship Panel and the Local Court
Queensland	*Guardianship and Administration Act 2000*	Guardianship and Administration Tribunal
South Australia	*Guardianship and Administration 1993*	Guardianship Board
Tasmania	*Guardianship and Administration 1995*	Guardianship and Administration Board
Victoria	*Guardianship and Administration 1986*	Guardianship and Administration List, Victorian Civil and Administrative Tribunal
Western Australia	*Guardianship and Administration 1990*	State Administrative Tribunal
New Zealand	*Protection of Personal and Property Rights Act 1988*	Court may appoint 'welfare guardian'

Typically, the legislation refers to the guardian acting in the consumer's best interests and/or the consumer's health and well-being, along with acting according to the consumer's wishes if these are known. Mental health (or sometimes guardianship) legislation may limit the guardian's capacity to consent to or refuse some psychiatric treatments (such as electro-convulsive therapy and psycho-surgery); it may be necessary to obtain authorisation from a guardianship authority or Mental Health Tribunal. This highlights the need for nurses to become familiar with the relevant mental health and guardianship legislation in their jurisdiction.

Negligence

To successfully sue in an action for negligence, the consumer (plaintiff)—the person who initiates the civil case—must satisfy on the balance of probabilities the following four legal elements:

1   The plaintiff (consumer) is owed a duty of care.
    This will usually be easily satisfied when the person is a consumer—see *Australian Capital Territory v Crowley and The Commonwealth of Australian and Pitkethly* (2012). There was no relationship of doctor and consumer or health-care provider and consumer between the mental health service and the consumer because at no stage did the mental health service undertake treatment or embark upon treatment of the consumer.

2   The duty of care is breached by an act or omission.
    See *Wang v Central Sydney Area Health Service* (2000) where a patient has refused medical treatment that is considered to be immediately necessary or wants to leave a health care facility contrary to medical advice, a health care provider has a duty to carefully explain the consequences of so doing.

3   Consequent upon the breach (causation), physical, psychological and/or financial harm results.
    The act or omission must cause loss or harm to the consumer—see *Smith v Pennington* (2016) where despite the breach being the failure of the health service to provide advice to the consumer's parents, the plaintiff could not prove that 'but for' the breach of duty the consumer would not have tried to hang himself in any event (that is, whether the parents were warned or not).

4   The resultant harm/injury was reasonably foreseeable in the circumstances.
    The harm or loss was reasonably foreseeable to a reasonable person (nurse) and not merely speculative or fanciful—see *Warner (by his tutor the Protective Commissioner) v State of Qld.* (2006) where an attendee at an emergency department, suffering from schizophrenia, absconded and later fell (query: jumped?) from a building. The court was unable to speculate as to the cause of death and hence the eventuality was not foreseeable as it was uncertain. (Note: the court found no breach of duty in any event.)

Duty of care and standard of care

What is the standard of care required and how is it ascertained? Nurses need to consider whether any acts or omissions could harm consumers. Their level of ability to do so equates to a standard of care of a nurse of their own level of expertise, knowledge and skill— see *Rogers v Whitaker* (1992). The ascertainment or measure of that standard is determined by the profession examining the circumstances under review. This 'test' is referred to as the 'Bolam test':

> A [health practitioner] is not negligent if he acts [sic] in accordance with a practice accepted at the time as proper by a responsible body of [the relevant health profession's] opinion even if others ... may adopt a different practice.

Sidaway v Governors of Bethlam Royal Hospital (1985) at p. 881

This 'test' for the standard required of a health practitioners has been legislated in each Australian jurisdiction (see Table 8.8).

TABLE 8.8 LEGISLATED STANDARD OF CARE TESTS IN AUSTRALIA

Jurisdiction	Act	Provision
Australian Capital Territory	*Civil Law (Wrongs) Act 2002*	s. 42
New South Wales	*Civil Liability Act 2002*	s. 50
Queensland	*Civil Liability Act 2003*	s. 22
South Australia	*Civil Liability Act 1936*	s. 41
Tasmania	*Civil Liability Act 2002*	s. 22
Victoria	*Wrongs Act 1958*	ss. 58, 59
Western Australia	*Civil Liability Act 2002*	s. 5PB
Northern Territory	Nil	Bolam test (Rogers v Whitaker (1992))

The law and confidentiality

At common law, medical and nursing notes and records (paper, electronic and otherwise produced) belong to the health service, although the information is owned by the consumer—see *Breen v Williams* (1996). For clarity, the Commonwealth has created a legislative scheme in relation to the issues of privacy and confidentiality, including health records and data.

BOX 8.3 HUNTER AND NEW ENGLAND LOCAL HEALTH DISTRICT V MCKENNA (2014)

A 42-year-old male consumer (Pettigrove) had a long history of mental health illness including schizophrenia. He was treated in the community of Echuca, Victoria. In July 2004, he was staying in NSW with his friend Stephen Rose. On the 20 July 2004, Rose became concerned about Pettigrove, who was experiencing 'physical jerks', and called an ambulance. Pettigrove was admitted to a hospital in Taree. Detained under the *Mental Health Act 1990* (NSW) for suicidal ideation, the following day Pettigrove was discharged to accompany Rose back to Echuca to be close to his family. This arrangement was done with the consent and understanding of the treating psychiatrist. That evening near Dubbo, Pettigrove killed Rose on the basis 'that something inside me said to do it'. Pettigrove

hanged himself in jail some two months later. Rose's family sued the health service for negligence.

The High Court found no negligence on behalf of the health service or hospital. The decision turned largely on s. 20 of the *Mental Health Act 1990* (NSW), which prescriptively states that a mentally ill person is *not* to be detained unless 'no other less restrictive care is appropriate and reasonably available'. The Court concluded that despite the risk that a mentally ill person might act irrationally following discharge, such harm caused by a consumer would be inconsistent with the duty under legislation; namely, not to restrict the liberties of consumers where there are less restrictive means of treatment available.

The Commonwealth Australian Information Commissioner (AIC), supported by the Office of the Australian Information Commissioner (OAIC), is responsible for administering the *Privacy Act 1988* (Cth). The Australian Privacy Principles (APPs), which are contained in schedule 1 of the Act, outline how most Australian Government agencies (for example, Medicare and health services and hospitals) and all private health service providers (APP entities) must handle, use and manage personal information.

The thirteen APPs are not prescriptive; each health-care service or hospital needs to consider how the relevant principles apply to its own situation. The principles cover:

- the open and transparent management of personal information, including having a privacy policy
- rules for the collection of solicited personal information and receipt of unsolicited personal information, including giving notice about collection
- how personal information can be used and disclosed (including overseas)
- maintaining the quality of personal information
- keeping personal information secure
- right for individuals to access and correct their personal information.

APP 12 requires an APP entity (for example, a health service) that holds personal information about an individual (for example, a consumer) to give the individual access to that information on request. There are limits, however. APP 12.3 lists ten grounds on which an organisation can refuse to give access to personal information, including where the organisation reasonably believes that:

- giving access would pose a serious threat to the life, health or safety of any individual (consumer), or to public health or public safety (APP 12.3(a))
- giving access would have an unreasonable impact on the privacy of other individuals (APP 12.3(b))
- the request for access is frivolous or vexatious (APP 12.3(c)).

Similarly, the New Zealand Privacy Commissioner's website (www.privacy.org.nz) provides information about the New Zealand *Privacy Act 1993* and a link to its twelve Privacy Principles. Note that only the Australian Capital Territory, New South Wales and Victoria have specific health information legislation, but all states and territories are bound by the Commonwealth legislation.

BOX 8.4 R (MRS) V BALLARAT HEALTH SERVICES (2007)

Mrs R (the applicant) requested details about any psychiatric and/or police records Ballarat Health Services held about her and any records relating to her thyroid condition. She wanted the information 'to establish and to enable herself to secure more evidence of claims of a conspiracy by her ex-husband and others'.

There were nineteen entries that were in dispute concerning a refusal by the health service to release the information.

The refusal of release of the information was upheld by the tribunal on a number of grounds, including:

REFLECTION QUESTIONS

- The information clearly contained information relating to the personal affairs of persons other than Mrs R.
- It was difficult to see how the released information could assist with her claims.

Although not relevant to the *R (Mrs) v Ballarat Health Services* (2007) case, another ground for non-disclosure could be if the release of information could seriously threaten the life or health of the consumer; for example, acerbate a consumer's suicidal ideation.

Some mental health legislation contains law about confidentiality and when information can be disclosed. For example, where a consumer does not consent to the disclosure of information to a carer, this must be respected; see, for example, s 288 (2)(a) of the *Mental Health Act (2016)* (Qld). However, there is some tension between carers' requests to be lawfully provided with more information and consumers' concern about protection of their rights to privacy and confidentiality (National Mental Health Consumer and Carer Forum, 2011).

Where information is unlawfully disclosed, consumers may sue pursuant to three possible legal causes of action:

- *breach of contract*—where information is innately confidential in nature, either expressly or impliedly (*Wright v Gasweld Pty Ltd* (1991))
- *breach of confidentiality*—where the information is:
  - confidential in nature
  - imparted in circumstances giving rise to an obligation of confidentiality
  - used without authorisation to the detriment of the consumer
- *negligence*—where the four principles of negligence can be proven (see above).

Finally, the Nursing and Midwifery Board of Australia's *Code of Professional Conduct for Nurses in Australia* (ANMC, 2008b) and *Code of Ethics for Nurses in Australia* (ANMC, 2008a) both outline the requirement for nurses to observe confidentiality in the course of their practice.

Failure to disclose information and negligence

Mental health consumers disclose the most intimate and confident information and histories; it is the essence of providing mental health care. As discussed in more detail below, confidentiality is a fundamental and paramount issue for nurses. The very nature of the role of mental health nurses means that some disclosures by consumers are of the most intimate and personal sort, some of which can be confronting. For example, a nurse working in forensic mental health may have a paedophile disclose an overwhelming sexual attraction towards a young person, or even a desire to kill that person. Legally, what is the nurse to do in this situation? Negligence applies to the failure to disclose information in such situations that result in foreseeable harm to a third party—see *Breen v Williams* (1996). A nurse may disclose sensitive and intimate information about another person beyond the therapeutic relationship if adverse or life-threatening consequences to another 'identified' party could result—see *Tarasoff v Regents of the University of California* (1976).

W v Egdell (1990) involved a psychiatric assessment by Dr Egdell of consumer W, who had been diagnosed with paranoid schizophrenia and detained for an unlimited period in a secure hospital after being convicted of manslaughter for killing five people. The doctor was asked by the consumer's solicitors to provide a report to support W's application of transfer to a less secure facility. The report did not support the removal and the consumer's solicitors continued with the judicial application, but without disclosure of the report. The doctor sent a copy of the report to two relevant authorities (one being the court determining the application). The consumer sought an injunction on the disclosure of the report and sued for breach of confidentiality. The court found that despite a duty of confidentiality, the doctor had an overriding duty to public safety to communicate with the proper authorities.

In *Smith v Jones* (1999) a sadistic rapist of prostitutes in a defined area of a Canadian city, while on bail, was ordered to consult a psychiatrist. Believing that communications were confidential, he advised the psychiatrist of his continued fantasies to kidnap, sadistically rape and murder prostitutes from the same location. Against the offender's lawyer's instructions not to disclose to the court such information, the psychiatrist tendered the evidence of the fantasies to the court (which he believed would be acted upon). On appeal, the court allowed the breach of confidentially as being in the public's interest and noted that health practitioners need to consider:

- clarity of the risk
- severity of the risk
- imminence of harm.

See also *Furniss v Fichett* (1958), *R v Lory* (Ruling 8) (1997) and *Hunter v Mann* (1974).

Ethics, privacy and confidentiality

'Privacy' is a broader notion than confidentiality and relates to all aspects of the therapeutic relationship, including consumer encounters (including whether an encounter has taken place) and the secrecy and security of information memorialised in physical, electronic and graphic records created as a consequence of these encounters (DeCew, 2000). Confidentiality is defined more narrowly as relating to the restriction of information to individuals belonging to a set of specifically authorised recipients (Allen, 2014). Hence, Bok (1982) characterised confidentiality as referring 'to the boundaries surrounding shared secrets and to the process of guarding these boundaries' (p. 119).

There exist good public policy reasons for the maintenance of consumer confidentiality. One reason is it accords with utilitarianism (or consequentialism). For nurses to be in the best position to diagnose and treat consumers, they need all the information that might be available and truthful answers to their clinical questions (Oakley, 1997; Bennett, 2007). Consumers are more likely to be honest, frank and open, particularly if the information is embarrassing and stigmatising (for example, mental health and substance misuse), if they feel that such disclosures will remain confidential—see *Hunter v Mann* (1974).

The ethical principle of autonomy is another principle-based argument supporting the notion of consumer confidentiality. Confidentiality is part of a consumer's autonomy, encompassing not just physical bodily integrity but also what other individuals know about their personal information. It goes to the consumer's autonomous integrity (Bok, 1982).

A final argument is based on promise keeping. There is an implicit promise between nurses and consumers to keep information secret; and when health practitioners breach confidentiality, they break this promise, which breaches the fidelity of the therapeutic relationship.

Breach of confidentiality

Two main ethical arguments are advanced in support of breaching a consumer's right to confidentiality: respect for autonomy and prevention of harm (even related to an 'innocent' third party).

The first is posited by Bok (1982), who advocates that if confidentiality is essentially based on respect for autonomy, potential victims have a right to know if they are at risk, so they can determine what they will do. It would be a contradiction to avoid breaching confidentiality when the breach is required to protect the autonomy of an unknown or innocent other individual.

The second is not just the protection of harm to others (see *Tarasoff v. Regents of the University of California* (1976)), but also related to the prevention of harm to the mental health consumer themselves; in the case of consumers with suicidal thoughts, non-disclosure may lead to a failure to protect the consumer.

A mental health nurse practitioner is working in a sexual health clinic. They are consulting with a married male consumer who is bisexual. The consumer advises that his wife is not aware of his bisexuality or his bisexual sexual encounters. The nurse practitioner orders blood tests for HIV/AIDS and hepatitis B status. The results return positive for both. At a post-testing consultation the consumer refuses to advise or permit the nurse practitioner to devolve this information to his wife.

1   From a legal or moral perspective. can the nurse practitioner breach confidence and inform the wife?

2   Does it make any difference legally or morally if the wife is also a consumer of the nurse practitioner?

3   Does it make any difference if the male consumer advises that he is having unprotected sexual activity with the wife and that to change to protected sexual activity would expose his bisexuality and cause the wife great pain, leading to a breakdown of the relationship? What if his wife has a history of suicide attempts when previous relationships have broken down?

See *PD v Dr Nicholas Harvey and Ors* (2003).

Professional boundaries: ethics and law

Maintaining appropriate boundaries between nurses and consumers is an ethical and legal matter, since consumers can be vulnerable to exploitation, and may be harmed when nurses fail to recognise the professional boundaries of their role. This is likely to be viewed as unprofessional conduct or professional misconduct by the nursing regulatory authorities (for example, AHPRA). For example, in *Nursing and Midwifery Board of Australia v Buckby* (2015), a mental health nurse was having a predatory sexual relationship with two consumers and was suspended from practice for seven years.

The potential damage to mental health consumers from inappropriate relationships with nurses was also the subject of the expert witnesses' evidence in *Southern Area Health Service v Brown* (2003). In this case, a student met a female consumer during his clinical placement and began visiting her in her home. Two psychiatric nurses caring for the consumer were aware of this, but failed to intervene. The nurses were in breach of their duty of care. The consumer successfully sued in negligence because of the harm she suffered from a sexual assault by the student.

The former Australian Nursing & Midwifery Council and the Nursing Council of New Zealand (2010) jointly developed *A Nurse's Guide to Professional Boundaries* to be used in conjunction with nurses' codes and practice standards; and this continues to be used in Australia. However, the Nursing Council of New Zealand (2012b) has since developed *Guidelines: Professional Boundaries*, taking into account particular contextual factors, including New Zealand's small population and cultural factors. Both regulatory authorities' guidelines continue to refer to the relevant codes.

The most relevant statement in the *Code of Professional Conduct for Nurses* is: 'Nurses promote and preserve the trust and privilege inherent in the relationship between nurses and people receiving care' (Australian Nursing and Midwifery Council, 2008b, p. 6); and recognises the particular vulnerability of people with mental illness. Principle 7 is the most relevant in the New Zealand *Code of Conduct*: 'Act with integrity to justify health consumers' trust' (Nursing Council of New Zealand, 2012a, p. 8); while the *Guidelines: Professional boundaries* (Nursing Council of New Zealand, 2012b) recognise the vulnerability of people with mental illness.

CRITICAL THINKING OPPORTUNITY

You are a recently graduated male registered nurse (RN) with postgraduate qualifications in mental health, and discover that a colleague has used health-care records to obtain a former consumer's phone number. A few months after the female consumer's discharge from hospital, your colleague has commenced a sexual relationship with the discharged consumer.

1   Which sections of the *Code of Professional Conduct for nurses in Australia* (Australian Nursing and Midwifery Council, 2008b) and *Code of Ethics for Nurses in Australia* (Australian Nursing and Midwifery Council, 2008a) have been breached?

2   What is your professional responsibility?

3   Has your colleague engaged in 'unprofessional conduct' or 'professional misconduct'?

SUMMARY

This chapter has introduced you to law and ethics in mental health nursing. Mental health legislation in Australian jurisdictions and in New Zealand has been utilised to show how mental illness is defined. It has been shown that these definitions have implications for whether people are subject to mental health law, including involuntary treatments and interventions in the community and health facilities. Diagnosis with a mental illness, as defined in the various Mental Health Acts, may affect a person's ability to be self-determining; and this has been examined from both legal and ethical points of view.

As well as providing an overview of ethical theories and principles, issues of particular relevance to mental health practice have been reviewed. These include ethical and legal aspects of consent, confidentiality and regulation of the profession.

It is evident that mental health practice occurs in a unique legislative framework: other areas of health care are not subject to the same statutory control of practice. Furthermore, the nature of mental illness poses particular challenges for mental health nurses' obligations to act both ethically and legally.

DISCUSSION QUESTIONS

1   Why is it important that legislation exists to govern the care of mentally ill people?

2   What are some differences between ethics and law in mental health-care contexts?

3   When should a person's individual freedom be restricted by law?

4   What are the potential benefits of psychiatric advance directives?

5   Why may there be tension between some carers' and mental health consumers' views about respecting confidentiality?

TEST YOURSELF

1   Consequentalism is also known and referred to as:

a   deontology

b   virture theory

c   teleology

d   principlism

2 Amoralism involves a nurse being:

   a confronted by a moral problem but not recognising it exists

   b indifferent, rejecting or absent with concern for morality in the circumstance

   c fixed or wedded to a position due to the primacy of their own moral position

   d in deliberate violation or breach of accepted ethical behaviour

3 Which is the most accurate answer? A consumer's consent to treatment can:

   a not be withdrawn once a consent form has been signed

   b be provided via three means (implied, expressed or in writing)

   c provide immunity from being sued for any act of negligence

   d be validly given if they are not too intoxicated

4 Which of the following is indicative of a person suffering from a mental health illness pursuant to the various Mental Health Acts? When they:

   a engage in sexually risky and promiscuous behaviour

   b engage in antisocial behaviour

   c are a member of a particular religious group who hold unusual and non-orthodox ideology

   d believe that they are the 'son of God'

USEFUL WEBSITES

Australian Government Department of Health: www.health.gov.au

Family Court of New Zealand—Mental health treatment: https://www.justice.govt.nz/family/court-ordered-treatment/mental-health-treatment/

Mental Health Foundation of New Zealand: www.mentalhealth.org.nz

Ministry of Health, New Zealand: www.health.govt.nz

National Mental Health Consumer and Carer Forum: www.nmhccf.org.au

Nursing and Midwifery Board of Australia: www.nursingmidwiferyboard.gov.au

Nursing Council of New Zealand: www.nursingcouncil.org.nz

Privacy Commissioner, New Zealand: www.privacy.org.nz

REFERENCES

Allmark, P. (1995). Can there be an ethics of care? *Journal of Medical Ethics*, 21(1), 19–24.

Armstrong, A. E. (2006). Towards a strong virtue ethics for nursing practice. *Nursing Philosophy*, 7(3), 110–124.

Aroskar, M. (1986). Are nurses' mindsets compatible with ethical practice? In P. Chinn (Ed.), *Ethical issues in nursing* (pp. 69–79). Rockville: Aspen Systems.

Arya, D. (2012). Compulsory treatment and patient responsibility. *Australasian Psychiatry*, 20(6), 472–477.

Australian Nursing and Midwifery Council (2006). *National competency standards for the registered nurse* (4th ed.). Retrieved from www.nursingmidwiferyboard.gov.au.

Australian Nursing and Midwifery Council (2008a). *Code of ethics for nurses in Australia*. Retrieved from www.nursingmidwiferyboard.gov.au.

Australian Nursing and Midwifery Council (2008b). *Code of professional conduct for nurses in Australia*. Retrieved from www.nursingmidwiferyboard.gov.au.

Nursing and Midwifery Board of Australia & Nursing Council of New Zealand (2010). *A nurse's guide to professional boundaries*. Retrieved from www.nursingmidwiferyboard.gov.au.

Beauchamp, T. (1978). Paternalism. In W. T. Reich (Ed.), *Encylopedia of bioethics* (pp. 1194–1201). New York: Free Press, London: Collier Macmillan.

Beauchamp, T., & Childress, J. F. (2013). *Principles of biomedical ethics* (7th ed.). New York: Oxford University Press.

Begley, A. M. (2005). Practising virtue: A challenge to the view that a virtue-centred approach to ethics lacks practical content. *Nursing Ethics*, 12(6), 622–637.

Benjamin, J. (2001). Between the subway and the spaceship ethics: Practical ethics in the twenty-first century, *Hastings Center Report*, 31(4), 24–31.

Bennett, R. (2007). Confidentiality. In R. Ashcroft, A. Dawson, H. Draper & J. McMillian (Eds.), *Principles of health care ethics* (pp. 325–332). Chichester: John Wiley and Sons.

Bentham, J. (1962). An introduction to the principles of morals and legislation (reprinted from 1789 ed.). In M. Warnock (Ed.), *Utilitarianism* (pp. 33–77). London: Fontana Library/Collins.

Berghmans, R., & van der Zanden, M. (2012). Choosing to limit choice: Self-binding directives in Dutch mental health care. *International Journal of Law and Psychiatry, 35*(1), 11–8.

Blum, L. (1980). Compassion. In A. O. Rorty (Ed.), *Explaining emotions.* Berkeley: University of California Press.

Bok, S. (1982). *Secrets: On the ethics of concealment and revelation.* Oxford: Oxford University Press.

Bowden, P. L. (1995). The ethics of nursing care and 'the ethics of care'. *Nursing Inquiry, 2*(1), 10–21.

Buchanan, A. (2009). *Justice and health care: Selected essays.* Oxford: Oxford University Press.

Burns, T., & Dawson, J. (2009). Community treatment orders: How ethical without experimental evidence? *Psychological Medicine, 39*(10), 1583–1586.

Callaghan, S., & Ryan C. J. (2012). Rising to the human rights challenge in compulsory treatment: New approaches to mental health law in Australia. *Australian and New Zealand Journal of Psychiatry, 46*(7), 611–620.

Childress, J. (1982). *Who should decide? Paternalism in health care.* New York: Oxford University Press.

Cooper, M. (1991). Principle-oriented ethics and the ethics of care: A creative tension. *Advances in Nursing Science, 14*(2), 22–31.

Crowden, A. (2004). *The debate continues: unique ethics for psychiatry. Australian and New Zealand Journal of Psychiatry, 38*(3), 111–114.

Curzer, H. (1993). Is care a virtue for health care professional? *Journal of Medicine and Philosophy, 18*(1), 51–69.

DeCew, J. (2000). The priority of privacy for medical information, *Social Policy and Practice, 1*(2), 213–234.

Everett, B. (2001). Community treatment orders: Ethical practice in an era of magical thinking. *Canadian Journal of Community Mental Health, 20*(1), 5–20.

Feinberg, J. (1971). Legal paternalism. *Canadian Journal of Philosophy, 1*(1), 105–124.

Feinberg, J. (1984). *Harm to others: The moral limits of the criminal law.* New York: Oxford University Press.

Finfgeld-Connett, D. (2008). Meta-synthesis of caring in nursing. *Journal of Clinical Nursing, 17*(2), 196–204.

Gaut, D. (1992). *The presence of caring in nursing.* New York: National League of Nursing Press.

Gilligan, C. (1982). *In a different voice.* Cambridge: Harvard University Press.

Gillon, R. (1995). Medical ethics: Four principles plus attention to scope. *Monash Bioethics Review, 14*(3), 23–30.

Hare, R. (1981). Moral thinking: Its levels, methods and point. Oxford: Clarendon Press.

Hart, H. (1963). *Law, liberty and morality.* Stanford: Stanford University Press.

Health Services Commissioner/Te Tiohau Hauora Hauatanga. (2009). *A Review of the Health and Disability Commissioners Act 1994 and Code Health and Disability Services Consumers' Rights.* Retrieved from http://www.hdc.org.nz/the-act--code/review-of-the-act-and-code-2009%2011/8/17.

Hodkinson, K. (2008). How should a nurse approach truth-telling? A virtue ethics perspective. *Nursing Philosophy, 9*(4), 248–256.

Jametone, A. (1993). Dilemmas of moral distress: Moral responsibility and nursing practice. *AWHONN Clinical Issues, 4*(4), 542–551.

Johnstone, M.-J. (2009a). *Alzheimer's disease, media representations and the politics of euthanasia: Constructing risk and selling death in an aging society.* Ashgate, Farnham, Surry.

Johnstone, M.-J. (2009b). *Bioethics: A nursing perspective* (5th ed.). Sydney: Churchill Livingstone.

Johnstone, M-J, (2013). *Alzheimer's disease, media representations and politics of euthanasia: constructing risk and selling death in an aging society.* Ashgate, Farnham, Surrey.

Johnstone, M-J (2016). *Bioethics: A nursing perspective* (6th ed.). Sydney: Churchill Livingstone.

Kerridge, I., Lowe, M., & Stewart, C. (2009). *Ethics and law for the health professions* (3rd ed.). Sydney: Federation Press.

Kerridge, I., Lowe, M. & Stewart, C. (2013). *Ethics and Law for the Health Professions* (4th ed.). Federation Press. Annadale, NSW, Australia.

Kisely, S., Campbell, L. A., & Preston, N. (2005). Compulsory community treatment and involuntary treatment for people with severe mental disorders. *Cochrane Database Systematic Review, 3,* CD004408.

Light, E. M., Kerridge, I. H., Ryan, C. J., & Robertson, M. D. (2012a). Community treatment orders in Australia: Rates and patterns of use. *Australasian Psychiatry, 20*(6), 478–482.

Light, E. M., Kerridge, I. H., Ryan, C. J., & Robertson, M. D. (2012b). Out of sight, out of mind: Making involuntary community treatment visible in the mental health system. *Medical Journal of Australia, 196*(9), 591–593.

Little, M. (1998). Care from theory to orientation and back. *Journal of Medicine and Philosophy, 23*(2), 190–209.

Little, M. (2001). On knowing the 'why': Particularism and moral theory. *Hastings Center Report, 31*(4), 32–40.

Lutzen, K., & da Silva, A. B. (1996). The role of virtue ethics in psychiatric nursing. *Nursing Ethics, 3*(3), 202–211.

Martin, R., & Nickel, J. (1980). Recent work on the concepts of rights. *American Philosophical Quarterly, 17*(3), 165–180.

McCarthy, J. (2006). A pluralist view of nursing ethics. *Nursing Philosophy, 7*(3), 157–164.

Mckie, A., & Swinton, J. (2001). Community, culture and character: The place of the virtues in psychiatric nursing practice. *Journal of Psychiatric and Mental Health Nursing, 7*(1), 35–42.

McSherry, B. (2008). International trends in mental health laws: Introduction. *Law in Context, 26*(2), 1–9.

McSherry, B., & Freckelton, I. (2013). *Coercive rights: Rights, law and policy.* Oxford: Routledge.

Mill, J. S. (1962). *Utilitarianism* (reprinted from 1861 ed.). In M. Warnock (Ed.), *Utilitarianism* (pp. 251–354). London: Fontana Library/Collins 251–342.

National Mental Health Consumer and Carer Forum (2011). *Privacy, Confidentiality & Information Sharing – Consumers, Carers & Clinicians.* Retrieved from https://nmhccf.org.au/sites/default/files/docs/nmhccf_pc_ps_ip.pdf.

Nussbaum, M. (2006). *Frontiers of justice; disability, nationality, species membership.* Cambridge: Harvard University Press.

Newham, R. (2015). Virtue ethics and nursing: On what grounds? *Nursing Philosophy, 16*(1), 40–50.

Nicaise, P., Lorant, V., & Dubois, V. (2013). Psychiatric advance directives as a complex and multistage intervention: A realistic systematic review. *Health and Social Care in the Community, 21*(1), 1–14.

Nursing Council of New Zealand (2012a). *Code of conduct.* Retrieved from www.nursingcouncil.org.nz.

Nursing Council of New Zealand (2012b). *Guidelines: Professional boundaries.* Retrieved from www.nursingcouncil.org.nz.

O'Reilly, R. (2004). Why are community treatment orders controversial? *Canadian Journal of Psychiatry, 49*(9), 579–584.

Oakley, J. (1997). The morality of breaching confidence to protect others. In L. Shotten (Ed.), *Health care law and ethics.* NSW: Social Science Press.

Oakley, J., & Hocking, D. (2001). *Virtue ethics and professional roles*. New York: Cambridge University Press.

Ozolins, J., & Grainger, J. (2015). *Foundations of healthcare ethics*. Sydney: Cambridge University Press.

Pellegrino, E. (1995). Toward a virtue-based normative ethics for the health professions. *Kennedy Institute of Ethics Journal, 5*(3), 253–277.

Powers, M., & Faddern, R. (2006). *Social justice: The moral foundations of public health and health policy*. New York: Oxford University Press.

Rawls, J. (1971). *A theory of justice*. Oxford University Press, Oxford.

Robertson, M., & Walters, G. (2014). *Ethics and mental health: The patient, profession and community*. Boca Raton: Taylor & Francis Group.

Sen, A. (2009). *The idea of justice*. London: Allen Lane/Penguin.

Silber, T. (1989). Justified paternalism in adolescent healthcare: Cases of anorexia nervosa and substance abuse. *Journal of Adolescent Health Care,* 10(6), 449–453.

Srebnik, D. (2005). Issues in applying advance directives to psychiatric care in the United States. *Australasian Journal on Ageing, 24*(1), S42–S45.

Swanson, J. W., Swartz, M. B., Elgogan, E. B., van Dorn, R. A., Wagner, H. R., Moser, L. A., Wilder, C., & Gilbert, A. R. (2008). Psychiatric advance directives and reduction of coercive crisis interventions. *Journal of Mental Health, 17*(3), 255–267.

Unwin, N. (1985). Relativism and moral complacency. *Philosophy, 60*(232), 205–209.

Volker, D. L. (2003). Is there a unique nursing ethic? *Nursing Science Quarterly, 16*(3), 207–211.

Weller, P. (2008). Advance directives and the translation of human rights principles in mental health law: Towards a contextual analysis. *Quarterly Mental Health Consumer, Carer and Community Forum*. Retrieved from www.law.monash.edu/centres/calmh/rmhl/docs/pw-mhcc-act-0508.pdf.

Weller, P. (2012). *New law and ethics in mental health advance directives*. Hove: Routledge.

WHO General Assembly (1991). *The protection of persons with mental illness and the improvement of mental health care*. Retrieved from http://www.un.org/documents/ga/res/46/a46r119.htm.

Wilder, C. M., Elbogen, E. B., Moser, L. L., Swanson, J. W., & Swartz, M. S. (2010). Medication preferences and adherence among individuals with severe mental illness and psychiatric advance directives. *Psychiatric Services, 61*(4), 380–385.

World Medical Association (2008). *World Medical Association declaration of Helsinki: Ethical principles for medical research involving human subjects* (rev. ed.). Retrieved from www.wma.net/en/30publications/10policies/b3/.

Young, R. (1986). *Personal autonomy. Beyond negative and positive liberty*. London: Croom Helm.

ACTS AND REGULATIONS

Adult Guardianship Act 1988 (NT)

Advanced Personal Planning Act 2013 (NT)

Bill of Rights Act 1990 (NZ)

Civil Law (Wrongs) Act 2002 (ACT)

Civil Liability Act 1936 (SA)

Civil Liability Act 2002 (NSW)

Civil Liability Act 2002 (Tas)

Civil Liability Act 2002 (WA)

Civil Liability Act 2003 (Qld)

Guardianship Act 1987 (NSW)

Guardianship and Administration Act 1986 (Vic)

Guardianship and Administration Act 1990 (WA)

Guardianship and Administration Act 1993 (SA)

Guardianship and Administration Act 1995 (Tas)

Guardianship and Administration Act 1986 (Vic)

Guardianship and Administration Act 2000 (Qld)

Guardianship and Management of Property Act 1991 (ACT)

Health Practitioner Regulation National Law Act (all states and territories)

Health Practitioners Competence Assurance Act 2003 (NZ)

Human Rights Act 2004 (ACT)

Mental Health (Compulsory Assessment and Treatment) Act 1992 (NZ)

Mental Health Act 2007 (NSW)

Mental Health Act 2013 (Tas)

Mental Health Act 2014 (Vic)

Mental Health Act 2014 (WA)

Mental Health Act 2015 (ACT)

Mental Health Act 2016 (Qld)

Mental Health Act 2016 (SA)

Mental Health and Related Services Act 1998 (NT)

Powers of Attorney Act 1998 (Qld)

Privacy Act 1988 (Cth)

Protection of Personal and Property Rights Act 1988 (NZ)

Wrongs Act 1958 (Vic)

CASES

Antunovic v Dawson (2010) 30 VR 355

Australian Capital Territory v Crowley and The Commonwealth of Australia and Pitkethly (2012) ACTCA 52

Breen v Williams (1996) 138 ALR 259

Burnett v Mental Health Tribunal [1997] ACTSC 310

Carter v Walker (2010) 32 VR 1

Furniss v Fitchett (1958) NZLR 39

Gillick v West Norfolk and Wisbech Area Health Authority (1985) 3All ER 402

Hart v Herron (1984) Aust Torts Rep 80–201

Hunter and New England Local Health District v McKenna (2014) HCA 44

Hunter v Mann (1974) 1QB 767

Kracke v Mental Health Review Board & Ors (General) (2009) VCAT 646.

Logdon v DPP (1976) Crim LR 121

M v Mental Health Review Tribunal & Ors (2015) NSWSC 1876

Nursing and Midwifery Board of Australia v Buckby (2015) WASAT 19

PD v Dr Nicholas Harvey and Ors (2003) NSWSC 487

PJB v Melbourne Health and Anor (Patrick's case) (2011) VSC 327

R (Mrs) v Ballarat Health Services (2007) VCAT 2397

R v Lory (Ruling 8) (1997) 1 NZLR 44

Re C (Adult: Refusal of Treatment)(1994) 1 All ER 819

Re J (No2) (2011) NSWSC 1224

Rogers v Whitaker (1992) 175 CLR 479

Schloendorff v. Society of New York Hospital, 105 NE 92 (NY 1914)

Sidaway v Governors of Bethlam Royal Hospital (1985) AC 871

Smith v Pennington (2016) NSWSC 1168

Smith v. Jones [1999] 1 SCR 455

Southern Area Health Service v Brown (2003) NSWCA 369

Tarasoff v. Regents of the University of California 17 Cal. 3d 425, 551 P.2d 334, 131 Cal. Rptr. 14 (Cal. 1976)

W v Edgell (1990) 1 ALL ER 835

Wang v Central Sydney Area Health Service (2000) NSWSC 515

Warner (by his tutor the Protective Commissioner) v State of Qld (2006) NSWSC 593

Watson v Marshall & Cade (1971) 124 CLR 621

White v The Local Health Authority & Anor (2015) NSWSC

Wright v Gasweld Pty Ltd (1991) 22 NSWLR 317

XX v WW and Middle South Area Mental Health Service (2014) VSC 564

Z v Mental Health Review Tribunal (2015) NSWCA 373

CHAPTER 9

Consumer and Carer Participation and Leadership

EVAN BICHARA,
SUSAN JOHNSON AND
IAN MUNRO

Acknowledgment

The authors would like to acknowledge the contribution of Isabell Collins and Wanda Bennetts who wrote this chapter in the second edition.

KEY OUTCOMES

AFTER READING THIS CHAPTER, YOU SHOULD BE ABLE TO:

- appreciate the perspectives of consumers and carers
- understand the issues related to consumer and carer participatin in mental health
- Identify the issues for consumers and carers in negotiating the mental health system
- Explain how consumer and caer participation leads to greater empowerment and open dialogue

KEY TERMS

- carer burden
- carer participation
- CHIME framework
- co-designing
- empowerment
- Open Dialogue
- peer support
- peer support networks (PIR)
- partners in recovery
- psychoeducation
- recovery colleges

Introduction

In this chapter the reader will gain insights from individuals who have experienced the mental health system either as a consumer or carer, as their lived experience is critical to the ongoing development of services that can provide effective care to those in need. Today, governments around the world are seeing the value in having a dialogue with consumers, not only about how they would like to see services run, but also about the design and day-to-day management of these services.

SECTION 1 CONSUMER INVOLVEMENT

EVAN BICHARA

IAN MUNRO

Current areas of work that have been expanded within the consumer movement are:

- co-designing
- recovery colleges
- peer support.

Co-designing

Co-design (also known as co-production) is the new buzz word within mental health ... so what does it mean? The Victorian Council of Social Services (2015) argues that co-designing new initiatives with people experiencing vulnerabilities engages professionals to begin initiatives with these people's experiences, perspectives, values, challenges and understandings. It involves finding ground-up or bottom-up solutions to many dilemmas or problems seen in the community.

Co-design changes the way professionals conceptualise or approach people's vulnerabilities in the pursuit of social change, because identifying someone as vulnerable often leads us to focus on their weaknesses and the need to protect them from possible harm. This intention is important and is rightly reflected in ethical protocols or guidelines for working with people. However, an overemphasis on vulnerability may underestimate the degree to which people can determine their visions for their own well-being or to effectively participate in decision-making processes. Focusing upon vulnerabilities can also underestimate an individual's resilience or their capacity to grow, to develop living skills, and to self-manage risk from their learning and employing coping strategies. This allows individuals to move forward in life, actively influencing their own environment to suit their needs.

Co-designing initiatives allows this to progress. It also invests people with dignity and values their input in becoming productive citizens within our community. Many people who have experienced profound trauma or disadvantage have clearly demonstrated significant resilience and a range of skills, which need to be recognised and respected in engagement initiatives from the start, allowing them to work alongside professionals in co-designing, planning, implementing and even evaluating activities, projects and programs together.

Co-designing involves fostering a sense of curiosity; to be open, honest and deeply inquisitive about people's lives. We need to forget the idea that expertise or professionalism means getting something right immediately or knowing all the answers. Professionals need to be inclusive of people's ideas, lived experience of illness and use of services within the community.

This approach to designing services is clearly supported by government policy. For example, in *Victoria's 10-Year Mental Health Plan* (Victorian Department of Health and Human Services, 2015b), the Victorian government has recognised the value and importance of co-design—that multiple sets of expertise and knowledge can enhance recovery through:

■ professional training and experience, research and evidence-based practice
■ personal experiences of distress and personal journals of recovery
■ personal experiences of caring for someone with mental illness (Victorian Department of Health and Human Services, 2015b, p. 18).

Co-design involves working alongside many vulnerable people experiencing mental health issues to create genuine effective interventions, services and programs that will work in the context of their lives and reflect their goals and values in life (Victorian Department of Health and Human Services, 2015b, p. 19).

This involves letting go of professional assumptions about consumers' perspectives and experiences, and, more importantly, actively and directly learning from what consumers say and do. Expertise, professional knowledge and research can then be considered in relation to group input—to add colour, insights and more importantly the possibilities of approaching realistic approaches to the social problems of specific groups. The partners in recovery (PiR) program is a case where a more consistent approach enables clearer outcomes for people living with severe illness, with measures reflecting the social determinants of mental health and well-being. PiR works towards better recovery-oriented outcomes for people living with complex needs. Better coordination of services improves both consumer outcomes and service efficiencies. System collaboration promotes collective ownership of consumer outcomes and system innovations (Grzelinska & Hayden, 2016, p. 35).

Co-design is different from traditional feedback methods that ask user groups to comment on their use of or the satisfaction with services that have already been planned or implemented. Co-design begins with people and looks at their experiences, perspectives, values, challenges and understandings as part of the service planning process. It looks beyond people's vulnerabilities, which can challenge the way service-providers work with people experiencing vulnerabilities.

MIND UK (2013) suggests that six principles provide the foundation for co-design:

1   *Taking an assets-based approach*—transforming the perception of people, so that they are seen not as passive recipients of services and burdens on the system, but as equal partners in designing and delivering services.
2   *Building on people's existing capabilities*—altering the delivery model of public services from a deficit approach to one that provides opportunities to recognise and grow people's capabilities and actively support them to put these to use at an individual and community level.
3   *Reciprocity and mutuality*—offering people a range of incentives to work in reciprocal relationships with professionals and with each other, where there are mutual responsibilities and expectations.
4   *Peer support networks*—engaging peer and personal networks alongside professionals as the best way of transferring knowledge.
5   *Blurring distinctions*—removing the distinction between professionals and recipients, and between producers and consumers of services, by reconfiguring the way services are developed and delivered.
6   *Facilitating rather than delivering*—enabling public service agencies to become catalysts and facilitators rather than being the main providers themselves (Slay & Stephens, 2013, p. 3).

Another example of co-design is the Croydon Service User Network (SUN) in the UK, which has been explicitly co-designed by psychiatrists and consumers (Slay & Stephens, 2013). SUN members participate in the running of the service, provide feedback, represent their groups at the SUN Steering Group and work alongside staff to help in the running of the groups. This ongoing connection between consumers and professionals allows for a blurring of roles, and for building greater trust and a sense of shared endeavour. All members are making a valuable contribution in running the network, organising group meetings or providing direct support to other members (Slay & Stephens, 2013, p. 7).

Recovery colleges

Recovery colleges, or recovery education centres, reinforce and allow people to focus on their strengths, rather than drawing attention to what is wrong with them, which can occur even with the best intentions of helping people to get better (Perkins et al., 2012). Recovery colleges use an education model for approaching recovery.

Established in 2013, the Mind Recovery College was the first recovery college in Australia. It operates on the basis of two ideas: that valuable knowledge and skills can be gained from first-hand experience of mental distress; and that learning can aid people to recover a life they value. The College's co-design approach means that people with personal experience of mental distress are involved in the design and delivery of courses and the running of the College, as well as participating in its activities (Mind Australia, 2012). The College began offering courses in 2013 and now presents more than 50 courses across seven campuses in Victoria and South Australia. The majority of these are run by people with lived experience of mental ill-health—46 per cent have personal experience and 11 per cent are carers or family (Parnell, et al., 2016).

Within recovery colleges people discover who they are and learn skills and tools to promote recovery, which allows them to understand the unique contributions they have to offer. Moving from a therapeutic to an educational approach carries with it a number of caring changes in its focus on relationships with people that are central to promoting effective recovery. The educational approach:

- helps people recognise and make use of their talents and resources rather than defining them through their problems, deficits or dysfunctions, as can be the case with therapy.
- supports people to achieve their goals and ambitions rather than focusing all activities as therapies.
- allows staff to become coaches who help people find their own solutions rather than defining problems and applying professional therapy.
- encourages people to choose their own courses and become experts in managing their own lives—rather than maintaining a power imbalance where professionals are the only experts (Perkins et al., 2012).

CRITICAL THINKING OPPORTUNITY

Through the weblink www.recoverycollege.org.au search for the recovery college within your area and find out what programs are running for consumers with a mental illness.

How do you think you could use some of these resources when you work with consumers and their carers who have a mental illness?

While recovery colleges have proven popular with consumers, they are not designed to replace specialist mental health assessment and treatment services or outreach support work. Rather, they are designed to complement specialist and community services.

Hardy (2016, p. 10) argues recovery colleges present a welcoming and inclusive service model, which is important in enabling people to find the confidence to attend and participate. Involvement in a recovery college helps people to find connection and support from others in their community. Hardy feels something powerful happens when people come together for the purpose of sharing their knowledge and experience to produce something of value for others. This is particularly evident in co-design workshops, where between ten and twenty participants are involved, usually for two to three hours. Participants often demonstrate the ability to discuss very personal and emotional experiences while retaining the ability to talk about elements that might be important in course design. Being able to simultaneously engage with emotional and cognitive functions provides the opportunity for reflection and understanding. This is especially true in an environment where individuals are able to hear the experiences and thoughts of others who have similar challenges in their recovery (Hardy, 2016).

This can create a partnership arrangement with the mental health service that allows the creation of many opportunities, including the reduction of costs through co-designed seminars or courses that decrease isolation or increase peer support, while at the same time offering a broad range of professional expertise. Importantly, recovery colleges create a network of social opportunities among peers and the general community, which reduces the social isolation for people experiencing mental illness.

Peer support

Peer support services are based on the belief that individuals who have lived experience relating to mental health, life-changing events, addictions or problem behaviours can relate to people experiencing the same problems and trying to deal with similar issues—as opposed to those who provide care and who have not had these same experiences (Hardy, 2016). People with such lived experience have worked as consumer advocates, consumer representatives and peer workers in the public mental health sector for the past two decades, but according to the authors of the NSW strategic plan, *Living well: A strategic plan for mental health in NSW 2014–2024*, do not always encounter positive acceptance (Hardy, 2016). Stigma and discrimination, sometimes subtle and sometimes obvious, can cause a divide between the peer workforce and other staff. Formal structures, policies and procedures that support the peer workforce and provide a development pathway are needed if government services are to realise their full potential (Hardy, 2016).

The inclusion of the peer support model has the potential to be a great value in service provision for government and not-for-profit providers in the mental health field. There has been a considerable growth in services by not-for-profit service providers. Mind Australia, for example, has developed a suite of residentially based services in Victoria, including peer-recovery committees, prevention and recovery case services, community-based residential recovery care, youth residential rehabilititation and supported accommodation services (Mind Australia, 2017). The impact of such programs has been greatly underestimated, yet they have played an important role in providing support for consumers. Everyone living with or experiencing a mental health issue has the right to access avenues to share their lived experience in a confidential, safe environment where they are heard, respected, honoured and understood (Centre of Excellence in Peer Support, 2015).

CRITICAL THINKING OPPORTUNITY

1   After reviewing Mind Australia's website (www.mindaustralia.org.au/need-help/mind-services-in-victoria/mind-victoria/residential-services.html) and the services that they offer to individuals and carers, what gaps do you think might remain?

2   What do you think might be a barrier to individuals wanting to seek assistance from Mind Australia?

It allows opportunities to understand and de-stigmatise mental health issues through the power of sharing information. It gives a renewed sense of self-respect, understanding and belonging to consumers through being part of a circle of a caring community. It allows people to rediscover themselves and possibly activate their own personal hidden resources enabling them to do greater things (Centre of Excellence in Peer Support, 2015).

SECTION 2   CARER LEADERSHIP AND PARTICIPATION

SUSAN JOHNSTON

Carer participation

The *National Standards for Mental Health Services* (Australian Government Department of Health, 2010) and the *National Standards for the Mental Health Workforce* (Australian Government Department of Health, 2013) set out the requirements for carer-inclusive practices in which carers are included in treatment planning decision-making and are actively involved in the development, planning, delivery and evaluation of services. Despite these standards, it is common for carers to feel excluded. According to the Australian Commission on Safety and Quality in Health Care (2014), carer-inclusive practice has not been universally implemented and remains a work in progress.

EVAN BICHARA, SUSAN JOHNSON AND IAN MUNRO

Evidence supports the participation of carers in collaboration with consumers and clinicians in planning mental health care to optimise outcomes (Wallcraft et al., 2011). However, carers commonly report experiencing feeling isolated and excluded (Eassom et al., 2014; Rowe, 2012; Victorian Department of Health and Human Services, 2015b). Carers report feeling marginalised, uninformed, disempowered, ignored, not respected or taken seriously and excluded from decision-making in Australian studies (Lawn & McMahon, 2015; Lawn et al., 2013). A *Carers' Recognition Act* was first passed in WA in 2004 and since then other Australian states and territories have passed legislation. The Victorian Government introduced a *Carers' Recognition Act* in 2012 (Victorian Government, 2013) and a new Mental Health Act in 2014 (Victorian Government, 2014). Under the *Carers' Recognition Act 2012* (Vic), carers are 'encouraged to take part in care planning and making decisions about care' (Victorian Department of Health & Human Services, 2012, p. 3). The Victorian *Mental Health Act 2014* (Victorian Government, 2014) requires service providers to involve carers in decisions about assessment, treatment and recovery, and to recognise, respect and support the carer's role. Professional attitudes to communication and engagement with carers was identified as a barrier to upholding the rights of carers in a systematic review by Rowe (2012). Establishment of the Mental Health Complaints Commission, in 2014, has provided carers with an avenue to ensure their voices are heard. Carers and organisations representing mental health carers, such as Tandem, have promoted the movement towards carer inclusive practice.

Carer burden

The role of 'carer' is commonly thrust upon family members for the first time by a crisis when their loved one first becomes unwell. Carers are 'often overwhelmed, confused, and fearful' (Lovelock, 2016, p. 15) and commonly experience 'demoralization, conflict, and self-blame' (McFarlane, 2016, p. 7). When medications are prescribed for people with serious mental illness it is commonly the role of the carer to ensure compliance and this can put the carer in the role of an enforcer.

> Lacking in knowledge and wanting their loved one to be better, carers often find themselves aligning with 'professionals' who appear to offer solutions. This dynamic often fractures the relationship between 'carer' and now 'consumer', further shattering the individuality and mutuality of their previous relationship. Ultimately this situation doesn't support the recovery journey.
>
> ———————————
> Lovelock (2016, p. 15)

The burden of caring commonly impacts negatively upon the mental and physical health of carers (Pinquart & Sorensen, 2003; Schulz & Sherwood, 2008). The carer burden of people diagnosed with a mental illness is higher than carers of people with somatic illnesses (Ampalam, Gunturu & Padma, 2012; Hastrup at al., 2011). The caring role can consume a person's life till they feel they have lost their former self-identity and they need to reconstruct their identity incorporating their caring role. 'Effects of the caring role include social isolation, loss of friendship, community disconnection and unemployment' (Lovelock, 2016, p. 16).

Participants of Family Peer Education Programs run by the Mental Illness Fellowship report being personally impacted by grief and loss, poor emotional and physical health, financial concerns and stigma (Lovelock, 2016). Both consumers and carers report experiencing disconnection, loss of hope, loss of identity, disruption of the meaning in their lives, and disempowerment (Lovelock, 2016). When family members lack knowledge and understanding of their loved one's condition, they can create unachievable demands and expectations, and become anxious, exasperated, demoralised or even hostile, putting the consumer at increased risk of relapse (McFarlane, 2016).

Carers have their own recovery journey to travel. Factors identified to be important to consumers in their recovery are hope, identity, empowerment, meaningful life and connection (Leamy et al., 2011; Mancini, Hardiman & Lawson, 2005). Peer support workers are found to increase hope, empowerment and social connectedness of consumers (Davidson et al., 2012; Repper & Carter, 2011; Walker & Bryant, 2013). Carers on their own recovery journey also need to be provided with hope, empowerment and connection. Lovelock (2016) recommends CHIME (Leamy et al., 2011) as a framework for supporting carers on their own recovery journey. Leamy and colleagues (2011) developed the conceptual framework based upon data from a systematic review and narrative synthesis on personal recovery in mental illness. The CHIME framework (**C**onnectedness; **H**ope and optimism about the future; **I**dentity; **M**eaning in life; and **E**mpowerment) comprises thirteen characteristics of the recovery journey and five identified recovery processes. Characteristics of the recovery journey are as follows:

Recovery is an active process

Individual and unique process

Non-linear process

Recovery as a journey

Recovery as stages or phases

Recovery as a struggle

Multidimensional process

Recovery is a gradual process

Recovery as a life-changing experience

Recovery without cure

Recovery is aided by supportive and healing environment

Recovery can occur without professional intervention

Trial and error process.

Leamy et al. (2011, p. 448)

Identified recovery processes:

Category 1: Connectedness

Peer support and support groups

Relationships

Support from others

Being part of the community

Category 2: Hope and optimism about the future

Belief in possibility of recovery

Motivation to change

Hope-inspiring relationships

Positive thinking and valuing success

Having dreams and aspirations

Category 3: Identity

Dimensions of identity

Rebuilding/redefining positive sense of identity

Overcoming stigma

Category 4: Meaning in life

Meaning of mental illness experiences

Spirituality

Quality of life

Meaningful life and social roles

Meaningful life and social goals

Rebuilding life

Category 5: Empowerment

Personal responsibility

Control over life

Focusing upon strengths

Leamy et al. (2011, p. 448)

Carer support groups

Carer support groups can provide the peer support needed to facilitate the carer's recovery journey (Reay-Young, 2000). Recently, carer peer workers have been employed by some clinical services to provide support to carers in their recovery journey. Organisations such as Tandem, MIND, SANE, ARAFMI and the MI Fellowship offer support to carers of people with a mental illness. Online forums are also available for carer peers to give and receive support.

In 2008, David Clark set up an online community named Wired into Recovery (WITR). Clark (2016) aimed to 'create an environment in which people can inspire and learn from each other and provide mutually beneficial support' and create hope, understanding and a sense of belonging.

Lisbeth Riis Cooper, co-founder of the Cooper Riis Healing Community (a non-profit psychosocial rehabilitation residential facility in the USA), shares her recovery story from a carer perspective on the Wired into Recovery website (Cooper, 2012). She says:

> *We aren't always the main character.* For many of us, it takes a little time to realize that our family members are ultimately responsible for their own recovery. In fact, taking personal responsibility is the key to recovery. By sharing stories, families help each other learn how to let go, how to trust, how not to enable (or disable) and, yes, how to let our family members stumble sometimes. We are not the stars of these recovery stories, but we can play supportive roles.

> *We are the main character in our own recovery story.* When a family member struggles with extreme emotional states, all family members struggle. Families need support and encouragement to work on their own recovery process to heal and find joy again. When families regain balance through self-care, they become more supportive and available to their family member as well.

Consider what it would be like to be a carer for a moment.

1   What might it be like to provide care to a loved one?

2   What information might you want?

3   Who do you gain this from?

4   How does privacy work here?

Family psychoeducation for empowering carers and reducing carer burden

Empowerment is the perception that a person has choices and control over the consequences in his or her life. When carers' concerns are ignored and they are excluded from decision-making it can lead to feelings of disempowerment. For the carer to have the optimal positive impact on the care recipient, they need to maintain their own well-being. Consequently, the promotion of carer-inclusive practice is crucial to improving the quality of care and consumer outcomes.

Yesufu-Udechuku and colleagues (2015) conducted a systematic review and meta-analysis of interventions to improve the experience of caring for people with severe mental illness and concluded that psychosocial interventions can decrease caregiver burden and psychological distress and to improve carer quality of life. Psychoeducation multi-family groups (PMFGs) have been recommended as an evidence-based intervention for psychosis that reduces relapse, enhances recovery and improves the lives of carers (Hayes, Harvey & Farhall, 2013; McFarlane, 2016). Multi-family group treatment (MFGT) is a similar approach: 'A main theoretical foundation of MFGT is that by increasing social network size and support by enabling families to benefit from each other's experiences in solving problems, better illness course and improved outcome occur' (Stuart & Schlosser, 2009, p. 435). However, family psychoeducation (FPE) is rarely offered by mental health clinical services in Australia (Hayes, Harvey & Farhall, 2013). Two clinical services have introduced FPE in Victoria and evaluations have been very positive (Hayes, Harvey & Farhall, 2013). Wellways is a community mental health support organisation that offers multi-family psychoeducation courses (including a specific course for families dealing with dual diagnosis) in many states in Australia. These courses are facilitated by carer peers. My family found attending one of these courses very beneficial.

Mental health nurses can play a role in recommending group family psychoeducation to empower carers with knowledge and provide them with connections to facilitate their recovery journey and enable them to take a more proactive role in shaping the mental health services of the future.

Risk–benefit analysis

Consumers and carers can be distressed by the adverse effects associated with psychotropic medications, and when consumers and carers are excluded from decision-making their concerns are often ignored. Families are usually highly motivated to protect their loved one from harm. Estimating the magnitude of the benefits and risks associated with a proposed treatment is very difficult for consumers, carers and health professionals. The problem of under-reporting of adverse medication events has been recognised (Australian Health Ministers' Advisory Council, 2009; Gonzales-Gonzalez et al., 2013) and this leads to risks of adverse effects being under-estimated. This can seriously bias the analysis of risk versus benefit of pharmacological treatments. Significant uncertainty surrounds any claims made by clinicians that the benefits of a proposed treatment will greatly outweigh the risks associated with the treatment (Frances, 2013). The lack of accuracy involved in estimating the magnitude of the risks of adverse effects is a serious concern. Consequently, there is a legitimate need for consumer and carer concerns about adverse effects to be taken into consideration in treatment planning—because they experience the consequences.

Australian Health Ministers' Advisory Council (2009) developed a *Framework for Reducing Adverse Medication Events in Mental Health Services* and recommended that consumers, carers and health professionals be encouraged to report adverse medication events. Mental health practitioners are advised to provide consumers and carers with possible adverse reactions including the possibility of adverse medication events occurring in the long term (Australian Health Ministers' Advisory Council, 2009). Further, 'consumers should be involved in making decisions about their medications, and their input should be highly valued and respected' (Australian Health Ministers' Advisory Council, 2009, p. 8).

The Victorian *Mental Health Act 2014* (Victorian Government, 2014) legislates the inclusion of carers and consumers in treatment planning and legitimates the making of decisions that involve a degree of risk, and this includes risk of relapse. Consumers with serious mental illness bear a heavy burden of adverse effects; the burden increases over the long term and it is debatable whether the benefits outweigh the risks (Gøtzsche, Young & Crace, 2015; Moncrieff, 2015). The impact of antipsychotics on dopamine receptors can exacerbate addictive behaviours leading to nicotine and caffeine addictions (de Haan et al., 2006) and pathological gambling (European Medicines Agency, 2016; Health Canada, 2015). When the concerns of consumers and carers to minimise the long-term harm associated with pharmacological treatment are overlooked in favour of prioritising relapse prevention at all cost, in risk-averse organisational cultures consumers and carers can feel disempowered, hindering their recovery.

Deegan (1996, p. 3) describes how being over-medicated feels:

> They kept telling us that these medications were good for us and yet we could feel the high dose neuroleptics transforming us into empty vessels. We felt like will-less souls or the walking dead as the numbing indifference and drug induced apathy took hold. At such high doses, neuroleptics radically diminished our personhood and sense of self.

Polypharmacy is widely practised in psychiatry with the associated increased risk of adverse effects due to drug-drug interactions (Kukreja et al., 2013). Epidemiologic studies provide evidence that some psychotropic medications are associated with an increased risk of aggression and violence (Lucire, 2016; Moore, Glenmullen & Furberg, 2010). This can have catastrophic consequences for consumers, carers and health professionals. Carers and consumers need to be empowered with unbiased information upon which to base decisions regarding treatment planning. According to Frances (2013, p. 90), when prescribing psychiatric medications, 'there is never a fair risk/benefit/cost calculus—the benefits are exaggerated, the risks minimized, the costs ignored.' Frances (2013, p. 90) claims that 'side effects and complications are measured perfunctorily and barely reported'. Further:

> Evaluations of benefits and harms are based on group data, which have to be applied to judgments for individual patients and can therefore be advisory only; the individual's subjective experience is crucially important to consider.

Gøtzsche et al. (2015)

RxISK (https://rxisk.org) is an independent drug safety website, run by medical experts, providing information on reported adverse events.

Pressure on availability of inpatient beds impacts upon the priorities of clinical services, which need to minimise risk of relapse and hospitalisation. This can be in conflict with the priority of consumers and carers to minimise the risk of side effects of the medications.

High rates of non-compliance with treatment among people with serious mental illness are reported in the literature (Aldridge, 2011). Consumers choose to stop taking medication for various reasons including the perception that the adverse effects outweigh the benefits. Abrupt withdrawal of antipsychotics can precipitate a withdrawal-related relapse (Moncrieff, 2006). Abrupt withdrawal of antidepressants can have very serious negative consequences. Coercing consumer to comply with prescribed treatment can impact negatively upon their sense of autonomy and result in consumers and carers feeling disempowered. 'Recovery involves regaining active control over one's life' (Aldridge, 2011, p. 5).

Aldridge (2011) recommends a planned non-adherence harm-reduction intervention that involves supporting those who make the decision to stop taking psychiatric medication by providing information on slow tapering to reduce the harm of abrupt withdrawal and supporting and monitoring the consumer during the withdrawal process; see, for example, the *Harm Reduction Guide to Coming Off Psychiatric Drugs* (Hall, 2007). The non-adherence harm reduction approach 'acknowledges the patient's ability to choose and learn from experience' (Aldridge, 2011, p. 2). According to Hall (2007, p. 6), 'the essence of any healthy life is the capacity to be empowered'.

After many years of paternalistic treatment, one of my loved ones moved to a different clinical service and was given the opportunity to make a decision that involved a degree of risk of relapse but offered him the chance to reduce the impact of serious medication side effects. I advocated on my loved one's behalf and quoted the relevant section of the Victorian *Mental Health Act 2014*: '11 (d) persons receiving mental health services should be allowed to make decisions about their assessment, treatment and recovery that involve a degree of risk' (Victorian Government, 2014, p. 21).

With some reluctance his wishes were respected and he felt empowered and hopeful. He has since made remarkably good progress in his recovery. A common theme that has emerged from lived experience stories of recovery is that regaining 'control over and input into one's life' (Scottish Recovery Network, 2006, p. 1) is crucial to recovery. According to Brown and Kandirikirira (2007, p. 9):

> Social influences on recovery included the flexibility and responsiveness of services to
> individual needs, the willingness of friends, family and community to encourage, enable
> and empower individuals to take risks; and the willingness and cooperation of others not to
> undermine individuals allowing them the right to self-determination.

A priority of the Victorian Department of Health and Human Services' *Strategic Plan* is 'Empowering patients, clients and carers':

> The freedom to make decisions that affect our lives is a fundamental right that each of us should
> enjoy. Exercising control supports self-esteem and preserves dignity and human rights.

Victorian Department of Health and Human Services (2015a, p. 32)

Changing an entrenched risk-averse organisational culture, with treatments based predominantly on the biomedical model, to a recovery-oriented, consumer- and carer-inclusive culture is going to take a long time, but progress is being made. A culture change to a recovery orientation will require services to move from 'a narrow focus on symptom reduction' (Perkins et al., 2012, p. 2) 'to thinking more broadly about options that enhance people's autonomy and self-determination in the ways their recovery is supported' (Mind Australia, 2012, p. 7).

Two National Health Service (NHS) Trusts in London published a position statement in which the issue of risk was discussed as follows:

> Risk is inherent in all mental health services and in Recovery-oriented services risk will remain. However it is sometimes necessary to take risks in order to learn and grow. A Recovery-oriented service will require a change in our emphasis from risk avoidance to constructive and creative risk taking. We must seek to differentiate between the risks that must be minimised (self-harm, harm to others) and the risks which people have a right to experience.

South London and Maudsley NHS Foundation Trust and South West London and
St George's Mental Health NHS Trust (2010, p. 19)

Social context

My experiences as a carer interacting with mental health clinical services are that the emphasis is on biomedical treatments and little attention is paid to the social context of people's lives, despite strong evidence of the impact of social factors influencing the development of mental distress. Contexts of adversity, trauma, abuse and racism greatly increase the risk of experiencing psychosis (Read & Dillon, 2013; Read, Mosher & Bentall, 2004). The focus of current services is on symptom reduction and medications. Scant attention is given to psychosocial interventions despite evidence supporting their efficacy.

Phillip Thomas is a UK psychiatrist who has worked in the NHS for over 20 years. Thomas (2015) emphasises the need to attend to the contexts of consumer' lives: 'People's contexts should be central to our understanding of psychosis and distress, yet far too often they are overlooked in the fruitless search for the biological origins of mental distress and technological solutions to its management' (Thomas, 2015, p. 27).

Parachute Crisis Respite Centres (CRCs) offer accommodation for people in psychiatric crisis as an alternative to an inpatient stay in a psychiatric hospital. Peer workers offer support in the centres. CRCs offer a safe, home-like, supportive environment where guests are taught to use new recovery and relapse prevention skills (Riverdale Mental Health Association, 2010). Alternative approaches to responding to people in crisis have shown good outcomes for consumers (Alexander at al., 2016). An evaluation of the Swedish Parachute Project found that 'it is possible to successfully treat FEP (First Episode Psychosis) consumer with fewer inpatient days and less neuroleptic medication than is usually recommended, when combined with intensive psychosocial treatment and support' (Cullberg et al., 2002, p. 276). Crisis Respite Services have been established in South Australia (SA Health, 2014). An evaluation by Zmudzki and colleagues (2016) found that consumers experienced improved satisfaction, quality of life, hope and belief in their potential to recover. Psychiatric hospital admissions and length of stay were reduced (Zmudski et al., 2016).

Carers witness their loved ones' distress when they are admitted as an involuntary consumer to a locked ward and are searching for alternatives that will offer a more peaceful environment. Crisis Respite Centres offer a feasible alternative.

Exploring an alternative model of crisis care: Open Dialogue

Open Dialogue was originally developed in West Lapland, Finland, in the 1980s. Open Dialogue is now the only model for all mental health treatment in this area. This area 'now has the best documented outcomes in the Western world' (Hetherington, 2015). Open Dialogue perceives psychosis as 'a temporary, radical, and terrifying alienation from shared communicative practices: a "no man's land" where unbearable experience has no words and no genuine agency' (Seikkula & Olson, 2003, p. 409). All psychiatric personnel, including nurses, are trained in family therapy or psychodynamic individual therapy, and all psychiatric crises are treated in a family- and network-centered manner by multidisciplinary crisis teams, mostly in the consumer's home (Aaltonen, Seikkula & Lehtinen, 2011). The person in acute distress is usually seen by the treating team, at the family home, along with all other important persons (that is, relatives, friends and other professionals) connected to the situation (Seikkula & Olson, 2003). Neither the consumer nor family is seen as the cause of psychosis or an object of treatment, but as 'competent or potentially competent partners in the recovery process' (Gleeson et al., 1999, p. 390, in Seikkula & Olson, 2003, p. 405). At two-year follow-up, 'it was found that 81 per cent of consumers did not have any residual psychotic symptoms and that 84 per cent had returned to full-time employment or studies. Only 33 per cent had used neuroleptic medication (Seikkula, Alakare & Aaltonen, 2011, p. 192).

Scandinavia, Russia, Germany, France and some states in the USA have introduced Open Dialogue (Hetherington, 2015). Peer-supported Open Dialogue (POD), a variant of the Open Dialogue model, will be piloted in four NHS trusts in the UK (Hetherington, 2015). The NSW Mental Health Commission also conducted a Forum on Open Dialogue (see 'Useful websites' at the end of this chapter). Many members of my carers' support group, including myself, are very impressed with the reported results of the use of Open Dialogue and have lobbied for its introduction in Australia.

ABOUT THE CONSUMER John and Mary's stories

John was admitted as an involuntary consumer to the inpatient unit after being visited by the Crisis Assessment Team who found him to be experiencing delusions and hallucinations, believing his parents to be imposters who are threatening him. John was frightened and timid, and admitted to having taken recreational drugs. Mary was told that her son's condition was caused by defective neurotransmitter functioning in the brain and that antipsychotics will relieve the symptoms.

John is traumatised by witnessing another consumer set himself on fire during his inpatient stay, and finds the high level of stimulation in the ward environment difficult to deal with. John is commenced on an antipsychotic medication, stabilised and discharged home.

John's father is very critical, hostile and domineering. John's functioning deteriorates. Mary witnesses her son's greatly increased appetite and weight, emotional blunting, decreased motivation, apathy and endless pacing (akathisia). John commences smoking and constantly craves nicotine and caffeine. Mary finds these changes very distressing and worries constantly about her son's poor quality of life and his long-term physical health. Mary expresses her concerns regarding these side effects, but her concerns are dismissed and ignored. Mary reports to the treating team that there has been a great deal of conflict in the family and she believes that this has had a very detrimental effect on John and that he needs to be in a more peaceful environment. The community mental health clinic treating team's focus is entirely on symptom reduction.

John decides to stop taking his medication gradually. Mary witnesses the return of her son's motivation, the cessation of the pacing and his appetite return to normal. However, after two months, John relapses and again becomes psychotic. John had to be coerced by Mary into taking his medication prior to this relapse because the distressing side effects made John reluctant to take the medication. After his relapse John is willing to regularly take his medication, without coaxing, having learnt from this experience. He no longer feels bullied into compliance. John attends the Community Mental Health Clinic and is commenced on Abilify (Aripirazole). Mary is told that

EVAN BICHARA, SUSAN JOHNSON AND IAN MUNRO

John will experience less restlessness (akathisia), lose weight and his mental state will improve to the point where he will be able to work in paid employment. Mary is told this medication may also cause increased agitation but this can be counteracted by giving Valium.

John's concentration improves and he no longer experiences delusions and hallucinations after the dose of Abilify is increased to above the recommended maximum dose. John begins exhibiting unprovoked rage, sudden, intermittent, aggressive verbal outbursts, something he has never done before. Valium causes John to be more disinhibited and his behaviour deteriorates. John also commences gambling obsessively and loses large sums of money. No connection is made by the treating team between the changes in behaviour and the high dose of Abilify. John's siblings witness the aggressive outbursts and are very frightened. John becomes estranged from all his family members and friends as they think the aggression is a symptom of his illness. Mary questions the safety of the treatment but the risk of aggression precipitated by this treatment is not acknowledged.

John is offered a scarce bed in a community residential psychosocial rehabilitation facility run by a non-clinical mental health community support organisation. He moves to the new location and changes treatment team. The new treating team listen to John and Mary and the Abilify is reduced slowly and he is commenced on an alternative antipsychotic. John's aggressive outbursts cease. John benefits from interaction with peers and a peer worker. He feels more connected and accepted. John is encouraged to be more independent and is empowered to make autonomous decisions, take more personal responsibility, set meaningful life goals and rebuild his identity. John's damaged relationships begin to heal. John and Mary both have restored hope in progress on their recovery journeys.

REFLECTION QUESTIONS

Discuss alternatives ways of addressing John's crisis.

1   What supports could you recommend for Mary?

2   What information could you provide to Mary to assist her in participating in treatment decisions?

3   How could John's family be helped to better cope with the stresses of having a family member with a serious mental illness?

SUMMARY

In this chapter students can develop insights into the inclusion of consumers' wishes into their day-to-day care, and how this has an impact upon their recovery. Through a variery of programs, consumers are assisting mental health professionals in the development and daily running of services. Their involvement is central to current mental health services.

The role of the carer is one that previously was omitted or ignored by mental health professionals, but today it is essential that their voices are heard, so they can gain information and nurses can learn from their wisdom about what strategies have been tried, been successful or failed for their loved one.

DISCUSSION QUESTIONS

1   How might you include consumers' thoughts and wishes into your care plan?

2   What are some of the personal biases that health-care individuals might have about including consumers' ideas into care plans?

3   What if any, do you think might be the benefits of including consumers' ideas about recovery into their care plan?

4   Carers often have a major role in providing care to consumers within the community; what information do you think they might require to be able to ensure this care is appropriate to the consumer?

5   What do you think your role might be in providing care to carers of consumers?

TEST YOURSELF

1   The inclusion of carers in mental health care can:

   a   improve carer and family well-being

   b   reduce carer stress and reduce their burden of care

   c   improve understanding of mental illness, treatments and services

   d   all of the above

2   Carer involvement can:

   a   reduce the incidences of relapse and improve adherence to treatment

   b   improve family functioning and increase periods of wellness

   c   improve the consumer's quality of life and social adjustment

   d   all of the above

3   Consumers have the right to contribute and participate as far as possible and may include:

   a   the development of mental health policy

   b   provision of mental health care

   c   representation of mental health consumer interests

   d   all of the above

4   Psychoeducation:

   a   improves family empowerment

   b   takes the place of other treatments

   c   is required for adherence with medication

   d   is only undertaken by trained psychotherapists

USEFUL WEBSITES

Inner South Family and Friends mental health-carers support group: http://ispaf.org/

Mental Health Carers Australia: www.mentalhealthcarersaustralia.org.au/

Mental Health Commission of NSW—Forum on 'Open Dialogue' crisis care: http://nswmentalhealthcommission.com.au/news/our-news/forum-on-open-dialogue-crisis-care

Mental Health Commission of NSW—The peer workforce: http://nswmentalhealthcommission.com.au/mental-health-and/the-peer-workforce

Mental Health Complaints Commissioner: www.mhcc.vic.gov.au/

Mental Illness Fellowship of Australia: www.mifa.org.au/

Mind Australia—Community resources for families and carers: https://www.mindaustralia.org.au/resources/families-and-carers.html

National Alliance on Mental Illness: www.nami.org

National Prescribing Service—Adverse Medicine Events Line: www.nps.org.au/contact-us/adverse-medicines-events

(1300 134 237)

Neami International—The importance of experience: www.neaminational.org.au/our-approach/peer-support-workers

RxISK: http://rxisk.org

SANE Australia—Families & carers: https://www.sane.org/families-carers

Tandem: https://tandemcarers.org.au

Wellways: https://www.wellways.org

YouTube—Open Dialogue: An alternative Finnish approach to healing psychosis: https://www.youtube.com/watch?v=HDVhZHJagfQ

YouTube—Open Dialogue presentation: New approaches to mental health services: https://www.youtube.com/watch?v=vRjk4_ybCqU&feature=youtu.be

REFERENCES

Aaltonen, J., Seikkula, J., & Lehtinen, K. (2011). The comprehensive Open-Dialogue approach in Western Lapland: I. The incidence of non-affective psychosis and prodromal states, *Psychosis, 3*(3), 179–191.

Aldridge, M. A. (2011). Addressing non-adherence to antipsychotic medication: A harm-reduction approach. *Journal of Psychiatric and Mental Health Nursing*, 1–12.

Alexander, M. J., Lindy, D., Munoz, A., Pessin, N., & Sadler, P. (2016). *Crisis as opportunity: Parachute NYC as a promising crisis alternative practice*. National Alliance on Mental Illness (NAMI) Convention, Denver. Retrieved from https://www.nami.org/getattachment/Get-Involved/NAMI-National-Convention/2015-Convention-Presentation-Slides-and-Resources/B-2-Crisis-as-Opportunity-Integrating-Peers-into-Crisis-Alternatives-in-Parachute-NYC.pdf.

Ampalam, P., Gunturu, S., & Padma, V. (2012). A comparative study of caregiver burden in psychiatric illness and chronic medical illness. *Indian Journal of Psychiatry, 54*(3), 239–243. http://doi.org/10.4103/0019-5545.102423.

Australian Commission on Safety and Quality in Health Care (2014). *Scoping study on the implementation of National Standards in Mental Health Services*. Sydney: ACSQHC.

Australian Government Department of Health (2010). *National standards for mental health services*. Retrieved from www.health.gov.au/internet/main/publishing.nsf/Content/CFA833CB8C1AA178CA257BF0001E7520/$File/serv3.pdf.

Australian Health Ministers' Advisory Council (2009). *Framework for reducing adverse medication events in mental health services*. Retrieved from https://www.health.gov.au/internet/main/publishing.nsf/Content/CE22F94BA006DC4FCA257D9300123435/$File/adverse.pdf.

Brown, W., & Kandirikirira, N. (2007). *Recovering mental health in Scotland. Report on narrative investigation of mental health recovery*. Glasgow:, Scottish Recovery Network. Retrieved from http://scottishrecovery.net/wp-content/uploads/2008/03/Recovering_mental_health_in_Scotland_2007.pdf.

Clark, D. (2016). *Wired into recovery*. Retrieved from www.recoverystories.info/wired-in-to-recovery/.

Centre of Excellence in Peer Support (2015). *Charter of peer support*. Retrieved from www.peersupportvic.org/peer-support-charter.

Cooper, L. R. (2012). *The power of storytelling*. Retrieved from www.recoverystories.info/the-power-of-storytelling-by-lisbeth-riis-cooper/.

Cullberg, J., Levander, S., Holmqvist, R., Mattsson, M., & Wieselgren, I.-M. (2002). One-year outcome in first episode psychosis patients in the Swedish Parachute project. *Acta Psychiatrica Scandinavia*, 106, 276–285.

Davidson, L., Bellamy, C., Guy, K., & Miller, R. (2012). Peer support among persons with severe mental illnesses: A review of evidence and experience. *World Psychiatry, 11*(2), 123–128.

de Haan, L., Booij, J., Lavalaye, J., van Amelsvoort, T., & Linszen, D. (2006). Occupancy of dopamine D2 receptors by antipsychotic drugs is related to nicotine addiction in young patients with schizophrenia. *Psychopharmacology, 183*(4), 500–505.

Deegan, P. E. (1996). Recovery and the conspiracy of hope. *Sixth Annual The MHS Conference of Australia and New Zealand* (pp. 1–14). Brisbane.

Eassom, E., Giacco, D., Dirik, A., & Priebe, S. (2014). Implementing family involvement in the treatment of patients with psychosis: A systematic review of facilitating and hindering factors. *BMJ Open, 4*(10). doi: 10.1136/bmjopen-2014-006108.

European Medicines Agency (2016). *Abilify*. Accessed from www.ema.europa.eu/docs/en_GB/document_library/EPAR_-_Procedural_steps_taken_and_scientific_information_after_authorisation/human/000471/WC500020172.pdf.

Frances, A. (2013). *Saving normal.* New York: Harper Collins.

Gleeson, J., Jackson, H., Stavely, H., & Burnett, P. (1999). Family Intervention in early psychosis. In P. McGorry & H. Jackson (Eds.), *The recognition and management of early psychosis* (pp. 380–415). Cambridge: Cambridge University Press.

Gonzalez-Gonzalez, C., Lopez-Gonzalez, E., Herdeiro, M. T., & Figueiras, A. (2013). Strategies to improve adverse drug reaction reporting: A critical and systematic review. *Drug Safety, 36*(5), 317–328. doi: 10.1007/s40264–013–0058–2.

Gøtzsche, P. C., Young, A. H., & Crace, J. (2015). Does long term use of psychiatric drugs cause more harm than good? *BMJ, 350*, h2435. http://doi.org/10.1136/bmj.h2435.

Grzelinska, V., & Hayden, R. (2016). A systems approach to improving mental health outcomes: Views from Partners in Recovery. Vicserv mental health conference, May 2016.

Hall, W. (2007). *Harm reduction guide to coming off psychiatric drugs.* Freedom Center and The Icarus Project. Retrieved from www.willhall.net/files/ComingOffPsychDrugsHarmReductGuide2Edonline.pdf.

Hardy, D. (2016). *Living well: A strategic plan for mental health in NSW 2014–2024.* Retrieved from http://nswmentalhealthcommission.com.au/mental-health-and/the-peer-workforce.

Hastrup, L. H., Van Den Berg, B., & Gyrd-Hansen, D. (2011). Do informal caregivers in mental illness feel more burdened? A comparative study of mental versus somatic illnesses. *Scandinavian Journal of Public Health, 39*(6), 598–607.

Hayes, L., Harvey, C., & Farhall, J. (2013). Family psychoeducation for the treatment of psychosis. *InPsch, 35*(2).

Health Canada (2015). Safety information for antipsychotic drug Abilify and risk of certain impulse-control behaviours . Retrieved from http://healthycanadians.gc.ca/recall-alert-rappel-avis/hc-sc/2015/55668a-eng.php.

Hetherington, J. (2015). Peer-supported Open Dialogue. *Therapy Today, 26*(10), 26–29.

Kukreja, S., Kalra, G., Shah, N., & Shrivastava, A. (2013). Polypharmacy in psychiatry: A review. *Mens Sana Monographs, 11*(1), 82–99.

Lawn, S., & McMahon, J. (2015). Experiences of family carers of people diagnosed with borderline personality disorder. *Journal of Psychiatric and Mental Health Nursing, 22*(4), 234–243. doi: 10.1111/jpm.12193.

Lawn, S., Walsh, J., Barbara, A., Springga, M. Y., & Sutton, P. (2013). The bond we share: Experiences of caring for a person with mental and physical health conditions. In R. Woolfolk & L. Allen (Eds.), *Mental disorders: Theoretical and empirical perspectives.* InTech.

Leamy, M., Bird, V., Le Boutillier, C., Williams, J., & Slade, M. (2011). A conceptual framework for personal recovery in mental health: Systematic review and narrative synthesis, *British Journal of Psychiatry, 199*(6), 445–452.

Lovelock, R. (2016). Recovery from a carer perspective new paradigm: Towards recovery hope, innovation and co-design. *Australian Journal of Psychosocial Rehabilitation.* Retrieved from www.vicserv.org.au/images/PDF/newparadigm_/2016-autumn-newparadigm.pdf.

Lucire, Y. (2016). Pharmacological iatrogenesis: Substance/medication-induced disorders that masquerade as mental illness. *Epidemiology, 6*, 217.

Mancini, M. A., Hardiman, E., & Lawson, H. (2005). Making sense of it all: Consumer providers' theories about factors facilitating and impeding recovery from psychiatric disabilities. *Psychiatric Rehabilitation Journal, 29*(1), 48–55.

McFarlane, W. R. (2016). Family interventions for schizophrenia and the psychoses: A review. *Family Process* doi:10.1111/famp.12235.

Mind Australia (2012). *Establishment of the mind recovery college: A concept paper.* Retrieved from www.recoverycollege.org.au/images/Articles/Mind_Recovery_College_Concept_Paper_2012.pdf.

Mind Australia (2017). *Residential services.* Retrieved from https://www.mindaustralia.org.au/need-help/mind-services-in-victoria/mind-victoria/residential-services.html.

MIND UK (2013). In Slay, J., & Stephens, L. (Eds.) (2013), *Co-production in Mental health: A literature review.* London: MIND for Better Mental Health, New Economics foundation.

Moncrieff, J. (2006). Does antipsychotic withdrawal provoke psychosis? Review of the literature on rapid onset psychosis (supersensitivity psychosis) and withdrawal-related relapse. *Acta Psychiatrica Scandanavia, 114*(1), 3–13.

Moncrieff, J. (2015). Antipsychotic maintenance treatment: Time to rethink? *PLoS Med, 12*(8), e1001861. doi:10.1371/journal.pmed.1001861.

Moore, T. J., Glenmullen, J., & Furberg, C. D. (2010). Prescription drugs associated with reports of violence towards others. *PLoS ONE, 5*(12), e15337. doi:10.1371/journal.pone.0015337.

Parnell, D., McInerney, M., Liebhaber, D., Chaffey, E., & Van Wierst, M. (Eds.) (2016). *Towards recovery, new paradigm.* Psychiatric Disability Services of Victoria.

Perkins, R., Repper, J., Rinald, M., & Brown, H. (2012). *Recovery colleges.* UK: Centre for Mental Health.

Pinquart, M., & Sörensen, S. (2003). Differences between caregivers and noncaregivers in psychological health and physical health: A meta-analysis. *Psychology and Aging, 18*, 250-267.

Read, J., & Dillon, J.(Eds.) (2013). *Models of madness: Psychological, social and biological approaches to psychosis* (2nd ed.). Hove: Routledge.

Read, J., Mosher, L. R., & Bentall, R. P. (Eds.) (2004). *Models of madness: Psychological, social and biological approaches to psychosis.* Hove: Routledge.

Reay-Young, R. (2000). Support groups for relatives of people living with serious mental illness: An overview. *International Journal of Psychosocial Rehabilitation, 5*, 56–80.

Repper J., & Carter T. (2011). A review of the literature on peer support in mental health services. *Journal of Mental Health, 20*(4), 392–411.

Riverdale Mental Health Association (2010). *Parachute NYC: A new RMHA program.* Retrieved from http://rmha.org/programs-and-services/parachute/.

Rowe, J. (2012). Great expectations: A systematic review of the literature on the role of family carers in severe mental illness, and their relationships and engagement with professionals. *Journal of Psychiatric and Mental Health Nursing, 19*(1), 70–82. doi: 10.1111/j.1365–2850.2011.01756.x.

SA Health (2014). *Crisis respite—Facility and home based. Summary service model.* Adelaide: Government of South Australia.

Schulz, R., & Sherwood, P. R. (2008). Physical and Mental Health Effects of Family Caregiving. *The American Journal of Nursing, 108*(9 Suppl), 23–27. Retrieved from http://doi.org/10.1097/01.NAJ.0000336406.45248.4c.

Scottish Recovery Network (2006). *Journeys of recovery: Stories of hope and recovery from long term mental health problems.* Glasgow: Scottish Recovery Network. Retrieved from http://scottishrecovery.net/wp-content/uploads/2008/05/JourneysofRecovery-August-2009.pdf.

Seikkula, J., Alakare, B., & Aaltonen, J. (2011). The Comprehensive Open-Dialogue Approach in Western Lapland: II. Long-term stability of acute psychosis outcomes in advanced community care Psychosis 3,3,192–204.

Seikkula, J. & Olsen, M. (2003) The open dialogue approach: Its poetics and micropolitics. *Family Process, 42*, 3, 403–418.

Slay, J., & Stephens, L. (Eds.), *Co-production in Mental health: A literature review.* London: MIND for Better Mental Health, New Economics foundation.

South London and Maudsley NHS Foundation Trust and South West London and St George's Mental Health NHS Trust (2010. *Recovery is for All. Hope, Agency and Opportunity in Psychiatry. A Position Statement by Consultant Psychiatrists.* London: SLAM/SWLSTG. Retrieved from http://www.rcpsych.ac.uk/pdf/recovery%20is%20for%20all.pdf.

Stuart, B. K., & Schlosser, D. A. (2009). Multifamily group treatment for schizophrenia. *International Journal of Group Psychotherapy, 59*(3), 435–440. http://doi.org/10.1521/ijgp.2009.59.3.435.

Thomas, P. (2015). *Psychiatry in context.* Monmouth: PCCS Books.

Victorian Council of Social Service (2015). *Walk alongside: Co-designing social initiatives with people experiencing vulnerabilities.* Melbourne: VCOSS.

Victorian Department of Health and Human Services (2015a). Department of Health and Human Services Strategic Plan. Retrieved from http://dhhs.vic.gov.au/about/strategic-plan/.

Victorian Department of Health and Human Services (2015b). *Victoria's 10-year Mental Health Plan.* Retrieved from https://www2.health.vic.gov.au/mental-health/priorities-and-transformation/mental-health-priorities-for-victoria.

Victorian Department of Health and Human Services (2016). *Working with consumers and carers.* Retrieved from https://www2.health.vic.gov.au/mental-health/working-with-consumers-and-carers.

Victorian Government (2013). *Carers Recognition Act 2012*, Version 2. Retrieved from www.legislation.vic.gov.au/domino/Web_Notes/LDMS/LTObject_Store/LTObjSt7.nsf/DDE300B846EED9C7CA257616000A3571/0F775B508CE892D9CA257B96000AE0F3/$FILE/12−10a002bookmarked.pdf.

Victorian Government (2014). *Mental Health Act 2014.* Retrieved from www.legislation.vic.gov.au/domino/web_notes/ldms/pubstatbook.nsf/f932b66241ecf1b7ca256e92000e23be/0001F48EE2422A10CA257CB4001D32FB/$FILE/14−026aa%20authorised.pdf.

Walker, G., & Bryant, W. (2013). Peer support in adult mental health services: A metasynthesis of qualitative findings. *Psychiatric Rehabilitation Journal, 36*(1), 28–34.

Wallcraft, J. A. N., Amering, M., Freidin, J., Davar, B., Froggatt, D., Jafri, H.,

Herrman, H. (2011). Partnerships for better mental health worldwide: WPA recommendations on best practices in working with service users and family carers. *World Psychiatry, 10*(3), 229–236.

Yesufu-Udechuku, A., Harrison, B., Mayo-Wilson, E., Young, N., Woodhams, P., Shiers, D., Kuipers, E., & Kendall, T. (2015). Interventions to improve the experience of caring for people with severe mental illness: Systematic review and meta-analysis. *British Journal of Psychiatry, 206*(4), 268–274. doi: 10.1192/bjp.bp.114.147561.

Zmudzki, F, Griffiths, A., Bates, S., Katz, I., & Kayess, R. (2016). *Evaluation of Crisis Respite Services: Final report.* Social Policy Research Centre, University of New South Wales. Retrieved from https://www.sprc.unsw.edu.au/media/SPRCFile/Crisis_Respite_Services_Evaluation__Final_Report.pdf.

PART 2

Challenges to People's Mental Health

Our understanding of what constitutes mental illness has significantly increased in the past few decades. We are now aware that mental illness and associated challenges in living with, and overcoming mental health issues, are very complex, impacting on virtually every aspect of a person's daily life—psychological, emotional, physical, social, cultural and spiritual. Individuals experiencing mental health challenges struggle to understand what is happening to them and what they can do to work through their illness experience. Families of those with a mental illness are also confronted with challenges of how to be there to support their loved one while trying to come to terms with what is happening to them.

As mental health nurses, it is incumbent on each one of us to be highly skilled and knowledgeable about the causation, symptom presentation, diagnosis and management of mental illnesses and be able to work in partnership with mental health consumers and their families as the person moves toward recovery.

Part 2 of this text introduces you to a range of mental health conditions that people may experience across the spectrum of the life-cycle including, mood and anxiety disorders, psychosis, personality disorders, eating disorders, alcohol, tobacco and other drugs and mental health challenges encountered by young people and the older person.

Therapeutic interventions used within the context of difference illness experiences are discussed with particular attention to the role of the nurse in engaging with the consumer and family in providing quality holistic and consumer-focused care.

CHAPTER 10

Mood and Anxiety Disorders

MARGARET MCALLISTER
AND WENDY CROSS

Acknowledgment

The authors would like to acknowledge the contribution of Gerry Dares who co-wrote this chapter in the second edition.

KEY OUTCOMES

AFTER READING THIS CHAPTER, YOU SHOULD BE ABLE TO:

- define the common terms related to mood
- state the distinguishing features of anxiety
- state the distinguishing features of depression
- distinguish between the different mood conditions
- discuss the management of a consumer with a mood condition.

KEY TERMS

- affect
- anxiety
- bipolar disorder
- cognitive behaviour therapy (CBT)
- depression
- dysthymia
- flight of ideas
- hypomania
- major depressive disorders
- mania
- mood
- resilience

Introduction

This chapter presents an overview of different mood disorders, focusing specifically on anxiety, depression and bipolar disorders. The chapter begins by exploring some of the complex features of mood before examining each of these three main disorders in some depth. Theories of causation and best available therapeutic interventions are discussed, as well as the role that mental health nurses can play in facilitating comfort, restoring homeostasis and promoting well-being and recovery.

What is mood?

A mood is simply the way a person feels, usually over an extended period of time. But understanding this is never simple. Feelings are the result of complex interplays between genetics, biological status (including hormone and neurotransmitter levels), psychological traits, social experiences, intellectual or cognitive reasoning and life circumstances (Bronson & Bronson, 2013).

Mood has a strong influence on behaviour. For example, if a person is feeling apathetic they are unlikely to exercise. Mood is also difficult to control. If a person feels sad or depressed, for example, it is not easy to simply put this feeling aside and get on with the business of work and social interactions. Moods are sometimes difficult to distinguish from one another. Consider the moods of delight and excitement, for example. You might be able to tell the difference between them in yourself, but would you be able to distinguish them in a young child, or perhaps a person with dementia?

People differ in their ability to give names to different moods. Their gender, age or life circumstances can also be factors—if they have suffered past traumas, for example, they may attribute an erroneous descriptor to their own moods, or to other people's moods. The term for an inability to give words to emotions is 'alexithymia' and is thought to be quite a common personality trait (Maclaren, 2006). Such people may have difficulty distinguishing between bodily sensations that are linked to emotions. Their repertoire of emotions may be limited to just a few, such as 'I'm happy' or 'I'm angry'. As you can imagine, with such a limited repertoire the person may not go on to develop good emotional intelligence, which can lead to emotional detachment from others.

Because moods are strongly linked to the endocrine and central nervous systems, they can sometimes be released in surges. In adolescence, for example, when a child's body is changing, the experience of labile (that is, rapidly swinging) moods is common. This is difficult for both the young person and those around them—such as parents, teachers and peers—to understand and accept. During menses, at menopause and during life crises when endocrine surges occur, emotional arousal can be extreme or unusual. A person bursting into laughter at the death of a loved one, for example, could be the result of a biologically induced mood fluctuation.

Moods can sometimes be unpredictable. While it is common to feel happy when events around us are positive, and sad when events are upsetting, there may be times when moods arise that are surprising and cause concern; for example, feeling blue for no discernible reason, feeling bursts of anger or feeling on edge without knowing why. When moods occur in an intensity that is uncomfortable, have a long duration and interfere with daily life, they may be identified as disordered.

As we know, hormones can be stimulated and released as a result of interactions within the social environment and this will of course have an impact on mood. Falling in love is a classic example: person meets person, feels an attraction and the mood of each is uplifted. They begin to feel happy, perhaps even euphoric. Such a state is said to be 'mood congruent'; that is, the mood is in keeping with the situation. It is understandable and seems quite normal. Sometimes, however, people can experience mood incongruence—the person who laughs during a sad experience is an example.

One final explanation about mood that is important for all clinicians to understand is the difference between mood and affect. When conducting a mental state examination, clinicians are trained to explore and identify a person's affect as well as their mood. As discussed, mood is the general enduring feeling state. In contrast, affect is the display of emotions that are generally more fleeting. For example, a person could have clinical depression and this is their enduring mood, but from time to time their affect may lift, particularly after interaction with people they love or with whom they are having a stimulating experience. In this case, the person may have a contented or even happy affect, but it does not last. Their depression is likely to intrude again at a later time.

CRITICAL
THINKING
OPPORTUNITY

In order to fully examine the difference between mood and affect, you could ask the following questions of a consumer:

1   How does your mood generally affect you?

2   Are there times during the day when your mood is less pronounced or when it changes?

MARGARET MCALLISTER AND WENDY CROSS

The questions raised in the 'Critical thinking opportunity' box are not easy to answer. However, it is important to gently persist with this line of questioning, or at least to be very observant of the person during interview to determine whether mood and affect interact. Incongruity between mood and affect may signal that changes are occurring, such as a depression that is gradually lifting. It can also be a signal to alert astute clinicians to situations of risk. For example, if a person says they are depressed in mood, but you observe that their affect is showing contentment or at least no signs of significant sadness, then this might indicate the possibility that the person has made a decision about self-harm and could be suicidal.

To remember the difference between mood and affect, it may be helpful to imagine these concepts as similar to the relationship between a season (mood) and the weather today (affect). Affect refers to immediate expressions of emotion, while mood refers to emotional experience over a prolonged period of time. This is similar to how mood and affect interact (also see Table 10.1).

TABLE 10.1 MOOD AND AFFECT COMPARED	
Mood	**Affect**
■ An enduring feeling state	■ Changes in emotion
■ When disordered it may be described as anxiety, bipolar disorder, cyclothymia, depression, dysthymia, major depressive disorder, mania etc.	■ May be described as guarded, sad, happy, frustrated, aroused, suspicious, angry, flat, blunted, vigilant etc.
■ May last for weeks, months or years	■ May last for hours or days

Anxiety

Dame Judi Dench, perhaps Britain's greatest actor, who has played roles as varied as Queen Elizabeth I, M in the Bond movies and Jean in the long-running series *As Time Goes By*, revealed a dream that she often has where she is on a stage, the curtain is about to go up and she can't remember any of her lines! 'I'm standing there, all dressed up, and whispering: "What do I say now?"' she says. 'It's awful, really, it's the big fear. The one that never goes away' (Adams, 2012). This is what anxiety can feel like: a deep sense of foreboding, a feeling that lingers and swells and comes back to you, regardless of rational argument and rebuttal. It is an emotion that all of us experience, but for some the emotion can be experienced to such a degree that it is distressing and disabling, and people are unable, without help, to control it.

A useful definition for anxiety is that it is a normal reaction that the body uses to respond with alarm to triggers. When it reaches extreme proportions it is abnormal, or disordered. For those aiming to work in mental health, there are three key features to ascertain, and thus to ask of the consumer:

1 *Intensity.* Does the anxiety match the circumstances, or is it extreme?
2 *Duration.* Does the anxiety last for long after the stressor has passed?
3 *Adequate response.* Does the mind and body respond in reasonable or extreme ways to the stressor causing the anxiety?

For example, an actor who feels butterflies in the stomach, dry mouth and worries that she will not remember her lines when standing in front of an audience could be seen as a person who is feeling anxiety that matches the circumstances. The symptoms affecting the mind ('Will I be able to remember my lines?') and the body (gastrointestinal constriction) seem reasonable and not extreme. When the curtain opens, the anxious actor takes to their position and begins their lines. Clearly the duration has not been long, and their functioning has returned. This is a picture of normal anxiety: an emotional force that motivates and prepares the person for peak performance.

Anxiety, like all moods, can run different courses for people. It can arrive sharply—sometimes without warning—or it can arise after a significant trauma and grumble away quietly until some unknown trigger releases it so that it quickly mounts to a crippling crescendo and then departs just as quickly. Anxiety disorders are highly prevalent mental health problems in the Australian community. Up to 14 per cent of the population experiences one type of the many anxiety disorders that are listed in the fifth edition of the *Diagnostic and Statistical Manual of Mental Disorders* (DSM 5) and 2–3 per cent of the population will be diagnosed each year (Australian Bureau of Statistics, 2007). Of all the mental health problems that are listed, anxiety disorders are the most common.

CRITICAL THINKING OPPORTUNITY

More women (17.9 per cent) than men (10.8 per cent) either experience an anxiety disorder or are diagnosed with a disorder, for a total of more than 2.3 million Australians (Slade et al., 2009).

1 Why do you think there is a distinction between genders?

2 When you consider the types of disorders listed in the DSM 5 (see below), which of these might be experienced more by women than men?

3 Which might be experienced more by men than women?

While termed a 'mental health problem', anxiety disorders affect the mind and the body equally. Emotional distress that is constant, surging or unpredictable is extremely difficult for the mind to tolerate. It is understandable that, as human beings, we all want to make sense or find some reason for the anxiety appearing in our lives, where the mind can begin to work illogically and the body responds behaviourally. Living with anxiety can be an ongoing battle where the person must cope with intermittent and unexpected adrenaline surges, waves of nausea, hot flushes and intrusive, irrational thoughts. It is little wonder, then, that some people who experience ongoing anxiety try hard to avoid the triggers that bring it on and minimise the symptoms through any means possible.

According to the DSM 5, there are twelve different disorders where anxiety is a primary feature, being intense, of long duration and extreme. The most common are listed first.

1 *Post-traumatic stress disorder (PTSD).* It is an unfortunate reality that trauma is a common experience in our society. This trauma could be significant and overwhelming such as experiencing the conflict of war or childhood sexual abuse, or it could be the result of repeated difficulties that are accumulated, and seemingly relentless. Examples include bullying, violent assaults or car accidents. Immediately following this trauma it is normal to feel anxiety and to need the support of others and a calming environment. But when a significant period of time lapses and the individual is still feeling the anxiety, being unable to sleep restfully and perhaps reliving the whole experience, PTSD may be diagnosed. In addition to these symptoms, individuals are often notably 'on edge', experience nightmares and seek to avoid any reminders associated with the trauma. When the person re-experiences the trauma (often in a nightmare or during a daydream) they can believe themselves to back on the battlefield or being raped again—they might scream and struggle, and remember whole scenes of horror. Finally, in the mind's attempt to protect the person from this re-traumatisation, people can often shut down,

becoming numb, dissociated and spaced out, and feel nothing. Given these impacts, PTSD, like many mental disorders, can fracture families and ruin lives.

2 *Social phobia.* This disorder involves anxiety in response to exposure to certain types of social or performance situations, often leading to avoidance behaviour. In comparison to the more dramatic PTSD, social phobia might appear innocuous, but being frightened every time a social situation presents itself is depleting on the body's resources and the mind's capacity to calm and coach. Being socially phobic, like any anxiety, is an uncomfortable feeling and a disabling condition. Too often people turn to substances like alcohol or drugs, which can lead to co-morbidity and make health-care management more complex.

3 *Generalised anxiety disorder (GAD).* This is a disorder that involves a generalised, persistent and excessive level of worry and anxiety of at least six months' duration. There is no panic, but rather the fear is 'free floating'—constantly there, not triggered by anything in particular and not occurring more in one context than another. Because GAD involves no rest from anxiety, it can leave the person feeling fatigued, irritable, and eventually helpless and depressed.

4 *Specific phobia.* This disorder is characterised by intense anxiety and then avoidance that is evoked by exposure to an object that in ordinary circumstances would not usually provoke such a degree of arousal. Examples of specific phobias are acrophobia (severe fear of heights), claustrophobia (irrational fear of no escape or being closed in), nyctophobia (severe fear of darkness), ophidiophobia (abnormal fear of snakes), arachnophobia (irrational fear of spiders) and trypanophobia (irrational fear of medical procedures).

5 *Panic disorder.* This is where the person experiences recurrent unexpected panic attacks; that is, there is a sudden, intense and overwhelming fearfulness, terror and sense of impending doom. The body typically reacts in alarm, stimulating the adrenal cortex and the sympathetic nervous system to secrete cortisol and adrenaline—to prepare to defend itself. Symptoms include shortness of breath, palpitations, chest pain and tingling.

6 *Agoraphobia.* Associated with panic disorder, agoraphobia (which literally means fear of the market place) is a condition where the person develops a fear of having a panic attack in a social place, which would be embarrassing and difficult to escape from, and this leads to avoidance. Different from social phobia, which is a fear of performing in public, this phobia is fear of being out in the open. A consequence of the avoidance is that people can lead very restricted lives, unable to leave their homes and becoming socially isolated and neglected.

7 *Acute stress disorder.* This is a condition where, immediately following a traumatic or terrifying event, the person feels overwhelming fear and helplessness. They may feel similar symptoms to PTSD such as repeatedly reliving the experience, ranging from feeling alert and overstimulated to numb and dissociative. They are essentially unable to function mentally or physically.

8 *Obsessive-compulsive disorder.* This involves the combined experience of obsessions—unwanted, intrusive and often irrational thoughts that are difficult to control—and compulsions, which are repetitive behaviours that need to be performed in an attempt to vanquish the distressing thoughts and relieve the anxiety. In this condition, anxiety is partially managed by the performance of ritualised behaviours and the repetitive thoughts, and when the compulsive behaviours or obsessive thoughts are blocked in any way, anxiety mounts.

9 *Agoraphobia without history of panic disorder.* Agoraphobia most often develops as a result of panic attacks. Often panic attacks occur in public and—through association—being in public becomes

fear-inducing itself. However, in a few cases agoraphobia has been known to develop independently and in the absence of a panic attack. The diagnosis of agoraphobia without history of panic disorder is made if there has not been a previous episode of panic associated with the agoraphobia. In this disorder there is an unpredictable fear of harm or embarrassment, rather than from fear of having a panic attack. There has been some debate over whether agoraphobia without history of panic disorder actually exists or whether it is a manifestation of other anxiety conditions.

10 *Anxiety disorder due to a general medical condition.* The main characteristic of this condition is experiencing significant anxiety as a direct result of a medical condition. The symptoms must be of a considerable intensity to exhibit prominent angst, panic attacks, obsessions and/or compulsions. There must be evidence (such as history, physical examination or laboratory tests) that the anxiety is the direct consequence of the medical condition.

11 *Substance-induced anxiety disorder.* The main features of a substance-induced anxiety disorder are prominent symptoms of anxiety due directly to the physiological effects of a substance. The onset of the condition must be in association with a substance and could include alcohol, medication, caffeine and/or toxins. For this condition the anxiety disorder can manifest either throughout the intoxication or during withdrawal of the substance. There must not have been a previous existing anxiety condition. A substance-induced anxiety disorder that commences during the withdrawal period may first display symptoms up to four weeks after discontinuing the substance.

12 *Anxiety disorder not otherwise specified.* This classification includes all those conditions where anxiety and/or phobia is a prominent feature and the symptoms and onset do not meet any other diagnostic category.

If you came across unfamiliar terms in this list, you may find it interesting to explore their meaning by searching for them on your preferred search engine.

CRITICAL THINKING OPPORTUNITY

Theories of causation of anxiety

The cause of anxiety disorders remains contentious. Are we born with the tendency to become anxious and for it to develop in intensity to an extent where it causes harm, or do we develop it over the course of our lives? This nature versus nurture debate introduces two main theories of causation: biological theories and learning theories. Such 'single-cause' theories have been criticised for a failure to appreciate the interaction between the mind and body as well as body and mind (Bourne, 2015). That is, an anxiety may start out because of a neuro-chemical deficiency, which leads to physical problems. Conversely, an anxiety that begins because of social or psychological trauma may then trigger neuro-biological changes. There are also other theories of causation: cognition, socio-ecological and interactions among them all.

The biological theory includes the following hypotheses:

■ *The evolutionary argument.* Humans have evolved over hundreds of thousands of years, and we remain predisposed to fear what our ancestors feared; for example, waking in fright at night for no reason could have performed an important safety function when we were cave-dwellers and vulnerable to predators (Hofer, 2015).

- *Genetic inheritance.* Current thinking in this area is that anxiety disorders have an element of inheritability, but that there is something more at play to explain why identical twins, who have the exact same genes, have varying expression of anxiety disorder. That is, where one twin may have a disorder, the other twin may either develop a different kind of anxiety disorder, or have no disorder over the course of their lives (Fraga et al., 2005). The thinking is that there may be epigenes that mediate genes and the environment, either switching on or off the expression of anxiety (Pembrey, Saffery & Bygren, 2014).
- *Altered brain biochemistry.* Neurotransmitters that are not flowing or being produced or absorbed correctly may linger in areas of the brain that stimulate the sympathetic nervous system so that it is constantly activating the fight or flight mechanism.

Learning theories, by contrast, suggest that anxiety disorders are acquired through learning by association, through reinforcement or through role modelling (Olson & Hergenhahn, 2015). For example, a child may develop a fear of water after experiencing a near-drowning event, and forever after associate water with danger, and so avoid swimming and other activities.

Cognition theories

The cognitive perspective of anxiety sees the behaviours apparent in anxiety disorder as the result of a chain of events whereby a trigger in the environment leads to the person thinking in distorted ways and this exacerbates anxious feelings and behaviours (Eysenck, 2014). For example, a person may need to make a public speech and begin to think or say to himself: 'I can't do this. It's going to be a disaster.' These thoughts then fuel anxious feelings and may lead to panic or avoidance.

Socio-ecological theories

These theories propose that the environment as well as social events can play a role in creating stress for individuals (Taylor, 2014). While some stress in one's life is necessary for motivating action, high levels of stress can lead to overload on the mind and body, depleting coping mechanisms and leading to stress breakdown. Sometimes stress breakdown is manifest in physical ways (such as illness) and other times it is manifest in psychological ways (such as anxiety).

Current general consensus is that it is likely that the development of an anxiety disorder involves a combination of these aspects (Daitch, 2011). Table 10.2 provides an overview of situations that contribute to the development of an anxiety disorder.

TABLE 10.2 SITUATIONS THAT CONTRIBUTE TO THE DEVELOPMENT OF AN ANXIETY DISORDER	
Physical	▪ Drugs; for example, nicotine, caffeine, prescription drugs, amphetamines, marijuana and cocaine ▪ Drug withdrawal ▪ Inadequate nutrition
Early childhood/family	▪ Genetics ▪ Childhood experiences and associations ▪ Role modelling ▪ Unsafe early childhood ▪ Parenting; for example, rewards and punishment, or sensitising

Social/ecological	■ Accumulative stress ■ Life events; for example, divorce or financial difficulties ■ Life changes; for example, changing jobs or schools or a natural disaster ■ School exams ■ Bullying ■ Punishment
Psychological	■ Coping strategies ■ Traits ■ Self-talk or thinking processes ■ Attributions ■ Anticipatory stress
Medical/psychiatric	■ Endocrine; that is, thyroid or adrenal ■ Chronic illness ■ Menopause ■ Cardiac ■ Eating disorders ■ Depression ■ Post-traumatic stress disorder

Therapeutic interventions

When to seek help for an anxiety problem can be difficult to determine, as people often vary in their self-management of anxiety. When the symptoms of anxiety are present, reasonably stable and not getting any worse, a person may decide an intervention is not necessary. In some cases these are anxiety episodes of short duration and they recede either on their own, or if the source of the episode is removed. For example, self-care strategies might be put into place to manage the anxiety of an upcoming exam, and once the exam is over the anxiety decreases. When anxiety is present in higher amounts, so that it interferes with a person's ability to perform their work or function socially, therapeutic intervention may be introduced.

There are four main approaches to treatment: medication, behavioural therapy, cognitive behaviour therapy and other counselling (of which there are many types). These are now examined in some depth.

Medication

Anti-anxiety medications, also called anxiolytics, are commonly prescribed when an anxiety disorder is diagnosed. It is widely understood that medications will not cure the anxiety disorder, but they can reduce the intensity of the symptoms, allowing the person to be able to concentrate, sleep and not be constantly ruminating over fears (beyondblue, 2017).

A range of types of anxiolytics is available. The challenge for the consumer and clinician is finding a drug that is able to be tolerated, with minimal side effects. Should one drug be ineffective, others can be trialled. These drugs include:

■ benzodiazepines, such as alprazolam (Xanax), which have the problem of leading to tolerance and dependence

- antidepressants, prescribed at a lower dose than for depression, such as escitalopram (Lexapro), which are quite well accepted with few side effects
- beta blockers, such as propranolol (Inderal), which have a useful side effect of minimising the anxious feeling without causing sedation, but may not produce as strong relief.

These medications can be very effective in reducing anxiety symptoms and should be looked at as a temporary measure until other psychotherapeutic interventions can be introduced to develop the person's ability to manage life stressors, and to think differently about triggers. Medications are not a cure for anxiety, but a useful adjunct to a holistic therapeutic approach (beyondblue, 2017).

Behavioural therapy

Anxiety can develop through associations after experiencing a specific, environmental stimulus, and thus breaking these associations through guided exposure can effectively sever the link between triggers and emotional response. The assumption in exposure therapy is that anxiety involves thinking and behaviour that have been learned, and through training they can be unlearned. Generally the therapies proceed in combination with medications and relaxation training. So, anxiolytics are prescribed to reduce fearfulness, which can impede learning. Then the individual is taught relaxation skills so they can use these instead of the habitual trains of thought or automatic behaviours they have learned to use when faced with the stressor. There are two common approaches:

- *Flooding* is an approach that involves extended immersion and exposure to the feared situation. The assumption is that anxiety will have a ceiling effect: it will reach a peak, and the person will realise that catastrophic things do not occur for them, and then the emotion will begin to subside. This technique has been used successfully for post-traumatic stress disorder.
- *Graduated exposure* is a technique in which the person is gradually exposed to the feared object, first through guided imagery and then through real-life experiences. During exposure, the person is encouraged to rehearse their newly learned skills of relaxation and positive self-talk as they experience the fearful image or event. Phobias are very successfully treated in this way.

Cognitive behaviour therapy

Cognitive behaviour therapy (CBT) is an approach that assumes that anxiety disorders involve thinking (cognition), feeling (emotion) and behaviour (actions such as avoidance). Thus, the aim of this therapy is to work to: change thinking patterns that have become habits; build up emotions that are the opposite of anxiety, such as relaxation and a sense of calm; and expand action patterns that may also have become habits (Wright, 2006).

The therapist takes an active role in working with the consumer to identify specific goals and target behaviours, and then in teaching the consumer to become more analytical about stressors in their environment, more reflective and alert to the moods that they are feeling, and more skilled in practising alternative ways of thinking and behaving. They use the ABC model:

- *A*: an antecedent event can occur (for example, a crowded room)
- *B*: the belief that elicits and triggers belief or self-talk (for example, 'I'm going to embarrass myself')
- *C*: and a behavioural consequence (anxiety or humiliation).

Critically, the consumer is encouraged to identify the irrational or negative self-talk that they are allowing, and to consciously challenge and replace these with more realistic and less extreme thoughts. So, in this example, the consumer might be encouraged to challenge the truth that they will definitely embarrass themselves, or to say to themselves, 'Well, so what? What if I don't do this perfectly? It's not the end of the world,' and so on. Typically this therapy is time limited and usually goals are achieved within 20 sessions.

Other counselling approaches

People who are anxious will frequently benefit from having someone to talk to. Numerous studies have shown that different forms of counselling are equally effective in producing positive results in the treatment of anxiety disorder, particularly when used in combination with the above approaches (Lambert, 2013).

While counselling traditions and styles differ, the common features of successful therapy are when the counsellor is able to develop trust, focus on the consumer and their uniqueness, empathise, be non-judgmental and offer alternative ways to view stressors. Alternative counselling approaches include:

- *Acceptance and commitment therapy (ACT)*. ACT is an approach that grew out of cognitive behavioural therapy and encourages people to identify their 'core values' and, rather than respond in extreme ways to anxiety, to notice the feelings and thoughts that develop. The consumer is encouraged to accept reactions and be present, choose a valued direction and take action (Harris, 2009).
- *Mindfulness-based cognitive therapy*: Mindfulness grew out of Eastern philosophies such as Buddhism that encourage acceptance and being present in the now, rather than thinking about the past or worrying about the future. In this approach, the consumer is encouraged to observe, tolerate and master thoughts and feelings. Staying in the moment can teach us that we can bear distress and also that moods and feelings ebb and flow. Consumers learn to meditate, which allows the mind to rest and become calm (Gunaratana, 2011).
- *Solution-focused therapy (SFT)*: SFT grew out of a criticism of conventional therapies that tended to be problem focused, attending more to what was going wrong with the consumer than what was going right, or could be going right. Instead of focusing on the past, and hypothesising about causes of anxiety, SFT focuses on the future. It is brief and goal directed, and uses specific questioning techniques to encourage the person to imagine their life with minimal distress, and to set short-term realistic goals that will help them to scale the problem down to size, and see themselves as capable and strong (Australian Institute of Professional Counsellors, 2007; McKergow & Korman, 2009).
- *Narrative therapy*: Similar to SFT, narrative therapy is also solution focused, but uses techniques such as storytelling, letter-writing, poetry and metaphors to encourage people to talk about their life story, and then ultimately to tell a new story about themselves. A narrative therapist will listen to and explore an individual's story with them to find out how the story restricts them in moving forward. Narrative therapy focuses on an individual's strengths of how they have previously overcome difficulties rather than on the negatives of a given situation (Seo et al., 2015).

Skilled nursing care

When a person feels overwhelmed by intense anxiety, they are very much in need of someone who can help them to feel safe, supported and protected from perceived or real stressors. If skilled mental health nurses are available, they can provide that support. They can also assist in dispensing and evaluating medications, providing timely education, and applying the principles of the therapeutic approaches discussed above to reduce symptoms and facilitate better coping. It is very important that mental health nurses also learn and practise the skills of professional counsellors; that is, be empathetic, non-judgmental, trusting and goal-directed.

ABOUT THE CONSUMER Penny's story

Penny is a 27-year-old single mother with an 8-year-old daughter. Penny has lived with the symptoms of anxiety since she was in high school. Penny says she started worrying constantly when she was in her final school years. She worried about how she looked, whether she was liked by other people and if she was smart enough to pass her Year 12 exams.

This led to many years where Penny stayed home because of the fear of what might happen if she went outside. During this time she complained of feeling stressed and constantly worrying about anything and everything. Soon after she graduated from high school she had a panic attack while in a public place and she has never forgotten this. Even though she seldom went out, she met someone and was able to have a child.

Since having her daughter, Penny has had to challenge her tendency to stay at home because she was too anxious to go out. To maintain as normal a life as possible, Penny tries to do all the things a 'normal' mother would do. These include walking her daughter to school every day, helping in the classroom, attending school concerts and doing weekend activities away from home. Penny says that if she did not have a child she would stay at home more and not have the current social circle she now has.

REFLECTION QUESTIONS

1 Why do you think Penny is anxious about leaving her home?

2 What supports can you think of that might be useful to Penny and her family?

3 What types of pharmacological and non-pharmacological interventions can you think of that might be helpful for Penny?

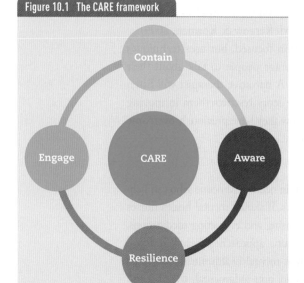

Figure 10.1 The CARE framework

Assessing a consumer's strengths and needs through clinical reasoning

The *International Classification of Diseases* (ICD) and *Diagnostic and Statistical Manual of Mental Disorders* (DSM) assist mental health workers to distinguish between normal anxiety and anxiety disorder, and then to identify which type of anxiety disorder may be occurring. In order to be able to identify signs and symptoms, mental health nurses need to be skilled at noticing, interpreting, responding and reflecting. Skilled nursing care also involves the ability to nurture, comfort and empower people so that they feel supported and capable of enduring a period of intense upset—whether this be physical, emotional, spiritual or (as in the case of anxiety) all three.

The CARE framework is a simple memory tool that can assist nurses to think strategically when it comes to anxiety care. The acronym stands for Contain, raise Awareness, build Resilience and Engage (McAllister & Walsh, 2003); see Figure 8.1.

Containing anxiety

There may be times when a person experiences levels of anxiety that are subjectively distressing, mounting and dangerously high. If they are raised any higher, the person may feel as though they are about to die, or will not be able to control themselves. During these times, external provision of control, safety and calmness are very important. If a person has tachycardia, is hyperventilating and perhaps crying or wailing, a firm, calming voice to provide reassurance and simple direction can be very effective:

Listen to my voice, Penny. Take some slow, deep breaths: in, two, three; out, two, three. Anxiety is taking over here. Listen to me so that we can calm it down.

In addition, removing the person from a noisy, cluttered environment into a space that is restful and low stimulus such as a darkened bedroom may be useful. Listening to a relaxation tape—particularly one that has been handmade by the mental health nurse, whose voice is recognisable and associated with trust—may assist the person to reach deeper into a calm state. Anxiolytic medication administered orally, intramuscularly, intravenously or rectally also can provide immediate relief and this is useful if the situation is disruptive and out of control.

Raising awareness using health education

In the verbal intervention above, you may have noticed the subtle use of health education. Penny has been reminded that this situation is simply the force of anxiety dominating her life at the moment. It isn't always going to be so powerful, and there are things that people can do to take back control and to minimise its impact. In the longer term, it will be important for Penny to develop insight into what triggers or exacerbates anxious feelings. These triggers can be reframed, managed in short doses, or avoided. In addition, Penny can learn ways to consciously minimise anxiety through bio-feedback (learning how to tell the body to relax when it wants to tense up) and self-talk (learning how to challenge and replace any irrational thoughts that feed the anxiety).

Of course, lengthy health education sessions during an anxiety surge are not appropriate. Any information provided at this time is unlikely to be heard and even less likely to be remembered. But when the person is calm and indicating a desire to learn more about their condition, there are a number of strategies that together you can consider:

1   engaging in dialogue about how to change the way anxiety operates
2   reading health-oriented literature
3   watching and then discussing relevant videos and films
4   listening and learning about mindfulness
5   practising deep muscle relaxation, breathing, yoga and meditation
6   engaging in physical activities that reduce tension and anxiety; for example, walking, swimming, tennis and having a massage
7   undertaking individual or group-based psychological therapies; for example, CBT, behavioural therapy, systematic desensitisation and exposure therapy

8 joining face-to-face support groups

9 employing internet-based information and support

10 using contingency planning—a useful conversation to have with a well consumer about anxiety is for them to consider what they will do should anxiety re-emerge in their lives. Will they call 000 as a first port of call? Or will they use some or all of the strategies they have learned through the therapeutic experience? If so, which ones, in which order, and why?

Building resilience

Resilience is the ability to bounce back from adversity. In the case of anxiety, it is highly likely that a person who has experienced one trauma in their life is going to experience future challenges or even more trauma. But it doesn't mean that anxiety disorders will be an inevitable consequence. Harnessing inner strengths, learning new coping skills, using therapeutic doses of effective medications, accessing counselling early and continuing to utilise available supports within the community are all ways that anxiety disorder can be kept at bay.

Nurses working in acute care or transition services may be the important lynchpin for introducing consumers to these resilience strategies. Thus, having an updated list of recommended resources available in your local community is a very important strategy.

Being engaging

Even though nurses are well known for being proficient at tasks and very busy people, skilled nursing care is not only about doing things for people. In many cases, it is also about knowing how to be there for someone, so that they can have someone to trust and rely upon when they are feeling distressed or alone, so that they can know who to turn to should they have questions or needs, and so that they can develop a connection with a positive role model. Simply by having access to a person who is willing to be present during an anxiety attack—to not judge, command or intimidate—can be the turning point that people need to change their lives and to take back control.

Anxiety can be very distressing to witness—especially if the person is externalising by crying or raging—but acceptance, calmness and being steadfast in your belief that it will pass are all powerful and contagious attributes. If you believe, perhaps the consumer will too.

Major depressive disorder

Major depressive disorder (MDD) is another major mood disorder, and a condition that has spread within society. According to the World Health Organization (WHO, 2012), depression occurs in 5 per cent of the general population. It has such wide variety in its impact and expression that probably every nurse, regardless of practice context, will regularly encounter it. In the clinical sense, MDD is much more than sad mood. According to the DSM 5, this clinical or major depression is characterised by five or more of these features being present over a two-week period:

- pervasive and persistent low mood
- low self-esteem
- loss of interest or pleasure in normally enjoyable activities
- weight loss
- insomnia or hypersomnia
- psychomotor agitation or retardation

- fatigue or loss of energy
- feelings of worthlessness
- diminished ability to think
- recurrent thoughts of death.

ABOUT THE CONSUMER John's story

John is a 40-year-old man who lives with his wife Susan and two children on a dairy farm that has been in the family for three generations. Susan recently raised concerns about John with her GP. John was not the sort of person who talked about his emotions, but she felt he was very depressed and that this had been going on for over a year. The farm had been running at a loss for several years. Over the last year, John had begun to take less care of farm maintenance. He was also drinking to excess and was generally non-communicative and sullen. After the visit she discussed her concerns with John. He admitted that something did not feel right inside himself and he reluctantly agreed to visit the GP.

On assessment the GP learned that John had been feeling low for over six months, and sometimes he felt that life would be easier if he was not around. He had no active plans for suicide. He said that physically he felt tired all the time, and yet had trouble getting to sleep at night, and in the mornings he would wake well before dawn. His appetite was poor, he was constipated, his blood pressure was 160/100 and his pulse was irregular at 90 bpm. John admitted that he felt it was his duty to keep the farm running, even though he really had no enthusiasm for it. He felt like he was in a dark, dark place and nothing, not even his children, made him feel happy.

REFLECTION QUESTIONS

1 Using your skills of clinical reasoning, how would you describe the impact of John's depression?

2 What would you suggest are his strengths and vulnerabilities?

Some medical disorders are associated with the development of depression, notably myocardial infarction, diabetes, adrenal disorders and cerebrovascular accident (CVA) (Egede, 2007). Depression can also occur during and following pregnancy. It is more common in women than men and the prevalence of depression (how long it endures) is greater for older people than it is for those who are young. Further, some prescribed medications can exacerbate or bring on depression. These include steroids and drugs of addiction such as alcohol and narcotics. Therefore, an astute nurse will appreciate that if they are working in cardiac, chronic disease self-management, pain clinics, palliative care, drug and alcohol or a dedicated mental health unit, many of their consumers could be suffering with depression as well as their diagnosed condition.

Unrelieved depression not only reduces people's *joie de vivre* (joy of living) and quality of life, but it can also lower their pain threshold, interfere with motivation and commitment to adhere to treatment plans, and increase the risk of self-harm and suicide.

Depression has an impact on every single part of a person's life: physically, emotionally, intellectually, spiritually, socially and behaviourally. People usually seek help for depression because they begin to realise that it is impacting negatively on their capacity and willingness to work, engage in hobbies, relate to people and do the things they normally enjoy. Even so, too many people suffer in silence with this major mental disorder. Some reports have suggested that only about 50 per cent of those who are experiencing clinical depression receive medical treatment for it (Commonwealth of Australia, 2010).

This disorder creates poor regulation of neurotransmitters such as dopamine and serotonin. It flattens emotion, and can deepen to the extent that the person can no longer even access tears, which can provide relief from sadness. Some people can become so depressed that they describe anhedonia (the absence of pleasure) and nihilism (a belief that they are nothing). In psychotic depression, the person can experience mood-congruent hallucinations, such as voices telling them they are worthless or bad, and delusions, such as that they are the devil, evil or inherently bad.

Perhaps because depression is so common in society, and so easily recognised, too many people wrongly believe that it is possible to simply 'snap out of it', or to stop indulging the negative feelings. These kinds of simplistic views are unhelpful to the person who is experiencing an extreme mood disorder. The negative judgments made by others in society about a person who is depressed may be taken to heart and deepen the person's sense of unworthiness or guilt, and they may begin to feel ashamed of themselves, and to feel as though the world might be better off without them in it. This is how a person with depression can become caught up in a vicious cycle of self-harm (Hawton, Saunders & O'Connor, 2012); see Figure 8.2.

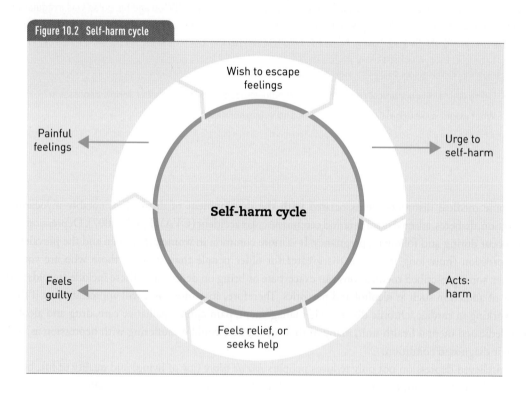

Figure 10.2 Self-harm cycle

Wish to escape feelings

Painful feelings

Urge to self-harm

Self-harm cycle

Feels guilty

Acts: harm

Feels relief, or seeks help

The person may endure very painful feelings of depression, emptiness or unworthiness. They may perceive that they are unable to bear such pain and have an urge to hurt themselves, either through acts of commission (like alcohol abuse, cutting, overdose or worse) or omission (neglect); and this can make them feel some initial relief but later lead to feelings of guilt for being weak or a burden on family or society, and so the pain returns and the cycle begins again.

Depending on one's attitude to mental disorder, ability to cope with disturbed moods, and faith in medicine and psychiatry, some people may dismiss depression as simply a reaction to stress, and so they may endure a protracted mental health issue when it could be more quickly relieved with a range of treatment approaches.

A person who is significantly depressed may lack energy and yet be unable to sleep well. They may have difficulty concentrating or focusing on a task. They may even begin to physically slow down, leading to slowing of gut motility and loss of appetite. The person may begin to think that they have a physical illness and may even become more sensitive to pain, noise and light. This impact on the neurological system is termed a 'neurovegetative state'. With all of these disorders of mood, much of the psychic pain that people endure is not always outwardly visible. People can be suffering, and suffering in silence and isolation.

Returning to the case study of John, the average age of onset for depression is 40 years and it is more common in people living in rural and remote settings, and when people have few close relationships or are divorced. Only about 50 per cent of people receive medical treatment for depression, probably because the symptoms are dismissed as a sign of weakness, or signs of stress that will soon pass, especially if you 'pull yourself together'. Unfortunately, this attitude is incorrect and people are very unlikely to recover quickly from serious depression without assistance. Untreated depression can last for six months to years. Further, having a major depressive episode increases the likelihood of having another: 50–60 per cent who have a single episode go on to have another; 70 per cent who have a second episode then have a third; and 90 per cent who have third episode have a fourth.

The consequence of allowing serious depression to go untreated is a worsening mental state, risk of self-harm, suicide or severe substance abuse.

John displays many of the signs and symptoms of major depression:

■ *Physical effects.* In psychiatric language, the physical effects of depression are known as neurovegetative features. They occur because the whole system begins to slow down. Gastric emptying is slowed or delayed, cognitive processes are slowed, sleep is often delayed or disturbed, there is anergia or lack of energy, and often people will complain of generalised body pain or discomfort.

■ *Behavioural effects.* In severe depression, people's movements can become so slowed that they are unable to move from bed to chair, and they may be unable to complete simple tasks without assistance. Risk for self-harm, substance abuse and suicide is high at 15 per cent.

■ *Emotional effects.* Obviously emotions are disturbed in depression. It is common for people to feel sad, pessimistic, worried, afraid, anhedonic and nihilistic. However, in some cases, particularly involving older people, emotional disturbance may be more agitated and fearful or paranoid than sad, and thus diagnosis can be delayed or confused with delirium and sometimes dementia.

■ *Intellectual effects.* Because cognitive processes are slowed, people can engage in poor decision-making or ruminate over concerns without taking any action to solve them. In severe depression, people may even experience disturbances in thought formation and processes to a delusional extent. In this case, psychotic depression would be diagnosed. The person may complain of thought withdrawal, the belief that they are actually dead, that they have no memories or that all of their children are gone. These mood-congruent delusions are very distressing, but respond well to available treatments.

■ *Social effects.* Depression is frequently socially invalidated; that is, people around may not understand the behaviour as depression and may think it is a sign of weakness and respond with impatience. As a result, untreated depression can lead to unemployment, loss of friends, social isolation and being judged and ignored.

■ *Spiritual effects.* When a person feels sad for a long period they may begin to develop a sense of unworthiness or guilt; they may become despondent that they will never get better and they may long for sanctuary, peace, calm or transcendence. Some people may seek solace or answers in religion, self-help books and psychics.

It is tempting to think that because MDD is associated with neurotransmitter dysfunction, a medication to balance out dopamine or serotonin deficiencies will provide a simple remedy. Unfortunately, antidepressant medication is rarely an effective treatment on its own. Like other mental health conditions, major depression requires a whole of person approach; that is, the management of biological, psychological and social factors. Between 50 and 85 per cent of people will have more than one episode of depression, and the average length of an episode is nine months (Parker & Manicavasagar, 2005). Since major depression can recur, it can occur in the context of other disorders, and it can last for lengthy periods, it is vital that the person develops a strong relationship with their clinician so that there can be ongoing support, motivation and consultation to minimise the side effects and enhance the acceptability of treatment.

Medications for the treatment of depression

The first line of treatment is prescription of selective serotonin reuptake inhibitors (SSRIs). These drugs inhibit the reuptake of neurotransmitters, specifically serotonin, allowing this mood hormone to remain longer in the central nervous system. For some reason, this leads to mood stabilisation. SSRIs tend to be better tolerated by the person than other types of antidepressant medication and only need to be taken in one dose per day. Examples include fluoxetine (Prozac) and paroxetine (Paxil).

Another type of commonly prescribed drug is serotonin noradrenaline reuptake inhibitors (SNRIs), which works by inhibiting the reuptake of noradrenaline as well as serotonin. These drugs are thought to produce fewer side effects (such as weight gain), but they also are more difficult to withdraw from, causing light-headedness, nausea and headache. Examples include duloxetine (Cymbalta) and desvenlafaxine (Pristiq).

The most well known but now the oldest antidepressant group is the tricyclic antidepressants (TCAs). Examples of these medications are amitriptyline (Tryptanol) and doxepin (Sinequan). These drugs act on a different pathway but also inhibit the reuptake of noradrenaline and serotonin; however, they also tend to have side effects such as sedation, dry mouth, blurred vision and constipation.

Psychological interventions

Psychological interventions such as CBT and mindfulness-based CBT, combined with medications prescribed for at least six months, are the most common and effective treatments for depression (Manicavasagar, Parker & Perich, 2011). Electro-convulsive therapy (ECT) is also regularly used, particularly in Australia, to treat depression that is not feasible to treat using medications, or if medications have failed to be effective.

Guided recovery programs and other recent advances

With the advent of the internet, the rise of the self-help movement and consumer engagement in care, exciting new programs promoting guided recovery from depression are becoming more widely available. These include Mood GYM, the Sadness Program and myCompass. There are also more recent medical interventions being trialled such as deep brain stimulation, repetitive transcranial stimulation, and bright light therapy.

Bipolar disorder

The final disorder of mood explored in this chapter is bipolar disorder and it occurs in 1–3 per cent of the population. This disorder was previously called manic depression. Bipolar means 'two poles' and refers to the experience of a disorder of mood that shifts between episodes of mania and depression (highs and lows). Mania is severe over-arousal, involving elation, excitability, irritability, grandiose ideas that can reach delusional intensity, over-production of ideas (flight of ideas) pressure of speech and sometimes disinhibited, disorganised and risky behaviours. A manic episode can last a few days to several months. During this experience, the person may find sleep difficult, and can be easily distracted and fail to complete tasks. They may dress inappropriately, and engage in risky or disinhibited behaviours that are not normal for them, such as over-spending, promiscuity, gambling or substance abuse.

People who experience mania usually also experience a depressive swing that either follows immediately after the manic episode, or following some period where the person's mood has returned to a normal baseline.

There are several types of bipolar disorder:

- *Bipolar I* involves a manic episode or mixed episode plus depressive episodes of varying lengths.
- *Bipolar II* involves a major depressive episode plus a hypomanic episode.
- *Cyclothymia* involves hypomanic symptoms plus depressive symptoms.

Abnormalities in the structure and function of some regions of the brain are associated with bipolar disorder, though it remains unknown as to whether this is an effect of the disorder, or a preliminary cause. Theories about causation, based on repeated studies, suggest that genetics plays a large role, while environment and exposure to stress also have an influence. Twin studies have consistently shown that when one identical twin has bipolar disorder, the other twin has a 40 per cent risk of also developing it. In fraternal twins, however, the risk reduces to 0–10 per cent (Kieseppa et al., 2004). Recent life events, interpersonal relationships and the experience of childhood trauma may add to the vulnerability posed by the genetic predisposition (Miklowitz & Chang, 2008).

According to the kindling hypothesis, when a person who is genetically predisposed to bipolar disorder experiences one stressful event and then another, the stress threshold at which mood changes occur becomes progressively lower, until episodes of bipolar disorder eventually start and recur without any seeming stressful trigger (Bender & Alloy, 2011).

In order to meet the criteria for bipolar disorder under the DSM 5, a person needs to be experiencing the following:

- feelings of euphoria, elation or irritability
- impulsive, high-risk behaviour
- aggressive behaviour
- increased energy and rapid speech
- fleeting, grandiose ideas
- decreased sleep
- decreased appetite
- difficulty concentrating or organising thoughts
- inflated self-esteem
- mood congruent delusions and hallucinations.

Therapeutic interventions

A combination of medication and psychological techniques is the recommended treatment, which can help to reduce the duration and intensity of an episode and may also prevent relapses. The medication most commonly used is a mood stabiliser, such as lithium. Anti-convulsant medications such as carbamazepine also have a mood stabilising effect. Some of the newer antipsychotic drugs are also useful in treating the delusions, hallucinations, agitation, sleeplessness and thought disorder that is seen in the severe episodes of either mania or depression. Examples include risperidone, olanzapine and quetiapine.

All of these drugs have side effects, most notably weight gain, high cholesterol and risk for diabetes. The psychological therapies that have been previously outlined in this chapter have been proven to be effective, in combination with these medications, in treating bipolar disorder.

Disorders of mood are the most common mental health problems and are found across all spectrums of society, and according to Lépine and Briley (2011) are becoming more prevalent. For mental health nurses to work effectively with people affected by anxiety, depression or elevated moods, they need to understand the connection between mind and body, empathise with how powerfully moods can strip away motivation, meaning and purpose in life, and learn strategies that will help a person regain hope, spirit and self-belief.

TOPIC LINK
See Chapter 18 for more on psychotherapy.

Care planning

The following is an example care plan for John, the consumer presented in this chapter. The areas of daily living that are considered include biopsychosocial factors and the plan is mapped out using the nursing process (assessment, planning, implementation and evaluation). Remember, the success is in the detail, so be specific about who, when and what in the collaborative plan; and never include someone in the plan if they were not consulted in the planning process. In addition, the care plan must be developed in line with the recovery framework, which is central to mental health service provision.

Date: [Today's date]						
Consumer's name: John			Case managers: Margaret and Wendy			
Areas of daily living	Assessment of current situation	Goal	Plan *(undertaken with consumer)*	Implementation	Who is responsible *(include only those who have been consulted in the planning process)*	Evaluation/ review date
Sleep	Initial insomnia Early morning waking Fatigue	To feel rested and to gain 6–8 hours' sleep	Explain to John that his depressed mood can impact on all of his bodily functions. To feel rested, he may benefit from all of the things that normally help his mood: working on the farm, being with his family etc. Liaise with doctor to identify an antidepressant medication that may also help with sleep. Learn and then establish a restful night-time ritual.	Generate a list of activities that will help him get exercise and then help him feel tired at night, rather than ruminative. John and his wife Susan to remember to take the medication as prescribed. Margaret to discuss with John and Susan practices they can implement to reduce night time stimulation and prepare for a good sleep.	John and Susan Medical team, John and Susan	30/01/2018 One week after beginning drug, monitor that side effects are tolerable.
Depressed mood	At risk of sense of worthlessness, self-harm and suicide	John to feel his life has meaning and that it is enjoyable.	Margaret and Wendy to work with John and family to understand using CBT, the negative triad (self, world and future) and ways to interrupt this negative cycle through exercise, activities, thought stopping, distraction and spiritual support.	John to accept that his mood will take time to lift. Margaret and Wendy to support and convey hope. John to identify a list and then engage in activities that will help reinforce his sense of worth and help him feel optimistic about the world and future. Suggest Men's Shed or farmer support group as a way to share burden and provide distraction from rumination.	Family, community, Margaret and Wendy	Six weeks later monitor if this is improving mood and sleep.

Alcohol misuse	Impacting on sleep, mood, appetite and thinking	John to moderate alcohol use to six standard drinks per week.	Wendy to work with John to find other ways to reduce stress and relax, and to use alcohol as a weekly bonus rather than a daily reward.	John to buy low-alcohol drinks. Limit alcohol to 2–3 evenings a week. Find alternatives to stress management.	Susan and John to work together	Six weeks later monitor alcohol intake and liver function test (LFT).
Inadequate nutrition	Poor appetite		Margaret to work with John and Susan to assess and alter diet to include high protein, easily digestible foods five to six times a day.	Multi-vitamins while appetite is poor. Protein shakes three times a day. Five vegetables per day; two fruit; three protein; 2 litres water	Susan to work with John to ensure dietary intake is acceptable.	John to regain 2 kg in one month.
Altered elimination	Constipation Slow gastrointestinal tract (GIT)	Resume normal bowel movements.	Understand that depressed mood can slow digestion and to avoid constipation increased fluid and perhaps a laxative will assist in resuming regularity.	Natural laxative twice a week.	John and Susan	Bowel comfort in one week
Risk of CVS dysfunction	Hypertensive Irregular pulse Stress	Vital signs in normal limits.	Understand mind–body interaction and effects of stress	Margaret to gently explain need for stress management and holistic well-being, including treatment adherence, exercise, acceptance, distraction, talking and support. Vital signs monitoring weekly.	John, Susan, Margaret and Wendy	If BP and pulse remain outside normal limits for two weeks, see GP for new treatment.

SUMMARY

Throughout this chapter you have learned that:

■ Mood is the way a person feels, usually subjectively and over a period of time, and has a strong influence on behaviour. In contrast, affect is the display of emotions that can be observed.

■ Anxiety is a normal response that the body uses to respond with alarm to triggers. However, when it reaches extreme proportions it is abnormal, or disordered. There are twelve different disorders where anxiety is a primary feature, being intense, of long duration and extreme.

- There are four main approaches to the treatment of anxiety: pharmacotherapy and non-pharmacotherapeutic interventions such as behavioural therapy, cognitive behaviour therapy and other counselling methods.
- Major depressive disorder (MDD) is another major mood disorder. Unrelieved depression not only reduces people's enjoyment and quality of life, but it can also lower pain threshold, interfere with motivation and commitment to adhere to treatment plans, and increase the risk of self-harm and suicide.
- Like other mental health disorders, major depression requires a whole of person approach; that is, the management of biological, psychological and social factors.
- Bipolar means 'two poles' and refers to the experience of a disorder of mood that shifts between episodes of mania and depression. A combination of medication and psychological techniques is the recommended treatment, which can help to reduce the duration and intensity of an episode and may also prevent relapses.

DISCUSSION QUESTIONS

1 Why do you think mood has an impact on behaviour?
2 What are the key differences between mood and affect?
3 What was the older term for bipolar disorder?
4 What framework needs to be considered when developing a care plan?
5 What treatment considerations are recommended for the treatment of bipolar disorder?

TEST YOURSELF

1 Medical conditions that are most commonly related to mood disorders include:
   a heart disease
   b endocrine disorders
   c renal disease
   d fractures

2 Common anxiety disorders include:
   a phobias
   b obsessive-compulsive disorder (OCD)
   c generalised anxiety disorder (GAD)
   d all of the above

3 Physical effects of depression include:
   a pain
   b anhedonia
   c diarrhoea
   d rumination

4 Which pharmacological treatments are most effective for mood disorders?
   a SSRIs
   b Anticonvulsants
   c Anxiolytics
   d All of the above

MARGARET MCALLISTER AND WENDY CROSS

USEFUL WEBSITES

Beyondblue: www.beyondblue.org.au

Black Dog Institute: www.blackdoginstitute.org.au/

Psychology Today—The ten coolest therapy interventions: Introduction: www.psychologytoday.com/blog/in-therapy/201001/the-ten-coolest-therapy-interventions-introduction

REFERENCES

Adams, T. (2012). Judi Dench: 'I never want to stop working'. *The Observer*, 14 October. Retrieved from www.guardian.co.uk/film/2012/oct/14/judi-dench-interview-skyfall.

Australian Bureau of Statistics (2007). *National survey of mental health and wellbeing: Summary of results*. Retrieved from www.abs.gov.au.

Australian Institute of Professional Counsellors (2007). *AIPC's therapies ebook*. Retrieved from www.awakening.com.au/download/certificate_library/COUNS101%20Big%20Picture/jj._Five_Therapies.pdf#page=36.

Bender, R. E., & Alloy, L. B. (2011). Life stress and kindling in bipolar disorder: Review of the evidence and integration with emerging biopsychosocial theories. *Clinical Psychology Review, 31*(3), 383–398.

Beyondblue (2017). *Medical treatments for anxiety*. Retrieved from https://www.beyondblue.org.au/the-facts/anxiety/treatments-for-anxiety/medical-treatments-for-anxiety.

Bourne, E. (2015). *The anxiety and phobia workbook* (6th ed.). Oakland: New Harbinger.

Bronson, P., & Bronson, R. (2013). *Moods, emotions, and aging: Hormones and the mind-body connection*. New York: Rowman & Littlefield.

Commonwealth of Australia (2010). *National Mental Health Report 2010*. Canberra.

Daitch, C. (2011). *Anxiety disorders: The go-to guide for clients and therapists*. New York: WW Norton.

Egede, L. (2007). Major depression in individuals with chronic medical disorders: Prevalence, correlates and association with health resource utilization, lost productivity and functional disability. *General Hospital Psychiatry, 29*(5), 409–416.

Eyesenck, M. (2013). *Anxiety: The cognitive perspective*. Hove: Lawrence Erlbaum.

Eysenck, M. (2014). *Anxiety and cognition: A unified theory*. UK: Taylor & Francis Ltd.

Fraga, M., Ballestar, E., Paz, M., Ropero, S. et al. (2005). Epigenetic differences arise during the lifetime of monozygotic twins. *Proceedings of the National Academy of Sciences of the United States of America, 102*(30), 10,604–10,609.

Gunaratana, H. (2011). *Mindfulness in plain English*. New York: Wisdom Publications.

Harris, R. (2009). *ACT made simple*. Oakland: New Harbinger Publications.

Hawton, K., Saunders, K. E., & O'Connor, R. C. (2012). Self-harm and suicide in adolescents. *The Lancet, 379*(9834), 2373–2382.

Hofer, M. (2015). New concepts in the evolution and development of anxiety. In H. Simpson, Y. Neria, R. Lewis-Fernandez & F. Scheier (Eds.), *Anxiety disorders: Theory, research and clinical perspectives.* (pp. 59–68). New York: Cambridge University Press.

Kieseppa, T., Partonen, T., Haukka, J., Kaprio, J., & Lönnqvist, J. (2004). High concordance of bipolar I disorder in a nationwide sample of twins. *American Journal of Psychiatry, 161*(10), 1814–1821.

Lambert, M. J. (2013). The efficacy and effectiveness of psychotherapy. In M. J. Lambert (Ed.), *Bergin and Garfield's handbook of psychotherapy and behavior change* (6th ed.) (pp. 169–218). New York: Wiley.

Lépine J-P., & Briley, M. (2011). The increasing burden of depression. *Neuropsychiatric Disease and Treatment, 7*(Suppl 1), 3–7.

Maclaren, K. (2006). Emotional disorder and the mind-body problem: A case study of alexithymia. *Chiasmi International, 8*, 139–55.

Manicavasagar, V., Parker, G., & Perich, T. (2011). Mindfulness-based cognitive therapy vs cognitive behaviour therapy as a treatment for non-melancholic depression. *Journal of Affective Disorders, 130*(1), 138–144.

McAllister, M., & Walsh, K. (2003). C.A.R.E: A framework for mental health practice. *Journal of Psychiatric and Mental Health Nursing, 10*(1), 39–48.

McKergow, M., & Korman, H. (2009). In between—Neither inside nor outside: The radical simplicity of solution-focused brief therapy. *Journal of Systemic Therapies, 28*(2), 34–49.

Miklowitz, D. J., & Chang, K. D. (2008). Prevention of bipolar disorder in at-risk children: Theoretical assumptions and empirical foundations. *Development and Psychopathology, 20*(3), 881–897.

Olson, M., & Hergenhahn, B. (2015). *An introduction to theories of learning* (9th ed.). New York: Routledge.

Parker, G., & Manicavasagar, V. (2005). *Modelling and managing the depressive disorders: A clinical guide*. New York: Cambridge University Press.

Pembrey, M., Saffery, R., & Bygren, L, (2014). Human transgenerational responses to early-life experience: Potential impact on development, health and biomedical research. *Journal of Medical Genetics*. 51(9): 563–572. doi:10.1136/jmedgenet-2014-102577.

Seo, M., Kang, H., Lee, Y., & Chae, S. (2015). Narrative therapy with an emotional approach for people with depression: Improved symptom and cognitive-emotional outcomes. *Journal of Psychiatric and Mental Health Nursing, 22*, 379–389.

Slade, T., Johnston, A., Teesson, M., Whiteford, H., Burgess, P., Pirkis, J., & Saw, S. (2009). *The Mental Health of Australians 2. Report on the 2007 National Survey of Mental Health and Wellbeing*. Canberra: Department of Health and Ageing.

Taylor, S. (2014). *Anxiety sensitivity: Theory, research, and treatment of the fear of anxiety*. New York: Routledge.

World Health Organization (2012). *Depression: A global public health concern*. Geneva: WHO.

Wright, J. (2006). Cognitive behavior therapy: Basic principles and recent advances. *Focus: Journal of Lifelong Learning in Psychiatry, 4*(2), 173–178.

CHAPTER 11

Psychosis and Psychotic Disorders

SIMON DODD AND
SANDY JEFFS

KEY OUTCOMES

AFTER READING THIS CHAPTER, YOU SHOULD BE ABLE TO:

- describe what is meant by the term 'psychosis'
- identify the clinical features of a psychotic disorder
- describe the phases model of psychosis
- describe the impact of stress in relation to developing psychotic disorders
- describe the settings where a nurse will care for those who experience psychosis
- describe the skills needed within the stages of the nurse–consumer relationship.

KEY TERMS

- clinical staging
- delusion
- hallucination
- negative symptoms
- plasticity of symptoms
- positive symptoms
- premorbid
- prodrome
- psychosis
- relapse
- thought disorder
- vulnerability

Introduction

This chapter introduces you to an understanding of what psychosis is, and its effects on a person. Within the scope of the chapter we focus on the schizophrenia spectrum of psychosis.

The term 'psychosis' has been used to describe conditions that affect the mind, where there has been a loss of contact with reality. There are difficulties with this definition as there are assumptions as to what is 'normal' and what is 'reality'. An operational understanding of psychosis should always include the context of the person who is experiencing the psychosis. We look for the experiences such as hallucination and delusions by asking: 'What has changed?' (the course) and 'Where is the harm?' (pathology). These questions give us the context of the experience, and give the clinician a mandate to help. In addition, psychosis can describe the intensity of some symptoms or conditions; for example, delusional beliefs are of a psychotic intensity, and depression may be so severe as to have active psychotic symptoms.

Psychosis

Psychosis is most likely to occur in young adults, and is not common. Nonetheless, around one to three out of every 100 people will experience a psychotic episode (Simeone et al., 2015; van Os et al., 2009), which makes psychosis more frequently occurring than diabetes in young people. Psychosis usually appears as impairment to social functioning (most obviously relationship difficulties with family and peers). This may then be followed by sub-threshold psychotic symptoms (illusions or transient psychotic symptoms) with the advent of more prominent symptoms gradually (or more rapidly in rare cases).

Most people experiencing psychosis for the first time make a good recovery from the experience (Bertelsen et al., 2008; Petersen et al., 2008). Significant Australian population surveys have shown that the presence of psychotic symptoms may be much more common than previously thought, especially in young people. In some studies, up to 50 per cent of teenagers surveyed had some sort of experience of hallucination, and 9.3 per cent had them 'often' (McGorry et al., 1995). In a more recent finding, 8.4 per cent of Australian adolescents were reported as having experienced hallucinations (Scott et al., 2009). Psychosis happens across the world: there are reports of psychotic illnesses in all cultures and socioeconomic groups (Chisholm et al., 2008).

Psychotic symptoms

To understand psychosis, it is useful to look at the most commonly occurring symptoms. These can be structured as positive and negative symptoms. Positive symptoms are the presence of psychotic symptoms: 'positive', in the sense that they present in the person's experience but should be absent (they include hallucinations, delusions and thought disorder). Positive symptoms are distortions and excesses of the person's normal functioning. The following are details of positive psychotic symptoms a person may experience:

- *Hallucinations.* A person may experience changes in their experience of external stimuli. This can take any form that the person senses, although is most often auditory (hearing noises or voices) or visual (seeing). It can also be olfactory (related to the sense of smell), tactile (touch) or gustatory (taste). This experience occurs in the absence of other stimuli or is considered an illusion (a misinterpretation of an existing stimuli such as a shadow at a window being perceived as a person). These experiences are often congruent with any delusional ideas that the person may have, and can be oppressive and very distressing.
- *Delusional ideation.* A person experiencing a psychotic episode may hold false beliefs. These are often distressing, usually egodystonic (in discord with the persons self-perception or ego), and usually experienced by the person as real. These experiences are powerful enough to change behaviour. Such people are so convinced of their delusion that the most logical argument cannot make them change their mind. Delusions are described usually in terms of the content, such as paranoid-type delusions (for example, another is trying cause harm or wishes them harm) or grandiose-type delusions (for example, they believe they are just about to win a lottery); or in terms of the form, such as delusions of reference (where the person believes that things unrelated to them are influencing or conveying messages to them; for example, the radio) or passivity phenomena (where a person believes that some aspect of themselves is under the control of others or something external to them).
- *Thought disorder.* Thoughts become confused and/or do not flow correctly. Often this is identified by the person's speech, which does not make sense or is jumbled. The person often has difficulty concentrating, following conversations or performing previously straightforward cognitive tasks (such as school or work tasks). Thoughts may also subjectively seem to race or be slowed.

- *Changed behaviour.* The person, in responding to internal reality, can act on their beliefs and experiences. This often does not appear rational to the observer, and can be dramatic and dangerous. It may also be described in terms of the person's affect.
- *Affect.* A person's expressed emotion may change for no apparent reason. Mood swings are common and the person may feel unusually excited or depressed.

Negative symptoms are symptoms that remove capacity from the individual. They refer to experiences that should be present, but are absent or reduced, such as amotivation (reduction in drive that has an impact on the ability to perform activities), alogia (reduction or absence of speech) or blunted affect (a reduction in expressed emotion). Commonly, people experiencing negative symptoms have significant impairment in motivation levels, leading to a general reduction in living skills. They may feel strange and cut off from the world, and have impaired capacity to function cognitively. People's emotions may appear flattened or blunted; that is, they experience subjectively less emotion than they used to or would have when 'well'.

Each person's experience is different, and must be understood in their personal context. Symptoms vary from person to person, and may change over time often in relation to various stressors the person is experiencing. In some cases, there can be significant changes in the severity of symptoms displayed in relation to the level of stress the person may be experiencing; this has been described as plasticity of symptoms in that they may shift and morph due to changes in stress. In fact, they may evolve across various diagnostic categories—such as disorganisation and irritability—that may be identified as related to paranoid ideation, but which over time become more easily identified as part of an elevated mood.

The classical presentation is of a person experiencing a slow and gradual deterioration in functioning, with a corresponding increase in active symptomology; this may occur over months and years. Such people will often not seek help until crisis and, when they do, it may be for reasons other than psychiatric.

There are various types of disorders that have psychosis as a primary signifier. Schizophrenia is the archetype, with various related types. The primary difference is between the length of experienced illnesses (brief psychotic disorder and schizophreniform disorder, for example) or the cause of the psychosis (substance- or medication-induced psychosis). Also, schizophrenia has subtypes that describe the course or content of the presentation (residual type or paranoid type, for example).

The most recent review of the *Diagnostic and Statistical Manual of Mental Disorders* (5th edition; DSM 5) has led to significant review of the classification of schizophrenia spectrum disorders. The DSM 5 raises the symptom threshold for schizophrenia so that the individual is required to exhibit at least two of the specified symptoms (compared to only requiring one in the previous version of the DSM). Additionally, the subtypes of schizophrenia have been defined by the predominant symptom during diagnostic assessment, and the classification includes the concept of a spectrum or gradient of psychopathology experience and now includes schizotypal personality disorder in this continuum. The DSM also allows for two single domain subtypes of disorder: catatonia and delusional disorder.

Stages of psychosis

McGorry and colleagues (1996) posit a model to understand the experience and progression of schizophrenia. It illustrates the various stages that a person experiences, from a premorbid 'normal' state to the onset of psychotic symptoms and recovery (see Figure 11.1). The model makes some assumptions

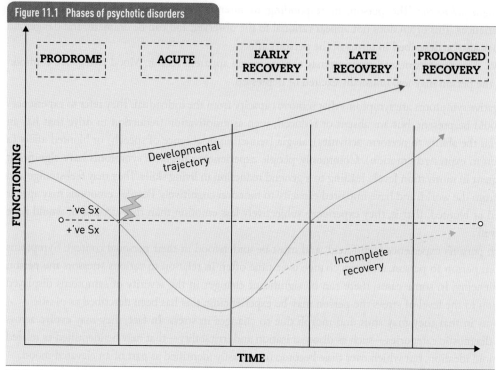

Figure 11.1 Phases of psychotic disorders

Note: Sx means 'symptoms'.

McGorry et al. (1996)

as to the inevitable nature of illness development. Note that the length of each phase varies from person to person, and that some people who experience psychosis do not go on to develop schizophrenia.

However, this model does not include the possibility of relapse, as discussed in the following five stages of a psychotic episode:

1 *Premorbid.* In this stage, there are no signs or symptoms of mental illness; rather, developmentally appropriate experiences and behaviours are the norm.

2 *Prodrome.* In clinical medicine, a prodrome refers to the early symptoms and signs of an illness that precede the characteristic manifestations of the acute, fully developed illness. Prodrome implies that the onset of an illness is inevitable. Prodrome in psychotic disorders essentially refers to the period of pre-psychotic disturbance, representing a deviation from a person's previous experience and behaviour. Generally, the early signs are vague and hardly noticeable. There may be changes in the way some people describe their feelings, thoughts and perceptions. In most cases, the prodrome is defined retrospectively once a diagnosis of psychotic disorder has been made. People who experience schizophrenia commonly have a long period of pre-psychotic prodromal symptoms, generally one to five years before the onset of psychosis (Larsen et al., 2000).

3 *Acute.* The acute phase is characterised by positive psychotic symptoms.

4 *Recovery and late recovery.* This phase begins when there is an initiation of treatment. The pattern of recovery varies from person to person. During the recovery phase, acute symptoms remit. Lieberman and colleagues (1993) report that the mean interval between initiating medication and achieving

maximum improvement was thirty-six weeks, with a median of eleven weeks. Up to 85–90 per cent of people with a first episode of psychosis will achieve a remission or partial remission of their positive psychotic symptoms within twelve months of initiation of treatment. During the late recovery phase, functional recovery occurs.

5 *Relapse*. The early course of schizophrenia and affective psychosis is turbulent and relapse prone, with up to 80 per cent of consumers relapsing within five years (Edwards et al., 2002). Psychosis is hypothesised to be caused by a variety of biological and psychological factors. These can be summarised in the stress vulnerability model of illness (see the following section). This model describes a person as having a set vulnerability to illness (in this case a psychotic illness), and when faced with excess stress the person suffers psychotic experiences. These experiences, if ongoing, may become persistent.

BOX 11.1 A CONSUMER'S LIVED EXPERIENCE OF PSYCHOSIS

When I was diagnosed with schizophrenia in 1976 it was seen back then as a virtual death sentence. The prognosis was dire. I was told by clinicians that with each episode of psychosis I had, I would go deeper into an unreachable madness, from which there was no recovery. There was no presumption of capacity—no thought that I would have the capability to achieve anything worthwhile in my life. I was a young graduate hoping to forge a future with meaningful work and an identity I was happy to own. However, with many admissions to psychiatric hospitals over the years I became embedded in the mental health system and the terrible pessimism that this instils in one's psyche. My world had fallen in a heap.

When a mind has a psychotic meltdown everything changes. The terror of such excruciating emotional distress leaves you with a fragile sense of self and a profound loss of self-belief. One feels like a distant alien in a threatening world. The grief is immense: you grieve for the loss of self, the loss of connectedness to the world, the loss of friends, the loss of opportunity, the loss of expectations and the loss of dignity. Doors close around you and the world is seen through a lens of abject failure: a failure to my friends and family, a failure to society and a failure in my own eyes. The overwhelming sense of hopelessness is profound and is compounded by a lack of self-confidence, which can cause you to retreat further into yourself. In many ways a mental illness infantilises you because you become dependent on others for a raft of supports. I rely on the government for my pension, my friends for support, the mental health system when I am unwell and my psychiatrist for ongoing therapy. One feels the eyes of the world look upon you full of judgment and fear, and you become a curiosity.

And then there are the voices; those peculiar creatures that inhabit my mind and barrage me with their persecution and abuse. One minute they are rambling and random, the next they are poignant and pointed; they can be cajoling and seductively persuasive, only to become pitiless and cruel. Their agenda is to destroy me or have me destroy myself. They warn me not to trust my friends or doctors, or anyone or anything that is a positive force in my life. The more miserable I am, the happier they are. Their rantings and ravings make it very difficult to concentrate on tasks or to have conversations with other people. When they are in full flight concentration is impossible. Sadly, relationships can be poisoned by voices while the wider world is perceived as a threatening place. There is a real struggle to make sense of things. Confusion reigns. Even making a small decision about which chair to sit in becomes a chore, let alone more demanding decisions.

Psychosis can engross you in its fantastical unreality generating paranoia and fear based on nothing tangible or real. And voices feed

SIMON DODD AND SANDY JEFFS

delusions and delusions feed voices. They are an indivisible force that casts a shadow over everything you do. Incongruent thoughts can fly through your mind like flighty birds. A stranger's voice erupts from my mouth and unfiltered thoughts tumble out. Wild beliefs that come from a small shard of truth, or from no truth at all, can spellbind you. There is a dream-like or nightmare-like sense associated with psychotic symptoms that gives weight to the experience. With my troubled mind I see strange creatures crawl on the walls. Tony Blair has implanted a microchip in my left ear and programmed it to delete my thoughts. I am Eve. I gave Adam the apple. I brought Original Sin into the world. My thoughts are being broadcast to the world; people can read my mind. My hockey coach is sending telepathic messages about me to George W. Bush and Condoleezza Rice. My evil oozes over everything and I mustn't let anyone touch me lest I contaminate them. The mirror is home to a hag who confronts me with the personification of the evil woman my voices tell I am. It is as though your mind is fragmented into a thousand pieces and your core has exploded. When one's inner world is already a hostile place, the last thing one needs is a hostile external world.

Admission to a psychiatric ward is a traumatic event that cannot be understated, especially if the admission is an involuntary one. Being locked up and losing a sense of control over your life is challenging. An overwhelming sense of disappointment grips you: *How did I end up in a place like this?* Then there is the fear factor of being in a threatening environment and not knowing who to trust. Doctors and nurses, who are complete strangers, will ask the consumer a raft of questions expecting them to tell everything. You don't know what to expect. This is a world like no other. You are already traumatised by your emotional distress, and you may have trauma as part of your childhood story, and now you are in a place which re-traumatises you. Staff need to remember that while a person may appear distracted and 'out of it', don't assume they are unaware or not taking in what is happening around them. People remember the asides clinicians have with each other while in their presence. Both kindness and cruelty are not forgotten.

Relapse

Relapsing into psychosis is always a blow to one's hope. You find yourself asking perplexing questions: *How did I let it happen again? How did I end up back in this situation? Am going to be always like this? Will I ever recover and be a 'normal' person doing 'normal' things? Why can't I be like everyone else with a job, friends and a future?* A relapse always brings a person face to face with the prospect of having a chronic illness, with being a hapless failure in the eyes of family and friends. And a relapse can come out of the blue. Just when you think things are picking up and you dare to dream, suddenly the psychosis has crept upon you and you are back to square one. It can seem like you are on a treadmill of madness that won't let you off. And with multiple admissions to a psych ward you feel you are in the revolving door between hospital and home. Relapses of illness make it very difficult to maintain employment, study or social activities. After each breakdown, the task to glue oneself back together is more and more problematic. Holding onto hope in the face of a chronic mental illness is a Herculean task.

Recovery

Recovery is a profoundly unique experience—a change to the way one sees oneself. It is a process deeply felt by all who enter its realm and not one that is easily or lightly attained. Each person's recovery will be different. Recovery might be getting out of bed for one morning of one week for one person, while another's recovery might be getting a full-time job. It is not a linear process. It may have twists and turns, and ups and downs that make it a harrowing experience. It is hard fought for some and one that comes after a long and fraught campaign to find meaning in life when all has seemed lost. There are setbacks and triumphs. Recovery is about self-understanding and about finding hope—a reason for getting out of bed. There is no right or wrong way to recover. My personal recovery is the opportunity to lead a meaningful and fulfilling life with or without ongoing episodes of illness, and is very different from clinical recovery which is much more about the absence of symptoms and functional impairment. I talk of recovering *with* my schizophrenia, not *from* it. I still live with its spectre. It is a constant. I go to bed to my voices every night. I harbour delusions that fester beneath the surface; a psychotic blow-out always feels imminent. I don't like to think of recovery as a singular, individuated project; it is done better when there is collaboration between the person, their treating teams and friends and family. It is done better when the person is not cut off and isolated. If I have learnt one thing from my battle with schizophrenia, it is that I cannot wage the war against it on my own.

In this brave new mental health world in which we talk about person-centred recovery it needs to be understood that while a person may be at the centre of their recovery, what surrounds that centre can strengthen or weaken it. When the centre cannot hold it needs to be supported. Sadly, not everyone is in that fortunate position to have their *team* to support them. Nor does a personalised recovery plan suit some when they don't have the necessary tools, ability or attitude to utilise in their recovery work. Everyone has to find their own balance and their own path to recovery, and a one-size-fits-all model is not going to help those who remain on the margins. Recovery is finding hope and living with possibilities again. And this can be kindled in someone with good treatment and good nursing.

Medication as a treatment should be used in conjunction with other supports. It is only a key that unlocks a door. What is behind that door and how it is treated is crucial to the person's well-being. Behind that door is a person with a heart, soul, hopes, dreams and aspirations, and a profound vulnerability. Medicating a person is not enough. You can medicate the brain but ultimately you have to talk to a mind. Treatment has to be of the whole person, not the components in isolation. The person has to be supported to live in the community and given skills to gain entry into the workforce or help them to retain a job. The loss of an identity is one

of the first casualties with the onset of an illness such as schizophrenia. Helping a person to build or rebuild their sense of self and an identity they are comfortable with is important. A person may lose the opportunity to enter the workforce or establish significant relationships. They may have their education interrupted or truncated. Helping the person to participate in creative activities can be a very empowering experience for them. A nurse can encourage someone to look at their options and find a path through their illness. But it must be done *with* the person not *for* the person. Encouraging someone to take risks is also important. Psychosis can shatter someone's confidence and cause them to withdraw from the world and not take risks because of a fear of failure or a fear of the unknown.

Medication

Medication is an ongoing problem because of the side effects. One cannot discount how overwhelming the effects of antipsychotic medication can be. The sedation, muddle-headedness, fuzziness, physical debilitation, lethargy, sexual dysfunction and loss of libido, a feeling of having one's thoughts depleted—all are impediments to taking medication. Weight gain is distressing because one feels powerless in the face of an ever-growing body. How we see ourselves in the mirror is important to our self-esteem, let alone how much of a hurdle being overweight is to being active. Antipsychotic medications are powerful drugs with powerful effects on a person's brain and body. Be sympathetic to someone's misgivings about medication and be especially mindful of how they are affecting a person.

The role of a nurse

Good nursing is a crucial ingredient for helping someone come to terms with being in a hospital setting or living with a mental illness in the community. Forming a therapeutic relationship can help someone develop trust in a setting that might otherwise seem hostile and impersonal. Breaching the barriers of psychosis is not easy and helping the person to emerge from a psychotic fog is something to aim for. If someone

SIMON DODD AND SANDY JEFFS

is overtaken with paranoia and suspicion, the nurse has to navigate this with patience and respectfulness, and not expect to engage with the person in a short time. In the acute clinical setting there might not be enough time to form a good therapeutic relationship, but a quality short-term relationship is better than nothing. Nurses are the ones who spend more time with the consumers and have the chance to form a good relationship with them. Trust is an issue and is not easily given to a nurse (or psychiatrist) in a clinical setting. Why would someone trust a nurse with their life story and emotional distress when they can't be sure they will see that nurse again? For many consumers, having to retell their story to an endless procession of staff can be frustrating and stressful. Sometimes people are too scared to talk about their feelings because they fear it may lead to an increase in medication. Nothing can go past spending time with someone, having a chat, finding out what they like to read, the music they like to listen to, or their favourite film. The basic humanity of validating a person and their experiences is essential to their dignity in a place where their dignity may have been compromised. Care, compassion, understanding and non-judgmental attitudes are key qualities necessary for good nursing. Consideration and thoughtfulness in staff can mean the difference between a good or bad experience of an admission, and can influence how a person would feel if they were faced with subsequent admissions to a psychiatric ward. Helping someone heal their broken mind is the role of good nursing.

Carers

Having an illness such as schizophrenia can make one dependent on family and friends for a home, social support and friendship, financial support and care when unwell. The relationship with one's carers can be rocky and difficult, especially if the illness is not under control. Our carers often don't have a choice in their role and they suffer their own difficulties in accepting their situation. They may lose friends and opportunities because they are caring for someone. Carers grieve for

their loved ones and what the mental illness has taken away from them. Everyone in a family is affected by someone's mental illness.

If friends are one's carers then one has to navigate the difficult territory between them being your friends and carers. I hate making my friends my jailers when I am unwell and need to be looked after day and night, day after day, week after week. It strains the friendship and puts them in an awkward position.

A consequence of being diagnosed with schizophrenia is that carers and friends, out of concern, can become over anxious about their loved one and inadvertently discourage them from taking risks because they fear they might crash and burn. Another outcome is being watched by loved ones for tell-tale signs of a relapse into madness. One feels the concerned gaze of friends and family upon oneself, and the pressure to live a measured life with no fluctuations of mood or behaviour is intensely felt. Carers' watchfulness is through worry for the well-being of the person they are caring for and is understandable, but it can become too attentive and oppressive. There is dignity in being able to take risks; how else can one see what one is capable of doing?

Trauma informed care

When someone presents at an acute psychiatric ward with auditory hallucinations and delusional thinking, you as a nurse will be crucial in helping them come to terms with their present situation. If the statistics are correct—with up 70 per cent of people who present to a mental health ward having experienced childhood trauma, sexual and physical abuse, severe neglect and/or domestic violence, or having witnessed terrorism or disasters—then nurses have to be aware that symptoms such as voices can be informed by these traumatic events. Rather than focusing on what is wrong with the person, perhaps it is worth asking: *What has happened to you to bring you here?* Their lived experience may have a very important part to play in the content of their voices and delusions. Historically, voices have been relegated to mere meaningless ramblings of madness, which had to be medicated away with powerful antipsychotic medication. If someone is hearing voices, don't dismiss them as unimportant. It is perhaps more validating for the person to have the content of their voices recognised by a nurse asking in a sympathetic manner what the voices are saying, how distressing they are, how the person feels about them, and is there a way we can work with you to help you manage the voices better? The voices might be saying something meaningful or drawing on events that have happened sometime in the person's life.

And don't forget that just being admitted to a psychiatric ward can be a traumatic experience in itself, or a re-traumatising event for people who already have trauma in their background. For a lot of people an admission to a psychiatric ward is often involuntary—they may not wish to be there. It takes a lot of reassurance to help someone to cope with the shock of what has happened. The human thing to do is sit to with the person and engage with them, and not to be afraid to talk about to them about their voices. Don't be afraid of them even if they are afraid of you. You can break down the barrier with non-judgmental kindness and by keeping in mind that they are most likely to be terrified and overwhelmed with what is happening to them.

REFLECTION QUESTIONS

1   What role can you play in alleviating anxiety during an admission to hospital for a person experiencing a psychotic episode?

2   How can you help a person remain hopeful during a traumatic psychotic experience?

The stress vulnerability model

There have been many aetiological models used to describe the causes of psychosis. The most useful model to understand these causes (aetiology) is the stress vulnerability model. This model was developed by Zubin and Spring (1977), and has been modified extensively to include psychosis and concepts of an area between wellness and illness that is in flux. The model also allows for many types of vulnerabilities and these will no doubt change as our understanding of the causes and course of the psychosis experience expands.

Our understanding of the effects of trauma have grown and it seems now a significant contributor leading to illness (Bechdolf et al., 2010; Bendall et al., 2013; Fusar-Poli et al., 2016; Varese et al., 2012), as well as a consequence of poor or inadequate treatment (Berry et al., 2013).

The model describes the impact of stress on different people with various degrees of vulnerability (see Figure 11.2). Importantly, stress changes and the impact of this change to stress also changes. If people are placed in a position whereby they exceed a threshold, they experience illness. The model is a useful psycho-educational tool, and is effective in normalising the experience of illness.

In this model, point A represents a person with a high capacity to manage stress. Point C represents a person with normal stress levels. Points B and F represent people who have some of sub-threshold psychosis experiences, and may or may not undergo a transition to illness, although these experiences may well be having an impact on the quality of life. Points D and E represent people experiencing frank psychotic symptoms.

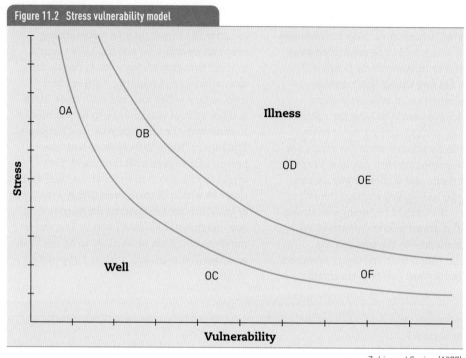

Figure 11.2 Stress vulnerability model

Zubin and Spring (1977)

It is important to note the dynamic nature of illness experiences. With a reduction of stress, the person may well dip beneath the threshold into 'wellness'. In addition, considering all human experience on a continuum from mental health to mental illness removes us from the false dichotomy of perfect health/profound illness.

The clinical staging model

The clinical staging model is a diagnostic model that is commonly used in medicine and has the benefit of offering different (potentially less costly and more benign) treatments depending on the stage of a person's illness. It defines the course of illness in terms of a continuum.

Various interventions can be chosen by the person (supported by their treating team) to prevent or delay progression from earlier to later stages of illness, and can be selected on the basis of defined risk/benefit, which will differ across different stages of illness. Table 11.1 details general interventions and nursing-specific interventions, which range from health promotion in the community to long-term hospital treatment for people with enduring illness.

TABLE 11.1 CLINICAL STAGING MODEL				
Clinical Stage	**Definition**	**Definition in phase model**	**Interventions**	**Nursing interventions**
0	Increased risk of psychosis No symptoms currently	Premorbid	Indicated prevention of first episode psychosis (FEP): ■ improved mental health literacy ■ family education, drug education ■ brief cognitive skills training	Mental health promotion based community mental health nursing
1a	Mild or non-specific symptoms of psychosis, including neurocognitive deficits; mild functional change or decline	Possible prodrome	Indicated prevention of FEP: ■ improved mental health literacy ■ family education, drug education ■ brief cognitive skills training	Mental health Promotion-based community mental health nursing
1b	Ultra-high risk of psychosis: Moderate but sub-threshold symptoms, with moderate neurocognitive changes and functional decline to caseness or chronic poor functioning (≥30 per cent drop in SOFAS* in previous 12 months OR <50 for previous 12 months)	Possible prodrome	Indicated secondary prevention of FEP: ■ psycho-education, formal CBT ■ active reduction of substance misuse ■ omega-3 fatty acids ■ antidepressant agents or mood stabilisers	Early intervention Community-based nursing
2	First episode of psychotic disorder: full threshold with moderate-severe symptoms, neurocognitive deficits and functional decline (GAF† 30–50) includes acute and early recovery periods	Acute and early recovery	Early intervention for FEP: ■ psycho-education, formal CBT ■ active reduction of substance misuse ■ atypical antipsychotic agents ■ antidepressant agents or mood stabilisers ■ vocational rehabilitation	Early intervention in hospital- and community-based early psychosis service

*Social and Occupational Functioning Assessment Scale
†Global Assessment of Functioning

SIMON DODD AND SANDY JEFFS

TABLE 11.1 CLINICAL STAGING MODEL (*CONTINUED*)

Clinical Stage	Definition	Definition in phase model	Interventions	Nursing interventions
3a	Incomplete remission from first episode of care	Late/incomplete recovery	Early intervention for FEP As for '2' but with additional emphasis on medical and psychosocial strategies to achieve full remission	Hospital- and community-based treatment
3b	Recurrence or relapse of psychotic disorder that stabilises with treatment but at a level of GAF, residual symptoms, or neurocognition below the best level achieved following remission from first episode	Late/incomplete recovery	Early intervention for FEP As for '3a' but with additional emphasis on relapse prevention and 'early warning signs' strategies	Hospital- and community-based treatment
3c	Multiple relapses, with objective worsening in clinical extent and impact of illness	Late/incomplete recovery	Early intervention for FEP As for '3b' but with emphasis on long-term stabilisation	Hospital- and community-based treatment with specialist recovery programs
4	Severe, persistent OR unremitting illness as judged by symptoms, neurocognition and disability criteria	Chronicity	As for '3c' but with emphasis on clozapine, other tertiary treatments, and social participation despite ongoing disability	Hospital- and community-based treatment with specialist recovery programs

Adapted from McGorry et al. (2006)

BOX 11.2 SETTINGS FOR MENTAL HEALTH NURSE CARE OF THOSE EXPERIENCING PSYCHOSIS

When we work with consumers, we know that the work that we do is important. In emergency departments around the country, particularly since the deinstitutionalisation of the large psychiatric facilities in the late 1980s (Coleborne & MacKinnon, 2006), there has been an increase in the contacts that health services can expect. In addition, the movement away from traditional inpatient facilities has forced modern nurses to change their practice, requiring them to become more flexible in the various settings available to their work practice.

In the inpatient unit—the traditional acute psychiatric setting—the length of stay of consumers has become noticeably shorter, with most rehabilitation and recovery programs now based in the community. The skills that the nurse uses in this setting in particular relate to containment and engagement. The person is usually very unwell and in crisis. This has led to a limiting of exposure to therapy for nurses specialising in the acute setting. However, the ward remains the setting in which most mental health nurses start their careers and where most nurses are employed (Patterson & Leeuwenkamp, 2008).

Today the principal setting is the community setting (that is, a clinic-based setting where the person visits a clinician), and is where most consumers will receive ongoing mental health care. The home setting, the person's place of residence, where the nurse is a visitor, is also significant. When a clinician visits a person in their own home, the nurse is privileged to experience their hospitality. Other settings may be described as 'neutral ground'. Examples of these include hospital emergency departments, police stations, cafés and parks. These environments give rise to issues of boundaries and confidentiality, but offer the benefit of empowering the person without intruding on the home.

1   Why do you think the clinical setting is the principal setting for mental health service provision?
2   Is the person's home a 'neutral' setting? Why or why not?

REFLECTION QUESTIONS

Applicability to the clinical practice setting

An understanding of the various psychoses is core to the majority of work that the modern mental health nurse does. In working with people who have experienced psychosis, we come to understand the global impact that this disorder has. All aspects of a person's life are damaged. From the interaction with loved ones at home to the most superficial contact at a corner shop, the experience of the outside world is changed, mostly to a darker truth. In Australian seminal studies, it appears that there has been a previously unthought-of levels of psychotic experiences in general community populations (McGorry et al., 1995).

It should be noted that there is a significant change in the therapy relationship, depending on the environment the person is seen in. The 'ownership' of a space has an impact on the engagement of the consumer and the relationship during the interview. This is a dynamic variable that does not become obvious until the person has been seen in an alternative environment. You cannot 'know' the person until you have seen them in their own place.

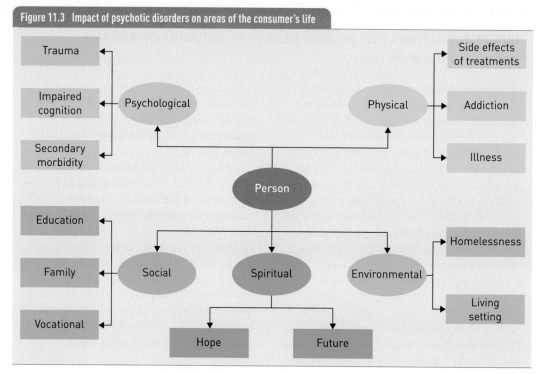

Figure 11.3   Impact of psychotic disorders on areas of the consumer's life

Knapp & Razzouk (2008)

The impact that these illnesses have on quality of life is also profound (Knapp & Razzouk, 2008) when we consider Figure 11.3, showing the areas in a person's life that are affected. The impact of psychosis on physical health is also significant. There are complex interactions between illness (the symptoms of psychosis contributing to behavioural disturbance), treatment (for example, the effects of neuroleptic medication on metabolic processes) and social factors (diet, exercise and high rates of smoking) that all contribute to a reduction in life expectancy of up to 20 years when compared to the general population (Lawrence, Hancock & Kisely, 2013).

Economically, the impact of schizophrenia and the psychoses is extensive. Mental illness, even within restrictive definitions, is still the seventh most expensive disease category in Australia (Williams & Doessel, 2008), and is responsible for 13 per cent of total burden of disease (Australian Institute of Health and Welfare, 2008, p. 224). Schizophrenia represented one-third of total costs, and ranked first in hospital costs within total mental health costs (Access Economics, 2008). When opportunity costs (lost earnings and carer's lost earnings) and intangible costs (distress, pain and suffering) are considered, it is clearly a major health issue. Effective early treatment has many compelling arguments, economically as well as clinically (Tsiachristas et al., 2016).

Skills you will use within the stages of the relationship

In day-to-day mental health care, the mental health nurse will have regular contact with consumers experiencing psychosis. In order to work with people with mental health problems, we must develop an ability to connect with them. There must be a balance between the distance that the experienced clinician must keep and the closeness that is necessary to understand and support the ill person. Various skills are required to help a person with psychosis. Many of these are not specific to psychosis, but are core skills when working with people with mental health issues. Because the environment the nurse works in is fluid, a framework to consider is depicted in Figure 11.4.

Connection

The main skill you will need is engagement: a development of the relationship such that some therapeutic work can be attempted. This process is essential to allow effective connection. The process of engagement may be healing in and of itself (Tait, Birchwood & Trower, 2003; Mitchell & Selmes, 2007). Practical actions are helpful at this time.

Working

Communication is essential in all stages, but comes to the fore when exploring the issues that the person is experiencing. This helps them in understanding the experience, and can assist in allowing consumers to formulate their experience. Also, because of the nature of the symptoms it is often difficult for consumers to communicate their needs effectively. Distress can be communicated in a variety of ways, and these are often not initially obvious.

We need to assist the consumer to develop a useful working relationship. This should give as much control for treatment to the consumer as is possible. This process of empowering is a balance between containing a person in personal crisis and encouraging that person to be in control. A sense of optimism is necessary in order to engender a sense of hope in the consumer. There is clear evidence that recovery is likely, and that psychosis is not the chronic sentence it may well have been in the past (Warner, 2009).

At this time, and as soon as possible, we should aim to connect the consumer to functional recovery. This reduces the damage done to the person's functioning environment and support systems, as well as providing positive benefits to the quality of life (Penn et al., 2011; Wunderink et al., 2013). Aim at symptom reduction, social reintegration and dealing with grief and loss.

Disengagement

Disengagement is about effectively connecting the person back into their own system, with appropriate supports and access to assistance in the event of recurring issues or increased stressors (Warner, 2009). This assumes that existing systems have been maintained. It may be necessary to assist the consumer in the development of new supports.

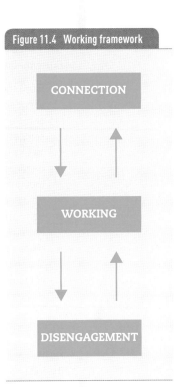

Figure 11.4 Working framework

ABOUT THE CONSUMER   Bahal's story

Bahal is a 17-year-old unemployed male of Turkish background living at home with his parents and older brother. Recently he was asked to leave school because of 'behavioural issues'. He was referred to your service by an ex-school counsellor at the request of his sister, who was 'worried he's going to kill himself or someone else'. Bahal is currently on a bond for driving without a licence and related charges. He is on a community order for recent threats towards police.

He presents as a slightly anxious but quite cooperative young man, quite unlike the way he is described by others. Bahal describes a number of difficulties dating back to a motor vehicle accident (when he was aged 11), when he was knocked over while crossing the road. He describes a brief loss of consciousness, but no fractures or bad bruising. There was no medical intervention at this time. His sister was unaware of this incident. Currently he describes the following:

■ Since the motor vehicle accident, he has experienced nightmares on average once a week, especially about an alien-like creature standing over him and looking at him. He wakes in fright. He also describes occasional experiences of his body levitating off the bed, and feeling strangled; and sometimes feels that something or someone enters his body, changing him (both his voice and appearance, making him behave 'unlike himself'). He fears that he may do something 'bad' to someone during these times.

■ He found academic work harder in secondary school. He was picked on by older children and bullied (he brought a knife to school because of this). He had few friends as 'they always let him down'.

■ He denies alcohol or substance use, but has had trouble with 'chroming' (sniffing solvent) in the past.

■ He hears vague calling of his name every three to four weeks.

■ Recently he has had some difficulties with his part-time work.

■ He has anxiety symptoms secondary to the above described stressors; for example, choking, chest pain, shortness of breath and feelings of fear (but no anxiety or panic in between incidents). He feels a lowering of mood secondary to these symptoms.

■ He complains of poor memory and becoming disorganised.

PAST PSYCHIATRIC HISTORY

He has seen the GP for 'nerves' in the past. He was treated with an antidepressant, but the duration or dosage of the treatment is unclear.

FAMILY HISTORY

His parents are practising Muslims who are not overly strict. He has a good relationship with his sister. He has a conflict with his brother, who tells Bahal that he is 'stupid' and needs help.

PERSONAL AND DEVELOPMENTAL HISTORY

He grew up in Australia. He had a normal birth and growth milestones. He describes himself as a healthy, 'good kid', a happy child. He deteriorated in secondary school, became isolated and picked on, got into fights, and became academically poor. He was a talented football player in the past (a professional was interested in him).

CURRENT SOCIAL CIRCUMSTANCES AND FUNCTIONING

He is living with parents and older brother. He has some friends, but cannot specify whom. He had a serious relationship with a girl for one-and-a-half years, but is currently single.

REFLECTION QUESTIONS

1   Psychosis affects the way a person interacts internally with the external environment. Using the latest research, how do you imagine this would affect Bahal's view of the future? How do you feel that you would respond to Bahal? What do you feel are the barriers and enablers for you to actively engage with Bahal? What issues around secondary morbidity should be considered for Bahal? How will you engage Bahal and his family in his care?

2   How would you prioritise care, ensuring Bahal's safety and the safety of others?

3   What are the cultural considerations for Bahal in terms of planning and implementing care?

4   Consider some of the diagnostic dilemmas and/or co-morbidities that may relate to Bahal's story. Who should you consult with in relation to your clinical assessment?

Care planning

The following is an example care plan for Bahal. The areas of daily living that are considered in the recovery framework and include biopsychosocial factors and the plan is mapped out using the nursing process (assessment, planning, implementation and evaluation). Remember, the success is in the detail, so be specific about who, when and what in the collaborative plan; and never include someone in the plan if they were not consulted in the planning process.

Date: [Today's date]						
Consumer's name: Bahal			**Consumer case manager: T. Player**			
Areas of daily living	**Assessment of current situation**	**Goal**	**Plan (undertaken with consumer)**	**Implementation**	**Who is responsible (include only those who have been consulted in the planning process)**	**Evaluation/ review date**
Mental health	Early signs of psychotic illness	Monitor and reduce impact of symptoms	Monitor early warning signs (EWS) of symptoms: feeling more agitated and pacing more; poor sleep; poor concentration.	Develop an early signs list and document this.	Bahal T. Player	23/03/18
			Action—if EWS are present' use distraction techniques.	Bahal to keep a list of early warning signs with him and a copy to be attached to the fridge door.	Bahal	Ongoing
	Distress and anxiety symptoms	Reduce impact of symptoms	Identify occasions and develop strategies for managing distress and monitoring triggers.	Use mindfulness techniques and diary for monitoring triggers and symptoms.	Bahal	Ongoing
Social	Unemployed since leaving school	Bahal wants to get a job	Look for potential volunteer jobs as a starting point. Liaise with vocation worker when available. Liaise with employment network groups for assistance.	Bahal will attend an appointment at the employment network service. Appointment will be arranged by T. Player.	T. Player and Bahal	23/03/18

Date: [Today's date]						
	Family relationships	Maintain family relationship	Use psychoeducation and initial family work to give appropriate information to his family as to Bahal's needs and current circumstances, including EWS and referral pathways.	Bahal's family will have access to information and support.	T. Player, Bahal and Bahal's family	23/03/18 Ongoing
	Legal issues related to court orders	Reduce legal issues and associated stresses	With Bahal's permission contact and engage legal services to support as appropriate.	Contact appropriate services.	Bahal and T. Player	23/03/18
	Cultural needs	Ensure Bahal's cultural needs are observed for and included in plan.	Discuss and support any cultural issues that Bahal may identify.	Speak with Bahal re cultural issues.	Bahal and T. Player	Ongoing
Biological	Assessment of physical needs	Identify any physical health issues and obtain baseline for them.	Discuss motivation, beliefs and ambivalence for adhering or not adhering to medication/ treatment.	Continue with regular appointments with T. Player.	T. Player and Bahal	Every two weeks
Environmental	Isolation and reduced social interactions	Minimise potential for isolation.	Explore membership to community groups related to Bahal's interests. Re-engage with local football club with a possibility of return to playing.	Develop a list of at least two interests for Bahal. Local football club address and trial day to be obtained by Bahal.	Bahal and T. Player	23/03/18
Substance using behaviours	History of substance use but none identified currently	Reduce the risks associated with substance use.	Monitor substance use and identify alternative methods for goal-obtaining behaviours (other than substance use).	Use appropriate motivational techniques and behavioural activation processes for Bahal to reduce chances of reuse of substances.	T. Player and Bahal	Each appointment
Risk behaviours	History of incidents involving threats towards others	Reduce incidents of risk behaviour.	Monitor and give alternatives for actions.	Work together to discuss alternatives to fear or stress induced by psychotic symptoms.	T. Player and Bahal	Each appointment

Nursing practice reflection

Young people who present with possible psychotic symptoms and complex family situations with multiple morbidities (or possible morbidities) are vulnerable to poor treatment. It is the responsibility and a privilege of the nurse to help them understand their experience in such a way to allow them to accept help and to begin recovery. Everyone has a right to be well and the nurse has a duty to assist and facilitate this task.

SUMMARY

In this chapter you have learnt that around three out of every 100 people will experience a psychotic episode. Nurses need to have an understanding of psychosis, and should always consider the context of the person who is experiencing the psychosis. Importantly, most people experiencing psychosis for the first time make a good recovery from the experience. A psychotic episode occurs in stages, and a useful model to understand the aetiology (causation) of psychosis is the stress vulnerability model. If the person is placed in a position whereby they exceed a threshold, they experience illness. The model is a useful psycho-educational tool, and is effective in normalising the experience of illness. Various skills are required to help a person with psychosis. Many of these are not specific to psychosis, but are core skills when working with people with mental illness. The skills you will use when working with people who experience mental illness are directed towards dealing with symptom reduction, social reintegration and grief and loss.

DISCUSSION QUESTIONS

1   What is meant by the term 'psychosis'?
2   What are positive and negative symptoms?
3   What is the clinical staging model?
4   What are the concepts of connection, working and disengagement involved in a therapeutic relationship?
5   What are the settings in which a nurse will care for those who experience psychosis?

TEST YOURSELF

1   The mental health nurse will use various skills to build a therapeutic relationship with a person who is experiencing psychosis. Using the working framework as a guide, the stages of building this working relationship are:
   a   beginning, middle and end
   b   connection, working and exit
   c   connection, working and disengagement
   d   beginning, working and disengagement

2 Select the statement that is correct for the receipt of ongoing mental health care for people who experience psychosis.

a Today, the principal setting is the hospital setting, and is where most consumers will receive ongoing mental health care.

b Today, the principal setting is the community setting (that is, a clinic-based setting where the person visits a clinician), and is where most consumers will receive ongoing mental health care.

c Today, the principal setting is the virtual setting (that is, an internet-based interactive setting where the person visits a clinician), and is where most consumers will receive ongoing mental health care.

d Today, the principal setting is the primary health setting (that is, a general practice-based setting where the person visits a clinician), and is where most consumers will receive ongoing mental health care.

3 The stress-vulnerability model is:

a the model that describes the impact of pressure on different people with various degrees of weakness

b the model that describes the impact of stress on different people with various degrees of the individual's resilience

c the model that describes the impact of the absence of stress on different people with various degrees of vulnerability

d the model that describes the impact of stress on different people with various degrees of vulnerability

4 From a consumers point of view which statement is most true?

a Good nursing is a crucial ingredient for helping someone come to terms with being in a hospital setting or living with a mental illness in the community. Forming a therapeutic relationship can help someone develop trust in a setting that might otherwise seem hostile and impersonal.

b Good nursing is demonstrated when the right medications are dispensed and that is how a therapeutic relationship is initiated.

c Nursing is considered 'good' when the nurse has provided care for that person for more than three days in a row.

d Forming a relationship with the person in care is the basis of good nursing.

USEFUL WEBSITES

Early Psychosis Prevention and Intervention Centre (EPPIC): http://oyh.org.au/our-services/clinical-program/continuing-care-teams/eppic-early-psychosis-prevention-intervention

Headspace: www.headspace.org.au

Orygen Youth Health: www.oyh.org.au

ReachOut.com: https://au.reachout.com/

SANE Australia— Psychosis: https://www.sane.org/mental-health-and-illness/facts-and-guides/psychosis

REFERENCES

Access Economics (2008). *Cost effectiveness of early intervention for psychosis* (pp. 1–49). Canberra: Access Economics.

Australian Institute of Health and Welfare (2008). *Australia's Health 2008*. Canberra: AIHW.

Bertelsen, M., Jeppesen, P., Petersen, L., Thorup, A., Ohlenschlaeger, J., le Quach, P., Christensen, T., Krarup, G., Jorgensen, P., & Nordentoft, M. (2008). Five-year follow-up of a randomized multicenter trial of intensive early intervention vs standard treatment for patients with a first episode of psychotic illness: The OPUS trial. *Archives of General Psychiatry*, 65(7), 762–771.

Bechdolf, A., Thompson, A., Nelson, B., Cotton, S., Simmons, M. B., Amminger, G. P. et al. (2010). Experience of trauma and conversion to psychosis in an ultra-high-risk (prodromal) group. *Acta Psychiatrica Scandinavica*, 121(5), 377–384.

Bendall, S., Alvarez-Jimenez, M., Nelson, B., & McGorry, P. (2013). Childhood trauma and psychosis: New perspectives on aetiology and treatment. *Early Intervention in Psychiatry*, 7(1), 1–4.

Berry, K., Ford, S., Jellicoe-Jones, L., & Haddock, G. (2013). PTSD symptoms associated with the experiences of psychosis and hospitalisation: A review of the literature. *Clinical Psychology Review, 33*(4), 526–538.

Chisholm, D., Gureje, O., Saldivia, S., Villalón Calderón, M., Wickremasinghe, R., Mendis, N., Ayuso-Mateos, J., & Saxena, S. (2008). Schizophrenia treatment in the developing world: An interregional and multinational cost-effectiveness analysis. *Bulletin of the World Health Organization, 86*(7), 542–551.

Coleborne, C., & MacKinnon, D. (2006). Psychiatry and its institutions in Australia and New Zealand: An overview. *International Review of Psychiatry, 18*(4), 371–380.

Edwards, J., Maude, D., Herrmann-Doig, T., Wong, L., Cocks, J., Burnett, P., Bennett, C., Wade, D., & McGorry, P. (2002). A service response to prolonged recovery in early psychosis. *Psychiatric Services, 53*(9), 1067–1069.

Fusar-Poli, P., Tantardini, M., De Simone, S., Ramella-Cravaro, V., Oliver, D., Kingdon, J. et al. (2016). Deconstructing vulnerability for psychosis: Meta-analysis of environmental risk factors for psychosis in subjects at ultra high-risk. *European Psychiatry, 40*, 65–75.

Knapp, M., & Razzouk, D. (2008). Costs of schizophrenia. *Psychiatry, 7*(11), 491–494.

Larsen, T., Moe, L., Vibe-Hansen, L., & Johannessen, J. (2000). Premorbid functioning versus duration of untreated psychosis in 1 year outcome in first-episode psychosis. *Schizophrenic Research, 45*(1–2), 1–9.

Lawrence, D., Hancock, K. J., & Kisely, S. (2013). The gap in life expectancy from preventable physical illness in psychiatric patients in Western Australia: Retrospective analysis of population based registers. *BMJ, 346*(1), f2539–f2539.

Lieberman, J., Jody, D., Geisler, S., Alvir, J., Loebel, A., Szymanski, S., Woerner, M., & Borenstein, M. (1993). Time course and biological correlates of treatment response in first episode schizophrenia. *Archives of General Psychology, 50*(5), 369–376.

McGorry, P. D., Edwards, J., Mihalopoulos, C., Harrigan, S. M., & Jackson, H. J. (1996). EPPIC: An evolving system of early detection and optimal management. *Schizophrenia Bulletin, 22*(2), 305–326.

McGorry, P., McFarlane, C., Patton, G., Bell, R., Hibbert, M., Jackson, H., & Bowes, G. (1995). The prevalence of prodromal features of schizophrenia in adolescence: A preliminary survey. *Acta Psychologica Scandinavia, 92*(4), 241–249.

McGorry, P., Hickie, I., Yung, A., Pantelis, C., & Jackson, H. (2006). Clinical staging of psychiatric disorders: A heuristic framework for choosing earlier, safe and more effective interventions. *Australian and New Zealand Journal of Psychiatry, 40*(8), 616–622.

Mitchell, A., & Selmes, T. (2007). Why don't patients attend their appointments? Maintaining engagement with psychiatric services. *Advances in Psychiatric Treatment, 13*(6), 423.

Patterson, T., & Leeuwenkamp, O. (2008). Adjunctive psychosocial therapies for the treatment of schizophrenia. *Schizophrenia Research, 100*(1–3), 108–119.

Penn, D. L., Uzenoff, S. R., Perkins, D., Mueser, K. T., Hamer, R., Waldheter, E. et al. (2011). A pilot investigation of the Graduated Recovery Intervention Program (GRIP) for first episode psychosis. *Schizophrenia Research, 125*(2–3), 247–256.

Petersen, L., Thorup, A., Oqhlenschlaeger, J., Christensen, T., Jeppesen, P., Krarup, G., Jorrgensen, P., Mortensen, E., & Nordentoft, M. (2008). Predictors of remission and recovery in a first-episode schizophrenia spectrum disorder sample: 2-year follow-up of the OPUS Trial. *Canadian Journal of Psychiatry, 53*(10), 660–670.

Scott, J., Martin, G., Bor, W., Sawyer, M., Clark, J., & McGrath, J. (2009). The prevalence and correlates of hallucinations in Australian adolescents: Results from a national survey. *Schizophrenia Research, 107*(2–3), 179–185.

Simeone, J. C., Ward, A. J., Rotella, P., Collins, J., & Windisch, R. (2015). An evaluation of variation in published estimates of schizophrenia

prevalence from 1990–2013: A systematic literature review. *BMC Psychiatry, 15*(1), 193.

Tait, L., Birchwood, M., & Trower, P. (2003). Predicting engagement with services for psychosis: Insight, symptoms and recovery style. *British Journal of Psychiatry, 182*(2), 123–128.

Tsiachristas, A., Thomas, T., Leal, J., & Lennox, B. R. (2016). Economic impact of early intervention in psychosis services: results from a longitudinal retrospective controlled study in England. *BMJ Open, 6*(10), e012611. Retrieved from http://dx.doi.org/10.1136/bmjopen-2016-012611. Retrieved from http://dx.doi.org/10.1136/bmjopen-2016-012611.

van Os, J., Linscott, R. J., Myin-Germeys, I., Delespaul, P., & Krabbendam, L. (2009). A systematic review and meta-analysis of the psychosis continuum: Evidence for a psychosis proneness-persistence-impairment model of psychotic disorder. *Psychological Medicine, 39*(2), 179–195.

Varese, F., Smeets, F., Drukker, M., Lieverse, R., Lataster, T., Viechtbauer, W. et al. (2012). Childhood adversities increase the risk of psychosis: a meta-analysis of patient-control, prospective- and cross-sectional cohort studies. *Schizophrenia Bulletin, 38*(4), 661–671.

Warner, R. (2009). Recovery from schizophrenia and the recovery model. *Current Opinion in Psychiatry, 22*(4), 374–380.

Williams, R. F., & Doessel, D. (2008). The Australian mental health system: An economic overview and some research issues. *International Journal of Mental Health Systems, 2*(1), 4.

Wunderink, L., Nieboer, R. M., Wiersma, D., Sytema, S., & Nienhuis, F. J. (2013). Recovery in remitted first-episode psychosis at 7 years of follow-up of an early dose reduction/discontinuation or maintenance treatment strategy: Long-term follow-up of a 2-year randomized clinical trial. *JAMA Psychiatry, 70*(9), 913–920.

Zubin, J., & Spring, B. (1977). Vulnerability: A new view of schizophrenia. *Journal of Abnormal Psychology, 86*(2), 103–126.

CHAPTER 12

Complexities and Rewards of Working with People with Personality Disorders

ROBERT TRETT
AND HALEY PECKHAM

Acknowledgment

The authors would like to acknowledge the contribution of Kate Cooke, Deb Dick and Catherine Bennett who co-wrote this chapter in the second edition.

KEY OUTCOMES

AFTER READING THIS CHAPTER, YOU SHOULD BE ABLE TO:

- appreciate the contested space of personality disorder and be able to consider a range of standpoints on the diagnosis
- appreciate dimensional perspectives to personality disorder in relation to recovery-focused care
- formulate nursing care approaches in the light of human adaptation to early attachment disturbance, trauma and neglect histories
- link such formulation to common factors approaches to providing evidence-informed nursing care to people meeting personality disorder criteria.

KEY TERMS

- attachment
- borderline personality disorder (BPD)
- coping
- mentalising
- neuroplasticity
- personality disorder (PD)
- psychotherapy
- recovery alliance theory of mental health nursing
- trauma

Introduction

The field of personality disorders (PD) is complex. People often suffer high levels of dysphoria, troubled relationships, chronic suicidal feelings, significant and sometimes lethal self-injury and gaining access to the mental health services required may itself be an ordeal. Throughout this chapter, Haley's story will illustrate the underlying troubles that people who may meet diagnostic criteria for PD cope with. This story provides insights into the sorts of early adverse experiences commonly associated with personality disorder. From the position of neuroscience, we draw attention to the adaptive qualities of the human brain, which, as the organ of the mind, makes adjustments in the interests of surviving long enough to procreate. This kind of survival, however, is not always in the best interests of well-being. We will see from Haley's account of psychotherapeutic treatment how the brain's neuroplastic capacity allows for new neural pathways to change in ways more compatible with well-being. We consider also how nurses may contribute to effective care, based on psychotherapeutic practice, and contend that relational healing is the core of this work. Throughout, we refer readers to psychotherapeutic practice in nursing (Trett & Peckham, in press) where we outline a cohesive common factors model for psychotherapeutic nursing.

ABOUT THE CONSUMER   Haley's story

I have never been diagnosed with personality disorder despite clearly meeting the diagnostic criteria for Borderline Personality Disorder at one time in my life. I intentionally stayed away from all professional intervention that could have led to that diagnosis and I'll discuss my reasons for this below. I self-harmed from the age of 17 until I was 30 with increasing severity, had very little sense of self and looked to others for information about who I was and what I was like and adjusted myself to fit what I perceived they wanted. I had intense and very turbulent interpersonal relationships, and a certainty that I would be abandoned in them, and I experienced my emotions with such burning intensity they rendered me unable to function reliably, if at all.

My lack of diagnosis was due to my intentional avoidance of psychiatric and medical services because I didn't believe doctors or psychiatrists could help me, and I didn't want a diagnosis because I didn't feel that I was ill. I had some insight into psychiatric services through my work so my opinion was informed. I believed and still believe that the issues and difficulties I had were a result of the experiences I had in childhood, so it didn't seem right to me to have a label saying that there was something intrinsically wrong with me when I felt that anyone would have had the difficulties I had if they had grown up in the in difficult environment I had grown up in. One of my major coping strategies was to shut down my emotions and lose myself in academic work. This has had some associated social and relational costs in my life, but has also afforded me the opportunity to study neuroscience and the concept of neuroplasticity.

Neuroplasticity has helped me to make sense of both the cause and cure of my difficulties. Neuroplasticity is a property of the brain that allows it to adapt to lived experience, subjective experience, and learn from it so that it can anticipate what may happen in the future and be ready and prepared for dealing with it. This is true whether you experience a safe and nurturing environment or an abusive or neglectful environment—your brain anticipates more of what it has already had.

Haley makes the point to us that mental health services may not be the first port of call for someone who is trying, on a daily basis, to cope with the problems generated by their historical experiences. Yet when things become too unstable to manage independently, people will attend emergency departments, doctor's surgeries or inpatient units in situational crises that may involve serious self-injury, high levels of suicidal impulsivity and generalised chaotic functioning. Sometimes people are highly conflicted about their need for help, comfort and connection to others. In turn, health services may act to confirm that comfort, care and human connection is not on offer. It is as if both parties share the conflicted space of PD, both acting on strong emotions and troubled relating styles rather than mutuality, compassion and trustworthiness. In relation to this we will cover issues relating to the compassion fatigue that nurses sometimes suffer in relation to PD and what we must do to take responsibility for our behaviour. We also investigate the ideas that inform the whole notion of PD and suggest a more sensitive way of formulating and understanding diagnosis. Finally we outline eight essential approaches to care for PD people.

ROBERT TRETT AND HALEY PECKHAM

ABOUT THE CONSUMER | Haley's story (continued)

Fear of abandonment and intense and volatile interpersonal relationships

I don't remember ever feeling warmth from or ever feeling wanted by my caregiver. At best I felt used, but mostly I felt that I was unwanted and a burden, and I often felt I was hated. I was scapegoated by my caregiver, while my family, grateful that the shrivelling ray of blame wasn't directed at them, passively accepted the situation. I was sometimes sent to school and told not to come home and I was frequently identified as being just like my absent and apparently abusive and inadequate parent. I spent a short time in foster care and lived out of home through various thoughtless and unhelpful arrangements made by social workers. At one point I stayed with a local friend and had to go home for meals. On every occasion I went home I was treated with hostility and contempt. My brief experience in foster care ended badly as I was thrown out, paradoxically because I was a pathologically good and compliant teenager. I believe my compulsion to cook and clean for my foster family, while being both polite and extremely grateful, left the biological children in the family feeling threatened and unnerved by my bizarre presentation. My experience of my family and of foster care was that no matter what I did or how hard I tried, I didn't belong, I didn't have a place and I was not worthy of a chance. After such profound experiences of rejection how could I anticipate anything other than abandonment in relationships?

My pervasive sense of shame permeated all of my relationships. I strenuously tried to be someone worthy and lovable, which involved presenting a false self as I knew I wasn't worthy and couldn't be loved. I was repeatedly and intensely attracted by some unconscious magic towards men who had also suffered trauma. I experienced a deep connection and a sense of belonging with these partners or boyfriends that was without question the very best feeling I had ever experienced in my life. In almost all of these relationships this intoxicating feeling of knowing and being known was usurped by our collective trauma and shame in the form of avoidance, aggression and addiction. Not having had any experience of empathy or emotional regulation, neither of us could provide any understanding, soothing or support to the other, or even hear each other over the deafening cries of our own unmet needs. The best feeling in the world became the worst feeling in the world. I couldn't give up—my early experiences had taught me to try harder to be what the other person needed me to be. My shame motivated me to earn love through understanding the other, through sex and through asking for nothing. I knew in my head that earning love wasn't possible, but I was compelled to try.

My relationships were intense, often dangerously volatile and wholly consuming. I could not function if my relationship was in jeopardy. They were always in jeopardy. My work and study were profoundly affected. I saw the end of every relationship as more evidence to confirm my basic unlovability, and the shame around hoping and trying but being met with the same bleak fact that I was unworthy precipitated a significant episode of self-harm each time a relationship ended.

Explanatory model for personality disorder

As indicated above, discussion of disordered personality involves entering a contested space. To ground discussion we commence with a brief review of how the idea of human personality might be conceptualised. Sarkar and Adshead (2012, p. 3) consider personality 'as a regulation of biopsychosocial factors in the service of good-quality survival of the individual within the particular constraints of their habitat and environment'. This is in essence an evolutionary perspective (Sarkar & Adshead, 2012). Personality is a combination of internal and social mechanisms that have evolved over time to regulate functioning in the service of surviving and thriving. In this model it is personality that regulates:

- individual levels of arousal, impulsivity and emotion
- self-directedness and self-soothing in response to survival challenges of stress and change

- reality testing
- an integrated sense of self over time
- social cooperativeness through verbal and non-verbal communications and predictable behaviour (Sarkar & Adshead, 2012, p. 4).

Personality disorder classification

Sarkar and Adshead's conceptualisation suggests that healthy personality relates closely to sound biopsychosocial regulatory mechanisms that adjust arousal, impulsivity, soothing and reality testing, permitting us to meet the demands of the social environment. Personality and identity are closely linked and develop healthily when secure attachment is established. It follows that PD is dimensionally opposite: conceptually it describes a state where the above regulatory mechanisms are impaired and identity is insufficiently formed. Most experts agree that this links closely to attachment failures, but as we will see below there is a range of views as to the role of abuse and neglect versus heritability factors in the genesis of poor attachment.

The above provides a non-judgmental position of PD. However, this definition is prone to misunderstanding. Colloquially, a disorder of personality is more likely to be understood as a defect in the *substance of a person*. It is this (mis)understanding that makes the term PD highly problematic as it implies an inner defectiveness of personhood, rather than a set of deficits that can be understood in the contexts of heritable vulnerability, adverse early experiences and related attachment failures.

Adverse family environments, poor attachment and vulnerable temperament are commonly associated with PD (Bandelow et al., 2005; Infurna et al., 2014; Infurna et al., 2016; Zanarini & Frankenburg, 1997). In particular, Infurna et al's (2016) study of 91 young people in Germany concluded the following childhood adversities:

1 childhood maltreatment, with sexual abuse and emotional abuse being most prominent, and emotional abuse defined as antipathy and neglect. Antipathy was the form of emotional abuse most prominent.
2 maladaptive family functioning including parental or carer responses to the child and overall quality of the family environment. Behavioural control, emotional involvement and communication were noted—not just attributable to one carer but reflecting the whole family system.
3 impaired parental bonding apparent in two main patterns; low care–high overprotection characterised by affectionless control; and low care–low overprotection characterised by neglectful parenting, low maternal care support and validation.

Within the overall PD classification, the diagnosis of Borderline Personality Disorder (BPD) emerged in DSM III (American Psychiatric Association, 1980). This was significant as BPD became the most validated of the many PDs classified in the DSM (Gunderson, 2009; Gunderson et al., 2011). Over time, many effective psychotherapeutic treatments were developed for BPD, improving the lives of those diagnosed with the disorder (Bateman & Fonagy, 1999, 2000; Clarkin et al., 2007; Giesen-Bloo et al., 2006; Linehan et al., 1991).

However, BPD is critiqued by a number of writers (Lawn & McMahon, 2015; Nicki, 2016; Proctor, 2010; Tyrer, 2009; Tyrer et al., 2011; Veysey, 2014). Feminist writers, as well as those with lived experience, have argued that BPD is pejorative in its explanatory model. They contend that the high levels of abuse and neglect suffered by most who have a BPD diagnosis is the better explanation for the negative affectivity and associated regulating mechanisms (such as self-harm, suicidal crises and interpersonal mistrust). These mechanisms, they argue, sit within a normal range of responses to real-world experiences of abuse and/or neglect. As the field of neuroscience progresses, it will become clearer how the experiences of abuse, neglect and traumatising attachments impinge on the developing brain and give rise to the common BPD symptoms of extreme emotional instability requiring extreme measures of self-soothing, such as substance use or self-harm.

Additionally, the gendered nature of the BPD diagnosis is criticised as a way of pathologising women's experiences of emotionality, self-destructiveness, rebelliousness, anger, sexuality and dependency, and that diagnosing personality disorder erroneously suggests *deficiency in personality* as the core problem, rather than an obvious real-world *experiences of victimisation* (Nicki, 2016).

We hold both a sceptical view of the term BPD, while maintaining respect for empirically supported BPD treatments that help many people. The approaches we describe below rely on such empirical literature.

Trauma experiences are overwhelmingly common in BPD, yet not present for all people. A small percentage of those diagnosed with BPD (less than 10 per cent) have no particular experience of trauma (Bandelow et al., 2005). In addition, twin studies show a remarkably higher heritability (Distel et al., 2008; Kendler et al., 2008; Torgersen et al., 2000). These factors, along with emerging neurobiological elements (Bandelow et al., 2005), and experiences of trauma and neglect common for many, must all be accounted for in an explanatory model of BPD.

As mentioned above, many experts (Fonagy et al., 2003; Gunderson & Links, 2008; Links, Ross & Gunderson, 2015) look to troubled early attachment as the genesis for any PD. Troubled attachment is easily understood in relation to abuse and neglect scenarios, but can also be explained by genetic factors such as heritable high impulsivity/low agreeableness (Kendler et al., 2008). Factors such as these are thought to prompt higher arousal in infants and young children. This in turn can prompt a mismatch in temperament between child and carer. In these cases, the carer feels unable to cope or respond adequately to their child's needs. Researchers (Gunderson et al., 2011; Zanarini, 2008) note that high levels of psychological pain, profound mistrust and sometimes hostility to attachment figures occur in families where these mismatches occur.

Regardless of origin, the shame, impossibility of love and unworthiness that Haley and others have experienced amounts to an enormous burden of subjective pain and adverse feelings of aloneness. Relationships are sought as a balm to the pain of aloneness, but these in turn trigger the early attachment dynamics. This creates an impossible bind and potentially a re-experiencing of a double bind in childhood where the biological drive to seek protection from attachment figures is foiled because the attachment figures are who the child may need the protection from. Put simply, when attachment yearnings activate, the unreliability and insecurity of early connections to others also activate. This involves a whole system of early experiences being effectively transmitted into present time, resulting in:

- naivety and inadequacy with regard to closeness–distance and ordinary day-to-day connecting and disconnecting (boundary and abandonment problems)
- expectation of emotional unpredictability and/or affectionless control by others
- accompanying fear of rejection and/or subjugation
- the repetition of sometimes negative coping mechanisms that control pain and can present as:
  - chronic suicidal feelings (death as an escape from pain)
  - self-harm urges

- anger/hostility
- explosive rage
- substance misuse
- emotional shutdown
- high risk-taking activities
- infliction of pain on self or others
- excessive self-control and restriction
- arbitrary shifts of focus to new directions or distractions.

Sometimes distractions can be positive and productive in the short term (as Haley outlines below). Times of positive distraction can also result in nurses mistaking apparent functionality as indicators of recovery. Distraction is not usually synonymous with recovery as it involves a defence rather than an adequate addressing of underlying needs for attachment, belonging and affiliation. People's full potential for participation within like-minded communities of friends, acquaintances, associates and fellow citizens is therefore not served by distraction. Distractions may, however, give respite from the intensity of emotional pain and associated efforts to control such pain. They can provide a space for all involved to regroup and figure out ways to build capacity for secure attachment and belonging.

Regardless of which of the above troubles may be active at any one time, all these difficulties are explainable in terms of adaptation to early experience—be this abuse and neglect or constitutional high impulsivity/low agreeableness. They do not need to be construed as indicating a personality deficiency. In fact, what we see is likely the person's best attempt at using their internal resources to survive and thrive.

Diagnosis

Despite the criticism that a PD diagnosis supports the idea of defective personality—rather than perfectly understandable adaptations to abuse, neglect and/or attachment injury—the diagnosis remains entrenched. Psychiatry itself, however, is critical of its classification system. Tyrer and colleagues (2009, 2011), critique the classification of PDs as follows:

- Separately classified PDs are merely arbitrary labels.
- There is poor differentiation between the various PDs.
- There is poor research evidence for some disorders, particularly passive- aggressive, avoidant, schizoid and narcissistic.
- There is high stigma attached to personality disorders, with the term PD often being used to indicate being untreatable.
- There are high degrees of co-morbidity between various categories of disorders, so much so that people can be diagnosed with more than one PD, or suffer symptoms better explained by psychotic or mood disorders (but due to treatment difficulties get labelled with PD).
- The diagnosis of PDs sets up an artificial dichotomy between those with a PD and those who do not meet diagnostic criteria, yet may suffer significant difficulty particularly in times of stress.

Despite criticisms such as these, the DSM 5 (American Psychiatric Association, 2013) made only slight modifications to the way PD is diagnosed within that system. These modifications were as follows:

- A newer hybrid dimensional-categorical approach was added to encourage further research into dimensional approaches.
- The DSM-IV's Axis I and Axis II were replaced with a single axis system.

- A category of 'PD not otherwise specified' was added to allow diagnosis where a number of symptoms characteristic of a personality disorder exist, but insufficiently to meet threshold for one of the specific disorders.

The categories of PD diagnosis remained unchanged:

- Cluster A ('odd, eccentric'): Paranoid, Schizoid and Schizotypal Personality Disorders
- Cluster B ('dramatic, emotional, erratic'): Borderline, Narcissistic, Histrionic and Antisocial Personality Disorders
- Cluster C ('anxious, fearful' cluster): Avoidant, Dependent and Obsessive-Compulsive Personality Disorder.

In the DSM 5 system, diagnosis is made on a categorical number count of symptoms (described for each category of PD). For a BPD diagnosis, five of nine possible symptoms must be observed frequently and intensely. The approach also permits clinicians to diagnose a range of separate PDs, even though, as Tyler suggests, the many overlapping criteria between these diagnoses calls into question their validity as distinct separate entities.

The World Health Organization's international classification of disease (ICD) approach to diagnosing PDs is growing more distinct from the DSM. With the expected release of the ICD-11 in 2017, the diagnosis of PD evolves from a categorical symptom count to a dimensional approach. Significantly, the various distinct PDs listed in the ICD-10 (similar to the DSM) will be reduced to single PD category. Severity will be assessed and dimensions classified (Tyrer, Reed & Crawford, 2015). This solves an essential problem with PD diagnosis, that of co-morbidity—the problem of there being many overlapping symptoms between various PDs (borderline, narcissistic, antisocial etc.) is solved by these disorders being collapsed into a single category.

The advance in this is that the diagnosis reflects a more cohesive description of human suffering. The regressive component is that this is still construed as a defect of personality rather than a coherent neurological-psychosocial 'best possible' adaptation to adverse early experiences.

Using the ICD-11, the diagnosis of PD will require the following:

- There is a pervasive disturbance in how an individual experiences and thinks about the self, others and the world, manifested in maladaptive patterns of cognition, emotional experience, emotional expression and behaviour.
- The maladaptive patterns are relatively inflexible and are associated with significant problems in psychosocial functioning that are particularly evident in interpersonal relationships.
- The disturbance is manifest across a range of personal and social situations (that is, it is not limited to specific relationships or situations).
- The disturbance is relatively stable over time and is of long duration. Most commonly, personality disorder has its first manifestations in childhood and is clearly evident in adolescence.

PD severity will be defined as Mild, Moderate or Severe, with a subcategory of Late Onset for those diagnosed who have no signs of personality disorder prior to the age of 25 (Tyrer, Reed & Crawford, 2015), and a sub-threshold category to be known as *personality difficulty* will be identified, referring to PD problems that arise in specific contexts (Fonagy, Campbell & Bateman, 2016). This is significant, in that the category of personality difficulties acknowledges that PD features in fact sit on a continuum from normal (non-disordered), through to levels of significant trouble and disability (defined as disordered). This idea of continuum is particularly to the fore in the description of five 'trait domains':

1   negative affective features, including distressing emotions such as anger, anxiety, self-loathing, irritability, vulnerability and depression

2   dissocial features, including disregard, manipulation and exploitation of others, callousness, poor empathy, hostility, ruthlessness, self-entitlement and aggression

3   disinhibition features, including impulsivity, risk-taking, irresponsibility, distractibility and recklessness

4   anankastic features, including perfectionism, perseveration, emotional constraint, stubbornness, deliberativeness, orderliness and concern with rules and obligations.

5   detachment features, including interpersonal distance, social withdrawal/indifference, isolation and poor attachment, intimacy and friendship avoidance that can extend to aloofness or coldness towards others, reserve and/or passivity, along with reduced experience of positive emotions and reduced pleasure.

Given that these trait domains are considered dimensionally rather than categorically, they describe various areas of trouble and difficulty that may be experienced, either alone or in combination. They are not intended as categories of disorder; rather, they are facets of personality that may apply to those who have no personality disorder but perhaps personality difficulty, brought to the fore by stressful occurrences (Tyrer, Reed & Crawford, 2015). Thus, these domain descriptions may be applicable to any of us to some extent. While limitations remain (see below), for someone diagnosed with a personality disorder or personality difficulty, the five domain traits may provide a language for clinicians, and those with lived experience to unpack specific areas of difficulty. If this is done without negative judgments, the descriptions may prompt a heuristic language that helps to further discern and describe presenting issues.

CRITICAL THINKING OPPORTUNITY

Given the contested space of PD, what is your stance in relation to PD and how might this inform the way you work with people who have a PD diagnosis?

Mid-point summary

The future of diagnosis points to a single category for personality disorder. We therefore use the category personality disorder (PD) over borderline personality disorder (BPD) in this chapter, except where BPD is being specifically referred to.

The PD field is a contested one. Feminist perspectives sit alongside attachment theories, neurobiology and the direct testimony of those with lived experience to influence how we might consider the explanatory models, classification and wider discourses relating to personality disorder.

PD diagnosis remains a long way from a social model that accounts for the many difficulties diagnosed people experience as common adaptations to adverse lived experience. The ICD-11 looks forward to a more cohesive approach to diagnosing PD, pointing clinicians to determining severity and assessing traits in a dimensional rather than categorical way. This nudges clinicians towards a more nuanced way of representing a person's particular difficulties.

ABOUT THE CONSUMER   Haley's story (continued)

Toxic shame, severe emotional dysregulation and extreme attempts to self-regulate

Those of us who have experienced interpersonal trauma or been abused, neglected or hurt by the very people who are supposed to care for us anticipate further hurt and trauma in our close relationships and develop a multitude of strategies to mitigate that anticipated pain. We may wish to become less reliant on relationships, seeking emotional regulation from substances or compulsive behaviours, and we may also be manipulative, defensive and aggressive within our relationships and lives, as it is the only way we know to get our needs met. I say this without any judgment. It was a tectonic shift for me to move from feeling like something that existed to meet the needs of others and not a person—where I both denied that I had needs and got them met indirectly and through subterfuge—to becoming a person in my own right with enough of a sense of self-worth and autonomy that I believed it was legitimate for me to have needs, and that I had the capacity to seek what I needed directly.

My early experiences in childhood shaped my sense of worth, purpose, selfhood, safety, autonomy and my emotional landscape, culminating in the constellation of difficulties that form the criteria for BPD: fragile sense of self, chronic emptiness, enduring fear of abandonment, extreme emotional instability and associated extreme forms of self-regulation, from dissociation to impulsive behaviours including self-harm.

The intense emotions and the behaviour of my caregiver terrified me. I became completely emotionally shut down. I dissociated as a matter of course. I did not lose time or a sense of continuity—I lost the capacity to speak, move or act. I would just wait until the storm was over. I resolved not to have emotions as I thought they were harmful to other people and I didn't want to perpetuate the harm that I felt had been done to me. However, my shut-down reaction was also harmful to myself and others, and it was incomplete. I was shut down until I got triggered by something and then I would both silently (but obviously) rage and then I would self-harm. I know now that my moods were extremely powerful and terrifying to be around, added to which my self-harming behaviour, which to me was a way of protecting everyone from my destruction, was experienced by others as an unspoken threat. I had no idea, but I would have been experienced as controlling and manipulative. At times I felt acutely suicidal and would not eat or move for a few days until it passed. I sometimes felt euphoric—unstoppable—and would spend an unusual amount of money on clothes or shoes. I had no way to experience my emotions safely and the idea of emotional regulation would have been beyond my understanding. I mostly felt flat and grey until I was triggered and then I would feel overwhelming rage and self-hate, which would inevitably end in self-harm. I had such contempt for myself in my head that cutting my arms felt completely right, validating and soothing. Self-harm was a tremendously effective means of regulating such extreme emotion.

Community support, social inclusion and 'family like affinity' (Nicki, 2016, p. 224) create a healing setting that is sometimes difficult to replicate in a public mental health system that has the power to coerce people to receive 'care' they do not wish to have. We acknowledge this difficult reality in the mental health services in Western economies such as Australia and New Zealand. Coercive mental health care is incompatible with the psychotherapeutic values we promote in this chapter. Care must be freely chosen for it to be effective—it cannot be coerced. However, many nurses will encounter people with PD in services where coercion is part of the care context. In the face of this we contend there is a clear practice responsibility for nurses to use best practices, to the best of their ability within the care setting in which they work. The choice of when, how and if to make use of what nurses offer always sits with the consumer. When consumers elect to make use of what nurses have to offer, this represents opportunities for us to give back something of value within what can be an iatrogenic system of care.

To give something meaning, multiple perspectives—arising from a shared language between nurse and the consumer—is required. This arises from nurses collaborating with the consumer to explore thoughts, ideas, emotions, memories, desires and meanings (to name a few) in a psychotherapeutic practice. We look now into some of the requirements and obstacles to these engagements.

Towards a shared understanding

Haley's harrowing account of adverse family life reminds us again of the adaptive nature of the symptoms that people diagnosed with PD present with. The perspective of the recovery alliance theory of mental health nursing (Shanley & Jubb-Shanley, 2007; Trett & Peckham, in press) suggests that the most important endeavour for nurses is to find a shared language that values the person's subjective experience and avoids objectifying labels.

ABOUT THE CONSUMER Haley's story (continued)

I did not know it at the time, but I now recognise that when I was triggered, I was triggered into shame, and my response to shame was to seriously hurt myself. I had been shamed for needing, shamed for wanting closeness, shamed for wanting love, shamed for making mistakes, shamed for thinking I could matter, shamed for not having 'reasonable' emotions, shamed for not being the right daughter, shamed for my lack of ability to love my caregiver or to be what was needed. Shamed for never being able to get it right even though I was caught in double binds where nothing right was possible. I was very shame prone! The narrative in my head was, 'You should know better; you should have learned by now. This is not for you; it's for the other children. You are not lovable. What were you thinking? Stop trying.' I cut myself to express the hatred and contempt I had for myself. Outwardly I was incredibly compliant and a pathologically good child that turned into a perfectionist and co-dependent adult who was constantly trying to fulfil a role in someone's life and earn their love.

Opportunities for being emotionally regulated by my caregiver and, as a consequence of that, learning how to emotionally regulate myself were catastrophically insufficient in my childhood. I experienced my emotions at high volume and with terrifying intensity. It is no wonder I shut them down wherever I could, and it's equally understandable that given my experiences, the pain and shame would erupt out of me and manifest in intense rage and self-loathing and an episode of self-harm. The hiding and devaluing of the self, associated with shame, may have protected me from more instances of being shamed. My submissive behaviours, which displayed my acceptance of my position as unworthy, unlovable and of no value, were protective, as I would not be inciting my caregiver to devalue me further. The shutting down of as much of my emotional life as possible was also adaptive. There was only room for one person's emotions in the household.

The language often used in psychiatry and psychology frameworks, while seeming harmless enough to many clinicians, may serve to activate the shame felt earlier in life. Words such as 'disturbance' and 'maladaptive' that continue in the most recent iterations of the diagnostic manuals (for example, ICD-11) can be easily construed as references to defects and serve to activate shame. Haley provides us with a different way to use language. Her approach formulates absence of internal worth, purpose,

ROBERT TRETT AND HALEY PECKHAM

selfhood, safety, autonomy and emotion as being shaped by earlier experiences, rather than defects of personality.

Using inquiry as the main approach, nurses can discover each person's particular experience and unique understanding of their troubles and vulnerabilities. With care, these can be compared to clinical understandings and create an intermingling of language and perspectives. This intermingling of experiences and concepts form a basis for a shared formulation.

Some, like Haley, will understand their issues to be the natural consequence of the experiences they have endured. Others will feel damaged beyond repair (Zanarini, 2008), and be less clear about the nature of their troubles in the first instance. Time will be needed to work through what they understand about themselves over many conversations. Over time, discussions may usefully cover:

- what the person understands to be the historical factors that led to present-day troubles
- the nature of vulnerabilities that seem to have existed from earliest memory to the current day
- coping methods, both positive and troubling, that are used to manage day-to-day difficulties
- impediments to social inclusion and access to peer support.

All this suggests that the gold standard for nurses is to combine empirical perspectives, including diagnostic frameworks, in a way that matches the language and sensibilities of the consumer and their circle of support. For any of it to work, it must be delivered in an atmosphere of compassion.

So what are the impediments to such a standard? Major problems are poor clinician attitudes and persistent discrimination that those with a PD diagnosis experience when presenting for help (Veysey, 2014). In their systematic, integrative literature review, Dickens, Lamont and Gray (2016) examined in detail nursing attitudes, behaviour, experience and knowledge of BPD. They showed nurses have reduced empathy, sympathy, optimism, intention to help, positive feelings and positive experiences alongside a higher desire for social distance, perception of dangerousness, strong negative feelings and indulgence in stigma inducing belittling or contradictory remarks; further, they show a consistently higher negative performance in relation to PD than members of other health disciplines (Dickens, Lamont & Gray, 2016). Nurses do not occupy this position alone—there is some evidence that these attitudes are shared with psychiatrists (Bodner et al., 2015). Psychiatrists, along with nurses, are significantly more negative about those with PD than psychologists and social workers. It may be of some small comfort that compared to psychiatrists, nurses rated more highly in their willingness to improve their professional skills.

Haley's experience in psychotherapeutic treatment was likely successful because it provided new and benevolent relational experience. She was treated as someone worthy of empathy, understanding, respect and care; someone who matters enough; and a real, autonomous individual. It is unthinkable that nurses who share the attitudinal impediments described above would be capable of creating the sort of confiding healing setting (Laska, Gurman & Wampold, 2014) that is required to support the sorts of changes that Haley speaks of.

So what structural solutions might mental health nursing collectively adopt? The first is that we need to acknowledge that in comparison with our allied health colleagues *we have a significant problem*. We then need to challenge a sentinel false belief. This false belief is that people with PD diagnoses have a level of self-control that people with other diagnoses do not have (Dickens, Lamont & Gray, 2016). The implication of this belief is that we suffer a collective misapprehension that people with PD diagnoses are in some way less deserving of care. At some level we believe, despite evidence to the contrary, that PD people can, through an act of will and without support, choose to function better. It pays us to reflect on this assumption: who would choose to self-harm if they had another effective way of calming themselves? Who would choose to manipulate others if they felt they could directly ask for and get what they need? Who would choose to be at the mercy of intense emotions if they could control the searing intensity of those emotions?

As mentioned above, nurses outrank psychiatrists in their willingness to improve knowledge, but we are cautious in suggesting knowledge acquisition as a sole solution. In addition to education, Dickens and colleagues (2016) place higher emphasis on supervision, more supportive ways of working, and informal peer support. As authors we remain uncertain as to all the factors required to turn around the therapeutic nihilism from which our profession suffers. Through our long experience in PD work as a mental health nurse and psychotherapist, respectively, we are convinced that compassion is a core requirement.

Much has been written on the power of compassion, both within nursing and in relation to PD (Bramley & Matiti, 2014; Krawitz, 2012; McCaffrey & McConnell, 2015; Raes, 2011). A standout factor from this literature is that to provide compassion to others, a capacity for self-compassion is required. For those of us lucky enough to have received compassion in our lives, there will be a lived experience and therefore an internal compassion template that can be called upon when working with others.

For others, a paucity of a lived experience of compassion places additional burden on a nurse who is expected know what this looks and feels like.

ABOUT THE CONSUMER Haley's story (continued)

My childhood experiences were with a caregiver who was extremely emotionally dysregulated. A tsunami of my caregiver's emotions determined my environment and what would happen to me. There was terrifying rage, blame and hostility, as well as dissociation, depression and despair that were no less terrifying. There were frequent swings between destructive and aggressive behaviour to suicidal behaviour, coupled with the crazy-making capacity to act completely normally when other adults were present. Unpredictably, there would be periods of calm and sometimes, rarely, I would be treated as though I was a friend or a confessor. I had a very clear message that I was responsible for creating these emotions in my caregiver.

How did I adapt in order to survive that environment? The experiences of being with someone unpredictable, and bigger and more powerful than me, who I feared but whose love I craved, shaped me to focus entirely and exclusively on them. I became exquisitely observant of and sensitive to another's moods and behaviours, and made every human effort to moderate both. My every act was an act of acquiescence or grovelling submission. I became hypervigilant of my caregiver and completely removed from my own experience. The feedback I got from my caregiver became my narrative of self. The way I was treated and used by my caregiver became my sense of worth and purpose. My caregiver's perception of me was my reality. It is not surprising that I couldn't name my emotions, couldn't articulate my needs and could only grasp a sense of who I was by proxy, through the way that someone else saw me. I felt like a ghost—as though my body was not made of substance so I could not effect change in the world. Without my caregiver present I genuinely did not know where to be or what to do. I couldn't even mentally frame the possibilities, much less act on them. When I first went into psychotherapy I repeatedly qualified every account of myself by saying, 'My [caregiver] wouldn't see it this way'. When I articulated myself, I felt as though I was lying or at least wrong. Other people's perceptions of me felt like facts, and my sense of who I was felt so insubstantial that if thought or spoke it would be crushed or blown away. I also had bodily experiences of feeling like my chair was being tipped back or as though a great weight was bearing on me.

ROBERT TRETT AND HALEY PECKHAM

So how might these troubles be best addressed? For some, personal therapy will help. For others, corrective experience in close adult relationships will make a difference. Various spiritual, political or recreational affiliations can create a sense of belonging, where compassion is experienced in the level of acceptance the person has within their circle. It is for individual nurses to consider how they may acquire lived experience of compassion should this be an issue; we raise these options as pointers for reflection.

In our opinion, the industrial machine-like nature that some mental health services expose nurses to on a daily basis makes a compassionate stance difficult. When this occurs, nurses' intentions need a reset—we must find a way to reconnect to a core compassionate stance. Cultural support for compassion within the organisational structures of health care is required to prompt both self-compassion and compassionate practice. As Bodner and colleagues (2015) suggest, joining together as peers or with a designated clinical supervisor may be the things that help nurses improve attitudes to those with PD. Our belief is that conscious effort to nurture compassion through peer support and supervision will achieve not only a compassionate stance, but also a state of trust that enables social learning. This capacity for trust can then be communicated in contacts with the people we work with; this is vital as trust is a touchstone for recovery (see below).

These factors together underpin the model for psychotherapeutic practice in nursing (Trett & Peckham, in press); we commend a person-centred humanistic nursing practice model as part solution to the negative views outlined in the studies above. A humanistic nursing practice applied to the field of PD joins the dots between:

1   the concept of PDs as diagnosable illnesses
2   the validation of the real-life experiences of those who would meet the criteria for PD, but find that way of conceptualising their difficulties alienating
3   a set of common mental health nurse practices that, consistent with Haley's lived experience of psychotherapy (below), provide people with a different sort of relationship—one that demonstrates compassion, creates trust and prompts new neural pathway development.

CRITICAL THINKING OPPORTUNITY

1   Have you encountered stigmatising, belittling or other negative responses from colleagues in relation to consumers with PD diagnoses?

2   What do you think drives these sorts of positions and how might you contribute to reducing the negativities some nurses express?

Pathways to change and self-knowledge

New studies into possible confounding factors that inhibit change in those with attachment-related problems have incorporated social learning theory and pedagogy to better understand the apparent rigidity of mind that is observed in those meeting PD criteria (Fonagy & Allison, 2014; Fonagy, Campbell & Bateman, 2016; Fonagy, Luyten & Allison, 2015). This rigidity is thought to include impairments in appreciating and adapting to changing social situations, understanding interpersonal occurrences, and updating beliefs about self and others based on real-world experiences. Rigidity and low trust lead to poor transmission of knowledge between people. This is due to preponderance of vigilance; in Haley's account she speaks of hypervigilance to her caregiver and her sense of self being rigidly subjugated to that person's reality. These sorts of experiences, established through adverse early life circumstances, leave the person rigidly closed off from the usual channels available within human culture to flexibly live, learn, thrive and change within community contexts. The person is instead unable to reality-test ideas, feelings and beliefs with others and in this state is closed off to knowledge and ideas that may naturally arise in the context of intimate relationships and broader affiliation within communities. In this way, the person is closed off from the usual learning journeys that most humans partake in daily, where sharing perspectives and advancing knowledge occurs naturally. It is as if a trifecta of wretchedness—a paucity of basic trust, a preponderance of vigilance and an accompanying rigidity of mind—leaves the person isolated, 'like my chair was being tipped back or as though a great weight was bearing on me'. This understanding points us to intentionally building trust as a primary approach to care. Research is still required to fully understand the therapeutic effects that intentional trust building might have, but we suggest the following approaches:

- an unmistakeable willingness on the part of the nurse to hear what is on the mind of the person
- a clear desire to share in meaning and sense making regarding mental processes
- the direction of effort to restoring agency and belief in self
- stepping outside a knowing, explaining and educating stance and entering a *not knowing* and *benign inquiry* stance
- the active linking of ideas, emotions, desires, memories and meanings to create a holistic sense of both the origins and the solutions to historical and present moment problems.

Psychotherapeutic practice

As noted above, empirically supported treatment approaches for personality disorder have flourished; these treatments are all talk-based psychotherapeutic approaches. They have contributed to clinical remission and significant hope for people suffering the effects of that disorder (Gunderson, 2009). Psychotherapeutic practice in nursing (Trett & Peckham, in press) forms a general basis for nurses to provide empirically supported care to those with PD. In addition to this, best practice in the PD field requires that we target the core difficulties experienced by people with PD (Bateman, Gunderson & Mulder, 2015), and remain focused on social capacity to take up life within a circle of friends and associates.

We outline below the additional factors that need to be considered arising from empirically supported PD-focused therapies. The empirical support for these approaches comes from a number of studies (Bateman & Fonagy, 1999, 2000; Clarkin et al., 2007; Doering et al., 2010; Giesen-Bloo et al., 2006; Linehan et al., 1991).

The specific psychotherapies outlined in these studies, in their pure form, are reserved to those who have severe and complex difficulties. They are usually provided in specialist services by clinicians, including nurses, who have specific training in those methods.

For those who are less severely impacted yet significantly troubled, a common factors approach will be sufficient (Bateman, Gunderson & Mulder, 2015). Nurses should feel confident to provide this type of care as studies show clinical remission of between 78 per cent and 99 per cent (Zanarini et al., 2012). In addition to these high rates of remission, recurrence of the disorder was limited to 36 per cent after two years and 10 per cent after eight years in one study (Zanarini et al., 2012) or 11 per cent after 10 years in another (Gunderson et al., 2011.)

The initial aims for psychotherapeutic treatment are to reduce life-threatening behaviour and improve levels of dysphoria related to thoughts, memories, fluctuating and often negative emotional states, emotional shutdown, interpersonal relating and issues of identity or sense of self.

ROBERT TRETT AND HALEY PECKHAM

Different sources have slightly different wordings, but a review of the key experts (Bateman, Gunderson & Mulder, 2015; Gunderson & Links, 2008; Links, Ross & Gunderson, 2015; McMain et al., 2009) suggests common ingredients. We adhere to the principles outlined in this literature while orienting our language to the idea that the troubles experienced by those diagnosable with PD are understandable adaptations to adverse experience and attachment failures, not defects of personhood.

BOX 12.1 EIGHT THERAPEUTIC TASKS

1 *Tend to emotional content reliably and actively:* As Haley experienced in her psychotherapy, a nursing approach involving active careful listening and concern for the person's difficulties is paramount. Very often difficulties involve delicate states of emotion that must not be explained away in Socratic linkages to 'maladaptive' thoughts and/or beliefs. Emotions and emotional experiences require empathic respect and validation (see the section 'Validation as core construct' later in this chapter). Nurses need to avoid reactivity to sometimes strongly expressed emotion (see the section 'Working with strong emotions' later in the chapter).

2 *Involve yourself in matters at hand:* The nurse actively engages in efforts to understand problems. Like Haley's therapist, the nurse errs on supporting the person's struggles to figure things out and steers clear of too many suggestions or, worse, listing off solutions that have little bearing on the person's knowledge, preferences or sensibilities.

3 *Focus on real-world relationship coping:* The nurse explores with the person how relationships, and importantly, the thoughts, feelings, ideas, desires and beliefs that are activated in interactions with others, can be best understood and coped with.

4 *Navigate misunderstandings:* There are almost always times when strong negative emotional experiences arise relating to the nurse's actions or inactions. It is supremely invalidating for nurses to interpret a person's complaints as being caused by their 'disorder' (see the section 'Supervision and the not knowing stance' later in this chapter). In these situations time should be spent exploring the following:

– What has happened?
– What has this meant in terms of their mental, physical and relational well-being?
– What is needed to repair the situation?

While it is not essential to agree with all perceptions, it is essential to validate underlying emotional experiences (see the section 'Validation as core construct' later in this chapter), and to avoid point–counterpoint discussions. These situations should not be managed too briskly, nor should they continue for too long. Real solutions that feel like the nurse has taken on board the person's perspectives must be found. Using the above three-part structure, coupled with a collaborative stance, should help to focus forward to solutions and avoid lasting therapy impasses. Nurses should apologise for causing offence, even when this was done unwittingly.

5 *Balance 'there and then' with 'here and now':* In line with the above, the focus for therapeutic practice is relatively 'here and now', rather than 'there and then'. This does not prohibit exploring past occurrences and difficulties, including painful memories relating to adverse past experiences. Subjective pain, originating from past adversity, needs validating in the present moment to prevent it growing in intensity (Zanarini, 2008).

Validating past pain is therefore done in a way that brings present focus. Typically nurses can ask: 'What's that like as we talk about it now'? 'What seems to help with this feeling now'?

Strong negative feelings that have a trauma component to them often feel endless when activated. To interrupt this, attention to the rise and fall of emotions is required: 'As we understand the effects of this together, what do you notice about the intensity of these feelings? Can we track this together right now? These feelings will come in waves. Let me know when this one reaches its peak and starts to subside.'

6 *Promote the person as an expert in their own experiences and a competent partner in managing risk:* The nurse's role is to support pre-existing strengths and competency, help discover new strengths and competencies, and support the person's decision making wherever possible (even when it may feel uncomfortable to the nurse). Through this the dignity of learning is upheld and risk is managed as a shared concern, involving the person as the number-one decision maker and their circle of support as the group who help keep things as safe as they can be.

The NHMRC guideline for personality disorder treatment (Australian Government, 2013) provides guidance to clinicians with a taxonomy for exploring lethality and chronicity factors. In this taxonomy, most situations suggest continuing outpatient therapeutic care focusing as best as possible on supporting survival strategies. Nurses should read this guideline in relation to risk management.

7 *Create predictability in the framework for care:* The frame for the work should be consistent and predictable with effort put in by nurses to giving notice of absences and predicting changes to schedules. It is also important to actively follow up if the person is unexpectedly absent, ensuring new appointments are made and the reasons for absences are explored in full. This is to create space for exploration of troubles that might have prompted non-attendance. Non-attendance is overtly considered in a problem-solving manner.

8 *Focus on mental process:* The above style of therapy is designed to help with interpersonal connection and real-world emotional support, through developing a partnership that favours reflecting on *states of mind* rather than *behaviour*. This is because states of mind rather than *urges to various actions* are the pathway to making meaning. By making mental states the focus, nurses help habituate a capacity for reflection. Mental state focus can be promoted as the best way to understand self and others. This means nurses' inquiries are directed to understanding life's struggles in terms of thoughts, feelings, ideas, desires, memories, beliefs and meanings. Nurses also draw attention to how the person may better understand others, in terms of their mental states.

The mechanism for achieving this sort of reflective functioning is the regulating effect of being listened to and taken seriously; in effect, the nurse holding the person's mind in mind (Fonagy & Bateman, 2006). As a result, the person experiences being helped fully and generously by the nurse. Together exploring troubles and searching for solutions to real-world troubles occurs. The skill is in orienting support towards making sense of how mental processes affect understanding of both self and others, and how these new understandings might result in real-world interpersonal activities. This is likely to be more effective than the more limiting practice of cheerleading changes in behaviour.

REFLECTION QUESTIONS

Many nurses feel they need to directly address the behaviours they observe PD people engaging in; this feels particularly urgent when behaviour is destructive or self-destructive.

1 What are your thoughts about remaining focused on the mental processes that might drive behaviour?

2 How might you maintain such a focus when your risk assessment suggests that you should exert control to prevent a consumer's engaging self-harm?

3 Is it ever necessary to take control over someone's destructive behaviours?

Summary

In summary, we return to Haley's story and our core contention that it is relational healing, applied by nurses in their work with people who may be diagnosed with PD, that makes the difference. The approach Haley outlines worked because of the plasticity of the human brain. The brain's original adaptations to adverse experiences, in the presence of heritable vulnerabilities, reflect a common experience of serious attachment failure. These adaptations are expressed in particular neural pathway developments. Healing relationships provide the experience of new possibilities and support change by overwriting the old habituations and biological imperatives that achieve survival, but for many also a life of pain and distress. The rerouting of pathways, arising from new relational experiences, orients the person to recovery of trust and, most importantly, to expanded capacity for social learning and citizenship within circles of like-minded peers, associates and more intimate friends.

ABOUT THE CONSUMER Haley's story (continued)

Relational healing

Following a death in my family, my tutors at university were sympathetic and supportive, and gave me a lot of leeway around my studies. I had the unexpected reaction of becoming enraged when this happened. It seemed to me that a death was a really ordinary thing to happen—sad and painful, but ordinary. Being given latitude as an adult because of this death made me feel crazy, when by contrast as a child I endured an extraordinary level of emotional violence that had been ignored, dismissed or invalidated by almost every adult I had told. The contrast in the understanding and sympathy I was being offered as an adult—which I didn't need—compared to how desperately I had needed an adult to see and stop what was happening to me as a child was maddening.

I entered psychotherapy shortly after this event. I was the most nervous and anxious that I had ever been in my life while I was waiting to see my psychotherapist for the first time. At some level I think I knew that I was so vulnerable that if this attempt to seek help didn't work out, the psychological and emotional impact on me would put me in danger. I was exceptionally lucky. My psychotherapist was wise, patient and skilled in doing very little beyond holding the most precious space for me to both find myself, and to risk trusting him. He gave me no indication of his approval or disapproval of me, which was incredibly uncomfortable as that was how I calibrated myself, but was also absolutely necessary for me to find myself beyond my fragility and not to repeat my eternal 'people pleasing' pattern. He also set no agenda for what we would speak about; in particular he did not direct me to talk about, or to try to stop, self-harming. He helped me to discover my feelings and allowed me the dignity of feeling them at the intensity and depth that they washed over me. He didn't try to silence them, tidy them up or to turn them into gold so I could be grateful for them. He did not deliver sickening platitudes. His tolerance of my emotion modelled tolerance to me, and his ability to sit with my distress rather than control me respected my autonomy, even when that was frightening, and it helped me to take responsibility for myself. Through consistent experiences of empathy, attunement, care and respect in psychotherapy I came to feel of value—that I could trust myself and my feelings, and that therapy was a place where I could take my intense emotion and it would be validated and therefore soothed. It was a place I discovered that relationships could be helpful and not just dangerous and exploitative.

Through a lens of neuroplasticity it seems to me that my childhood experiences of relationship left me learning not to trust, not to share my vulnerability with anyone and to emotionally self-regulate alone by self-harming. I see all of these strategies as being highly adaptive to the situation in which they were forged. Relationships were not safe—in fact they posed the greatest danger that I faced—so every strategy that turned me away from relationships was protective and adaptive. I would extend this understanding to other so-called 'maladaptive' coping strategies of substance use, eating disorders and compulsive behaviours. However, I didn't want the effects of my childhood to last my whole life. The strategies I learned that protected me as a child denied me any chance of building a healthy relationship as an adult. It wasn't a case of just having to find the right person. The harm that had been done to me I carried into relationships with my mistrust, avoidance and fear.

To change that devastating repetitive pattern of relating required me to have a new experience of relationships so my neuroplastic brain could have the opportunity to learn something different. What I needed to learn was how to experience my emotions differently, how to be soothed, how to feel safe and how to reach out and how to relate healthily. I understood the words but had no idea of what that actually looked like in action. Like anything we learn, the new skill develops through experience, and is improved with practice. The new neural pathways are enhanced with repetition. I needed thousands of experiences in psychotherapy of moving from an emotionally dysregulated state to an emotionally regulated state, and fortunately that was my experience in psychotherapy. Eventually that neural pathway became so practised I could self-soothe by bringing to mind my psychotherapist: what he might say to me or how I might feel if he were with me. This new experience of relationship in the context of psychotherapy opened me up to all the benefits there are in healthy relating; chiefly, emotional regulation and with it increased self-worth, trust, authenticity, acceptance and respect.

Having had this new experience, I could carry it into the world as a healthier anticipation of relationships. I am doing that, and in a journey that is not without disappointments, frustration and fear, I do anticipate healthier relationships and I am having healthier relationships too. I wouldn't meet criteria for BPD on 95 out of 100 days, I'm not mentally ill, I don't think I ever was and while I'll always be vulnerable when I am emotionally overwhelmed and dysregulated, I make decisions about relationships, work and play that robustly support my emotional health.

Working with strong emotions

People sometimes express strong emotions. These can reflect a state of mental over-arousal involving a temporary loss of capacity to reflect on self and other. The best response to this is for the nurse to validate these feelings, to show an unmistakable desire to connect, and to empathise with and be curious about the feelings. In dealing with a range of negative emotions, particularly anger or hate, this requires active grounding in compassion; it is a complex and difficult task and often requires debriefing and support for the nurse in the aftermath. When done well it introduces a novel response: instead of experiencing another person seeking to control their negative affects through proscription, the person experiences someone keen to remain connected and interested to understand how this emotion has come about. Instead of someone trying to control their feelings, there is interest in knowing something about the feelings and, furthermore, support for self-knowledge through discovering what has happened to prompt the strength of feeling and what that might mean.

This may mean the nurse introducing additional soothing so the person has the chance to slow down their thoughts and de-arouse their emotions.

Other activity may include clarifying and apologising for the unintended effects of conversations that may have prompted sensitivities or offence. The point here is to convey that causing offence is the last thing nurses want to do, and yet sometimes it happens through ordinary human lack of awareness, clumsiness or inattention.

Point–counterpoint transactions are to be avoided at all costs as they will likely re-escalate arousal levels. The nurse's purpose is to lower arousal so that meanings may be more easily explored. As soothing is established, the nurse tries to reactivate a reflective space that explores related mental processes: 'What triggered this emotion? Have thoughts sped up and as they slow down can we focus on understanding them better? What beliefs about self and other have been activated? What do you make of all this? Do urges to any particular actions arise? What might these mean for how to manage things over the next few hours/days?'

This doesn't mean that nurses should place themselves in physical danger; the intention is to provide a place where all feelings including negative ones can be explored and understood. Interventions—such as saying 'Could you please stop shouting at me as all this is preventing me being able to think. I need to be able to think clearly so I can work out how to best help you'—can reorient the person to reducing escalations. Sometimes creating space and a quiet environment will help. If the nurse needs to leave the scene then s/he should always come back to attempt re-engagement when things feel safer.

Meaning making in the therapuetic relationship

Many psychotherapeutic ideas centre on using the therapeutic relationship as a place where past feelings and other related mental states can be interpreted. Therapists practising from this approach wait for issues from the person's past to be prompted in some way in the therapeutic relationship. Attempts then are made to prompt 'insight' by using interpretation that invites the person to work through things in a way that helps them experience past difficulties differently in the therapeutic relationship. This approach suggests that new experiences in therapy are the primary factor to achieving change.

This method is not a first-line approach for most with PD. We suggest nurses steer clear of considering that complexity in the therapeutic relationship reflects earlier relationship issues. Particularly, nurses should refrain from interpreting occurrences within nurse–consumer relationship as being repetitions of early childhood dynamics or adverse experiences.

This is because interpretations such as these, while seeming accurate, can easily backfire:

- The person may find interpretations disorienting due to them not according with their memories or ideas of early relationships.
- They may seem irrelevant to someone who is struggling to figure out what solutions might exist for real-life problems, rather than think their past experiences.
- It may feel insulting to the person that the nurse assumes s/he knows the depths of adversity experienced in the past and is in some special position to make up for such losses. People who have experienced terrible adversity can find well-intentioned but misguided interpretations as making light of their past pain.

Working with change

Therapy is expected to prompt change, but a change orientation can elicit fear and misunderstanding if not handled well. Two factors are at play with regard to change:

1 The person struggling with PD is also very often struggling with an impossible dilemma: 'I need to change, but I can't change'. Both these are indisputable facts. Their contradictory nature causes ambivalence, stress and sometimes hopelessness. It is hard to contemplate two truths that sit side by side when they appear so contradictory.

2 Due to early adverse experiences, many people learn to adapt to the external situation and have little sense of personal agency. Haley illustrates this in her story. This means that truth is derived from context rather than a consistent set of internal values, ideas and positions on life. Ironically, given the general reputation of PD consumers of being non-compliant, this results in an over-compliance when therapy goals are being set. The trouble is that context of a therapeutic relationship is very different from the contexts people find themselves in in everyday life. In a different context, the person finds themselves complying with a different set of ideas. These may be in complete conflict with the therapeutic goals set in the therapeutic context.

This context-derived sense of self explains why there is an impression that many PD people are non-compliant to goals. The more accurate picture is that commitments to change, honestly made in the context of a therapeutic relationship, may have little meaning in the rest of the person's life.

Despite these complexities, change goals are important. They should be broad enough to capture the core difficulties of PD, while specific enough to be visible and meaningful in the real world.

Goals provide the therapy with structure and direction; the work is given due urgency and direction not because of time rationing factors (although these may also exist in the specifications of some organisations nurses work for) but rather because of the need to relieve core troubles that lead to chronic suicidal feelings, self-harm, interpersonal crises and accompanying distress.

A hierarchy of goals taken from the general psychiatric model of treatment (Links, Ross & Gunderson, 2015) provides a structure to goals nurses might suggest. These are outlined in clinical language here, but all discussion of goals needs to adhere to the shared language principle rather than being laden with clinical jargon.

- six-week goal—less stress and dysphoria
- six-month goal—a reduction in the frequency and severity of self-destructive, high-risk-taking and suicidal or self-harm urges with an increase in problem-solving responses and self-familiarity/understanding
- twelve-month goal—improved interpersonal functioning with better ability to discern and respond fittingly to others' feelings and ideas, along with increased self-confidence in relationships.

These goals are not intended as an off/on switch. They should not be accompanied by tick boxes. Acknowledgment should be made that the person is not expected to have all these things achieved perfectly and on time. They are a guide for both parties and progress is best considered as a continuum. Instead of tick boxes, a Likert scale may be more appropriate.

Initially the nurse will hold more commitment to these goals, but over time by coming back and discussing progress dimensionally, and using a solution-focused perspective, psychotherapy will be structured around measurable progress. This helps prevent prolonged periods of directionless interactions.

Supervision and the not knowing stance

Much is stated on the importance of clinical supervision in mental health nursing practice. Supervision is a place for collegial and senior level support to nurses. Just as good treatment in this field is focused on supporting the person's capacity to reflect on self and other, supervision supports the reflective capacity of the nurse.

Particularly vital in supervision is exploring self-states in relation to the work, as well as the nurse's capacity to maintain their compassion. The supervisor's use of a 'not knowing explorative stance' can model the framework required for successful treatment. The 'not knowing explorative' stance is where the supervisor is one where the trained supervisor projects a 'naive curiosity'. The key questions for the nurse centre on whether the style and qualities of interaction with the person are conducive and on track with the meta goals in relation to reflection, reduction in dysphoria, reduction in risks and increases in effectiveness and confidence in real-world relationships.

Hold clinical reviews to pick up on the more specific question as to how therapy is tracking against the expected six-week, six-month and twelve-month goals. If they are not, what factors need to be considered and how can the work best be supported by the team and organisation? Any changes to treatment, particularly in relation to increasing or decreasing intensity of contact, need to be carefully thought through and introduced to the person and their family/circle of support with due care and reassurance.

This asks questions about the consumer's mental processes in relation to real-world occurrences (for example, thoughts, ideas, emotions, memories, desires, beliefs and meanings). Through exploring these, the person is supported to create their own meaning.

Validation as core construct

Core to the above approaches is the notion of validation. As it is such a core capability in all evidence-based PD treatment approaches, we outline here some of its pedigree and meanings.

As a technique, validation arose in Marsha Linehan's ground-breaking treatment for BPD, dialectical behaviour therapy (Linehan, 1993). It arises in consideration of the acceptance versus change dynamic (see the section 'Towards a shared understanding' earlier in the chapter). Linehan describes acceptance as a radical position: 'the therapist's willingness to find the inherent wisdom and "goodness" of the current moment and the participants in it, and to enter fully into the experience without judgment, blame, or manipulation' (Linehan, 1993, p. 109). Validation is a strategy arising from this stance. It seeks out the 'wisdom, correctness, or value in the individual's emotional, cognitive, and overt behavioural responses … believing in the patent's inherent ability to get out of the misery that is her life and build a life worth living' (Linehan, 1993, p. 99).

In Bateman and Fonagy's metallization-based treatment (MBT), validation is endorsed as a way of exploring the person's internal experiences and working out ways to consider alternative experiences that arise from reflections on self. 'If the patient says I am a fool … reassuring … that he is not a fool will be ineffective and simply make him feel misunderstood, but saying something like you have never appeared like a fool to me but tell me what makes you say that at the moment is both validating and offers an alternative perspective' (Bateman & Fonagy, 2006, p. 161).

World-renowned BPD researcher Mary Zanarini (2008, p. 510) describes validation as an essential technique to lessen subjective pain: 'Patients need to feel that someone understands their pain and is neither frightened nor disgusted by it'.

Care planning

You are a nurse in a community care team. Haley is seeing you once per week for twelve months.

Care Plan 1

	Haley's viewpoint	Haley's desires	Mutual goals/ plan	Agreed approach	Review
Working alliance	I'm not at all sure that you can help me as you can't really understand my issues in a way that could assist me change anything.	I don't want judgments or you trying to control me and I am not going to conform to your ideas of what I should be like.	I don't know what can help me. I don't want to self-harm but it's the only way I can control things and if you want me to stop it that leaves me with no way of coping. Given you said you want to meet regularly with me, I am willing to see you each week for a while and see if there is something you can help me with.	We take time to figure out together what might help. Rather than try focusing on stopping self-harm, we'll see what we can make of feelings or events that might have prompted self-harm impulses, or indeed other things that might seem important. We work out together, step by step, what might help.	In six weeks we will talk about this plan and see how things are going. Our aim is to check if things feel they're heading in the right direction. An indicator for this might be less stress overall, or less intensity in negative emotions. It won't be necessary for these indicators to be occurring at 100 per cent. Our aim will be to gather impressions, as a way to understand what might be helping and what we have learned from the process at that point. From there we can work out if there is anything we need to adjust in the plan.
Coping focus	I don't know how to cope with things in my life.	I could just end up trying to please you. It happens to me sometimes—I end up conforming to others' expectations. This helps me to cope, but I end up disgusted with myself and then I self-harm. I want something else but I don't know what is possible.	If we explore what's on my mind I might figure something out about all this. That may help my negative feelings. I need help to identify times when it feels like I am conforming to others rather than exploring things for myself. We don't know what will happen from this in terms of coping, but we agree to invest the time to find out.	We meet once a week for around 50 minutes to explore the possibilities. We'll let each other know if scheduling changes are required. We start from a place of not knowing and see what can be figured out together. If self-harm starts to increase in frequency or intensity for any reason, we talk about it to see if something is occurring here that is prompting this. We then see if we can adjust things in a way that helps.	
Self-responsibility control	Self-control is helped by self-harm.	I don't know how to think about what I want. It's too hard.	We can talk about what I might want, but if things become too difficult I'll need to change the subject or stop the session.	Control will ultimately rest with Haley. Nurse's role is to prompt joint exploration but not direct it. Haley's role is to use the space to make sense of things that come up for her.	

ROBERT TRETT AND HALEY PECKHAM

1 How would you prioritise Haley's needs from a psychotherapeutic practice perspective?

2 Validation is ubiquitous to good outcomes in the PD field, but what do you validate when all you see is self-destructive behaviour?

3 What factors might indicate Haley is establishing a therapeutic alliance with you?

4 From the psychotherapeutic perspective, what are the most important qualities for you to bring to the therapeutic alliance with Haley?

TEST YOURSELF

1 What is the key difference between diagnosing PD using the DSM 5 and the forthcoming ICD-11?

a The DSM 5 provides better differentiation of diagnoses

b The DSM 5 outlines PD symptoms better than the ICD-11

c The ICD-11 has a single PD diagnosis and specifies severity and traits

d The ICD-11 is more flexible and nuanced

e The DSM 5 is more scientifically valid

2 Use of distraction can be helpful but can also hinder treatment because:

a respite from emotional pain can also lead to denial

b attachment needs are not well served through distraction

c distractions cause everyone to get complacent about PD problems

d participation and citizenship is required for PD people to properly recover

e establishing secure attachment and reducing suffering requires due attention and support

3 Negative attitudes among nurses working with PD consumers is:

a a highly misunderstood problem caused by **splitting** behaviours

b higher among nurses and psychiatrists than social workers and psychologists

c understandable given the pressure nurses are under

d best solved by educating nurses about PD

e to be raised by nurse-managers as a performance issue

4 The initial engagement period between a nurse and someone who may have a PD requires:

a assessing if the consumer meets diagnostic criteria

b reassurance that self-harm and depression is usually due to childhood sexual abuse and requires systematic desensitisation treatment

c creating a nursing care plan that articulates risks and how these can be reduced over time

d attending to issues of trust, alliance building and creating a predictable framework for care

e reassurance that the person isn't defective because PD is a heritable condition

USEFUL WEBSITES

Helpful videos

Dr Nancy McWilliams talks to Project Air Strategy about personality disorder: https://www.youtube.com/watch?v=3_W9dr7TNAs

Peter Fonagy—How breakdowns in trust impede ability to mentalize: https://www.youtube.com/watch?v=SM6mNNOWpeE

Mentalization-based treatment training video with Anthony Bateman—Not knowing stance: https://www.youtube.com/watch?v=BZl4OtQvDDg

'Back from the edge'—Borderline Personality Disorder: https://www.youtube.com/watch?v=967Ckat7f98

Early intervention for young people with BPD (borderline personality disorder)—Prof Andrew Chanen: https://www.youtube.com/watch?v=vmjytXKsziY

'Hope and optimism for BPD in Australia'—A/Prof Sathya Rao https://www.youtube.com/watch?v=Ie8lbaolKF8

REFERENCES

American Psychiatric Association (1980). *Diagnostic and statistical manual of mental disorders* (3rd ed.). Washington, DC: APA.

American Psychiatric Association (2013). *Diagnostic and statistical manual of mental disorders* (5th ed.). Washington, DC: APA.

Australian Government (2013). *Clinical practice guideline for the management of borderline personality disorder*. National Health and Medical Research Council. Retrieved from https://www.nhmrc.gov.au/_files_nhmrc/publications/attachments/mh25_borderline_personality_guideline.pdf?

Bandelow, B., Krause, J., Wedekind, D., Broocks, A., Hajak, G., & Rüther, E. (2005). Early traumatic life events, parental attitudes, family history, and birth risk factors in patients with borderline personality disorder and healthy controls. *Psychiatry Research*, *134*(2), 169–179.

Bateman, A. W., Gunderson, J., & Mulder, R. (2015). Treatment of personality disorder. *The Lancet*, *385*(9969), 735–743.

Bateman, A., & Fonagy, P. (1999). The effectiveness of partial hospitalization in the treatment of borderline personality disorder: A randomised control trial. *American Journal of Psychiatry*, *156*, 1563–1569.

Bateman, A., & Fonagy, P. (2000). The effectiveness of psychotherapeutic treatment of personality disorder. *British Journal of Psychiatry*, *177*, 138–143.

Bateman, A. and P. Fonagy (2006). *Mentalization based treatment for borderline personality disorder a practical guide*. New York, Oxford.

Bodner, E., Cohen-Fridel, S., Mashiah, M., Segal, M., Grinshpoon, A., Fischel, T., & Iancu, I. (2015). The attitudes of psychiatric hospital staff toward hospitalization and treatment of patients with borderline personality disorder. *BMC Psychiatry*, *15*(1), 2.

Bramley, L., & Matiti, M. (2014). How does it really feel to be in my shoes? Patients' experiences of compassion within nursing care and their perceptions of developing compassionate nurses. *Journal of Clinical Nursing*, *23*, 2790–2799.

Clarkin, J., Levy, K. N., Lenzenweger, M., & Kernberg, O. F. (2007). Evaluating three treatments for borderline personality disorder: A multiwave study. *American Journal of Psychiatry*, *164*, 922–928.

Dickens, G., Lamont, E., & Gray, S. (2016). Mental health nurses' attitudes, behaviour, experience and knowledge regarding adults with a diagnosis of borderline personality disorder: Systematic, integrative literature review. *Journal of Clinical Nursing*, *25*, 1848–1875.

Distel, M. A., Trull, T. J., Derom, C. A., Thiery, E. W., Grimmer, M. A., Martin, N. G., & Boomsma, D. I. (2008). Heritability of borderline personality disorder features is similar across three countries. *Psychological Medicine*, *38*(9), 1219–1229.

Doering, S., Horz, S., Rentrop, M., Fischer-Kern, M., Schuster, P., & Benecke, C. (2010). Transference focused psychotherapy v. treatment by community psychotherapists for borderline personality disorder: Randomised controlled trial. *British Journal of Psychiatry*, *196*, 389–395.

Fonagy, P., & Allison, E. (2014). The role of mentalizing and epistemic trust in the therapeutic relationship. *Psychotherapy*, *51*(3), 372–380.

Fonagy, P., & Bateman, A. W. (2006). Mechanisms of change in mentalization based treatment of BPD. *Journal of Clinical Psychology*, *62*(4), 411–430.

Fonagy, P., Campbell, C., & Bateman, A. (2016). Update on diagnostic issues for borderline personality disorder. *Psychiatric Times*, *33*(7), 1.

Fonagy, P., Luyten, P., & Allison, E. (2015). Epistemic petrification and the restoration of epistemic trust: A new conceptualization of borderline personality disorder and its psychosocial treatment. *Journal of Personality Disorders*, *29*(5), 575–609.

Fonagy, P., Target, M., Gergely, G., Allen, J. G., & Bateman, A. W. (2003). The developmental roots of borderline personality disorder in early attachment relationships: A theory and some evidence. *Psychoanalytic Inquiry*, *23*(3), 412–459.

Giesen-Bloo, J., van Dyck, R., Spinhoven, P., van Tilburg, W., Dirksen, C., van Asselt, T., & Arntz, A. (2006). Outpatient psychotherapy for borderline personality disorder: Randomized trial of schema-focused therapy vs transference-focused psychotherapy. *Archives of General Psychiatry*, *63*, 649–658.

Gunderson, J. G. (2009). Borderline personality disorder: Ontology of a diagnosis, *American Journal of Psychiatry*, *166*, 530–539.

Gunderson, J. G., & Links, P. S. (2008). *Borderline personality disorder A clinical guide* (2nd ed.). Washington DC: American Psychiatric Publishing.

Gunderson, J. G., Stout, R., McGlashan, T. H., Shea, M. T., Morey, L. C., Grilo, C. M., & Skodol, A. E. (2011). Ten-year course of borderline personality disorder, psychopathology and function from the collaborative longitudinal personality disorder study. *Archive of General Psychiatry*, *166*, 827–837.

Infurna, M. R., Brunner, R., Holz, B., Parzer, P., Giannone, F., Reichl, C., & Kaess, M. (2016). The specific role of childhood abuse, parental bonding, and family functioning in female adolescents with borderline personality disorder. *Journal of Personality Disorders, 30*(2), 177–192.

Infurna, M., Parzer, P., Giannone, F., Resch, F., Brunner, R., & Kaess, M. (2014). Childhood adversity, bonding and family functioning: Is there a specific association with borderline personality disorder in adolescents? In *3rd ESSPD Conference on Borderline Personality Disorder and Allied Disorders.*

Kendler, K. S., Aggen, S. H., Czajkowski, N., Røysamb, E., Tambs, K., Torgersen, S., & Reichborn-Kjennerud, T. (2008). The structure of genetic and environmental risk factors for DSM-IV personality disorders: A multivariate twin study. *Archives of General Psychiatry, 65*(12), 1438–1446.

Krawitz, R. (2012). Behavioural treatment of severe chronic self-loathing in people with borderline personality disorder. Part 2: self-compassion and other interventions. *Australasian Psychiatry, 20*(6), 501–506.

Laska, K., Gurman, A., & Wampold, B. (2014). Expanding the lens of evidence-based practice in psychotherapy: A common factors perspective. *Psychotherapy, 51*(4), 467–481.

Lawn, S., & McMahon, J. (2015). Experiences of care by Australians with a diagnosis of borderline personality disorder. *Journal of Psychiatric and Mental Health Nursing, 22*(7), 510–521.

Linehan, M. M. (1993). *Cognitive-behavioral treatment of borderline personality disorder.* New York: Guilford Press.

Linehan, M. M., Armstrong, H. E., Suarez, A., Allmon, D., & Heard, H. L. (1991). Cognitive-behavioural treatment of chronically parasuicidal borderline patients. *Archive of General Psychiatry, 48*, 1060–1064.

Links, P. S., Ross, J., & Gunderson, J. G. (2015). Promoting good psychiatric management for patients with borderline personality disorder. *Journal of Clinical Psychology, 71*(8), 753–763.

McCaffrey, G., & McConnell, S. (2015). Compassion: A critical review of peer-reviewed nursing literature. *Journal of Clinical Nursing, 24*, 3006–3015.

McMain, S. F., Links, P. S., Gnam, W. H., Guimond, T., Cardish, R. J., Korman, L., & Streiner, D. L. (2009). A randomised trial of dialectical behaviour therapy v. general psychiatric management for borderline personality disorder. *American Journal of Psychiatry, 166*, 1365–1374.

Nicki, A. (2016). Borderline personality disorder, discrimination, and survivors of chronic childhood trauma. *International Journal of Feminist Approaches to Bioethics, 9*(1), 218–245.

Proctor, G. (2010). BPD: Mental illness or misogyny. *Therapy Today, 21*(2), 16–21.

Raes, F. (2011). The effect of self-compassion on the development of depression symptoms in a non-clinical sample. *Mindfulness, 2*, 33–36.

Sarkar, J. and G. Adshead (2012). The nature of personality disorder. *Clinical Topics in Personality Disorder.* London, Royal College of Psychiatrists, 3–20.

Shanley, E., & Jubb-Shanley, M. (2007). The recovery alliance theory of mental health nursing. *Journal of Psychiatric and Mental Health Nursing, 14*, 734–743.

Torgersen, S., Lygren, S., Øien, P. A., Skre, I., Onstad, S., Edvardsen, J., & Kringlen, E. (2000). A twin study of personality disorders. *Comprehensive Psychiatry, 41*(6), 416–425.

Trett, R., & Peckham, H. (in press). Psychotherapeutic practice in mental health nursing. In K. Edward & I. Munro (Eds.), *Mental health nursing dimensions of praxis* (3rd ed.). Melbourne: Oxford University Press.

Tyrer, P. (2009). Why borderline personality disorder is neither borderline nor a personality disorder. *Personality and Mental Health, 3*, 86–95.

Tyrer, P., Crawford, M., Mulder, R., Blashfield, Farnam, A., Fossati, A., & Reed, G. (2011). The rationale for the reclassification of personality disorder in the 11th revision of the International Classification of Diseases (ICD-11). *Personality and Mental Health, 5*, 246–259.

Tyrer, P., Reed, G., & Crawford, M. (2015). Classification, assessment, prevalence, and effect of personality disorder. *Lancet, 385*, 717–726.

Veysey, S. (2014). People with a borderline personality disorder diagnosis describe discriminatory experiences. *Kotuitui: New Zealand Journal of Social Sciences, 9*(1), 20–35.

Zanarini, M. (2008). Reasons for change in borderline personality disorder (and other axis II disorders). *Psychiatric Clinics of North America, 505–515.

Zanarini, M. C., & Frankenburg, F. R. (1997). Pathways to the development of borderline personality disorder. *Journal of Personality Disorders, 11*(1), 93–104.

Zanarini, M., Frankenburg, F., Reich, B., & Fitzmaurice, G. (2012). Attainment and stability of sustained symptomatic remission and recovery among patients with borderline personality disorder and axis II comparison subjects: A 16 year prospective follow-up study. *American Journal of Psychiatry, 169*, 476–483.

CHAPTER 13

Eating Disorders

LEANNE JAVEN, ALAN MOORE AND ALYSON MARCHESANI

Acknowledgment

The authors would like to acknowledge the contribution of Michelle Snell and Hayley Bennett who wrote this chapter in the previous edition.

KEY OUTCOMES

AFTER READING THIS CHAPTER, YOU SHOULD BE ABLE TO:

- describe the key features of anorexia nervosa, bulimia nervosa, binge eating disorder, other specified feeding and eating disorder, and unspecified feeding and eating disorder
- discuss the significant impact these disorders can have on the physiological and psychological health of consumer
- understand the role of the nurse in assessment and management of eating disorders
- identify evidence-based approaches to treatment
- understand that developing a therapeutic relationship with sufferers of eating disorders is fundamental to their recovery process.

KEY TERMS

- anorexia nervosa
- binge eating disorder
- body mass index
- bulimia nervosa
- exercise
- other specified feeding and eating disorder
- purging
- re-feeding
- restriction
- unspecified feeding and eating disorder

Introduction

In this chapter, we focus on several common eating disorders; however, it is important to note that in the fifth edition of the American Psychiatric Association's (2013) *Diagnostic and Statistical Manual of Mental Disorders* (DSM 5) there are additional feeding and eating disorders that you may see in clinical practice, whether these be in the inpatient, outpatient or community settings. Understanding both the psychological and physiological aspects of eating disorders is necessary for the successful treatment of these challenging conditions.

Specific eating disorders

Eating disorders discussed in this chapter are anorexia nervosa, bulimia nervosa, binge eating disorder, other specified feeding and eating disorder, and unspecified feeding and eating disorder.

Anorexia nervosa

Anorexia nervosa (AN) has over the years been documented in various medical writings predominantly regarding the physical and mental health of young women and more recently of young men. According to the DSM 5 criteria, to be diagnosed as having AN a person must display:

- persistent restriction of energy intake leading to significantly low body weight (in context of what is minimally expected for age, sex, developmental trajectory and physical health)
- either an intense fear of gaining weight or of becoming fat, or persistent behaviour that interferes with weight gain (even though significantly low weight)
- disturbance in the way one's body weight or shape is experienced, undue influence of body shape and weight on self-evaluation, or persistent lack of recognition of the seriousness of the current low body weight.

Within AN diagnostic criteria it is important to note there are two subtypes: binge-purging (self-induced vomiting or misuse of laxatives, diuretics or enemas) and restricting (weight loss primarily through dieting, fasting and/or excessive exercise) (American Psychiatric Association, 2013).

CRITICAL THINKING OPPORTUNITY

1   What are the nursing considerations for someone suffering from AN?

2   How and why might you involve family members in the care management, shared decision making and discharge planning of those who experience AN?

Bulimia nervosa

Bulimia nervosa was first documented in medical writings in the late 1970s, again as an eating disorder predominantly seen in young women, manifesting as marked disturbances in the mental and physical health of the individual. Bulimia nervosa (BN) is characterised by frequent episodes of binge eating followed by inappropriate compensatory behaviours such as self-induced vomiting to avoid weight gain. Currently, in order to receive a diagnosis of BN an individual must engage in recurrent episodes of binge eating, experience feelings of loss of control over eating during the binges, employ recurrent inappropriate behaviours to compensate for the caloric input (such as vomiting, laxative abuse, strict dieting or strenuous over-exercise) and have a sense of self that is unduly influenced by their body shape or weight. The bingeing and compensatory behaviours must occur at a specified frequency and not occur exclusively during an episode of AN.

ABOUT THE CONSUMER   Bec's story

Bec is a 34-year-old married woman working full-time as an analyst for a large corporation. She lives with her husband in their own home. She was referred by her GP and presented to an outpatient eating disorders specialist service for an assessment. On assessment, Bec presents with an eighteen-year history of eating disorder symptoms with co-morbid depression/anxiety. Currently her eating disorder symptoms take the form of a significant fear of fatness, where she equates becoming fat with 'being a pig'. She has body image distortion, but nevertheless shows some insight—'I think I look terrible. I'm too thin because I'm sick'—and understands that being this thin is a threat to her health.

She describes being preoccupied with shape, weight and eating, spending much of her time thinking about food, worrying about her weight and shape, or worrying about what she might eat or how she might burn up calories. She has a typical pattern of excessive dietary restraint and also reports consuming large quantities of water, up to 6 litres daily. Bec tends to avoid high-calorie food such as fatty foods and high carbohydrate dense foods. She denies calorie counting, but is very aware of the calorie content of most things; she denies weighing herself frequently; she admits to intermittent vomiting; and she denies using laxatives, but in the past has taken over-the-counter diet pills. She reports exercising regularly, spending large periods of time swimming and going to the gym. A recent blood test shows that she has an electrolyte imbalance. Bec and her husband have been trying to start a family for the past four years without success and Bec feels guilty because she has been advised by her GP that her inability to conceive is likely in the context of her longstanding eating disorder diagnosis; despite this her GP has referred her to a fertility specialist.

Her husband of six years has been very supportive and caring, but more recently he has advised that he does not know how much longer he can endure her behaviour and as such their relationship is becoming increasingly strained. He works full-time in the corporate world and is often away on business.

REFLECTION QUESTIONS

1   How might you work collaboratively with Bec to develop a recovery-oriented treatment plan?

2   How might you continue to engage Bec if she decides treatment is unhelpful?

3   How would you maintain links with the various professionals working with Bec?

4   Bec presents to the specialist eating disorder outpatient department for review and expresses suicidal ideation in the context of continuing weight restoration. What would you do?

5   How might you reduce the risk of deterioration?

Binge eating disorder

The essential feature of binge eating disorder (BED) is recurrent episodes of binge eating that occur on average at least once a week for three months. An episode of binge eating is defined as eating in a discrete period of time an amount of food that is larger than most people would eat in a similar period of time under similar circumstances. An occurrence of excessive food must be accompanied by a sense of lack of control and marked distress. Severity is based on the frequency of episodes (American Psychiatric Association, 2013).

Other specified feeding and eating disorder

This category applies to a presentation in which symptoms of clinical distress and impairment of functioning are present, and which are characteristic of a feeding and eating disorder, but do not meet the full criteria for the disorders mentioned above. OSFED includes atypical anorexia nervosa (AAN), subthreshold BN, subthreshold BED, purging disorder and night eating disorder (American Psychiatric Association, 2013).

Unspecified feeding and eating disorder

Unspecified feeding and eating disorder (USFED) 'applies to presentations in which symptoms characteristic of a feeding and eating disorder that cause clinically significant distress or impairment in social, occupational, or other important areas of functioning predominate but do not meet full criteria for any of the disorders in the feeding and eating disorders diagnostic class' (American Psychiatric Association, 2013, p. 354).

Early recognition

Individuals with an eating disorder may present in a variety of ways including a deterioration in behaviours, cognition and physical health that may not be identified by the individual as an eating disorder. Consider evaluating an individual for a possible eating disorder who presents with the following:

- electrolyte disturbance
- amenorrhea/menstrual irregularities
- gastrointestinal complaints
- oral and dental symptoms
- seizures
- rapid weight loss
- changes in behaviour such as social isolation and avoidance of meal times with family
- lowering of mood with or without suicidal ideation
- obsessive behaviours
- changes in food preferences
- low self-esteem
- fatigue
- negative body image (National Eating Disorders Collaboration, 2015).

BOX 13.1 THE SCOFF QUESTIONNAIRE

Early detection in consumers with unexplained weight loss improves prognosis and may be aided by use of the SCOFF questionnaire, which uses five simple screening questions and has been validated in specialist and primary care settings (Luck et al., 2002). The questionnaire has a sensitivity of 100 per cent and specificity of 90 per cent for AN. Though not diagnostic, a score of 2 or more positive answers highlights the need for a more detailed assessment and history taking.

S—Do you make yourself **S**ick because you feel uncomfortably full?

C—Do you worry you have lost **C**ontrol over how much you eat?

O—Have you recently lost more than **O**ne stone (6.35 kilograms) in a three-month period?

F—Do you believe yourself to be **F**at when others say you are too thin?

F—Would you say **F**ood dominates your life?

An answer of 'yes' to two or more questions warrants further questioning and more comprehensive assessment.

A further two questions have been shown to indicate a high sensitivity and specificity for bulimia nervosa. These questions indicate a need for further questioning and discussion:

1   Are you satisfied with your eating patterns?

2   Do you ever eat in secret?

Hill et al. (2010)

Multidisciplinary assessment

A multidisciplinary assessment is necessary to determine whether the consumer has an eating disorder and then to recommend the best treatment options. Increasingly, nurse practitioners are taking a leading role in the assessment process; however, dietetics, psychology and medicine are also involved in providing a comprehensive assessment.

Incorporated in the assessment process are the presenting problem, psychiatric history, forensic history, medication, use of alcohol and other drugs (AOD), family history including genogram, developmental/personal history, mental state examination, risk assessment, physical assessment (vital signs; in particular lying/standing blood pressure and heart rate, height, weight, body mass index and electrocardiogram), current and past medical history, summary, and nursing care requirements. Specifically, the nurse should assess:

- *physical health*—using a systems approach; including cardiovascular, respiratory, gastrointestinal and central nervous system health, along with general health concerns and a general examination
- *anthropometry*—lowest weight, highest weight, desired weight, consumer's perception, and contributing factors to weight fluctuations
- *biochemistry*—full blood examination, urea and electrolytes, calcium, magnesium and phosphate, glomerular filtration rate, thyroid function test, liver function tests, iron studies, vitamin D, folate, B12, and zinc
- *physical health considerations*—appetite, concentration, energy, sleep, hair, nail and skin integrity, gastrointestinal symptoms, bowel function, menstrual cycle, body composition and bone mineral density scan
- *diet history*—current intake and eating disordered behaviours (compensatory behaviours, weight control measures and the consumer's view of their diet).

Possible differential diagnosis

It is important that any other illness presentations and/or organic conditions that may cause weight loss are excluded before an eating disorder diagnosis is made. Some alternatives to consider include:

- endocrine disorders
- mood disorders
- anxiety disorders
- psychotic disorders
- substance abuse
- tumours
- cancers.

Re-feeding syndrome

Re-feeding syndrome is understood to be due to the switch from fasting gluconeogenesis to carbohydrate-induced insulin release, triggering rapid intracellular uptake of potassium, phosphate and magnesium to metabolise carbohydrates (Kohn, Madden & Clarke, 2011). This, on top of already low body stores of electrolytes due to starvation, can lead to rapid onset of phosphataemia, hypomagnesia and hypokalemia. In addition, insulin-triggered rebound hypoglycaemia can occur, exacerbated by depleted glycogen stores (Hay et al., 2014).

TABLE 13.1 HEALTH COMPLICATIONS SECONDARY TO EATING DISORDERS

Due to weight loss	Due to purging behaviours
Cardiovascular: hypotension, bradycardia, postural tachycardia, arrhythmias, syncope (fainting) and sudden deat	**Gastrointestinal**: inflammation and enlargement of salivary gland, gastric and oesophageal erosion, and gastric rupture
Dermatological: dry skin, hair loss, lanugo (fine downy hair on body) and oedema	**Dental**: discolouration and significant erosion of dental enamel, particularly of front teeth
Endocrine: amenorrhoea, lowered oestrogen, lowered follicle-stimulating hormone and lowered luteinising hormone	**Metabolic**: severe electrolyte disturbances, particularly lowering of potassium, magnesium and chloride
Skeletal: osteopenia, osteoporosis and associated fractures	**Dermatological**: abrasions to knuckles of hands (from induced vomiting)
Haematological: anaemia, low B12, low white blood cell count, lowered platelets, low magnesium, lowered zinc levels, low calcium, low sodium and low phosphate	
Gastrointestinal: abdominal pain, bloating, nausea, delayed gastric emptying, constipation and/or diarrhoea	
Thermoregulatory: hypothermia (may mask serious infection)	

Berkman, Lohr and Bulik (2007)

Risk factors for developing re-feeding syndrome include the degree of malnutrition the consumer presents with and their ability to adapt to the changes. The greater the degree of malnutrition, the greater the risk of abnormalities (Hay et al., 2014). Significant disturbance in electrolyte levels (outside of the norm) and blood sugars can result in multi-system organ failure; in particular, cardiac and respiratory failure, which requires experience and expertise in the field to manage the risks safely and effectively.

Electrolyte shifts generally occur after the first forty-eight hours of re-feeding and may present as late as three to five days after feeding starts. Re-feeding syndrome is more commonly seen in the hospital setting for severe AN and where consumers have significant weight loss in a short time-frame due to severe restriction of nutritional intake.

High-risk consumers have one or more of the following:

- body mass index (kg/m^2): <16
- unintentional weight loss: >15 per cent in the past three to six months
- little or no nutritional intake: >10 days
- low levels of potassium or magnesium before feeding

At-risk consumers have two or more of the following:

- body mass index: <18.5
- unintentional weight loss: >10 per cent in the past three to six months
- little or no nutritional intake: >5 days
- history of alcohol misuse, drugs, including insulin, chemotherapy, antacids or diuretics.

Mild- to moderate-risk consumers are defined as any consumer who has had little or no nutritional intake for >5 days.

Current RANZCP clinical practice guidelines (Hay et al., 2014) recommend commencing re-feeding at 6000kJ/day. This should be increased by 2000kJ/day every two to three days until an adequate nutritional intake to meet the person's needs for weight restoration is reached.

This regime should be supplemented by phosphate at 500mg twice daily and thiamine at least 100mg daily for the first week, and thereafter as clinically indicated for people at high risk of re-feeding syndrome. Each service should have a protocol and policy to adhere to.

The most important factors in preventing re-feeding syndrome are a heightened awareness of the syndrome, and regular monitoring of the person's clinical status, including physical observations and biochemical monitoring (Hay et al., 2014).

Evidence-based approaches for the treatment of eating disorders

The general principles of treatment for all eating disorders have been described by Hay and colleagues (2014):

- Involve family, carers and significant others in treatment and to gain collateral information.
- The least restrictive treatment is the first option.
- Utilise a recovery-oriented model.
- Use a person-centred approach.
- Adopt a collaborative, multidisciplinary team approach with nursing, medical, psychology and nutrition input.
- Health practitioners need to be culturally aware of the consumer's beliefs and values, and how that may influence their presentation.

There is moderate research to suggest that individuals, who are under the age of 18 years and living at home with their family, can benefit from engaging in the *Maudsley Family Based Treatment* program. The Maudsley approach is an intensive outpatient treatment, where parents play an active role in helping their child regain weight. There are three phases to the treatment, usually conducted within fifteen to twenty sessions over the course of twelve months—with parents gradually handing the control back to the adolescent and encouraging the adolescent to re-establish a healthy self-identity. The Maudsley Family Based Treatment program is offered to families of children with a relatively short period of illness, usually less than three years in duration (Lock and LeGrange, 2013).

Specialist therapist-led approaches for adults show the most promising outcomes, specifically *Cognitive Behavioural Therapy–Enhanced* (CBT-E), which was developed by Christopher Fairburn throughout the 1970s and 1980s. Originally intended for bulimia nervosa specifically, it was eventually extended to all eating disorders (Fairburn, 2008). There are shortcomings in the literature, making robust comparisons between psychological treatments difficult.

CBT-E refers to a 'transdiagnostic personalised psychological treatment for eating disorders'. It was developed as an outpatient treatment for adults, but there is an intensive version for day patient and inpatient settings (Dalle Grave, 2012). CBT-E has four stages. Stage one focused on gaining a mutual understanding of the person's eating problem and helping them modify and stabilise their eating pattern. The emphasis is on education and addressing concerns about weight. Stage two is related to formulation, review and planning the next stage. Stage three is focused on addressing concerns about body shape and eating, while addressing the consumer's ability to deal with day-to-day events. Stage four relates to maintaining changes, managing setbacks and recovery (Fairburn, 2008). The effective therapeutic relationship within CBT has been described in similar terms, focusing on both the tasks/goals and the clinical alliance and such an alliance makes change possible.

Other individual therapies include interpersonal psychotherapy, specialist supportive clinical management (SSCM) and cognitive remediation therapy. These are still being researched for their efficacy, and are briefly discussed here.

Interpersonal psychotherapy is an evidence-based treatment for eating disorders, primarily bulimia and binge-eating disorders. The main reason for this is that consumer with eating disorders can present with significant interpersonal difficulties that appear to contribute to maintenance of the illness. Some may predate the illness, while others may be the result of the illness. The treatment has three phases usually over four to six months. The first phase is to engage the consumer, the second phase is to develop the focus of the treatment based on the interpersonal problems identified, and the third is to ensure change and long-term recovery (Murphy et al., 2012).

Specialist supportive clinical management (SSCM) is an outpatient treatment that can be offered to individuals of low weight. The treatment was developed for a psychotherapy trial for AN as a comparison treatment to CBT-E and interpersonal psychotherapy (IPT). It combines features of clinical management and supportive psychotherapy and addresses the core symptoms of AN, including low weight, restrictive eating patterns and compensatory behaviours. The treatment focuses on normal eating and weight restoration, providing education and information, while also addressing broader life issues (McIntosh, 2015).

Cognitive remediation therapy (CRT) for AN targets cognitive style rather than focusing on weight and shape. It consists of mental exercises aimed at improving cognitive strategies, thinking skills and information processing, with the aim of exercising connections in the brain in the hope of improving function (Tchanturia & Lock, 2011). CRT is a brief individual intervention run over eight to ten sessions and encourages consumers to consider the ways in which they think and behave (Tchanturia, Lloyd & Lang, 2013).

Regarding bulimia nervosa and binge eating disorder, the first line of treatment in adults is individual psychological therapy. The best evidence is for CBT-E (Hay et al., 2014). Where access to a therapist is delayed, it is suggested that evidenced-based self-help manuals can be utilised.

Though it is often difficult to achieve a therapeutic relationship with consumers suffering from an eating disorder, it is important to consider the stage of change, motivation and medical status of the consumer. As the illness crosses a number of disciplines, including nursing, psychiatry, medicine and dietetics, it is also important to provide a multidisciplinary approach to care and treatment. A number of studies have shown that the therapeutic alliance may be one of the most important arenas in the treatment of eating disorders (Constantino et al., 2005; Zaitsoff et al., 2015).

Consumers with eating disorders in the general hospital

Many consumers with eating disorders present to general hospital emergency departments or via a medical admission before they are seen by specialist eating disorder services. The presenting signs and symptoms may include electrolyte disturbance, cardiac changes or an unexplained collapse. Some consumers also present to gastroenterology or clinical nutrition outpatient departments with symptoms such as weight loss or vague gastric symptoms.

When the consumer presents in a medical setting, it is important that their psychological needs are catered for and that they are not simply medically stabilised and discharged before having an adequate mental health assessment—and, if indicated, a treatment plan. In the outpatient setting it is equally as important for clinicians to consider an eating disorder diagnosis and provide a mental health assessment rather than proceed to endless physical investigations and interventions.

Often an inpatient medical setting is the first opportunity for the consumer and their family to be engaged in a therapeutic alliance; the Consultation Liaison Psychiatry Service (available in public hospitals) is notable in this regard. The importance of close liaison between the medical and psychiatric teams is the subject of the Management of Really Sick Patients with Anorexia Nervosa (MARSIPAN) Report (Royal College of Psychiatrists Physicians & Pathologists, 2014).

Supporting consumers with their recovery while in a medical setting can be challenging but necessary at many junctions of eating disorders.

Inpatient versus outpatient treatment

Outpatient treatment is the first line in the management of AN, whereas hospitalisation is primarily reserved for situations of acute medical instability and weight restoration for severely underweight consumers. Consumers that present with significant co-morbidities including self-harm and suicide ideation should be considered for a general acute psychiatric admission.

When hospitalisation is indicated as a result of a severe and enduring eating disorder, consumers usually respond best to a collaborative agreement setting achievable goals, such as medical rescue, weight gain and reducing compensatory behaviours (i.e.: self-induced vomiting, misuse of laxatives and/ or excessive exercising). The primary focus of hospitalisation is on enhancing their quality of life and maintaining hope. As always, it is important to include family members and significant others in the decision-making process regarding treatment options (i.e.: self-induced vomiting, misuse of laxatives and/or excessive exercising). When making a decision about feeding against the person's will, short-term and long-term implications should be considered, as many individuals with longstanding eating disorders have experienced negative inpatient care (Hay et al., 2014). The potential adverse effects on the therapeutic alliance and recovery also needs to be considered. The short-term weight gain response of voluntary consumers with AN has been shown to be comparable to those admitted involuntarily. Evidence also indicates that many who are treated on an involuntary basis later agree that treatment was necessary and have remained therapeutically engaged (Hay et al., 2014).

The therapeutic relationship underpins the person's active engagement in their care even when that care is to be provided to the person involuntarily. The 'crucial dimensions of active engagement for adherence may be patient optimism about the usefulness of treatment, meaningful involvement in therapy, patient interest in understanding their illness and realistic perceptions of the therapist (Thompson & McCabe, 2012).'

Therapeutic alliance

Therapeutic alliance has long been acknowledged as a significant predictor in the effectiveness of response to treatment across a variety of treatments and disorders (Arnow et al., 2013; Horvath et al., 2011), as well as predicting treatment drop-out, response rates and consumer outcomes (Pereira et al., 2006). However, more recently studies have explored its relationship with consumer recovering from a range of eating disorders. Stiles-Shields and colleagues (2016) noted that establishing a therapeutic relationship is pivotal in the treatment and recovery of anorexic consumers, while acknowledging that developing and maintaining such a relationship can be particularly challenging, leading to staff frustration and exhaustion.

Therapeutic alliance is about the relational bond that develops between a consumer and clinician via collaborative work, trust and open communication, while endeavouring to establish and accomplish mutual treatment goals (Bordin, 1979; McCance & McCormack, 2016).

Therapeutic alliance has been shown to prevent premature treatment drop-out in eating disorder inpatient settings, improve compliance (Sly et al., 2013) and reduce symptoms at the end of treatment and follow-up (Stiles-Shields et al., 2013), as well as aid weight recovery (Bourion-Bedes et al., 2013).

Waller, Evans and Stringer (2012), in a study on the use of a therapeutic alliance during the early stages of CBT for treating eating disorders, identified that it resulted in a therapeutic alliance that was equal or superior to that achieved in psychotherapy for a general range of disorders, and the consumer rated the therapeutic alliance in CBT highly.

One potential method of developing a therapeutic alliance is through the development of a mutual treatment plan with the consumer and their family. However, it is not an easy task as many consumers (and sometimes their families) prefer to deny, minimise or medicalise their symptoms, which should be viewed as part of the illness and not as an obstruction by the consumer or their family. A successful therapeutic relationship requires the nurse to have high-quality communication and interpersonal skills and also to be able to build rapport and trust with the consumer (Silverman, Kantz & Draper, 2016; McCance & McCormack, 2016). Without a trusting, therapeutic nurse–consumer relationship, the treatment and recovery of people with eating disorders can be unnecessarily impeded and prolonged (Stiles-Shields et al., 2013; Stiles-Shields et al., 2016).

Pharmacotherapy

There is limited evidence for use of psychotropic agents for consumers with eating disorders. Prescribing for co-morbid conditions such as anxiety and mood disorders ideally is left until it is apparent that symptoms are not primarily related to starvation.

Low doses of antipsychotics like Olanzapine may be helpful for severely anxious consumers with obsessive eating ruminations; however, further research is necessary as to the efficacy of this approach.

Adults with BN and BED may be offered a trial of antidepressants. Selective serotonin reuptake inhibitors (SSRIs) are the drugs of choice, specifically Fluoxetine, where early response is a strong predictor of effectiveness (Taylor, Paton & Kapur, 2015).

Antidepressant drugs may be used for the treatment of adolescents; however, they are not considered as first-line treatment and monitoring of suicide risk is indicated. As with all medications, there is a risk of side effects; in particular, a prolonged QTC interval. ECG monitoring should be instigated if the prescription of medication is warranted. There is no evidence to suggest prescribing medications can reverse bone mineral density loss.

When prescribing, one needs to apply the quality use of medicine approach and the principles of the National Medicines Policy (Quality Use of Medicines, 2016).

TOPIC LINK
See Chapter 15
for more on
Psychopharmacology.

Care planning

The following is an example care plan for Bec, the consumer presented in this chapter. The areas of daily living that are considered include biopsychosocial factors and the plan is mapped out using the nursing process (assessment, planning, implementation and evaluation). Remember, the success is in the detail, so be specific about who, when and what in the collaborative plan; and never include someone in the plan if they were not consulted in the planning process.

Date	Assessment	Treatment goals	Implementation	Person responsible	Evaluation
	Medical instability	Medical rescue Biochemical, haematological and cardiac stability	Monitor vital signs: heart rate, blood pressure (lying/standing), temperature twice daily Daily blood pathology ECG	Nurse and treating doctor	Daily
	Falls risk	Prevention of falls	Supervision and use of wheelchair; may need constant observation	Nurse and treating doctor	Daily
	Excessive water intake	Adequate fluid intake as per dietary requirements	Fluid balance chart Follow meal plan and fluid intake	Nurse and treating doctor	Daily
	Low body weight	Safe weight restoration	Dietician assessment Commence meal plan Monitor compliance Supervise weighing twice weekly in gown pre-breakfast post-void Observe and monitor for re-feeding syndrome	Nurse	Daily
	Electrolyte derangement history; intermittent vomiting	Stabilisation	Daily bloods, meal plan adherence and supplementation as required	Nurse and treating doctor	Daily
	History of excessive exercise	Minimise energy expenditure	Close observation Use of wheelchair if necessary	Nurse and consumer to work together on goals	Daily
	Consumer has history of taking diet pills	Reduce compensatory behaviours	Search consumer belongings on admission and return from leave	Nurse, treating doctor and consumer to work together on minimising access to diet pills	Daily
	Eating disorder cognitions: body image disturbance and fear of weight gain	Address eating disorder cognitions	Group and individual therapy	Treating team in collaboration with the consumer	Daily
	Inadequate nutrition	Work towards regular eating: food groups, portion size and variety Address eating behaviours	Meal plan and dietetic psychoeducation	Nurse and dietician	Daily Weekly dietetic group

Date	Assessment	Treatment goals	Implementation	Person responsible	Evaluation
	Anxiety/ Depression	Stabilise symptoms	Further assessment Medication if warranted Psychological intervention as needed Ongoing monitoring: risk assessment/MSE	Nurse / Doctor	Daily Twice weekly ward round meetings
	Minimal family support and understanding	Family engagement	Psychoeducation Family intervention Meal support therapy with family involved Refer to family therapy and support groups	Nurse and treating doctor	Daily to weekly
	Eating disorder with anxiety and depression	Relapse prevention	Ongoing specialist eating disorder treatment Medical support from local GP Consider AMHS	Nurse and treating doctor	Daily to weekly

SUMMARY

It is important to understand that eating disorders are complex mental illnesses that result in significant medical complications and therefore nurses play a pivotal role in the care of consumers presenting with these conditions.

It is also common for consumers to present with co-morbid mental health disorders such as anxiety, depression and personality disorders, so when creating a care plan, consider evidence-based treatment for all diagnoses.

Eating disorders have a significant impact on people's lives and thus when working with consumers and their significant others, it is essential to be mindful of their stage of change and work collaboratively with them to improve overall health and well-being.

DISCUSSION
QUESTIONS

1   What is a typical medical presentation with a consumer suffering from bulimia nervosa?

2   What pharmacological treatment has been indicated for bulimia nervosa and binge eating disorder?

3   What is the evidence based treatment approach for adolescents suffering from anorexia nervosa?

4   What could be alternative differentials that may on first sight present as similar to that of an eating disorder?

TEST YOURSELF

1   What is a typical medical presentation with a consumer suffering from bulimia nervosa?
    a   gum disease
    b   hypokalaemia
    c   Russell's signs
    d   bloating

2   Which specific SSRI pharmacotherapy treatment has been indicated for bulimia nervosa and binge eating disorder?
    a   Paroxetine
    b   Fluvoxamine
    c   Sertraline
    d   Fluoxetine

3   What is the evidence-based therapy for adolescents?
    a   psychotherapy
    b   cognitive behavioural therapy
    c   Maudsley Family Based Treatment program
    d   interpersonal therapy

4   Low doses of antipsychotics like Olanzapine may be helpful for
    a   severely anxious consumer with obsessive eating ruminations
    b   severely anorexic people
    c   severely dehydrated people with AN
    d   people where anxiolytics have not worked

USEFUL WEBSITES

Academy for Eating Disorders (USA): www.aedweb.org

Australia & New Zealand Academy for Eating Disorders: www.anzaed.org.au

Eating Disorder Hope: www.eatingdisorderhope.com

Eating Disorders Victoria: www.eatingdisorders.org.au

 and www.howfaristoofar.org.au

International Association of Eating Disorders Professionals Foundation: www.iaedp.com

National Eating Disorders (USA): www.nationaleatingdisorders.org

National Eating Disorders Collaboration: http://nedc.com.au

NSW Health—Centre for Eating and Dieting Disorders: www.cedd.org.au/?id=1

Western Australia Department of Health—Centre for Clinical Interventions: www.cci.health.wa.gov.au/resources/mhp.cfm

LEANNE JAVEN, ALAN MOORE AND ALYSON MARCHESANI

REFERENCES

American Psychiatric Association (2013). *Diagnostic and statistical manual of mental disorders.* (5th ed.; DSM 5). Washington: American Psychiatric Association.

Arnow, B. A., Steidtmann, D., Blasey, C., Manber, R., Constantino, M. J., Klein, D. N., Markowitz, J. C., Kocsis, J. H. (2013). The relationship between the therapeutic alliance and treatment outcome in two distinct psychotherapies for chronic despression. *Journal Consult of Clinical Psychology, 81*(627).

Berkman, N., Lohr, K., & Bulik, C. (2007). Outcomes of eating disorders: A systematic review of the literature. *International Journal of Eating Disorders, 40*(4), 293–309.

Bordin, E. (1979). The generalizability of the psyhcoanalytic concept of the working alliance. *Psychotherapy Theory Research and Practice, 16,* 252–260.

Bourion-Bedes, S., Baumann, C., Kermarrec, S., Ligier, F., Feillet F., Bonnemains, C., Guillemin F., & Kaubuth, B. (2013). Prognostic value of early therapeutic alliance in weight recovery: A prospective cohort of 108 adolescents with anorexia nervosa. *Journal of Adolescent Health, 52,* 344–350.

Constantino, M. J., Arnow, B. A., Blasey, C., & Agrad. W. S. (2005). The association between patient characteristics and the therapeutic alliance in cognitive behavioural and interpersonal therapy for bulimia nervosa. *Journal of Consulting and Clinical Psychology, 73*(2), 203–211.

Dalle Grave R. (2012). *Multistep cognitive behavioural therapy for eating disorders.* Maryland: Jason Aronson.

Fairburn, C. G. (2008). *Cognitive behaviour therapy and eating disorders.* New York: Guildford Press.

Hay, P., Chinn, D., Forbes, D., Madden, S., Newton, R., Sugenor, L., Ward, W. (2014). Royal Australian and New Zealand College of Psychiatrists clinical practice guidelines for the treatment of eating disorders. *Australian & New Zealand Journal of Psychiatry, 48*(11), 1–62.

Hill, L. S., Reid, F., Morgan, J. F., & Lacey, J. H. (2010). SCOFF: The development of an eating disorder screening questionnaire. *International Journal of Eating Disorders, 43*(4), 344–351.

Horvath, A. O., Del Re, A. C., Fluckiger, C., & Symonds, D. (2011). Alliance in individual psychotherapy. *Psychotherapy, 48,* 9–16.

Kohn, M. R., Madden, S., & Clarke, S. D. (2011). Refeeding in anorexia nervosa: Increased safety and efficiency through understanding the pathophysiology of protein calorie malnutrion. *Current Opinion in Pediatrics, 23,* 390–394.

Lock, J., & LeGrange, D. (2013). *Treatment manuel for anorexia nervosa—a family based approach.* (2nd ed). London: Guilford Press.

Luck, A. J., MorganLuck, J. F., Reid, F., O'brien, A., Brunton, J., Price, C., Perry, L & Lacey, J. H. (2002). *The SCOFF questionnaire and clinical interview for eating disorders in general practice: comparative study.* Bmj, 325(7367), 755–756.

McCance, T., & McCormack B (2016). Person centred practice framework. In B. McCormack & T. McCance, *Person centred practice in nursing and health care: Theory and practice* (pp. 36–59). Wiley Blackwell.

McIntosh, V. (2015). Specialist supportive clinical management for anorexia nervosa: Content analysis, change over course of therapy, and relation to outcome. *Journal of Eating Disorders, 3*(1), 1.

Murphy, R., Straebler, S., Basden, S., Cooper, Z., & Fairburn, C. G. (2012). Interpersonal psychotherapy for eating disorders. *Clinical Psychology and Psychtherapy, 19*(2), 150–158.

National Eating Disorders Collaboration (2015). *Understanding the warning signs.* Retrieved from www.nedc.com.au/recognise-the-warning-signs.

Pereira, T., Lock, J., & Oggins, J. (2006). Role of the therapeutic alliance in family therapy for adolescent anorexia nervosa. *International Journal of Eating Disorders, 39* (98), 677–684.

Quality Use of Medicines (2016). Retrieved 18 August 2016 from www.health.gov.au.

Royal College of Psychiatrists Physicians & Pathologists (2014). *MARSIPAN Management of really sick patients with anorexia nervosa.*

Silverman, J., Kantz,S., & Draper J (2016). *Skills for communicating with patients* (3rd ed.). CRC Press.

Sly, R., Morgan, J. F., Mountford, V. A., & Lacey, J. H. (2013). Predicting premature termination of hospitalised treatment for anorexia nervosa: The role of therapeutic alliance, motivation, and behaviour change. *Eating Behaviours, 14*(2), 119–123.

Stiles-Shields, C., Touyz, S., Hay, P., Lacey, J. H., Crosby, R. D., Rieger, E., Bamford, B. H., & LeGrange, D. (2013). Therapeutic alliance in two treatments for adults with severe and enduring anorexia nervosa. *International Journal of Eating Disorders, 46*(8), 783–789.

Stiles-Shields, C., Bamford, B., Touyz, S., LeGrange, D., Hay, P., & Lacey, H. (2016). Predictors of therapeutic alliance in two treatments for adults with severe and enduring anorexia nervosa. *Journal of Eating Disorders, 4*(13), 1–7.

Taylor, D., Paton, C., & Kapur, S. (2015). *The Maudsley prescribing guidelines in psychiatry* (12th ed.). Oxford, UK; Wiley-Blackwell.

Tchanturia, K., & Lock, J. (2011). Cognitive remediation therapy for eating disorders: Development, refinement and future directions. *Behavioural Neuroscience, 6,* 269–287.

Tchanturia, K., Lloyd ,S., & Lang, K. (2013). Cognitive remediation therapy for anorexia nervosa: Current evidence and future research directions. *International Journal of Eating Disorders, 46*(5), 492–495.

Thompson, L., & McCabe, R. (2012). The effect of clinician patient alliance and communication on treatment adherence in mental health care: A systematic review. *BMC Psychiatry, 12,* 87.

Waller, G., Evans, J., & Stringer, H. (2012). The therapeutic alliance in the early part of cognitive behavioural therapy for eating disorders. *International Journal of Eating Disorders, 45,* 63–69.

Zaitsoff, S., Pullmer, R., Cry, M., & Aime, H. (2015). The role of the theraputic alliance in eating disorder treatment outcomes: A systematic review. *Eating Disorders, 23*(2), 99–114.

CHAPTER 14

Alcohol, Tobacco, Other Drugs and Co-occurring Disorders

NAOMI CRAFTI AND
VICTORIA MANNING

Acknowledgment

The authors would like to acknowledge the contribution of Gylo Hercelinskyj, who wrote this chapter in the previous edition.

KEY OUTCOMES

AFTER READING THIS CHAPTER, YOU SHOULD BE ABLE TO:

- describe the types of psychoactive substances that lead to a range of mental health and associated problems
- understand the typical patterns and prevalence of co-occurring disorders
- assess people for alcohol and other drug problems
- have a clear understanding of models of treatment of substance use disorders and how they apply to people with co-occurring disorders
- articulate models of recovery for mental health and alcohol and other drug use.

KEY TERMS

- addiction
- substance use disorders
- dependence
- co-occurring disorders
- recovery

Introduction

According to the Australian Institute of Health and Welfare (2016), the six disease groups causing the greatest burden of disease in Australia in 2011 were cancer, cardiovascular diseases, mental health disorders, substance use disorders, musculoskeletal conditions and injuries. Together these diseases were found to contribute 66 per cent of the total burden. Of these conditions, mental health and substance use disorders had the greatest impact of all in the younger age groups, late childhood, adolescence and adulthood to age 49 (Australian Institute of Health and Welfare, 2016).

There is a significant overlap between the use of psychoactive substances and the experience of mental health symptoms, and this is a complex and dynamic relationship. Thus, individuals who start to experience psychiatric symptoms may 'self-medicate' to dampen down these unpleasant experiences. Similarly, individuals who experiment with a range of illicit drugs may experience short- or longer-term psychological and mental health consequences. There may be individuals who are susceptible to both substance dependence and to mental illness as a result of adversities they experience early in life or as a consequence of a range of traumas. And there is evidence that there is a dynamic relationship where substance use and mental health symptoms can prolong and worsen over time. After reading this chapter, you will be able to understand the nature of the relationship between different kinds of substance misuse and mental health problems (with some additional information on the pattern and prevalence of substance misuse and abuse). You will also deepen your understanding about the ways that problems are recorded for co-occurring substance misuse and mental illness. The chapter will also offer information related to the prevalence (commonness) and patterns of co-occurring disorders, also called 'dual diagnosis'. Finally, the chapter will provide an overview of how to access treatment options for clients in your care within the context of the recovery model.

Typical patterns and prevalence of co-occurring disorders

There has been much debate on the label assigned to individuals with a concurrent mental health and substance use disorder. Whilst 'dual diagnosis' and 'co-morbidity' have been the dominant terms used in the US, UK and Australia, recognition that they are overly simplistic, medicalised and potentially stigmatising (Guest & Holland, 2011) has led to the wider adoption of terms such as co-existing or co-occurring disorders.

TOPIC LINK ■

See Chapter 10 for more on mood and anxiety disorders

     There is wide variation in the prevalence of co-occurring disorders reported in the Australian literature. This is due to differences in study method (for example, epidemiological versus clinical studies), the setting that reflects chronicity (for example, hospitalised versus community treatment settings), the way in which the disorder is operationalised and assessed (for example, structured diagnostic criteria versus problematic use), the data collection method (for example, research interview versus case audit review) and the time-frame adopted (for example, lifetime or past twelve months), to name a few. Nonetheless, the 2007 National Survey on Mental Health and Well-being (Teesson, Slade, & Mills, 2009) indicates that 35% of individuals meeting DSM-IV criteria for a substance use disorder (31% of men and 44% of women) have at least one co-occurring affective or anxiety disorder, representing nearly 300,000 Australians. Furthermore, of the 183,900 Australians who used alcohol or other drugs almost daily, 63% had a 12-month mental health disorder. Interestingly, 21.4 per cent of those with an affective disorder and 33.5 per cent of those with an anxiety disorder also had a substance use disorder. Co-occurring disorders are more prevalent among individuals attending health care services, since the presence of multiple disorders increases the likelihood that an individual will seek treatment (Berkson, 1946).

Patterns of co-morbidity

Among alcohol and other drugs (AOD) treatment populations, the most common mental health issues mirror those in the general population (that is, anxiety and depression); however, the rates of post-traumatic stress disorder (PTSD) and personality disorders (particularly borderline and antisocial personality disorder) are elevated by comparison to the general population (Deane, Kelly, Crowe, Coulson, & Lyons, 2013; Dore, Mills, Murray, Teesson, & Farrugia, 2012; McKetin, Lubman, Lee, Ross, & Slade, 2011; Manning et al, 2008). A US study found that up to 71% of individuals in residential AOD services had an DSM-IV Axis I disorder (Mortlock et al., 2011). Similarly, among those consumers attending mental health services, the substance use reflects patterns observed in the general population; that is, most commonly tobacco, alcohol, cannabis and stimulants (Bizzarri et al., 2016; Hunt, Malhi, Cleary, Lai, & Sitharthan, 2016a). However, rates of substance use tend to be higher among individuals with more severe mental illnesses—that is, schizophrenia and bipolar affective disorder (Drake, Mueser, & Brunette, 2007; Hunt, Malhi, Cleary, Lai, & Sitharthan, 2016b). Consequently, mental illness co-morbidity in AOD services is generally very common.

Addictive substances and co-morbidity

In this section, we will highlight the main substances that are used in Australia and internationally, and consider the kinds of mental health problems that may be experienced by users of these substances.

Alcohol

Alcohol consumption in Australia is widespread and associated with a large number of sporting, recreational and cultural activities. Findings from the National Health Survey conducted in 2014-15 indicate that 80.6% of Australians aged 18 years and over had consumed alcohol in the past year (ABS, 2016). A further 8.2% had consumed alcohol 12 or more months ago, and 10.7% had never consumed alcohol. Higher rates of alcohol consumption in the past year were also reported among males than females (85.6% versus 75.7%). However there is evidence that alcohol use is declining among younger populations, with two-thirds (66.2%) of all 15-17 year olds having never consumed alcohol compared to just 49.1% in 2011. However key findings from the 2016 National Drug Strategy Household Survey (NDSHS) suggest there are now fewer people drinking alcohol in quantities that exceeded lifetime risk guidelines (17.1%, down from 18.2% in 2013). The rates of past-month binge-drinking (i.e., consuming 5 or standard drinks on a single drinking occasion) has declined in those aged 18–24 from 47% in 2013 to 42% in 2016. Although, more people in their 50s were consuming 11 or more standard drinks in one drinking occasion in 2016 than in 2013. The most estimates in the prevalence of problematic alcohol, from the National Survey of Mental Health and Wellbeing in Australia indicated that around 20% of Australians meet lifetime criteria for alcohol misuse (i.e., abuse or dependence) on DSM-IV (Teesson et al, 2010).

Similar rates of alcohol use are observed in New Zealand. The most recent national health survey conducted in 2012/2013 indicated that 79% of adults (approximately 2,833,000 individuals) aged 15+ years had consumed alcohol in the past 12 months, with higher rates among men than women (84% versus 76%) (Ministry of Health, 2016). Approximately one in five (20.8%) residents aged 15 and above were identified as hazardous drinkers (based on a score of 8 or more on the alcohol use disorders identification test). However higher rates of hazardous drinking were reported among Maori (31.1%) or Pacific Peoples (23.6%) relative to European (21.9%) or Asian (6.7%) respondents (Ministry of Health, 2016). Alcohol, which is inherently depressant in nature, is associated with elevated rates of depressive symptoms, which may be resolved after weeks of abstinence in many but not all drinkers. However, depression is not the only form of mental disorder associated with alcohol use disorder: alcohol use disorder is also associated with anxiety and other less widespread mental health problems.

ABOUT THE CONSUMER   *John's story*

John is a 27-year-old man who lives in his own apartment and has successfully held down a job as an electrician since he completed his apprenticeship. However, he has started having a few days off work, citing colds and flu symptoms as the reason. But that is not the real reason—he has felt apathetic and has not wanted to leave the house. He has lost interest and motivation in his hobbies, his friends and in his family. A black mood has descended on him and it has taken away his energy and his vitality, and he does not want to spend time with other people. While he used to enjoy a drink with his friends, he now drinks at home, most nights, and instead of beer down at the pub, he is now drinking a couple of cans of strong cider and even neat vodka. He finds that it helps at the time, in the long evenings and sleepless nights, but when he wakes up the 'black dog' has returned and he feels worse than ever. He does not think that he has an alcohol problem, but knows that something is not right. He has drifted too far away from his friends and his brother to talk to them, and now he is worried that it is affecting his work.

NAOMI CRAFTI AND VICTORIA MANNING

1 Should John be encouraged to seek help?

2 If so, what kind of help would he need?

Stimulants

Stimulants increase the functioning of the central nervous system, speeding up the process of sending messages between the brain and other parts of the body. Stimulants include tobacco/nicotine, caffeine, amphetamines/methamphetamines (such as dexamphetamine or dexies and ice or crystal meth) and cocaine. The short-term effects of stimulant use include increased alertness and energy, increased confidence and less need for sleep. This combination of behaviour is sometimes referred to as being 'wired'. Stimulants can also increase heart and breathing rates, increase blood pressure, reduce appetite, cause the pupils to dilate and produce agitation and insomnia (Queensland Health, 2010).

Some stimulants, particularly amphetamines/methamphetamines and cocaine, can cause irrational, impulsive and aggressive behaviour. This behaviour may be coupled with paranoid thoughts and delusions. Stimulants can trigger psychotic episodes and studies have shown that in certain individuals this may result in chronic physical and mental illness (Ciccarone, 2011; Courtney & Ray, 2017).

Nicotine

Nicotine addiction (as a result of smoking tobacco) is a worldwide health issue. The World Health Organization (WHO) has estimated that by 2020 as many as 10 million people will die prematurely each year from tobacco related disease (World Health Organization, 2005). Largely because of national tobacco control policies and programs, the prevalence of smoking in Australia has declined over the past three decades and is currently among the lowest of any nation. In 1991, 24.3 per cent of the Australian population reported smoking daily and this had reduced to 12.8 per cent in 2013 (Australian Institute of Health and Welfare, 2014). Despite this, smoking tobacco still represents one of the greatest burden of disease of all behavioural risk factors, and tobacco is responsible for approximately 15,000 deaths in Australia every year and has significant social and economic costs (Australian Institute of Health and Welfare, 2016). New Zealand has witnessed a decline in the smoking, where the percentage of adults who smoke at least monthly has fallen from 20% in 2006/07 to 16% in 2015/16, particularly among those aged 15-17 where it fell from 16% to 6%. Among Māori New Zealanders, almost 39% reported smoking, with around one-third of smokers (36%) doing so daily. The New Zealand government has a goal for the country to be smokefree by 2025 where the targets are for daily smoking to fall to 10%, 19% and 11% among Māori, Pacific and non-minority adults' respectively (Ministry of Health, 2016).

Smoking has been implicated in many life-threatening illnesses including cancer, heart disease, stroke and chronic obstructive pulmonary disease. Smoking adversely effects both the mother and foetus during pregnancy and the health effects of passive smoking (tobacco smoke in the environment) on both children and adults is well documented (Royal Australian College of General Practitioners, 2009).

According to the 2010 National Drug Strategy Survey report:

> [C]ompared with non-smokers, smokers were more likely to rate their health as being fair or poor, were more likely to have asthma, were twice as likely to have been diagnosed with or treated for a mental illness, and were more likely to report high or very high levels of psychological distress in the preceding 4-week period.

(Australian Institute of Health and Welfare, 2011, p. 22)

Caffeine

While not generally considered problematic, caffeine is the most commonly used mood-altering drug in the world. It is most often consumed as coffee, tea, cola nut, cacao pod, guarana and mate. According to the Australian Bureau of Statistics (2012), 46 per cent of the Australian population consumes coffee, while tea is consumed by 38 per cent of people. In addition to coffee, tea and cola drinks, about 70 per cent of soft drinks contain caffeine, as does dark chocolate and coffee ice cream. A high proportion of New Zealanders (73%) are exposed to caffeine each year from the consumption of coffee, tea, cola type soft drinks, chocolate and foods containing these ingredients (Thomson & Schiess, 2010). Many over-the-counter medications, including analgesics and weight-loss products, also contain significant amounts of caffeine.

Caffeine is associated with several psychiatric syndromes, such as caffeine intoxication, caffeine withdrawal, caffeine dependence, caffeine-induced sleep disorder and caffeine-induced anxiety disorder (American Psychiatric Association, 2013). Studies have shown that caffeine consumption can increase health risks for cancer, heart disease, foetal abnormalities and impairments in cardiovascular function and sleep (Higdon & Frei, 2006, Temple et al 2017). Therefore, people with various conditions such as generalised anxiety disorder, panic disorder, insomnia, urinary incontinence and pregnancy are often advised to reduce or eliminate caffeine intake. Energy drinks are caffeinated beverages designed to enhance alertness. By 2006, there were over 500 brands of energy drink available around the world. Around a decade ago, energy drinks became a popular mixer with alcohol and in 2003 'ready to drink' alcohol energy drinks (AEDs) were introduced to the Australian market (Pennay et al., 2011). In a pilot study of young Australians, it was found that some people consumed eight or more AEDs on a typical night out. Wakefulness and increased energy were the primary benefits of AEDs, according to this sample, while others limited their consumption to avoid unpleasant consequences, such as sleep disturbance, severe hangovers, heart palpitations and agitation (Pennay & Lubman, 2012).

Methamphetamines

Methamphetamine is a man-made stimulant drug which is a more potent form of the drug amphetamine. There are three main forms of methamphetamine: methamphetamine powder ('speed'), methamphetamine base ('base') and crystalline methamphetamine ('crystal' or 'ice' or 'P' as it is more commonly known in New Zealand). Ice is the most pure form, followed by base than speed. The 'high' experienced from ice and base is much more intense than from speed and is associated with powerful responses, including the subsequent comedown or 'crash'. The potential for dependence (addiction) and chronic physical and mental problems is far greater for ice than for other forms of methamphetamine. While the latest Australian figures show no significant rise in methamphetamine use in 2013 (stable at around 2.1 per cent of the adult population of Australia), the use of speed fell from 51 per cent to 29 per cent of all methamphetamine users and the use of ice more than doubled from 22 per cent in 2010 to 50 per cent of all methamphetamine users in 2013 (Australian Institute of Health and Welfare, 2014). Recent methamphetamine users also used the drug more frequently in 2013 compared to 2010, and 25 per cent of ice users reported using the drug weekly compared to only 2.2 per cent of those using speed (Australian Institute of Health and Welfare, 2014). These statistics partially explain the increased visibility and adverse events associated with methamphetamine use currently. Recent users of methamphetamines were twice as likely to report high or very high levels of psychological distress and twice as likely to report being diagnosed or treated for a mental illness in the past twelve months, compared with non-recent users (Australian Institute of Health and Welfare, 2014).

In New Zealand, 1.1% of adults reported the use of amphetamines in the past year in 2016/2016 (New Zealand Ministry of Health, 2016). Amphetamine use was higher among younger age groups, primarily those aged 25-34 years (1.6%), compared to (.3%) in 55-64 year olds, and among males (1.7%) than females (.6%) and Maori adults were 3.4 times more likely to have used amphetamines in the past year compared to non-Maori's (Pacific peoples did not differ to non-pacific adults). However recent government statistics show that overall numbers of methamphetamine users in New Zealand have been dropping with only 0.9% (26,400 people) using the drug once or more in 2014/15, down from 2.2% in 2009. The use of ice is associated with brain and mental health conditions, including ruptured blood vessels in the brain, memory loss, indecision, depression and psychosis. These drugs can cause paranoia and hallucinations and the user may also become aggressive and violent (Dunn, Proudfoot, & Barry, 2011, Petit et al, 2012). There has been a significant increase in the risky practice of 'bingeing' on ice, according to the Ecstasy and Related Drugs Reporting System (Sindicich & Burns, 2011) and evidence suggests that binge use patterns are associated with increased mental and physical harm, including psychotic symptoms (Sindicich & Burns, 2011). Frequent use of methamphetamine can cause amphetamine-induced psychosis, increased risk of suicide, violent behaviour, tolerance and dependence. Dependent users are around three times more likely to experience psychotic symptoms compared with non-dependent users of the drug (Australian Institute of Health and Welfare, 2016).

Dependence on methamphetamine is more likely to be associated with either injecting or smoking, in contrast to either oral or intranasal methods of administration. Further, both injecting and smoking methamphetamine are associated with more frequent use, need for treatment, higher levels of risky behaviour and other poor health and mental health problems (Australian Institute of Health and Welfare, 2016).

Certain groups are more likely to report using methamphetamines recently compared to the general population, including those living in remote/very remote areas, youth populations, Aboriginal and Torres Strait Islander people, Maori people, those who are unemployed, or single people and certain occupational groups (for example, shift workers; (Australian Institute of Health and Welfare, 2016) Kirkpatrick et al 2009., Degenhardt et al., 2016; Oliveira et al., 2015;New Zealand Ministry of Health. 2016). In addition, methamphetamine use is more than six times higher among people experiencing high or very high levels of psychological distress compared to the general population. In 2015, methamphetamine was the most commonly reported illicit drug used by people entering the Australian prison system in the previous twelve months, increasing from 37 per cent in 2012 to 50 per cent in 2015 (Australian Institute of Health and Welfare, 2016).

Hallucinogens

Hallucinogenic drugs are drugs that change the way a person perceives the world. Hallucinogens affect all the senses, altering cognitions and emotions. They can cause a person to hallucinate—seeing or hearing things that do not exist or are distorted. There are many different kinds of hallucinogens, including LSD (lysergic acid diethylamide), PCP (phencyclidine), magic mushrooms (psilocybin), ketamine and mescaline (peyote cactus) (Australian Drug Foundation, 2011).

The effects of hallucinogens can last several hours and vary considerably, depending on the specific type of hallucinogen. Some of the typical effects of hallucinogens are feelings of euphoria, a sense of relaxation and well-being, hallucinations and distorted perception, disorganised thoughts, confusion and difficulty concentrating, thinking or maintaining attention, anxiety, agitation, paranoia and feelings of panic, dizziness, blurred vision, loss of coordination, increased breathing rate, increased heart rate and blood pressure, irregular heartbeat, palpitations, nausea and vomiting, increased body temperature and sweating (which may alternate with chills and shivering) and numbness (Australian Drug Foundation, 2011).

Feelings of panic, paranoia and fear associated with a 'bad trip' can lead to risky behaviour that can cause injury, such as running across a busy street. Some people may experience a drug-induced psychosis after using hallucinogens. This can occur after a single dose or long-term use. The psychosis is usually characterised by hallucinations, delusions and bizarre behaviour and can last for several hours or longer for some people.

According to the most recent National Drug Strategy Household Survey, in 2013, 9.4 per cent of Australians aged over 14 years had used hallucinogens (other than cannabis and ecstasy) at some stage in their life (Australian Institute of Health and Welfare, 2014). The 2007/2008 New Zealand Alcohol and drug use survey indicated that 3.2% of adults had used a hallucinogenic drug (LSD/DMT/other synthetic hallucinogens, naturally occurring hallucinogens, ketamine, or ecstasy) in the past year. LSD and other synthetic hallucinogens were most commonly used, with 1.3% of the adult population aged 16–64 years having used these drugs in the past year (New Zealand Ministry of Health, 2010).

Cannabis

Cannabis is the most widely used illicit drug in Australia and New Zealand. Approximately one-third of Australians (35 per cent) report having used cannabis at least once in their lives, while 10.2 per cent reported having used cannabis in the past twelve months (Australian Institute of Health and Welfare, 2014). In New Zealand, 11% of adults (15% of men and 8% of women) aged 15 or over reported using cannabis in the previous year (New Zealand Ministry of Health, 2015). Cannabis produces a sense of calmness and relaxation, with other positive effects including euphoria, perceptual and time distortion, and emotional intensification. Cannabis use can also result in negative reactions, including depression, paranoia, anxiety and panic attacks (Lubman & Baker, 2010). Reductions in brain regions (hippocampus and amygdala) associated with psychosis and depression and related cognitive deficits have been shown in long-term heavy cannabis users (Yücel et al., 2008).

Recent research has found that not only are people at risk for schizophrenia more likely to try cannabis, but using cannabis may also increase the risk of developing symptoms of schizophrenia (Gage et al., 2017). In addition, chronic cannabis use impacts negatively on the course of illness, severity of psychotic symptoms, frequency of psychotic relapse, treatment outcome and adherence to treatment for those diagnosed with psychosis (Lubman & Baker, 2010).

A number of epidemiological studies have also shown increased levels of depression in regular cannabis users, although the association is modest and the direction of causality is unknown (Lev-Ran et al., 2014). However, qualitative studies have found that young people report using drugs (mainly cannabis) to cope with mood or anxiety disorders, suggesting the need for treatment approaches that address both mental health and drug use (Lubman & Baker, 2010).

Opioids

According to the 2014 Australian *National Drug Strategy Household Survey*, less than1 per cent of people in Australia aged 14 years or older had used heroin in their lifetime and 0.1 per cent in the previous twelve months. This proportion has decreased significantly since 2010, the time of the previous survey (Australian Institute of Health and Welfare, 2014). According to the National Drug and Alcohol Research Centre (Sindicich & Burns, 2011), there were 360 opioid overdose deaths in 2007, 500 in 2008, 612 in 2009, and 705 in 2010. Increases in overdose deaths occurred in all of the major states, but were most marked in Victoria where such deaths increased 133 per cent from 73 in 2001 to 170 in 2008. Most of these deaths were due to heroin, but an increasing number have recently been due to pain-relieving prescription opioid drugs. Most deaths involve men in their early thirties (Roxburgh & Burns, 2012). For every fatal overdose, there are many more non-fatal overdoses. Non-fatal overdoses can result in severe physical and mental damage. In New Zealand heroin has a low prevalence relative to other countries. The most recent estimates are that there are 29,200 opioid and sedative users of which 2000 are estimated to be dependent and 27,200 casual users (McFadden Consultancy, 2016).

Many heroin users come from families in which one or more family members use alcohol or drugs excessively or have mental health problems. Often heroin users have had health problems early in life, behavioural problems beginning in childhood and low self-esteem. Among opioid-dependent adolescents, a 'heroin behaviour syndrome' has sometimes been described. This syndrome consists of depression (often with anxiety symptoms), impulsiveness, fear of failure, low self-esteem, low frustration tolerance, limited coping skills and relationships based primarily on mutual drug use (American Psychiatric Association, 2013).

Pharmaceuticals

Pharmaceutical drug abuse involves both over-the-counter medications and the misuse of prescription drugs. The main groups of over-the-counter products that may be abused by consumers include cough mixtures that contain dihydrocodeine, analgesics that contain codeine, products containing pseudoephedrine, beta2-agonists (for example, salbutamol inhalers) and products that contain sedating antihistamines. The groups of prescription drugs most commonly used for their psychoactive and pleasurable effects rather than medical purposes are anti-anxiety medications such as benzodiazepines, anti-depressants, and drugs of addiction including codeine, pethidine and morphine (Dobbin, 2014). Other prescription and over-the-counter medications that are used, though to a lesser extent include performance and image enhancing drugs such as anabolic steroids, laxatives, diuretics and herbal products that claim to alter metabolism

In the 2013 Australian *National Drug Strategy Household Survey*, pharmaceutical use referred to use of these medications for non-medical purposes; that is, the use of pharmaceutical drugs to induce or enhance a drug experience, enhance performance or for cosmetic purposes (Australian Institute of Health and Welfare, 2014). According to this survey, 4.7 per cent of people aged over 14 years reported recent use of pharmaceuticals for non-medical purposes. The pharmaceuticals most likely to be used in the previous twelve months were pain killers/analgesics, while use of tranquillisers/sleeping pills was the second most misused pharmaceutical drug type (Australian Institute of Health and Welfare, 2014). A recent paper on global rates of opioid analgesic use highlights dramatic increases in both Australia and New Zealand in the years 2001-2003 and 2011-2013(Berterame et al, 2016).

Benzodiazepines are generally prescribed to provide short-term relief of anxiety symptoms; however, if used for longer than prescribed, they can increase anxiety and also cause severe depression. At higher doses, people taking benzodiazepines are at risk of engaging in impulsive or unsafe behaviour and memory deficits. In addition, taking benzodiazepines with other prescribed or illicit drugs, particularly other depressants (alcohol, opiates or methadone), can lead to overdose or even death (Royal College of Psychiatrists, 2013).

Steroids

According to a 2014 Australian national study of regular injecting drug users, the proportion of this sample reporting using steroids at some stage in their lifetime was 6 per cent (Australian Institute of Health and Welfare, 2014). However, an Australian Crime Commission report (2013) found that approximately two-thirds of young men who began injecting drugs in the previous three years were using steroids. They also reported that the number of steroid detections at the Australian border had increased by 74 per cent in 2009–10. The number of steroid detections increased 7.2 per cent from 2014–15 to 2015–16, indicating that this is an burgeoning problem (Australian Australian Criminal Intelligence Commission, 2017). Anabolic-androgenic steroids are a synthetic form of testosterone and, when combined with exercise and diet, can increase muscle size and strength. The harms associated with steroid use range from acne and increased body hair to increased appetite, water retention and sleeplessness. There are also potential harms associated with unsafe injecting practices, such as sharing or reusing needles (Dunn, 2013).

Steroid users also report mental health issues such as increased aggression or 'roid rage' and changes in mood. There is also some evidence to suggest that people using steroids can develop a dependence on this drug and continue use, despite negative effect (Dunn, 2013).

Determining drug effects

The effects of a drug on an individual are idiosyncratic and depend on characteristics such as an individual's size, weight and health status, how regularly they use the drug and for how long they have taken the drug. The effects also depend on the amount taken, the route of administration and whether or not other drugs have been consumed at the same time (Australian Drug Foundation, 2011) .

In his book *Drug, Set and Setting: The Basis for Controlled Intoxicant Use*, (Zingberg, 1984) argues that it is not possible to understand drug use and the effects or outcomes of the drug experience unless you take into account the interrelationship of factors to do with the drug, the environment and the individual. The factors considered important by Zinberg are shown in Table 14.1.

One example of the enormous influence of the social setting and of social learning on drug use referred to by Zingberg (1986) comes from the Vietnam War. It was estimated that at least 35 per cent of enlisted men from the USA tried heroin while in Vietnam and that 54 per cent of these became addicted to it. When the extent of the use of heroin by soldiers in Vietnam became apparent, the army feared 'Once an addict, always an addict', and treatment and rehabilitation centres were set up in Vietnam. These programs were total failures. Often servicemen used more heroin in the rehabilitation programs

TABLE 14.1 FACTORS IN ZINBERG'S THEORY OF DRUG USE

The drug	The environment	The individual
■ The purity	■ Where	■ Gender
■ The route of administration (injected, snorted, smoked, etc)	■ With whom	■ Age
■ Dosage (how much)	■ What time	■ Health
■ With what other drugs	■ How	■ Expectations of the experience
■ Price	■ Safety of setting	■ Previous experience
■ Availability	■ Peer influence	■ Mood
■ Legality	■ Cultural factors	■ Tolerance
■ Form of the drug (capsules, home-bake, powder, etc)	■ Influence of advertising	■ View of oneself
	■ Media influence	■ Family background
	■ Poverty of setting	■ Genetic factors
		■ Beliefs/attitudes

than when on active duty. However, only 12% of veterans who had been addicted whilst serving in Vietnam, were addicted at some point during the three years after returning to the USA (Robins, 1993)). Apparently, it was the abhorrent social setting of the Vietnam war that led men who ordinarily would not have considered using heroin to not only use it but also to become addicted to it. However, once they returned to the USA, the improved environmental conditions resulted in far fewer addicted servicemen.

The challenges and harms associated with co-occurring disorders

Individuals with co-occurring disorders are more likely to experience a range of harms including a more severe, complex and active course of illness and a poorer long-term prognosis. Research suggests they have a higher risk of suicide and relapse, and a history of trauma, cognitive impairment and physical health complications. In terms of social issues, they are more likely to experience isolation, stigmatisation and interpersonal relationship difficulties, have more contact with the justice system and experience unstable housing and unemployment and financial difficulties (Kelly & Daley, 2013; Marel et al, 2016). As a consequence, individuals with co-occurring disorders tend to be heavier users of a range of health and welfare services: general practitioners, ambulance services and emergency departments; more frequent and longer episodes of inpatient treatment and hospitalisation; and greater use of housing, unemployment, welfare and criminal justice services (Cosci & Fava, 2011).

Engagement in and, retention in treatment as well as health and related outcomes are often compromised in clients with co-occurring disorders relative to those with a mental health or substance use disorder alone (Cosci & Fava, 2011; Rowles, Ellington, Tarr, Hertzer, & Findling, 2015;). Of particular concern is that clients can be turned away from treatment, with mental health issues a barrier to accessing AOD treatment, and ongoing AOD use a barrier to accessing mental health services. As a result, such individuals often fall 'through the cracks' or are 'ping-ponged' between services. To combat the challenges faced by clients navigating their way through the service system, the Australian government initiative 'No wrong door' provides consumers with multiple points of entry. The policy recognises that every door in the health care system (for example, primary care, mental health, AOD and family support services) is the 'right' door to getting help, and that each service has responsibility for providing care or referral to an appropriate service to meet the needs of the client (Croton, 2005).

In New Zealand, the Te Tāhuhu New Zealand Mental Health and Addiction Action Plan 2005-2015 outlines a high-level strategic framework to guide existing and future priority actions in terms of policy and service provision. The focus is on improving recovery and wellness for people, families, and communities affected by mental illness and addiction (New Zealand Ministry of Health, 2006).

What constitutes a substance use problem?

While the use of any psychoactive substance can potentially cause harm, not all substance use is harmful. The harm that is caused by substance use can be physical, psychological, social, financial or legal. It can be experienced by the user of the substance or by their friends, family, co-workers or the wider community. The chemical nature of a particular substance and its 'addictive' properties are not the only features of drug use that determine the potential for harm. Likewise, whether or not a substance is legally available is only moderately associated with its potential to cause harm. Prescription and over-the-counter medications are frequently associated with harmful use, and tobacco and alcohol are associated with the greatest overall harm (Nutt, 2012).

Substance use can be categorised according to behavioural patterns of use, with the key criteria being the amount taken and the effect on the person. The spectrum of drug use ranges from no use to dependent use of one or more drugs. Further, a person can have different patterns of use with different drugs (for example, someone could be a situational user of cannabis and an experimental user of ecstasy). Drug use patterns are as follows:

- *Experimental use*—A person 'tries out' a particular drug. Young people often experiment with drugs out of curiosity. Experimental use tends to be random and occurs mostly in social situations. There is no evidence to support the 'slippery slope theory' that experimentation leads to dependence

- *Recreational use*—A person uses one or more drugs in a deliberate or controlled way. Sometimes called social drug use, recreational use can occur very occasionally, every weekend or several times a week. Both licit and illicit drugs can be used recreationally. An example might be someone who uses ecstasy at a dance party two or three times a year, or has the occasional cigarette at a party but not at other times.

- *Situational use*—A person uses drugs to cope with the demands of particular situations. This pattern of use is associated with psychological triggers or habitual patterns of behaviour and can be a risk factor for dependent use; for example, having a glass of red wine after work when feeling stressed.

- *Intensive use*—A person consumes a heavy amount of drugs over a short period of time, or continuously uses a drug over a number of days or weeks. This pattern of consumption is also referred to as 'binge use'. An example of binge use might be an ice/amphetamine user who consumes a large quantity over one weekend, but then doesn't use again for several weeks.

- *Dependent use*—With dependent use an individual feels that they have little or no control over their drug use. They feel compelled to use in order to feel normal or to cope. Often called 'addiction', drug dependence is the result of prolonged, regular use of increasing amounts of the drug (Department of Health, 2012).

Diagnosis and classification

There are two main systems for the classification of substance use disorders: the *Diagnostic and Statistical Manual of Mental Disorders* (DSM), published by the American Psychiatric Association; and the *International Classification of Diseases* (ICD), published by the World Health Organization. Each of these systems provides diagnostic criteria for substance use disorders. Although similar, there are differences in these two systems that can be confusing. What is called 'substance use disorder (mild, moderate or severe) in the DSM 5 is called 'harmful use' in the ICD110. It is recommended that clinicians be familiar with the diagnostic system used within their service.

Generally, a diagnosis lists a particular substance and the related disorder, which might be intoxication, withdrawal, abuse, harmful use or dependence. There are also disorders that may be 'induced' by the substance, which can include symptoms of depression, anxiety or psychosis (Queensland Health, 2010).

A landmark epidemiological study by Anthony, Warner, and Kessler (1994), investigating drug dependence among Americans aged 15 to 54 years, found that about one in four (24 per cent) had a history of tobacco dependence, about one in seven (14 per cent) had a history of alcohol dependence, and about one in thirteen (7.5 per cent) had a history of dependence on an inhalant or controlled drug. About one-third of tobacco smokers had developed tobacco dependence and about 15 per cent of drinkers had become alcohol dependent. Among users of the other drugs, about 15 per cent had become dependent. This study was one of the first to refute the 'hijacked brain' hypothesis, because it showed that a minority of people who use substances become dependent, and that most of those who do report dependence at some stage in their life have overcome it. The authors also concluded that many more Americans aged 15 to 54 years have been affected by dependence on psychoactive substances than by other psychiatric disorders, which have been accorded a higher priority in mental health service delivery prevention and research. Epidemiological studies would suggest that the same is true in Australia (Australian Institute of Health and Welfare, 2016).

Harm minimisation

Prohibitionist approaches, while providing short-term decreases in the impact of particular substances, have been shown to have little long-term effect on either the prevalence or harm associated with a particular substance. As a result, more recent prevention and treatment approaches in Australia focus on supply reduction, demand reduction and harm reduction (Ministerial Council on Drug Strategy, 2004).

The website of the International Harm Reduction Association defines harm reduction as 'policies, programs and practices that aim primarily to reduce the adverse health, social and economic consequences of the use of legal and illegal psychoactive drugs without necessarily reducing drug consumption' (Wodak, 2014).

This philosophy does not imply that clinicians should ignore a client's attempts to reduce or cease their substance use, however, the intervention emphasises reducing negative impacts independently of changes in consumption. Examples of harm minimisation strategies include:

- providing access to clean injecting equipment and education (needle and syringe programs)
- drink-driving interventions
- detoxification programs
- opioid substitution treatment programs
- encouraging safer means of drug ingestion
- skill development programs.

It is important to emphasise that harm minimisation is a framework that can incorporate both abstinence-oriented and harm-reduction approaches, and provides a spectrum of supports and interventions to individuals, families and communities.

Prevention/early intervention is a significant part of any harm-minimisation approach and the provision of treatment services. Prevention refers to 'measures that prevent or delay the onset of drug use as well as measures that protect against risk and prevent and reduce harm associated with drug supply and use' (Ministerial Council on Drug Strategy, 2004, p. 22). Prevention/early intervention includes education and the provision of accurate information about drug use to users and the training of teachers, youth and health workers in early detection and intervention.

Aetiology of co-occurring disorders

In a seminal paper by Mueser and colleagues (1998) there are four basic models proposed to explain the elevated rates of co-occurring substance use and mental health problems:

- *Secondary psychopathology model*—where substance use causes some cases of mental health problems, possibly in individuals with a pre-existing vulnerability. They go on to argue that certain substances (such as LSD and cannabis) can cause transient psychotic episodes and may also precipitate longer-term psychiatric disorders.

BOX 14.1   'EQUASY' VERSUS ECSTASY

Professor David Nutt was appointed chairman of the UK Government's Advisory Council on the Misuse of Drugs (ACMD) in 2008. In 2009, he published an editorial in the *Journal of Psychopharmacology*, comparing the harms caused by horse-riding with the effect of taking ecstasy or cannabis. 'Equasy'—a fictitious addiction to horse riding—was calculated to result in one serious adverse event approximately every 350 exposures (based on available data), compared with the risk of taking ecstasy, estimated at one serious adverse event approximately every 10,000 exposures. As a result of this and other comments on the harms caused by legal and illegal drugs, Nutt was sacked by the then Home Secretary.

In *Drugs—Without the Hot Air* (2012), Nutt puts the case for an evidence-based scientific approach to drugs. He shows how we can quantify the overall harms of a drug, addressing issues from direct danger of death, through to environmental, financial and family factors, to obtain a true indication of the overall effect of a drug. Nutt argues that we need to use this information, based on fact not fear, to make informed decisions regarding drug use, and policymakers can likewise take a rational approach to legislation. A disconnect between governments' need to appear tough on drugs on the one hand, and a rational evidence-based approach to drugs legislation and treatment, has led to arguably damaging consequences for both individual drug users and the community.

- *Secondary substance abuse model*—where mental disorders may cause some substance disorders, again more likely in vulnerable individuals. There are two variations on this: the 'self-medication hypothesis' according to which substances are used to ease mental health symptoms (there is weak evidence for this); and the 'general dysphoria theory' based on the idea that substances will, at least temporarily, ease various kinds of distress and unhappiness that have their origins in mental health problems.
- *Common factors model*—the 'common cause' factors advanced have been genetic, neuro-cognitive, family-based, social and environmental, but there has been little convincing evidence collected in favour of any of these common cause models.
- *Bidirectional model*—although there is generally little research in favour of this mutually sustaining relationship, there is evidence that PTSD is associated with subsequent development of substance use disorders, which in turn can worsen the severity of the PTSD symptoms.

Models of care and treatment for co-occurring disorders

AOD treatment more broadly encompasses a wide range of approaches, including brief intervention, counselling, detoxification, rehabilitation and case coordination. As a chronic and relapsing condition, there is no 'quick-fix' for alcohol or drug dependence. Treatment can be expected to last several months or years and entails multiple modalities and approaches. For example, an alcohol-dependent client may undergo a period of medically assisted withdrawal in an inpatient setting, followed by outpatient counselling or a period of residential rehabilitation, while a client with co-occurring bi-polar effective disorder may receive more intensive case management following detoxification. The following section provides a brief overview of addiction treatment approaches with a focus on those shown to be effective with clients with co-occurring disorders There are three distinct models of care described in the literature for working with this population.

1 *Sequential treatment*—this is where one condition (usually the condition considered to be the primary underlying condition) is treated before the other (for example, treating the stimulant use disorder and when that is resolved treating the PTSD).
2 *Parallel treatment*—this is when both the AOD and mental health conditions are treated simultaneously but with the two treatments provided independent of each other (for example, treatment for opioid-dependence by specialist AOD services and treatment for bi-polar affective disorder by mental health services).
3 *Integrated treatment*—this is where both the AOD and mental health conditions are treated simultaneously by the same clinician, treatment provider or service, where the relationship between the two conditions can be considered and addressed during treatment and where multiple treatment approaches may be combined (for example, psychotherapy and pharmacotherapy).

Integrated approaches are considered to be superior to other models of care (that is, parallel or sequential) where disorders are treated with separate treatment plans. With integrated care, a variety of interventions are typically offered, including individual, group, family, residential and pharmacological approaches. Integrated programs minimise the risk of clients falling through the gaps between different service providers. According to a review of effective models of care for comorbid mental illness and illicit substance use conducted by NSW Ministry of Health (2015), the most effective models (i.e., those with at least a 'good' or 'moderate' level of evidence) include:

(1) Assertive community treatment (ACT), which is an intensive, multidisciplinary approach, where professionals provide outreach care to difficult to engage clients at risk of psychiatric hospitalisation. It specifically targets those with severe psychiatric disorders and a history of psychiatric hospitalisations (including homeless populations). Assertive outreach is considered a critical component of treatment given that clients with severe co-occurring disorders patients often struggle to manage linkages between services. Other common characteristics of ACT models are small caseloads (e.g., 10 clients per clinician), daily team meetings and 24-hour coverage by the treatment team.

(2) Integrated dual diagnosis treatment, which includes multidisciplinary, intensive case management teams; stage-appropriate treatment; integration of mental health and substance use treatment; individual and group modalities; time unlimited services and assertive outreach.

(3) Case management/care co-ordination where professional staff e.g., social workers coordinate care for complex/severely unwell psychiatric patients (including homeless populations). It typically entails comprehensive assessment of client need, the development and delivery of a care plan, with emphasis on communication, consultation and inter-agency working, assertive referral and support. Having a single point of contact reduces burden on the individual to navigate their way through the broader treatment system, thereby reducing the chances of them 'falling through the gaps'.

(4) The combined psychosis and substance use program (COMPASS model) is an 'integrated shared care' model in the UK which integrates treatment both at the level of the clinician and service. Both AOD and mental health conditions are addressed simultaneously by the mainstream mental health clinician.

(5) The comprehensive, continuous, integrated system of care (CCISC model) is the recommended model of care among homeless clients in the US. Program components include residential treatment,

TOPIC LINK
See Chapter 19 for more on case management.

medical care, counselling, psychiatric/psychological evaluation, recreational and vocational services, as well as comprehensive discharge planning.

Irrespective of the model of care, at a client level there needs to be a strong focus on engagement and continuing support, effective linkage across a diverse range of specialist agencies and community organisations, individually tailored interventions and a phased approach to change. Treatment must be guided by a comprehensive assessment with ongoing review based on assertive community work and effective case management.

What is the evidence that treatment is effective?

A substantial evidence base now indicates that once in specialist treatment for alcohol and/or drug problems, many individuals with AOD dependence improve (that is, reduce or cease use). To date, there have been three national longitudinal outcome studies conducted in Australia. The first is Australian Treatment Outcomes Study (ATOS), which recruited 825 heroin users entering opiate substitution treatment (methadone or buprenorphine) and residential rehabilitation. The sample was followed up at three months and one, two, three and eleven years (Teesson, Havard, Ross, & Darke, 2006; Teesson et al., 2017; Teesson et al., 2008). A significant reduction in heroin use in the month prior to interview was observed between baseline (99 per cent) and at one year (41 per cent), which was maintained at three-year (34 per cent) and eleven-year (24.8 per cent) follow-up (Teesson et al., 2008). As well as positive changes in AOD use, reductions in criminal involvement and improvements in general physical and mental health were also reported, although co-morbid depression was associated with poorer outcomes (Teesson et al., 2015).

The Methamphetamines Treatment Evaluation Study (MATES) recruited 360 methamphetamine or amphetamine users from community-based detoxification and residential rehabilitation services (McKetin et al., 2012) with both one- and three-year follow-ups, and reported similar findings to ATOS. Recovery in the MATES study was defined as continued abstinence, with reported rates of 33 per cent at the three-month follow-up, 14 per cent at the one-year follow-up and only 6 per cent at the three-year follow-up (McKetin et al., 2012).

Most recently, the Patient Pathways project recruited 796 AOD clients, of which 29 per cent were in long-term residential treatment, 44 per cent in acute withdrawal services and 27 per cent in outpatient delivered treatment (Lubman et al., 2016). Marked improvements in AOD use were observed at the 12-month follow-up, with just over half of the sample (52 per cent) achieving treatment success (that is, reliably reduced the frequency of their primary drug of concern in the month prior to assessment, or had been abstinent over this period), and 30.5 per cent of the retained sample achieved abstinence from all drugs of concern (Manning et al., 2017). A sizeable proportion of all three study cohorts had mental health issues (25–75 per cent in ATOS, 38–63 per cent in MATES and 55 per cent in Patient Pathways), so taken together, the findings provide evidence on the effectiveness of treatment for clients with co-occurring disorders.

Treatment of substance use disorders

There are numerous ways in which the treatment for substance use disorders can be delivered that have proven to to be effective. This includes multiple treatment types (e.g., detoxification, out-patient counselling and residential rehabilitation) and multiple psychosocial approaches (e.g., CBT, mindfulness based relapse prevention). The choice of treatment depends largely on the severity of the substance use problem and other related issues such as social stability, mental health, treatment history etc...), however effective treatment typically involves a combination of these and often requires multiple episodes of care.

Brief interventions

Brief interventions use talk-based therapies to support behaviour change, and include a suite of interventions ranging from a few minutes of simple, but structured, advice to 60 minutes of counselling, often with repeat (usually up to four or five) consultations. Brief interventions typically include psychoeducation motivational interviewing and counselling (Donoghue, Patton, Phillips, Deluca, & Drummond, 2014; Glass et al., 2017; Kaner et al., 2007 ; Saitz, Palfai, & Cheng, 2014). Brief interventions can be delivered by different practitioners in community settings; for example, GPs, practice nurses, health visitors, dieticians and other primary health care professionals in the normal course of their work as well as specialist workers. There is strong evidence to support the effectiveness of brief interventions in the treatment of alcohol problems in both primary care and specialist settings (Shand, Stafford, Fawcett, & Mattick, 2003) however, the literature indicates that they are less effective with clients with co-occurring disorders, who likely require a longer, more intensive treatment duration (Kaner, Brown, & Jackson, 2011).

Detoxification

Detoxification is a period of medical treatment when an individual is helped to overcome physical and psychological dependence on an addictive substance. The aim of detoxification is to help the client get to a drug-free state, prevent acute symptoms of withdrawal through mediation (for example, seizures) and manage common withdrawal symptoms (for example, sleep disturbance) physical and psychiatric disorders (Hayashida, 1998). Detoxification can be completed in both inpatient (that is, residential withdrawal) and outpatient (that is, non-residential withdrawal) settings and is often the start of the treatment journey for those who are dependent on substances.

Rehabilitation

Rehabilitation occurs in a residential (that is, inpatient) setting, with long-stay programs typically lasting between six and twelve months (NSW Health, 2000), or in non-residential (outpatient) settings, where programs run for around six to twelve weeks. The primary therapeutic approaches include the 12-step model, therapeutic community and cognitive-behavioural therapy-based interventions (European Monitoring Centre for Drugs and Drug Addiction, 2015). Extended periods of stabilisation and rehabilitation are particularly suited to clients with severe mental health issues, who are socially excluded, have poor educational and social skills, are unemployed or are experiencing housing instability (NSW Health, 2000). There is an ongoing lack of funding for residential rehabilitation beds in Australia and therefore therapeutic day rehabilitation programs (sometimes referred to as 'Dayhabs') are becoming more common. These typically require daily attendance for 6-8 weeks after detoxification treatment, however to date they have been subjected to limited evaluation.

Counselling/psychosocial interventions

Most psychosocial interventions are delivered on an outpatient basis, with face to face one-to-one or group sessions held weekly-to fortnightly and range from several weeks to several months. However, the following psychological approaches often feature in rehabilitation as well. Of the multiple psychological treatment approaches used in the treatment of substance use disorders, the dominant approaches are cognitive behavioural therapy (CBT), relapse prevention and motivational interviewing (MI). However, while clinical trials deliver interventions in their purest form (that is, in isolation and without other interventions), real-world clinicians typically draw on a 'tool box' of different techniques and interventions (for example, MI during the early stages to increase treatment readiness, followed by CBT or mindfulness to strengthen thought processes and related behaviours, followed by relapse prevention to help maintain positive behaviour change and prevent relapse). Much of the evidence base for the treatment of substance use disorders with psychosocial interventions has been generated from rigorous randomised controlled trials, which typically exclude individuals with severe mental health disorders. However, there is a growing body of literature on psychosocial interventions specifically for individuals with specific combinations of co-occurring disorders (Kelly & Daley, 2013; Kelly, Daley, & Douaihy, 2012; Marel et al., 2016).

E-health interventions

E-health refers to the provision of health services (information and interventions) through the internet and related technologies (for example, mobile applications). It has revolutionised health care by overcoming many of the barriers to face-to-face treatment, such as poor accessibility, poor availability, geographical restraints, stigmatisation, wait-times and the cost of treatment. Many e-health services, such as online counselling, provide free, 24/7 accessibility, anonymity and greater convenience to a broader client base by reaching under-resourced regional and rural areas, and more women (Garde, Manning, & Lubman, 2017). A recent review of studies examining telemedicine interventions highlights the promising role for technology in assessing, treating and supporting individuals to recover from substance use disorders (Marsch, Carroll, & Kiluk, 2014., Lal & Adair, 2014).

Integrated treatment approaches

Integrated treatment refers to the simultaneous treatment of two or more conditions (for example, mental health and substance use disorder) and the use of multiple treatments or approaches such as combined pharmacotherapy and psychosocial interventions. As such, integrated treatment typically entails a multidisciplinary team (for example, nurses, psychologists, social workers and case managers). Integrated treatment should be comprehensive, assertive, focus on both rehabilitation and harm-reduction, adopt a long-term perspective and use multiple, evidence based therapeutic modalities like MI and CBT. Studies suggest integrated treatment approaches aimed at reducing both psychological distress and problematic substance can be effective with co-morbid populations (Deady et al, 2016., Kelly & Daley, 2013). An example of an integrated treatment is Depression & Alcohol Integrated & Single-focused Interventions (DAISI), examined in a trial that compared nine sessions of depression-focused therapy with alcohol-focused therapy, integrated therapy using CBT and a brief integrated intervention in a sample of 284 individuals with coexisting depression and alcohol problems (Baker et al., 2014) at six, twelve, twenty-four and thirty-six months. The findings of the trial were that integrated treatment of depression and problematic alcohol use was associated with a greater reduction in drinking days and level of depression than a single-focused (depression or alcohol) intervention. However, a recent systematic review of integrated approaches for clients with severe mental illness and substance use disorders found no evidence to support the use of an integrated model, and reported that the quality of the evidence was poor (Hunt et al., 2013).

Aftercare, peer-support and mutual aid

In both the AOD and mental health field there has been a shift away from an acute care model to a model of sustained recovery management, nested within a broader recovery-oriented system of care. This system includes free and widely available peer-support and mutual-aid groups such as Alcoholics Anonymous (AA), Narcotics Anonymous (NA), SMART recovery and other self-help groups that can offer social support, positive role models and a sense of meaning and purpose. AA has received by far the greatest research attention in the mutual-aid area, with a review (Kaskutas, 2009) concluding that the evidence for AA effectiveness is strong in terms of the magnitude of its dose-response, consistency, temporal relationship (attendance being predictive of abstinence) and plausibility (mechanisms of action predicated on theories of behaviour change). Indeed, attendance at mutual aid was associated with improved outcomes for clients with alcohol as their primary drug of concern in the patient pathways study (Manning et al., 2017). Self-help groups may not be suitable for clients with certain co-occurring conditions (for example, social anxiety disorder and clients experiencing delusions), particularly in groups with a heavy spiritual philosophy such as AA's 12-step recovery program. Many individuals with co-occurring disorders take medication to manage their mental health symptoms and this has meant they encounter a lack of empathy and acceptance in some traditional mutual aid groups. Groups such as Dual Recovery Anonymous (DRA) now exist and adopt a dual focus fellowship with a mission to bring the benefits of mutual aid to persons recovering from co-occurring disorders. A review and synthesis of studies examining a similar group in the USA, 'Double Trouble', concluded that group participation has both direct and indirect effects on several important components of recovery: drug/alcohol abstinence, psychiatric medication adherence, self-efficacy for recovery, and quality of life (Magura, 2008). For clients with co-occurring disorders, 12-step groups have been shown to reduce both substance use and mental health problem severity, and helped them stay in recovery (Bergman et al, 2014)

Pharmacotherapy

There is an established evidence-base on the pharmacological treatments for some substance use disorders. Dependence on heroin is effectively managed through opiate substitution medications such as methadone and buprenorphine (suboxone). These medications have pharmacological properties that prevent the users from going in to withdrawal and help to stabilise the client. Clients can remain on prescribed medications (a maintenance program) or can slowly reduce their dosage if they wish to be drug-free. A Cochrane review strongly supports their effectiveness in the treatment of heroin dependence (Mattick, Breen, Kimber, & Davoli, 2014) in terms of retention in treatment, a reduction in use of illicit opioids and improved social functioning. However, successful opiate pharmacotherapy programs involve more than just prescription of medication, with adjunctive counselling/psychosocial interventions a core part of international treatment guidelines (European Monitoring Centre for Drugs and Drug Addiction, 2014; Gowing, Ali, Dunlop, Farrell, & Lintzeris, 2014; Kampman & Jarvis, 2015; Carroll & Weiss, 2016). For benzodiazepine dependence, clients generally receive a prescribed equivalent dose of benzodiazepine with a dosage that is tapered down slowly until they are drug-free (Parr, Kavanagh, Cahill, Mitchell, & Young, 2009). There remains limited evidence in terms of pharmacological treatments for other illicit drugs; however, for alcohol common medications used include Acamprosate, which reduces cravings through altering the levels of certain brain chemicals or receptors; Naltrexone, which reduces the rewarding effects of alcohol; and Dislufiram, a deterrent drug that causes unpleasant effects such as sweating, headache, dyspnoea, flushing, sympathetic overactivity, palpitations, nausea and vomiting when alcohol is consumed. For a review of pharmacotherapy, behavioural and psychosocial therapies and their combination for specific combinations of mental health and substance use disorders, see Kelly et al. (2012). In the context of mental health, pharmacotherapy is overseen by a medical practitioner or psychiatrist as there can be serious interaction effects with prescribed medications for mental health disorders as well as non-prescribed drug use. Finally, not all clients are suitable candidates for pharmacotherapy, such as those with certain medical conditions, including liver dysfunction and hepatitis.

■ TOPIC LINK

See Chapter 15 for more on psychopharmacology.

Assessment of AOD problems

Nurses make up the largest profession within the mental health workforce and are therefore likely to have the greatest impact on the identification and early intervention of substance use disorders, particularly through the use of routine screening and assessment in clinical settings. Presentations where there are marked psychosocial complications, wide fluctuations in mental state or frequent requests for medications (for example, analgesics and anxiolytics) should prompt screening for substance use disorders. With respect to alcohol, familiarity with standard drinks and consumption guidelines to reduce health risks is desirable when working with this population. Although currently under review, the most recent National Health and Medical Research Council (2009) consumption guidelines are that for healthy men and women, drinking no more than two standard drinks on any day reduces the lifetime risk of harm from alcohol-related disease or injury (long-term risk). Furthermore, to reduce the risk of injury on a single drinking occasion, healthy men and women should drink no more than four standard drinks (short-term risk). A standard drink in Australia contains 10g of alcohol (equivalent to 12.5mL of pure alcohol) and examples include a 285ml middy of lager, a small 100ml glass of wine and a nip (30ml) of spirits. When assessing alcohol consumption consider the following:

- quantity (number of standard drinks per day)
- frequency (drinking days each week)
- patterns of use (for example, binge episodes on weekends).

The alcohol use disorders identification test (AUDIT) is a ten-item screening tool developed by the World Health Organization (WHO) to assess alcohol consumption, drinking behaviours and alcohol-related problems. A score of 8–15 is considered to indicate hazardous or harmful alcohol use, where simple advice focused on the reduction of hazardous drinking is most appropriate. A score of 16–19 is considered to indicate medium-level alcohol problems that warrant brief counselling and continued monitoring. A score of 20 indicates potential alcohol dependence, warranting further diagnostic evaluation. There are shorter versions of the AUDIT available; for example, the three-item AUDIT-C (Bush, Kivlahan, McDonell, Fihn, & Bradley, 1998) to detect problematic use, as well as other measures such as the CAGE (Ewing, 1984) or the Fast Alcohol Screening Test (Hodgson, Alwyn, John, Thom, & Smith, 2002). To assess other substance use, the Alcohol, Smoking and Substance Involvement Screening Test (ASSIST), developed for the World Health Organization (WHO), is commonly used in primary and general medical care settings (World Health Organization ASSIST Working Group, 2002).. The ASSIST questionnaire assesses frequency of substance use both over the lifetime and over the past three months across nine categories of substances (tobacco products, alcohol, cannabis, cocaine, amphetamine-type stimulants, inhalants, sedatives/sleeping pills, hallucinogens and opioids), with a linked brief intervention.

The diagnostic criteria for substance use disorder are listed below. The presence of two or three symptoms leads to a diagnosis of 'mild substance use disorder', four or five symptoms to 'moderate substance use disorder' and five or more to a diagnosis of 'severe substance use disorder'.

DSM-5 substance use disorder:

1 failure to fulfil major role obligations
2 physically hazardous
3 recurrent social or interpersonal problems
4 tolerance (needing more frequent or larger quantities)
5 withdrawal
6 using more/for longer than intended
7 persistent desire or unsuccessful attempts to control substance use
8 excessive time spend obtaining, using or recovery from effects
9 reduced social, occupational or recreational activity
10 continued use despite physical or psychological problems
11 craving or strong desire to use a substance.

Areas of enquiry within a broader assessment of AOD use would include the following in addition to assessment of quantity and frequency of use:

- route of administration (for example, oral, snorting, smoking, injecting)
- age of first use
- most recent use (indication of drug-induced mental health disorder)
- pattern of use now and recently (poly-drug use and substitution)
- features of dependence
- consequences of use (for example, physical, psychological, social, vocational, and forensic)
- past treatment
- periods of abstinence
- reasons for use
- goals, intentions and readiness to change substance use
- mental state examination—evidence of poor self-care, intoxication (for example, slurred or rapid speech, consumer appearing sedated), impulsivity/disinhibition, irritability, hallucination and cognitive impairment
- physical examination—signs of intoxication (for example, pupil dilation or restriction), withdrawal (for example, tremors, sweating and shivering), liver disease (for example, jaundiced) and evidence of injecting drug use (needle track marks and infections).

Overall principles of treatment for individuals with co-occurring disorders

TOPIC LINK
See Chapter 13 for more on the therapeutic alliance.

- Use a non-judgmental empathic and encouraging approach when assessing substance use history to avoid under-reporting or defensive responses as therapeutic alliance is one of the strongest predictors of outcome.

- Use local names/terms for substances—for example, ice or shard (for methamphetamine), weed, pot, choof or ganja (for cannabis) and smack or harry (for heroin).

- Adopt a holistic approach, addressing related issues (relationship difficulties, housing instability and a lack of vocational skills training or employment) by enhancing problem-solving and communication skills.
- Explore and increase understanding of the link between their mental health and their alcohol or other drug use.
- Consider harm-reduction framework, recognising that for some abstinence may not be a realistic goal—at least in the short term or until their medication or mental health condition is more stabilised.
- Negotiate treatment goals, a treatment plan and treatment options.
- Adopt a longitudinal treatment approach, reassessing the patient's progress and adjusting interventions as needed over time.
- Involve family members and other carers in the assessment and treatment plan as they can provide round-the-clock support to the client in between therapy sessions or periods of hospitalisation.
- Improve family members' and carers' understanding of mental health and substance use disorders, and ensure they are supported.
- Try to keep patients engaged in treatment as long as possible since longer treatment is associated with better outcomes, particularly for those with high severity and complexity
- Treatment must be guided by a comprehensive assessment and ongoing review based on assertive community work and effective case management.

ABOUT THE CONSUMER Jenny's story

Jenny is a user of amphetamines who has experienced significant and growing problems with voices and hallucinations. She has been involved in different forms of substance use since adolescence, but it is amphetamine – and particularly methamphetamine – use that has really triggered her mental health problems.

It took her a long time before she was willing to attend a specialist AOD service and her initial experiences of them were not particularly helpful as the counsellor was not able to address the frightening voices she was hearing. Whilst she did not think she was mentally ill she felt she was heading in that direction.

It was only when she was later directed to an integrated service – where both mental health and drug problems were dealt with jointly, and where there was a strong peer support group, that she felt she was able to make some progress.

Although she still experiences cravings and occasional episodes of mental health problems, she is now stabilised on her medication and is well on the road to recovery. She has her life back and is studying for a degree at university and has strong career ambitions. She still needs her medication and is now a major force behind the support group, but life is positive for Jenny and she has a future that she cherishes and is excited about.

REFLECTION QUESTIONS

1 How would having an understanding of the relationship between mental health symptoms and substance use help Jenny?

2 In addition to the counselling Jenny received, what else could have contributed to her recovery?

NAOMI CRAFTI AND VICTORIA MANNING

ABOUT THE CONSUMER   Ewan's story

Ewan is a nursing student who did reasonably well in his first year of studies, although his social life had expanded and involved not only a few heavy nights each week, but also regular sessions of cannabis smoking with his friends in the evening. He became increasingly apathetic and detached from his studies, and started to experience some strange and unwelcome thoughts, although both alcohol and cannabis helped him to overcome these. At the start of his second year, he virtually stopped attending lectures, became increasingly detached from his friends and tended to spend long sessions at home smoking cannabis in his room. Whenever he stopped, the voices would come back and he was convinced that his friends were plotting against him. After some weeks, his girlfriend became so worried that she called an ambulance and Ewan was taken to a short-stay psychiatric ward for assessment.

REFLECTION QUESTIONS

1   As Ewan's health care worker, what steps do you need to take to identify what the underlying issues are?

2   What your initial aims would be around his mental health symptoms?

3   How you would start to develop a care and treatment plan for him?

Recovery

In a review of the evidence around recovery in mental health, Leamy, Bird, Le Boutillier, Williams, and Slade (2011) used the acronym CHIME to describe the common characteristics of the recovery experiences of individuals with mental health problems, based on their review of the evidence from recovery studies. CHIME represents the common characteristics of the successful studies: Connectedness, Hope, Identity, Meaning and Empowerment. This is consistent with the recovery model advanced by Deegan (1997) as a peer champion and advocate, who argued that a recovery model does not focus on remission but on transcendence—in other words, recovery is about well-being and quality of life, and a focus on positive engagement and activities. A similar model has been advanced in the AOD field by White and Evans (2013) who argue that 'recovery is more than remission—more than the subtraction of alcohol or drug use and/or related problems from an unchanged life'(White & Evans, 2013). There are two key principles to a recovery model: first, that most of the journey happens outside of treatment services; and second, that recovery is a personal and ongoing journey of transformation and change, based on a sense of hope and purpose.

The principles of recovery intervention apply to people with co-occurring disorders and will involve clinicians in three core tasks:

1   Developing a therapeutic relationship based on hope, respect and the shared belief that meaningful recovery is possible

2   Providing evidence-based treatments for the effective management of symptoms and to build the personal resources and supports to enable the client to engage effectively in the community

3   Assertively linking the client to community supports and resources that will help to build positive social networks and meaningful and rewarding activities

(Best 2012)

In addition, there is also growing evidence base about community mutual aid support groups for individuals with both mental health and substance use disorders (Zweben & Ashbrook, 2012). In the USA, there are a number of organisations that have emerged for those with a dual diagnosis, with Double Trouble in Recovery (DTR) and Dual Diagnosis Anonymous (DDA) the most prominent. One of the critical next steps in the development of a recovery model will be integrating AOD and mental health recovery resources in local communities and challenging the stigma and discrimination experienced by those with a co-occurring disorder.

The recovery agenda also necessitates a new treatment and staffing model for specialist dual diagnosis staff based on the underlying principles of recovery—a model built on hope, connectedness, empowerment and meaningful activities. What this means is that workers have to be aware of the resources in their community and be prepared to assertively link clients with community groups in the domains of mutual aid, peer support, recreational activities and vocational support, as a core part of their work. It also means every dual-diagnosis worker becoming an active advocate of recovery, challenging stigma and discrimination, and being a visible and attractive champion for recovery contagion in the community.

CRITICAL THINKING OPPORTUNITY

1   How could my work become more recovery-oriented?

2   Do I involve clients and their families sufficiently in establishing care plans and treatment plans?

3   Is my team working in a way that is recovery-focused? How would I be able to judge how effectively the principles of recovery are being implemented in my service?

4   What role could clients of your service play in establishing and maintaining a recovery focus?

Care planning

The following is an example care plan for Ewan, one of the clients presented in this chapter. The areas of daily living that are considered include biopsychosocial factors and the plan is mapped out using the nursing process (Assessment; Planning; Implementation; Evaluation). Remember, the success is in the detail, so be specific about who, when and what in the collaborative plan; and never include someone in the plan if they were not consulted in the planning process.

Date: [Today's date]						
Client's name: Ewan Case Manager:						
Areas of daily living	Assessment of current situation	Goal	Plan (undertaken with client)	Implementation	Who is responsible (including only those who have been consulted in the planning process)	Evaluation/ review date

| Mental health | 1. Ongoing assessment of psychiatric symptoms
2.Treatment of mental health disorder | 1. Develop rapport and trust with patient
2. Ewan will participate in treatment of psychiatric disorder | 1. Arrange for regular assessment of mental health
1. Provide explanation for ongoing assessment
2.1 Ewan will take prescribed medication
2.2 Ewan will attend psychiatrist consultations visits
2.3 Ewan will be given consistent opportunities to make decisions in his treatment planning | 1. Contact nurse to review Ewan's mental state every two hours
2.1 Ewan will be given information and education regarding benefits and side effects of medication regime
2.1 Ewan will be given information and education to enhance awareness of symptoms of mental illness and identify possible triggers
2.2 Nurse to ensure that Ewan has assistance to attend appointments with psychiatrist
2.3 Nurse will encourage Ewan to participate in all decisions made regarding treatment of his mental illness
2.3 Nurse will assist Ewan in identifying other people he would like to be involved in his treatment
e.g. Ewan's girlfriend /family members/significant others | 1.1 Contact nurse
1.2 Psychiatrist
2.1 Contact nurse
2.2 Nurse responsible for administration of pharmacotherapy
2.1 Treating Psychiatrist
2.2 Nurse to escort Ewan to treating Psychiatrist room whilst an inpatient
2.3 Contact nurse Treating Psychiatrist
2.3 Contact Nurse
2.3 Treating Psychiatrist | 1.Ongoing/Daily
Ongoing/Daily
48 hours
Ongoing/Daily |
| Social | 1. Minimal social supports and withdrawal from friendship groups
2. Withdrawal from engagement in university studies. At risk of failing | 1.1 Ewan to identify friends he is willing to reconnect with who can support is recovery
2. Support Ewan in Contacting Student Welfare and Nursing | 1.1 Ewan to write a list of five friends he is willing to contact by phone/social media
1.2 Ewan to be given information on appropriate Peer Support group/s
2.1 Assist Ewan in finding contact details for University staff.
2.2 Identify and arrange any documentation that can support Ewan's case for special consideration. E.g. sickness certificate. Letter from consulting psychiatrist | 1.1 Nurse will assist and encourage Ewan to develop this list
1.1 Nurse will arrange for Ewan to access computer and /or phone to make contact with identified supports
1.2 Nurse and or Social Worker to provide details of Peer Support Group/s and comprehensive information of benefits of linkage
2.1 Nurse to assist access to social worker
2.2 Contact treating psychiatrist and request sickness certificate and support letter | 1.1 Contact Nurse/ Social Worker
1.1 Nurse/ social worker/ occupational therapist
1.2 Nurse or social Worker
Or Member of Peer Support Group to visit Ewan whilst in hospital
2.1 Social Worker
2.2 Nurse/treating psychiatrist | 24 hours
24-48 hours
24-48 hours
4/5 days
4/5 days |

Biological	1. Physical health assessment 2. Ensure adequate food and fluid intake	1.1 Ewan to have physical health check up with General Practitioner (GP) including liver function test 2. Ewan to drink 8 glasses of water and eat three nutritious meals daily	1.1 Ewan to have an identified GP who he trusts and who can provide ongoing support 2.1 Nurse to observe and encourage food and fluid intake. 2.2 Nurse to explain importance of maintaining hydration and nutrition in recovery from AOD use and mental health problems	1.1 Determine if Ewan has an identified GP that he has a positive relationship with. If not assist Ewan in locating a bulk billing GP near where he lives or possibly on University campus GP Practice 2.2 Nurse to meet with Ewan to provide information on importance of fluid and nutrition. 2.2 Nurse to encourage Ewan to cook and prepare his own meals	1 Nurse 2 Nurse	One week Ongoing
Environmental	Housing	1. Ensure Ewan has safe and secure housing to return to when discharged	1. Assess Ewan's housing arrangements and identify if he is at risk of homelessness	1. Ask Ewan about his housing situation and identify any risks	1. Nurse or arrange social worker to discuss this with Ewan and possible links to housing services	1. 24 – 48 hours
Substance using behaviours	1. Assess presence of withdrawal from alcohol and cannabis 2. Harm reduction information and education on alcohol and cannabis u	1.1 Complete alcohol withdrawal scale 1.2 Assess for signs of withdrawal from cannabis 2.1 Reduce the range of harms associated with drug use including exacerbation of mental health problems	1.1 Explanation of implementation of alcohol withdrawal scale and assessment of cannabis withdrawal signs. Provide information regarding options for alleviating discomfort in relation to withdrawal experience if present. 2.1 In collaboration with Ewan develop a range of strategies to reduce harms related to drug use. Practical strategies that Ewan is willing to implement	1.1 Assess need for medication to prevent withdrawal seizures and address symptoms in relation to alcohol withdrawal. 1.2 Assess Provide information and education regarding responding to withdrawal of cannabis 2.1 In collaboration with Ewan identify the range of actual and potential harms related to his alcohol and cannabis use 2.2 Explore with Ewan strategies he has used that have minimised harms re drug use in past and offer other strategies that Ewan may be willing to try.	1.1 & 1.2 Nurse/ prescribing doctor 2. Nurse	Within 24 hours of admission 7 days

Risk behaviours	1. Assess risk of suicide and/or self harm	1. Identify suicidal ideation and level of risk	Completion of risk assessment	1.1 Complete risk assessment tool in collaboration with Ewan 1.2 If necessary develop a safety plan or respond to level of risk	Nurse	Daily (minimum)

SUMMARY

There is limited research on the prevalence of co-occurring mental health and substance use problems in the Australian and New Zealand context. However, it is well-established that their co-occurrence is the rule rather than the exception. There is also a gradually emerging evidence base on the effectiveness of integrated treatment models and interventions, although much of this has come from the USA and UK. Despite this, there has been a shift in government policies both within and beyond Australasia to educate and empower professionals in the broader health and welfare system, so that they can recognise and respond to the multiple needs of individuals with co-occurring disorders. There has also been increasing acknowledgment of the benefits of consumer and carer involvement in shaping appropriate treatment and support programs as part of the transition to a recovery-oriented approach.

DISCUSSION QUESTIONS

1   Do you think classifying drugs as either 'legal' or 'illegal' is relevant to their effects on mental health and subsequent treatment?

2   Mental health problems can lead to increased drug use and vice versa. From a recovery perspective, does it matter which came first? Why or why not?

3   Should people with co-occurring disorders be prevented from accessing the same treatment facilities as people with either a mental health or substance use problem only?

4   Can a person who has been diagnosed with a co-occurring mental health and substance use problem ever be considered 'recovered'?

5   How will a recovery model change the way co-occurring mental health and substance use disorders are perceived in the community and the impact of stigma on treatment seeking?

TEST YOURSELF

1   Which statement below best describes psychoactive drugs?

a   Any natural or synthetic chemical substance that comes from outside the body, crosses the blood brain barrier, and alters mood, perception or brain functioning

b   Any natural or synthetic chemical substance that comes from outside the body, crosses the blood brain barrier and has an effect similar to our natural neurotransmitters

c   Any natural or synthetic chemical substance that crosses the blood-brain barrier, has an effect similar to our natural neurotransmitters and alters mood, perception or brain functioning d any natural or synthetic chemical substance that comes from outside the body, crosses the blood-brain barrier, has an effect similar to our natural neurotransmitters, and alters mood, perception or brain functioning

2 Drugs may be classified according to their:

    a therapeutic purpose

    b source or chemical grouping

    c legal status

    d effect they have on the central nervous system

    e all of the above

3 Which of the following statements is incorrect?

    a An individual's age, gender and health all have an effect on the drug taken.

    b The effect of an individual's drug use is unrelated to where they use or whether they use alone.

    c The effect of an individual's drug use is related to the individual's expectations about the effects of the drug.

    d The effect of a drug is related to the amount of the drug taken, the route of administration, frequency of dosing, drug interactions, and the half-life of the drug.

4 Addiction develops when:

    a drug use is increased to maintain the euphoric effects or to avoid dysphoria or withdrawal

    b drug using individuals commit drug-related offences

    c the individual experiences cravings

    d the individual's drug use causes intoxication

USEFUL WEBSITES

Alcohol and Drug Foundation—Drug facts: www.druginfo.adf.org.au

Australian Community Support Organisation (ACSO): www.acso.org.au

Australian Drug Information Network (ADIN): www.adin.com.au

Counselling Online: www.counsellingonline.org.au

Gambler's Help: www.gamblershelp.com.au

Royal Women's Hospital—Women's Alcohol and Drug Service (WADS): www.thewomens.org.au/health-professionals/maternity/womens-alcohol-and-drug-service

Self Help Addiction Resource Centre (SHARC): www.sharc.org.au

Turning Point: www.turningpoint.org.au

REFERENCES

Aase, D. M., Jason, L. A., & Robinson, W. L. (2008). 12-step participation among dually-diagnosed individuals: A review of individual and contextual factors. *Clin Psychol Rev, 28*(7), 1235-1248. doi:10.1016/j.cpr.2008.05.002

Abou-Saleh, M. T. (2006). Substance use disorders: Recent advances in treatment and models of care. J Psychosom Res, 61(3), 305-310. doi:10.1016/j.jpsychores.2006.06.013

American Psychiatric Association. (2000). Diagnostic and Statistical Manual of Mental Disorders (4th ed.). Washington, DC.

American Psychiatric Association. (2013). Diagnostic and statistical manual of mental disorders (5th ed.). Arlington: American Psychiatric Association.

Anthony, J. C., Warner, L. A., & Kessler, R. C. (1994). Comparative epidemiology of dependence on tobacco, alcohol, controlled substances, and inhalants: Basic findings from the National Comorbidity Survey. Exp Clin Psychopharmacol, 2(3), 244-268.

Australian Bureau of Statistics. (2012). Australian Health Survey: First Results, 2011-12. Canberra: Australian Bureau of Statistics.

Australian Crime Commission. (2017). Illicit Drug Data Report 2015-16. Canberra.

Australian Drug Foundation. (2011). Hallucinogens: How drugs affect you. Melbourne: Australian Drug Foundation.

Australian Institute of Health and Welfare. (2011). 2010 National Drug Strategy Household Survey report. Drug statistics series no. 25. Cat. no. PHE 145. Canberra: AIHW.

Australian Institute of Health and Welfare. (2014). National Drug Strategy Household Survey detailed report: 2013. Drug statistics series no. 28. Cat. no. PHE 183. Canberra: AIHW.

Australian Institute of Health and Welfare. (2015). Trends in methylamphetamine availability, use and treatment, 2003–04 to 2013–14. Canberra: AIHW.

Australian Institute of Health and Welfare. (2016). Australian Burden of Disease Study: impact and causes of illness and death in Australia 2011. Australian Burden of Disease Study series no. 3. Cat. no. BOD 4. Canberra: AIHW.

Baker, A. L., Kavanagh, D. J., Kay-Lambkin, F. J., Hunt, S. A., Lewin, T. J., Carr, V. J., & Connolly, J. (2010). Randomized controlled trial of cognitive-behavioural therapy for coexisting depression and alcohol problems: Short-term outcome. Addiction, 105(1), 87-99. doi:10.1111/j.1360-0443.2009.02757.x

Baker, A. L., Kavanagh, D. J., Kay-Lambkin, F. J., Hunt, S. A., Lewin, T. J., Carr, V. J., & McElduff, P. (2014). Randomized controlled trial of MICBT for co-existing alcohol misuse and depression: Outcomes to 36-months. Journal of Substance Abuse Treatment, 46(3), 281-290. doi:http://dx.doi.org/10.1016/j.jsat.2013.10.001

Bergman, B. G., Greene, M. C., Hoeppner, B. B., Slaymaker, V., & Kelly, J. F. (2014). Psychiatric Comorbidity and 12-Step Participation: A Longitudinal Investigation of Treated Young Adults. Alcoholism: Clinical and Experimental Research, 38(2), 501-510.

Berkson, J. (1946). Limitations of the application of fourfold table analysis to hospital data. Biometrics, 2(3), 47-53.

Best, D. (2012). Addiction Recovery: A movement for social change and personal growth in the UK. Brighton: Pavilion Publishing.

Bizzarri, J. V., Casetti, V., Panzani, P., Unterhauser, J., Mulas, S., Fanolla, A., . . . Conca, A. (2016). Risky use and misuse of alcohol and cigarettes in psychiatric inpatients: A screening questionnaire study. Compr Psychiatry, 70, 9-16. doi:10.1016/j.comppsych.2016.05.011

Bush, K., Kivlahan, D. R., McDonell, M. B., Fihn, S. D., & Bradley, K. A. (1998). The AUDIT alcohol consumption questions (AUDIT-C): An effective brief screening test for problem drinking. Ambulatory Care Quality Improvement Project (ACQUIP). Alcohol Use Disorders Identification Test. Arch Intern Med, 158(16), 1789-1795.

Carroll, K. M., & Weiss, R. D. (2016). The role of behavioral interventions in buprenorphine maintenance treatment: a review. American Journal of Psychiatry, appi-ajp.

Cosci, F., & Fava, G. A. (2011). New clinical strategies of assessment of comorbidity associated with substance use disorders. Clin Psychol Rev, 31(3), 418-427. doi:10.1016/j.cpr.2010.11.004

Croton, G. (2005). Australian treatment system's recognition of and response to co-occurring mental health and substance use disorders - A submission to the 2005 Senate Select Committee on Mental Health. Retrieved from Wangaratta:

Deady, M., Mills, K., Teesson, M., Kay-Lambkin, F., Ross, J., Baillie, A., & Subotic, M. (2016). How do we best treat comorbid substance use and mental disorders?: Evidence-based approaches to integrated treatment.

Deane, F. P., Kelly, P. J., Crowe, T. P., Coulson, J. C., & Lyons, G. C. (2013). Clinical and reliable change in an Australian residential substance use program using the Addiction Severity Index. J Addict Dis, 32(2), 194-205. doi:10.1080/10550887.2013.795470

Deegan, P. E. (1997). Recovery and empowerment for people with psychiatric disabilities. Soc Work Health Care, 25(3), 11-24. doi:10.1300/J010v25n03_02

Degenhardt, L., Sara, G., McKetin, R., Roxburgh, A., Dobbins, T., Farrell, M., . . . Hall, W. D. (2017). Crystalline methamphetamine use and methamphetamine-related harms in Australia. Drug and alcohol review. Drug Alcohol Rev, 36(2), 160-170.

Department of Health. (2012). New directions for alcohol and drug treatment services: A roadmap. Melbourne: Victorian Government.

Dobbin, M. (2014). Pharmaceutical drug misuse in Australia. Australian Prescriber, 37, 79-81.

Donoghue, K., Patton, R., Phillips, T., Deluca, P., & Drummond, C. (2014). The effectiveness of electronic screening and brief intervention for reducing levels of alcohol consumption: a systematic review and meta-analysis. J Med Internet Res, 16(6), e142.

Dore, G., Mills, K., Murray, R., Teesson, M., & Farrugia, P. (2012). Post-traumatic stress disorder, depression and suicidality in inpatients with substance use disorders. Drug Alcohol Rev, 31(3), 294-302. doi:10.1111/j.1465-3362.2011.00314.x

Drake, R. E., Bartels, S. J., Teague, G. B., Noordsy, D. L., & Clark, R. E. (1993). Treatment of substance abuse in severely mentally ill patients. Journal of Nervous and Mental Disease, 181(10), 606-611.

Drake, R. E., Essock, S. M., Shaner, A., Carey, K. B., Minkoff, K., Kola, L., . . . Rickards, L. (2001). Implementing dual diagnosis services for clients with severe mental illness. Psychiatric Services, 52(4), 469-476. doi:10.1176/appi.ps.52.4.469

Drake, R. E., Mueser, K. T., & Brunette, M. F. (2007). Management of persons with co-occurring severe mental illness and substance use disorder: Program implications. World Psychiatry, 6(3), 131-136.

Dunn, M. (2013). More young men using steroids but do they know the harms? Retrieved from https://theconversation.com, 1/07/2013

Dunn, M., Proudfoot, H., & Barry, R. (2011). A quick guide to drugs and alcohol. Retrieved from Sydney, N.S.W:

Essock, S. M., Mueser, K. T., Drake, R. E., Covell, N. H., McHugo, G. J., Frisman, L. K., . . . Swain, K. (2006). Comparison of ACT and standard case management for delivering integrated treatment for co-occurring disorders. Psychiatric Services, 57(2), 185-196. doi:10.1176/appi.ps.57.2.185

European Monitoring Centre for Drugs and Drug Addiction. (2014). Residential treatment for drug use in Europe, EMCDDA Papers. Retrieved from Luxembourg:

Ewing, J. A. (1984). Detecting alcoholism. The CAGE questionnaire. Jama, 252(14), 1905-1907.

Farrell, M., Howes, S., Bebbington, P., Brugha, T., Jenkins, R., Lewis, G., . . . Meltzer, H. (2001). Nicotine, alcohol and drug dependence and psychiatric comorbidity. Results of a national household survey. British Journal of Psychiatry, 179, 432-437.

Gage, S. H., Jones, H. J., Burgess, S., Bowden, J., Davey Smith, G., Zammit, S., & Munafo, M. R. (2017). Assessing causality in associations between cannabis use and schizophrenia risk: A two-sample Mendelian randomization study. Psychol Med, 47(5), 971-980. doi:10.1017/s0033291716003172

Garde, E. L., Manning, V., & Lubman, D. I. (2017). Characteristics of clients currently accessing a national online alcohol and drug counselling service. Australasian Psychiatry, 0(0), 1039856216689623. doi:doi:10.1177/1039856216689623

Glass, J. E., Andréasson, S., Bradley, K. A., Finn, S. W., Williams, E. C., Bakshi, A.-S., . . . Saitz, R. (2017). Rethinking alcohol interventions in health care: a thematic meeting of the International Network on Brief Interventions for Alcohol & Other Drugs (INEBRIA). Addiction Science & Clinical Practice, 12, 14.

Gowing, L., Ali, R., Dunlop, A., Farrell, M., & Lintzeris, N. (2014). National guidelines for medication-assisted treatment of opioid dependence (2014). Retrieved from Canberra: http://www.nationaldrugstrategy.gov.au/internet/drugstrategy/Publishing.nsf/content/AD14DA97D8EE00E8

CA257CD1001E0E5D/$File/National_
Guidelines_2014.pdf

Griffiths, R. R., Juliano, L. M., & Chausmer, A. L. (2003). Caffeine pharmacology and clinical effects. In A. W. Graham, T. K. Schultz, M. F. Mayo-Smith, R. K. Ries, & B. B. Wilford (Eds.), Principles of Addiction Medicine, Third Edition (pp. 193-224). Chevy Chase, MD: American Society of Addiction Medicine.

Guest, C., & Holland, M. (2011). Co-existing mental health and substance use and alcohol difficulties – why do we persist with the term "dual diagnosis" within mental health services? Advances in Dual Diagnosis, 4(4), 162-172. doi:doi:10.1108/17570971111197175

Hamilton, M., King, T., & Ritter, A. (2004). Drug Use in Australia: Preventing Harm (2nd Ed.). Melbourne: Oxford University Press.

Hawton, K., Sutton, L., Haw C., Sinclair, J., & Deeks, J. J. (2005). Schizophrenia and suicide: Systematic review of risk factors. The British Journal of Psychiatry, 187(1), 9-20. doi:10.1192/bjp.187.1.9

Hayashida, M. (1998). An overview of outpatient and inpatient detoxification. Alcohol Health Res World, 22(1), 44-46.

Hodgson, R., Alwyn, T., John, B., Thom, B., & Smith, A. (2002). The FAST Alcohol Screening Test. Alcohol Alcoholism, 37(1), 61-66.

Horsfall, J., Cleary, M., Hunt, G. E., & Walter, G. (2009). Psychosocial treatments for people with co-occurring severe mental illnesses and substance use disorders (dual diagnosis): A review of empirical evidence. Harv Rev Psychiatry, 17(1), 24-34. doi:10.1080/10673220902724599

Hunt, G. E., Malhi, G. S., Cleary, M., Lai, H. M., & Sitharthan, T. (2016a). Comorbidity of bipolar and substance use disorders in national surveys of general populations, 1990-2015: Systematic review and meta-analysis. Journal of Affective Disorders, 206, 321-330. doi:10.1016/j.jad.2016.06.051

Hunt, G. E., Malhi, G. S., Cleary, M., Lai, H. M., & Sitharthan, T. (2016b). Prevalence of comorbid bipolar and substance use disorders in clinical settings, 1990-2015: Systematic review and meta-analysis. Journal of Affective Disorders, 206, 331-349. doi:10.1016/j.jad.2016.07.011

Hunt, G. E., Siegfried, N., Morley, K., Sitharthan, T., & Cleary, M. (2013). Psychosocial interventions for people with both severe mental illness and substance misuse. Cochrane Database of Systematic Reviews(10), Cd001088. doi:10.1002/14651858.CD001088.pub3

Kampman, K., & Jarvis, M. (2015). American Society of Addiction Medicine (ASAM) National Practice Guideline for the use of medications in the treatment of addiction involving opioid use. J Addict Med, 9(5), 358-367. doi:10.1097/adm.0000000000000166

Kaner, E. F., Beyer, F., Dickinson, H. O., Pienaar, E., Campbell, F., Schlesinger, C., . . . Burnand, B. (2007). Effectiveness of brief alcohol interventions in primary care populations. Cochrane Database of Systematic Reviews(2), Cd004148. doi:10.1002/14651858.CD004148.pub3

Kaner, E. F. S., Brown, N., & Jackson, K. (2011). A systematic review of the impact of brief interventions on substance use and co-morbid physical and mental health conditions. Mental Health and Substance Use, 4(1), 38-61. doi:10.1080/17523281.2011.533449

Kaskutas, L. A. (2009). Alcoholics Anonymous effectiveness: Faith meets science. J Addict Dis, 28(2), 145-157. doi:10.1080/10550880902772464

Kelly, T. M., & Daley, D. C. (2013). Integrated treatment of substance use and psychiatric disorders. Social work in public health, 28(0), 388-406. doi:10.1080/19371918.2013.774673

Kelly, T. M., Daley, D. C., & Douaihy, A. B. (2012). Treatment of substance abusing patients with comorbid psychiatric disorders. Addict Behav, 37(1), 11-24. doi:10.1016/j.addbeh.2011.09.010

Lal, S., & Adair, C. E. (2014). E-mental health: a rapid review of the literature. Psychiatric Services, 65(1).

Leamy, M., Bird, V., Le Boutillier, C., Williams, J., & Slade, M. (2011). Conceptual framework for personal recovery in mental health: systematic review and narrative synthesis. British Journal of Psychiatry, 199(6), 445-452. doi:10.1192/bjp.bp.110.083733

Lev-Ran, S., Roerecke, M., Le Foll, B., George, T., McKenzie, K., & Rehm, J. (2014). The association between cannabis use and depression: A systematic review and meta-analysis of longitudinal studies. Psychol Med, 44(4), 797-810. doi:doi:10.1017/S0033291713001438

Lubman, D. I., Allen, N. B., Rogers, N., Cementon, E., & Bonomo, Y. (2007). The impact of co-occurring mood and anxiety disorders among substance-abusing youth. Journal of Affective Disorders, 103(1-3), 105-112. doi:10.1016/j.jad.2007.01.011

Lubman, D. I., & Baker, A. (2010). Cannabis and mental health - management in primary care. Aust Fam Physician, 39(8), 554-557.

Lubman, D. I., Garfield, J. B. B., Manning, V., Berends, L., Best, D., Mugavin, J. M., . . . Allsop, S. (2016). Characteristics of individuals presenting to treatment for primary alcohol problems versus other drug problems in the Australian patient pathways study. BMC Psychiatry, 16(1), 250. doi:10.1186/s12888-016-0956-9

Magura, S. (2008). Effectiveness of dual focus mutual aid for co-occurring substance use and mental health disorders: A review and synthesis

of the "Double Trouble" in recovery evaluation. Substance Use and Misuse, 43(12-13), 1904-1926. doi:10.1080/10826080802297005

Mangrum, L. F., Spence, R. T., & Lopez, M. (2006). Integrated versus parallel treatment of co-occurring psychiatric and substance use disorders. Journal of Substance Abuse Treatment, 30(1), 79-84. doi:10.1016/j.jsat.2005.10.004

Manning, V., Garfield, J. B., Best, D., Berends, L., Room, R., Mugavin, J., . . . Lubman, D. I. (2017). Substance use outcomes following treatment: Findings from the Australian Patient Pathways Study. Australian and New Zealand Journal of Psychiatry, 51(2), 177-189. doi:10.1177/0004867415625815

Manning, V., Strathdee, G., Best, D., Keaney, F., McGillivray, L., & Witton, J. (2002). Dual diagnosis screening: preliminary findings on the comparison of 50 clients attending community mental health services and 50 clients attending community substance misuse services. Journal of Substance Use, 7(4), 221-228. doi:10.1080/14659890215691

Marel, C., Mills, K. L., Kingston, R., Gournay, K., Deady, M., Kay-Lambkin, F., . . . Teesson, M. (2016). Guidelines on the management of co-occurring alcohol and other drug and mental health conditions in alcohol and other drug treatment settings (2nd edition). Retrieved from Sydney, Australia:

Marsch, L. A., Carroll, K. M., & Kiluk, B. D. (2014). Technology-based interventions for the treatment and recovery management of substance use disorders: A JSAT special issue. Journal of Substance Abuse Treatment, 46(1), 10.1016/j.jsat.2013.1008.1010. doi:10.1016/j.jsat.2013.08.010

Mattick, R. P., Breen, C., Kimber, J., & Davoli, M. (2014). Buprenorphine maintenance versus placebo or methadone maintenance for opioid dependence. Cochrane Database of Systematic Reviews(2), Cd002207. doi:10.1002/14651858.CD002207.pub4

McKetin, R., Lubman, D. I., Lee, N. M., Ross, J. E., & Slade, T. N. (2011). Major depression among methamphetamine users entering drug treatment programs. Medical Journal of Australia, 195(3), 51.

McKetin, R., Najman, J. M., Baker, A. L., Lubman, D. I., Dawe, S., Ali, R., . . . Mamun, A. (2012). Evaluating the impact of community-based treatment options on methamphetamine use: Findings from the Methamphetamine Treatment Evaluation Study (MATES). Addiction, 107(11), 1998-2008. doi:10.1111/j.1360-0443.2012.03933.x

Mills, K. L., Lynskey, M., Teesson, M., Ross, J., & Darke, S. (2005). Post-traumatic stress disorder among people with heroin dependence in the Australian treatment outcome study (ATOS): prevalence and correlates. Drug Alcohol

Dependence, 77(3), 243-249. doi:10.1016/j.drugalcdep.2004.08.016

Ministerial Council on Drug Strategy. (2004). The National Drug Strategy: Australia's integrated framework 2004-2009. Retrieved from http://www.nationaldrugstrategy.gov.au/internet/drugstrategy/publishing.nsf/Content/5EAED77A78166EB5CA2575B4001353A4/$File/framework0409.pdf

Ministry of Health. (2010). Drug Use in New Zealand: Key Results of the 2007/08 New Zealand Alcohol and Drug Use Survey. Wellington: Ministry of Health.

Ministry of Health. (2016). Annual Update of Key Results 2015/16: New Zealand Health Survey. Wellington: Ministry of Health.

Morse, G. A., Calsyn, R. J., Dean Klinkenberg, W., Helminiak, T. W., Wolff, N., Drake, R. E., . . . McCudden, S. (2006). Treating homeless clients with severe mental illness and substance use disorders: Costs and outcomes. Community Ment Health J, 42(4), 377-404. doi:10.1007/s10597-006-9050-y

Mortlock, K. S., Deane, F. P., & Crowe, T. P. (2011). Screening for mental disorder comorbidity in Australian alcohol and other drug residential treatment settings. Journal of Substance Abuse Treatment, 40, 397-404.

Moyer, A., Finney, J. W., Swearingen, C. E., & Vergun, P. (2002). Brief interventions for alcohol problems: A meta-analytic review of controlled investigations in treatment-seeking and non-treatment-seeking populations. Addiction, 97(3), 279-292.

Mueser, K. T., Drake, R. E., Turner, W., & McGovern, M. P. (2006). Comorbid substance use disorders and psychiatric disorders. In W. R. Miller & K. M. Carroll (Eds.), Rethinking Substance Abuse (pp. 115-133). New York: Guilford Press.

Mueser, K. T., Essock, S. M., Drake, R. E., Wolfe, R. S., & Frisman, L. (2001). Rural and urban differences in patients with a dual diagnosis. Schizophrenia Research, 48(1), 93-107. doi:http://dx.doi.org/10.1016/S0920-9964(00)00065-7

National Health and Medical Research Council. (2009). Australian guidelines to reduce health risks from drinking alcohol. Retrieved from Canberra: http://www.nhmrc.gov.au/_files_nhmrc/publications/attachments/ds10-alcohol.pdf

NSW Health. (2000). Mental health and substance use disorder service delivery guidelines. Retrieved from North Sydney:

NSW Ministry of Health. (2015). Effective models of care for comorbid mental illness and illicit substance use: Evidence check review. Retrieved from NSW, Australia:

Nutt, D. (2012). Drugs – without the hot air. Retrieved from England:

Pennay, A., Cameron, J., Reichert, T., Strickland, H., Lee, N. K., Hall, K., & Lubman, D. I. (2011). A systematic review of interventions for co-occurring substance use disorder and borderline personality disorder. Journal of Substance Abuse Treatment, 41(4), 363-373. doi:10.1016/j.jsat.2011.05.004

Pennay, A., & Lubman, D. I. (2012). Alcohol and energy drinks: a pilot study exploring patterns of consumption, social contexts, benefits and harms. BMC Res Notes, 5, 369. doi:10.1186/1756-0500-5-369

Petit, A., Karila, L., Chalmin, F., & Lejoyeux, M. (2012). Methamphetamine Addiction: A Review of the Literature. Journal of Addiction Research, 1(6). doi:doi:10.4172/2155-6105.S1-006

Pray, M. E., & Watson, L. M. (2008). Effectiveness of day treatment for dual diagnosis patients with severe chronic mental illness. Journal of Addictions Nursing, 19(3), 141-149. doi:10.1080/10884600802306008

Queensland Health. (2010). Queensland Health Dual Diagnosis Clinical Guidelines. Retrieved from

Rowles, B. M., Ellington, A., Tarr, A., Hertzer, J. L., & Findling, R. L. (2015). Comorbidity and treatment in substance use disorders. International Public Health Journal, 7(2), 179-190.

Roxburgh, A., & Burns, L. (2012). Accidental drug-induced deaths due to opioids in Australia, 2008. Retrieved from Sydney:

Royal Australian College of General Practitioners. (2009). Smoking Cessation Pharmacotherapy: An update for health professionals. Retrieved from Melbourne:

Royal College of Psychiatrists. (2013). Benzodiazepines. In R. C. o. Psychiatrists (Ed.).

Saitz, R., Palfai, T. P., & Cheng, D. M. (2014). Screening and brief intervention for drug use in primary care: the ASPIRE randomized clinical trial. Jama, 312(5), 502-513.

Schafer, I., & Najavits, L. M. (2007). Clinical challenges in the treatment of patients with posttraumatic stress disorder and substance abuse. Curr Opin Psychiatry, 20(6), 614-618. doi:10.1097/YCO.0b013e3282f0ffd9

Scott, H., Johnson, S., Menezes, P., Thornicroft, G., Marshall, J., Bindman, J., . . . Kuipers, E. (1998). Substance misuse and risk of aggression and offending among the severely mentally ill. The British Journal of Psychiatry, 172(4), 345-350. doi:10.1192/bjp.172.4.345

Sewell, R. A., Ranganathan, M., & D'Souza, D. C. (2009). Cannabinoids and psychosis.

International Review of Psychiatry, 21(2), 152-162. doi:10.1080/09540260902782802

Shand, F. L., Stafford, J. A., Fawcett, J., & Mattick, R. P. (2003). Guidelines for the Treatment of Alcohol Problems. Retrieved from Canberra:

Sindicich, N., & Burns, L. (2011). Australian Trends in Ecstasy and related Drug Markets 2010. Findings from the Ecstasy and Related Drugs Reporting System (EDRS). Australian Drug Trend Series No. 64. . Retrieved from

Teesson, M., Havard, A., Ross, J., & Darke, S. (2006). Outcomes after detoxification for heroin dependence: Findings from the Australian Treatment Outcome Study (ATOS). Drug Alcohol Review, 25(3), 241-247. doi:10.1080/09595230600657733

Teesson, M., Marel, C., Darke, S., Ross, J., Slade, T., Burns, L., . . . Mills, K. L. (2015). Long-term mortality, remission, criminality and psychiatric comorbidity of heroin dependence: 11-year findings from the Australian Treatment Outcome Study. Addiction, 110(6), 986-993. doi:10.1111/add.12860

Teesson, M., Marel, C., Darke, S., Ross, J., Slade, T., Burns, L., . . . Mills, K. L. (2017). Trajectories of heroin use: 10-11-year findings from the Australian Treatment Outcome Study. Addiction. doi:10.1111/add.13747

Teesson, M., Mills, K., Ross, J., Darke, S., Williamson, A., & Havard, A. (2008). The impact of treatment on 3 years' outcome for heroin dependence: findings from the Australian Treatment Outcome Study (ATOS). Addiction, 103(1), 80-88. doi:10.1111/j.1360-0443.2007.02029.x

Teesson, M., Slade, T., & Mills, K. (2009). Comorbidity in Australia: findings of the 2007 National Survey of Mental Health and Wellbeing. Australian and New Zealand Journal of Psychiatry, 43(7), 606-614. doi:10.1080/00048670902970908

Thomson, B. M., & Schiess, S. (2010). Risk profile: Caffeine in energy drinks and energy shots. Retrieved from Wellington:

Todd, J., Green, G., Harrison, M., Ikuesan, B. A., Self, C., Pevalin, D. J., & Baldacchino, A. (2004). Social exclusion in clients with comorbid mental health and substance misuse problems. Soc Psychiatry Psychiatr Epidemiol, 39(7), 581-587. doi:10.1007/s00127-004-0790-0

White, W., & Evans, A. (2013). Defining recovery: A review of recent efforts. Drug and Alochol Review.

Wodak, A. (2014). Definition and evidence for harm reduction. Alcohol and alcoholism, 49(Suppl1), i30-i30.

World Health Organization. (2005). WHO framework convention on tobacco control. Geneva: WHO Retrieved from www.who.int/tobacco/framework/WHO_FCTC_english.pdf.

World Health Organization. (2009). Guidelines for the psychosocially assisted pharmacological treatment of opioid dependence. World Health Organization, Department of Mental Health and Substance Abuse.

World Health Organization ASSIST Working Group. (2002). The Alcohol, Smoking and Substance Involvement Screening Test (ASSIST): development, reliability and feasibility. Addiction, 97(9), 1183-1194.

Yücel, M., Solowij, N., Respondek, C., Whittle, S., Fornito, A., Pantelis, C., & Lubman, D. I. (2008). Regional brain abnormalities associated with long-term heavy cannabis use. Arch Gen Psychiatry, 65(6), 694-701. doi:10.1001/archpsyc.65.6.694

Zingberg, N. E. (1984). Drug, set and setting: The basis for controlled intoxicant use. New Haven: Yale University Press.

Zweben, J. E., & Ashbrook, S. (2012). Mutual-help groups for people with co-occurring disorders. Journal of Groups in Addiction and Recovery, 7(2-4), 202-222. doi:10.1080/1556035X.2012.705700

CHAPTER 15

Psychopharmacology

CHRIS ALDERMAN AND
KAREN-LEIGH EDWARD

KEY OUTCOMES

AFTER READING THIS CHAPTER, YOU SHOULD BE ABLE TO:

- recount important elements of the history of psychotropic drug development
- understand the place of drugs in the treatment of mental disorders
- describe important pharmacokinetic and pharmacodynamic processes and the ways in which these govern drug action
- discuss the means by which drugs can cause iatrogenic harm
- outline the various major classes of psychotropic drugs and the ways these are applied in the treatment of mental disorders.

KEY TERMS

- adherence
- concordance
- drug interaction
- extrapyramidal
- pharmacodynamics
- pharmacokinetics
- pharmacotherapy
- psychotropic drug
- quality use of medicines
- rechallenge
- recovery
- refractory

Introduction

It is likely that various forms of mental disorders have impacted upon humankind as long ago as the prehistoric era. Ancient people would usually attribute unusual behaviours or mental disturbances to an external influence such as demonic possession. As the biological basis for mental disorders has become better understood, treatment strategies that influence the elementary basis for mental illness increasingly have become a major focus for management. These biological interventions are a primary focus in treatment interventions. It is now axiomatic that the use of medicinal drugs (medications), also referred to as pharmacotherapy, is fundamental in the treatment of a large proportion of all cases of mental disorders. Drugs that exert their primary effects by influencing mental processes are often referred to as psychotropic drugs or agents (or just plain psychotropics). In contemporary practice, all nurses involved in the management of people with mental disorders need to have a practical, working understanding of the clinical pharmacology of psychotropics—this discipline is sometimes referred to as clinical psychopharmacology. Underpinning this is a requirement to have an applied understanding of the principles that critically influence psychotropic drug action: the pharmacokinetics and pharmacodynamics of drugs that will ultimately govern the expression of both therapeutic actions and adverse drug effects. These critical principles are discussed in more detail later in this chapter.

Hippocrates (460–370 BCE) is widely regarded as the clinician who conceived many basic tenets that remain applicable in modern medicine, even in contemporary times. He proposed that mental illness was caused by an imbalance of internal chemical forces, in line with the modern paradigm of a biological basis and internal locus for mental disorders (that is, rather than attribution to external influences). Despite the basically correct nature of his predictions, the foundations of neuroscience did not become sufficiently developed to allow further understanding of the biological basis for mental illness until many centuries had elapsed. In modern times, the treatments that are used for the management of mental disorders are usually broadly categorised as either psychological or biological. Psychological therapies include cognitive therapy, behavioural therapy, psychoanalysis and many others. These approaches are primarily oriented around counselling, are effective for many mental disorders, and in fact are the preferred treatment in some situations. Furthermore, it is increasingly evident that psychological therapies can be used with benefit in combination with biological treatments.

On the other hand, biological treatment for mental disorders can take a number of forms, but always involves the use of some form of physical intervention that can directly influence neurological disposition, function or even structure; for example, some forms of drug therapy are associated with neuroplasticity–neurological remodelling, such as that seen in depression and antidepressant medications. A neurotrophic hypothesis suggests that the opposing effects of stress and antidepressant drugs are mediated by modulation of kinase activity, resulting in neurological changes (Krystal et al., 2009).

A substantial proportion of treatment provided for the management of mental disorders is now delivered as psychotropic pharmacotherapy, and in many parts of the world much of this treatment is now prescribed by clinicians who are not psychiatrists (mostly general practitioners or primary care physicians). Indeed, the relatively simple access to pharmacotherapy and the aggressive promotion of medicinal drug products by multinational pharmaceutical companies have led commentators to call for caution in relation to the widespread use of pharmaceutical treatment options, citing the 'pathologisation' of everyday problems as a basis for advocacy of inappropriate use of psychotropic agents (Frances, 2013).

A brief history of psychotropic drugs

Arguably the most significant developments in the evolution of psychotropic drugs have origins in the early 1950s, an era that saw the introduction of the first truly effective psychotropic drugs. These included chlorpromazine and haloperidol as treatments for psychosis, and the tricyclic antidepressants (TCAs) and non-selective monoamine oxidase inhibitors (MAOIs) for affective disorders. These agents were truly revolutionary developments in the management of mental illness, because until that time there were no effective drug therapy options for the widespread conditions that they have been used to treat. Not long after this, the benzodiazepines were introduced into clinical practice. Probably the most famous of these was marketed as Valium (after the Latin *vale*, denoting 'strong' or 'well'). Diazepam would eventually become the most prescribed drug of all time. Although the benzodiazepines have had a controversial history, these agents are actually much safer than many other agents that are widely used in the community (for example, non-steroidal anti-inflammatory drugs, or NSAIDs). Benzodiazepines actually replaced barbiturates as treatment for anxiety and insomnia, and are much safer than the barbiturates.

As a result of a resolution in the US Senate in late 1989, the 1990s came to be known as the 'decade of the brain', an initiative of the US Library of Congress and National Institute of Mental Health (USA) to enhance public awareness of the benefits of brain research. Since 1990, many significant developments in psychopharmacology have followed, resulting in the introduction of impressive new treatment options for most major mental disorders. These include the atypical (new generation) antipsychotics, and the arrival of the selective serotonin reuptake inhibitors (SSRIs) and other new generation antidepressants. The range of treatment options now available for use in psychiatry has expanded so dramatically that the discipline of psychopharmacology has become enormously specialised and complex. Instead of working with a rather small range of drugs, prescribers now work with a vastly expanded range of options, emphasising the benefits of multidisciplinary team care in decision-making for consumers.

New classes of antidepressants and atypical antipsychotic drugs, as well as the novel use of drugs not traditionally used as psychotropic agents, all profoundly impact upon the treatment of mental illness. Prescribers and nurses need to understand a large range of complex drugs that have an evolving profile of adverse effects and drug interactions. An example of this change is the complexity of choice in prescribing the drug treatment of major depression (see Table 15.1).

TABLE 15.1 DRUG THERAPY FOR MAJOR DEPRESSION (AUSTRALIA), 1990 AND 2012		
Treatment options 1990	**Treatment options 2012**	
Tricyclic antidepressants	**Tricyclic antidepressants**	**Selective serotonin reuptake inhibitors**
Amitriptyline	Amitriptyline	Citalopram, escitalopram
Clomipramine	Clomipramine	Fluoxetine
Desipramine	Dothiepin	Fluvoxamine
Dothiepin	Doxepin	Paroxetine
Doxepin	Imipramine	Sertraline
Imipramine	Nortriptyline	Vortioxetine
Nortriptyline	Trimipramine	**Serotonin and noradrenaline reuptake inhibitors**
Protriptyline	**Monoamine oxidase inhibitors**	Venlafaxine/desvenlafaxine
Trimipramine	Phenelzine	Duloxetine
Monoamine oxidase inhibitors	Tranylcypromine	**Other antidepressants**
Phenelzine	Moclobemide	Bupropion
Tranylcypromine	**Noradrenaline reuptake inhibitors**	Mirtazapine
	Reboxetine	Agomelatine

Medicinal drug use in context

In the early 1990s the National Mental Health Policy and Plan was adopted in Australia, with the objective of providing a blueprint for the future delivery of mental health services. The strategy promoted the mental health of the Australian community, and sought to prevent the development of mental health problems and mental disorders, where possible. Additionally, the initiative aimed at reducing the impact of mental disorders on individuals, families and the community. In addition to the National Mental Health Policy and Plan is the Pharmaceutical Benefits Scheme (PBS), which was first introduced as a limited scheme in 1948 to provide free medicines for pensioners. Today the PBS provides access to a range of medicines at government subsidised prices that would otherwise be unaffordable. In common with Australia, the Government of New Zealand (NZ) invested in developing infrastructure targeted at optimising the safe and effective use of medicines within the NZ community. The Pharmaceutical Management Agency of New Zealand (PHARMAC) determines the range of medicines and related products that are subsidised for use in the community and in public hospitals. On the website dedicated to PHARMAC, consumers and clinicians can locate information related to medicine brand changes, media releases related to medicines, information sheets for medicines and the pharmaceutical schedule (see the 'Useful websites' section at the end of this chapter). The work of PHARMAC includes the development and implementation of public information campaigns, monitoring expenditure and usage patterns of drugs, and facilitating access to drugs with limited availability of data from clinical trials. The roles undertaken by PHARMAC include management of the schedule of government-subsidised community pharmaceuticals, and promoting optimal use of medicines.

For both Australia and NZ, government policy is based on the primary premise that effective drug treatments should be available, accessible and affordable. In Australia, this is consistent with the area of focus for the National Medicines Policy (Department of Health and Ageing, 2010); see Table 15.2.

	TABLE 15.2 FUNDAMENTAL ELEMENTS OF AUSTRALIA'S NATIONAL MEDICINES POLICY
a	Timely access to required medicines at a cost affordable to individuals and the community
b	Medicines of appropriate quality, safety and efficacy
c	A responsible and viable medicines industry in Australia
d	Achievement of quality use of medicines (QUM): — judicious selection of treatment options — appropriate selection of a suitable medication regimen, if considered necessary — safe and effective use of medications through monitoring, minimising misuse — ensuring that patients/carers have knowledge and skills to use medicines safely.

Additionally, the policies aim to facilitate timely access to required medicines at a cost affordable to individuals and the wider community, while ensuring that medicines meet appropriate quality, safety and efficacy standards. Australia's national strategy for quality use of medicines (QUM; Department of Health and Ageing, 2002) was designed to embrace the use of all medicines, including prescription, non-prescription and complementary therapies, with five key principles:

1 recognition of the primacy of consumers and their views
2 the notion of partnership between key participants (for example, between providers and consumer, and between providers)
3 the need for consultation and collaboration in the design, implementation and evaluation of QUM initiatives
4 support for existing QUM activities and initiatives
5 the need to adopt and embrace system-based approaches that foster an environment and behaviours that support QUM.

Many aspects of the work of nurses and other health workers involved in mental health address key elements of QUM, including:

■ judicious selection of management options (considering the place of medicines in treating mental disorders and maintaining health, and recognising the possibility that no treatment or a non-drug treatment may be most appropriate)

- appropriate selection of a suitable medication, if necessary; this will involve consideration of the clinical condition, risks and benefits associated with treatment options, the dosage and duration of treatment, coexisting illness, other therapies, monitoring considerations, and costs for the individual, the community and the health system as a whole
- safe and effective use of medications through monitoring, minimising misuse, and ensuring that the consumer or their carer has the knowledge and skills to use medicines appropriately.

CRITICAL THINKING OPPORTUNITY

1   How should nurses use QUM principles to optimise treatment outcomes for those with mental disorders?

2   What are the positive and negative roles played by the pharmaceutical industry in the QUM effort?

Medication-related problems

An understanding of medication-related harm that focuses exclusively on adverse drug reactions and drug–drug interactions does not allow an appropriately rich insight into the nature and scope of the problems that may be related to psychotropic pharmacotherapy. A medication-related problem (MRP) is any undesirable event experienced by the consumer that involves or is suspected to involve drug therapy, potentially interfering with desired outcomes. The most widely adopted system for categorisation of medication-related problems is that developed by Strand and colleagues (1990), who proposed eight categories of medication-related problems to define circumstances where people may be exposed to actual or potential medication-related harm. The eight categories of MRP used in this system are outlined in Table 15.3, with examples.

TABLE 15.3 CATEGORISATION OF MEDICATION-RELATED PROBLEMS

Category	Description	Example
Indication without drug therapy	There is an indication for medication use, but consumer is not receiving a drug for the indication	Person experiencing benzodiazepine withdrawal is not prescribed prophylactic pharmacotherapy
Drug use without indication	Person is taking a medication for which there is no medically valid indication	Person continues antipsychotics after episode of delirium resolves
Improper drug selection	Person has a medication indication but is taking the wrong drug	Person with history of ischaemic heart disease is prescribed tricyclic antidepressant
Sub-therapeutic dosage	Person has a medical problem that is being treated with too little of the correct medication	Insufficient dose of antipsychotic agent during exacerbation of psychotic illness
Over-dosage	Person has a medical problem that is being treated with too much of the correct medication	Person is prescribed a large dose of an antidepressant drug: the magnitude of the dosage does not create additional benefit but predisposes them to adverse effects
Adverse drug reaction (ADR)	Person has a medical problem that is the result of an ADR or adverse effect	Person develops tremor as a result of treatment with an antidepressant
Drug interaction	Medication–medication, medication–laboratory or medication–food interaction	Elevated serum methadone concentration with toxicity secondary to fluvoxamine treatment
Failure to receive a drug	Medical problem resulting from not receiving medication intended as part of designed treatment	Disabled person is prescribed a drug but cannot attend the pharmacy to have the prescription filled

Strand et al. (1990)

Nurses and the medicines management pathway cycle

The delivery of psychotropic drug therapy is complex, and clinicians from a single discipline cannot address all of the essential elements involved. The complex interplay related to medications for consumers include such activities as decision to treat, followed by prescribing, reviewing, issuing, administering, monitoring and communicating. The complexity of the medication management process is represented in Figure 15.1.

Figure 15.1 The medicines management pathway cycle

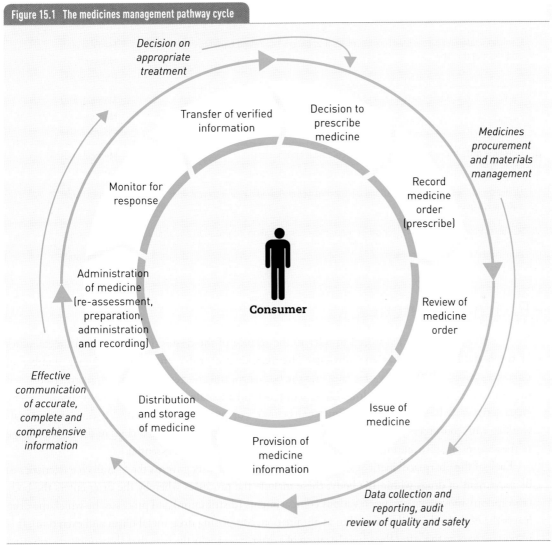

Courtesy of the Society of Hospital Pharmacists of Australia, Melbourne

Nurses are one group of key professionals involved in the administration, monitoring and prescribing of psychotropic drugs in the treatment of people with mental illness. There may be some overlap between the professional roles of nurses and those of other professional groups, emphasising the need for effective communication and, at the foundational level, a sound understanding of the pharmacokinetics and pharmacodynamics of drugs. Examples of roles for various professional groups are outlined in Table 15.4.

CHRIS ALDERMAN AND KAREN-LEIGH EDWARD

TABLE 15.4 PROFESSIONAL ROLES IN MEDICINES MANAGEMENT AND PSYCHOTROPIC PHARMACOLOGY

Professional role in medicines management	Health-care worker
Recognise or identify need for pharmacotherapy Prescribe and/or facilitate safe prescribing in accordance with legislation	Medical staff Nurses Pharmacists
Monitor for adverse effects and efficacy	Medical staff Nurses Pharmacists
Communicate and discuss with consumers and carers regarding benefits and risks of therapy	Medical staff Nurses Pharmacists
Participate in audits or research and investigations to advance knowledge	Medical staff Nurses Pharmacists
Combine drug therapy with non-pharmacological approaches	Medical staff Nurses
Understand, contribute and manage co-morbid general medical or surgical and substance use issues	Medical staff Nurses
Act as authoritative resource for other team members needing information about drugs	Pharmacists
Administer treatment to consumer	Medical staff Nurses

Pharmacokinetics

Pharmacokinetics is the term used to refer to the science of the disposition of drugs and metabolites in the body. Each drug has an individual pharmacokinetic profile that derives from a number of influences governing the entry of a drug into the body, reversible movements between internal sites, and the ultimate elimination of the drug. Drug action is fundamentally influenced by the pharmacokinetic characteristics (which are described in detail below). For nurses and other health-care professionals working with consumers in the context of prescribed and non-prescribed medicines or drugs, knowledge of the absorption, distribution, metabolism and elimination of drugs is essential.

Each of the pharmacokinetic parameters associated with a drug governs the overall characteristics of its movement of drugs within the body; these include the processes whereby the drug enters the body (absorption), movements between various compartments (distribution) and processes by which the drug leaves the body (collectively referred to as elimination, comprising drug metabolism and excretion). It is important to note that after the administration of a drug, it is usually the case that absorption, distribution and elimination actually occur simultaneously to some degree, at least for part of the duration of drug effects. By understanding the individual pharmacokinetic parameters of a drug, it is possible to have a rational basis for treatment decisions such as the optimum administration route, dose magnitude and frequency of administration.

A relatively recent development that is particularly relevant to the sciences fundamental to the pharmacokinetics of psychotropics (and indeed, other drugs) is referred to as *pharmacogenomics*. It is now understood that a person's genotype (the fundamental genetic makeup unique to that individual) can have a profound influence upon the expression of that person's phenotype (the physical expression of the influences of the genotype), meaning that the extent to which a person's genetic disposition is expressed in proteomics—the production and expression of proteins. As these proteins can include enzymes and other compounds that have a critical influence upon drug absorption and elimination, it is clear that the science of pharmacogenomics will be increasingly influential in our understanding of drug action. Moreover, it is clear that different phenotypes are concentrated among specific ethnic populations, paving the way for the science of 'ethnopharmacology', implying that a person's racial background may form the basis for estimating the magnitude and nature of an individual's response to a specific drug therapy.

CRITICAL THINKING OPPORTUNITY

1   Why is knowledge of the absorption, distribution, metabolism and elimination of prescribed and non-prescribed medicines or drugs essential for nurses and other health-care professionals?

2   Why has the contemporary nature of working with pharmacotherapy become so complex for health-care professionals?

3   What are medication-related problems (MRPs) and what is the nurse's role in minimising these?

Drug administration and absorption

Most drugs only produce a therapeutic effect after entering the systemic circulation and accessing the site of action. To do this, medication must be absorbed (undergo absorption) and move across a barrier structure and into the body's internal environment. Sometimes the route of administration involves direct introduction into the systemic circulation (for example, intravenous administration)—this may be because the agent is poorly absorbed after oral administration, or because intensified effects or rapid onset of action is needed. For most situations, the best route is oral administration, because of convenience, reliability and tolerability, and this is the route most commonly used for the administration of psychotropic drugs. After oral administration, a drug dissolves in the gastrointestinal fluids and absorption across the gut mucosa takes place. The drugs then diffuse into small blood vessels close to the gut lining.

These blood vessels form part of the hepatic portal circulation system, and from here drugs are transported directly to the liver prior to entry into the general systemic circulation. For some drugs, most of the orally administered dose is chemically modified into metabolites before accessing the systemic circulation. In this situation the drug is said to *undergo a significant first pass effect*, and only a relatively small proportion of the drug reaches the site of action. If oral administration is not practical or possible, the drug may be administered parenterally—for example, injected directly into a vein or other sites, such as intramuscularly or subcutaneously—where absorption into the general circulation follows. Intravenous administration usually results in faster onset and greater intensity of effect. In some cases (for example, depot formulations of antipsychotic drugs), intramuscular injections are deliberately formulated for slow release from the injection site, in order to achieve sustained action.

Drug distribution

'Drug distribution' is the term that describes reversible movements of drugs within the body, usually from one compartment to another. Drugs that are poorly soluble in water are usually distributed to sites outside of the general circulation. Drugs produce their therapeutic effects by binding to a receptor, and psychotropic drugs act as receptors in the central nervous system. Drug distribution to extravascular sites (located or occurring outside a blood or lymph vessel) is reversible—eventually the drug distributes back into the plasma, from which it will be eliminated. If a drug is extensively distributed to sites outside of the plasma, the plasma concentration does not truly reflect the total amount of drug in the body. The term 'volume of distribution' is used to describe that imaginary volume that would be consistent with the known amount of drug in the body, and the observed concentration in the plasma.

Drug metabolism and elimination

Metabolism (where the drug is converted into a different chemical, called a metabolite) is necessary because most drugs are organic chemicals and are poorly soluble in water. To allow drug excretion, the drug needs to undergo structural conversion to a new chemical compound, which is more soluble in water. Drug metabolism occurs in a number of sites, but the most important of these is the liver (see Figure 15.2). Metabolism usually (but not always) results in the creation of a metabolite with less pharmacological activity than the parent compound. Drug metabolism often involves several steps; these may involve oxidation and glucuronidisation. Under certain circumstances the activity of enzymes involved in drug metabolism is increased, and metabolism will occur at a faster rate (known as hepatic enzyme induction). In these situations the plasma level of the drug may be reduced relative to ordinary circumstances. Hepatic enzyme induction most commonly occurs as a result of the effects of another chemical from outside of the body (called an inducing agent). For example, cigarette smoking significantly increases the rate of metabolism for a number of drugs (including caffeine and clozapine), causing decreased plasma levels. Some may decrease hepatic drug metabolism (known as hepatic enzyme inhibition) and cause drug interactions resulting in increased serum concentrations and clinical effects (for example, clozapine toxicity after concurrent administration of fluvoxamine).

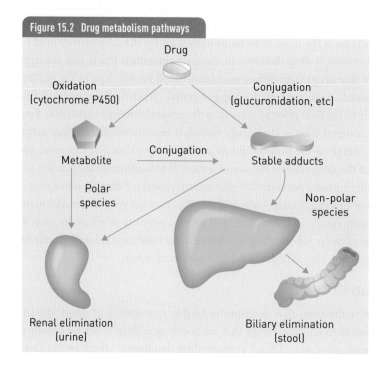

Figure 15.2 Drug metabolism pathways

Drug

Oxidation (cytochrome P450)

Conjugation (glucuronidation, etc)

Metabolite

Conjugation

Stable adducts

Polar species

Non-polar species

Renal elimination (urine)

Biliary elimination (stool)

The two major mechanisms by which drugs are eliminated from the body are by renal excretion and metabolic elimination. *Elimination* is the term used to refer to the various ways in which a drug irreversibly leaves the body. *Excretion* involves the irreversible transportation of the drug out of the body's internal environment.

Renal drug excretion

The kidneys are the principal organs for the ultimate elimination of drugs from the body. Drug elimination may be achieved through filtration at the glomerulus in the kidney, with the drug excreted into the urine. Drugs can be actively secreted into the urine, and also reabsorbed from the filtrate back into the systemic circulation, and thus renal clearance of drugs essentially reflects the composite of filtration, secretion and reabsorption. For some drugs, the great majority of the dose is excreted by the kidneys. A decline in renal function will cause increased drug levels and toxicity.

Elimination half-life

The elimination half-life of a drug is the time required for the plasma concentration to decrease by 50 per cent from an original value. If the plasma level decreases from 100 mg/L to 50 mg/L after a period of 24 hours, then the apparent half-life of the drug is said to be 24 hours. Steady-state plasma concentrations are not attained until the drug has been administered for a period of time approximately equivalent to five or six times the half-life of the drug. Similarly, the time taken to remove almost all of a drug from the body after a single dose (or after stopping a maintenance dose) is about five or six times the half-life.

CRITICAL THINKING OPPORTUNITY

1   Why are most drug doses administered by the oral route, and when might an alternative route be used?

2   What are the most common clinical circumstances where altered drug metabolism results in changes to the outcomes of treatment?

3   What is the elimination half-life?

Pharmacodynamics

Pharmacodynamics is the name of the discipline that is the basis to understand the *effects* of drugs in the body. A drug's pharmacodynamic characteristics include the mechanisms of *action* (either therapeutic or harmful) and the *effects observed* when the one drug is used in combination with others. The science of pharmacodynamics is complementary to that of pharmacokinetics and consumer-specific factors such as age, genetics, body mass and co-morbid illnesses which need to be considered by the nurse, as these aspects can have a profound effect on the pharmacodynamics of a drug. Consideration of the pharmacodynamic characteristics of drugs can be used to implement treatment intended for greatest therapeutic benefit with minimum likelihood of unwanted reactions.

Receptors

The effects of most drugs are mediated through interaction with cellular structures called receptors. Many psychotropic drugs produce their primary effects by influencing neurotransmission. Neurons (nerve cells, including those in the brain) are fundamentally comprised of dendrites, a cell body and axon terminals.

The dendrite collects a signal from another neuron and translates it to the cell body. The signal then moves to the axon terminals where it is transmitted to another neuron. The information is transmitted via chemicals called neurotransmitters, which are released and traverse the synaptic cleft (the space between two neurons) and ultimately interact with receptors on the dendrites of another neuron. The process is repeated from neuron to neuron.

Different functions and neuronal systems are dependent upon various neurotransmitters and receptors to function. For example, the neurotransmitter acetylcholine interacts with muscarinic and nicotinic receptors, influencing memory function and aspects of autonomic nervous function. Dopamine and serotonin play critical roles in the brain, modulating mood, cognition, appetite and many other critical functions: these neurotransmitters and their various receptor subtypes are key targets for mediating drug actions (both therapeutic and adverse effects) for many psychotropic drugs. Compounds such as hormones or neurotransmitters are the chemicals that would normally bind to receptors and alter the rate, extent or nature of a physiological function. Drugs that produce similar or synergistic effects to the endogenous compound found in nature are referred to as *agonists*, and those that produce an opposite effect are *antagonists*. For many psychotropic drugs, sub-classes of a number of receptors exist, and under certain circumstances a drug may act as both a receptor agonist and antagonist. Table 15.5 lists some common neurotransmitters, their receptors and their functions.

TABLE 15.5 NEUROTRANSMITTERS, RECEPTORS AND FUNCTIONS

Neurotransmitter	Receptors	Function
Acetylcholine	Muscarinic (M1-M5) and nicotinic	Memory function, sensory processing, motor coordination and autonomic nervous system
Norepinephrine	Alpha1 and alpha2, beta1, beta2 and beta3	Central nervous system, sensory processing, cerebellar function, sleep, mood, learning, memory and anxiety
Dopamine	D1–D5	Motor regulation, reinforcement, olfaction, mood, concentration and hormone control
Serotonin (5-HT)	5-HT1–5-HT8	Emotional processing, mood, appetite, sleep, pain processing, hallucinations and reflex regulation
Glutamate	NMDA (N-methyl-D-aspartic acid)	Memory and excitory function in the central nervous system
Gamma aminobutyric acid (GABA)	GABA	Major inhibitory neurotransmitter in the central nervous system
Histamine	H1 and H2	Sleep, sedation and temperature regulation

Edward & Alderman (2013)

Factors influencing drug response

There is a considerable range of factors that determine the response to a given dose of a particular drug administered to an individual person—it is often said that no two people will respond exactly alike to the same treatment. Some of the inter-individual variations are explained by differences in drug disposition that are generated by pharmacokinetic factors that influence the serum concentrations, duration of effect and intensity of peak action (see Table 15.6). Even so, many other pharmacodynamic factors will also exert a key influence upon the response to treatment.

TABLE 15.6 EXAMPLES OF PHARMACOKINETIC FACTORS INFLUENCING DRUG RESPONSE

Factor	Example
Age	Children and older people may be particularly sensitive to the effects of drugs, and may respond differently despite a similar serum concentration.
Co-morbid disease states	Drug response may depend on the characteristics of the disease state being treated: advanced or chronic conditions may not respond in the same fashion. Some disease states predispose the consumer to drug effects not otherwise seen; for example, people with HIV may be more susceptible to adverse effects of some drugs.
Psychological factors	Psychological factors may have a profound effect upon drug response, but the basis for this is poorly understood. People with chronic pain may achieve better pain relief after treatment of depression. The administration of a product with no active ingredient (a placebo) may generate a measurable clinical response, or effects that are reported by a consumer (both adverse effects and therapeutic effects). Placebo response in clinical trials involving psychotropic drugs is high, creating complications in the interpretation of the findings of these studies.

In some cases, the dose of a drug that is used with the aim of creating a therapeutic benefit is not noticeably different from that which can produce potentially lethal adverse effects. These agents are commonly referred to as drugs of *low therapeutic index*, and must be used with particular caution for consumers who are otherwise predisposed to drug-related problems.

Adverse drug reactions and drug interactions

All drugs are associated with a degree of risk for adverse effects, sometimes referred to as side effects or adverse drug reactions (ADRs). A basic profile of ADRs is generally established in clinical trials before the marketing of a drug, but not all reactions are elucidated at this stage and are subsequently understood during the post-marketing surveillance process. This is important because subjects in clinical trials do not necessarily completely represent the broader population that a drug will be used for later; for example, older people, children, pregnant women and people with multiple medical co-morbidities generally are under-represented in clinical trials.

ADRs may be related to the mechanism by which the drug produces its therapeutic effects. In this context, the drug administered for a therapeutic effect may produce a response of unexpected or excessive intensity (for example, hypoglycaemia with insulin). In other situations, ADRs arise through pharmacological effects unrelated to the intended therapeutic actions of the drug (for example, anticholinergic effects associated with some antidepressants). In some cases, the risk of an ADR for an individual person cannot be predicted from a prior knowledge of the drug's pharmacology. 'Idiosyncratic' ADRs may be relatively minor (for example, mild pruritic skin rash after administration of morphine), but in some cases these reactions can be very serious indeed. Examples of idiosyncratic ADRs of major significance include hepatitis or jaundice, exfoliative skin rashes and blood dyscrasias. Most idiosyncratic

1 What are agonists?

2 What are the factors that determine the response to a given dose of a particular drug administered to an individual person?

CRITICAL THINKING OPPORTUNITY

ADRs are reproducible upon rechallenge, a very undesirable outcome if in relation to a serious ADR, emphasising the need for clear documentation of previous adverse drug reactions in medical records.

ADRs are more likely among those treated with more drugs; older people (who are often treated with multiple drugs) are at special risk for adverse drug reactions.

When the effects of one drug are altered by another, this is referred to as a drug interaction. Pharmacodynamic drug interactions occur when pharmacological effects shared by both drugs cause additive actions; for example, when two sedatives are combined, the subsequent extent of central nervous system suppression may be profound. Drug interactions also result from changes in the pharmacokinetics of one drug caused by another, usually where the effect of one drug changes the rate of elimination of another. This type of interaction often happens when the administration of a drug alters the hepatic metabolism of another agent, but it can also result from changes to renal elimination. Drug interactions are most likely to be clinically relevant when the medications are of low therapeutic index (for example, anticonvulsants, opioids, warfarin or lithium).

Prescribing and nurse practitioners

Prescribing medications is no longer the sole domain of medical practitioners and dentists. Prescribing rights have been extended to other health-care professionals such as nurse practitioners (NPs). This health-care reform is a way to improve the excellence and access of health-care services to consumers while simultaneously increasing consumer choices within health-care settings. The Nurse Prescribing and Initiating Classification builds upon work undertaken by the National Nursing and Nursing Education Taskforce (N3ET) in 2005 that examined nurse practitioner prescribing in Australia (Lenhardt et al., 1997; Sessler, 2001). Specifics such as drug dosage, drug indications and special precautions vary within Australia from state to state and territory. Different prescribing programs have been developed to enable nurses (including enrolled nurses) and midwives to initiate treatment with a limited range of medicines in each state and territory. However, at present, only nurse practitioners (and midwife practitioners in NSW) are authorised to independently prescribe medications (Edward & Alderman, 2013). In New Zealand, nurse practitioners also practise independently and in collaboration with other health professionals. In addition, they prescribe medicines within their own area of speciality, similar to the case as seen in Australia.

Administration and drug calculations

Drug calculations are an important aspect of nursing practice. There is great variation in undergraduate curricula relating to drug calculations, especially for psychotropic drugs. On the whole, and for many students, the education related to drug calculations is not comprehensive.

Drug calculations need to be accurate each time of potential administration. Important aspects of basic drug calculations relate to basic mathematical skills, knowledge of the correct drug calculation formulae and practice in a clinical setting. The metric system was introduced in New Zealand and Australia in 1969 and 1970, respectively. This system of measurement is also known as the International System of Units (SI). Basic units in this system include weight (gram), liquids (litre) and length (metre); with the symbols 'g', 'L' and 'm', respectively. Common variations to these measurements are one-millionth (micro), one-thousandth (milli) and one thousand times (kilo, such as kilogram in weight measurement and kilometre in length measurement).

Drug calculation formulae

You will need to organise your drug calculations information using the desired dose, concentration and volume on hand. You need to follow drug formulae when you begin your calculations as follows:

Example 1

The consumer is prescribed fluoxetine for their mood disorder at a dose of 20 mg BD. You have available in stock fluoxetine solution where the concentration is 20 mg/5 mL. What is the volume to be given to the consumer?

Answer: 5 mL BD

Example 2

The consumer is prescribed venlafaxine XR for depression and prescribed 75 mg per day in divided doses (at breakfast and dinner). You have in stock 37.5 mg capsules. What is the volume to be given to the consumer?

Answer: 1 capsule BD

Important aspects of psychotropic pharmacotherapy

Although effective, non-drug treatments including psychotherapies and electro-convulsive therapy (ECT) are used in the management of mental disorders, psychotropic pharmacotherapy is also widely used and is an effective treatment strategy in many cases. Detailed coverage of drug treatment in mental health is beyond the scope of a general resource such as this text, but a brief discussion of the medications used in the treatment of various important types of mental disorders is provided below.

Drug treatment for psychosis

Psychosis is a serious condition that requires a holistic management approach. Drug treatment is the cornerstone of therapy: the agents used are referred to by a variety of names (for example, major tranquillisers and neuroleptics), but the term 'antipsychotic drug' is the most appropriate, reflecting the purpose for which the drugs are prescribed and the appropriate means by which response to treatment can be assessed.

The antipsychotic drugs have their origins in the early 1950s, an era that saw the introduction of drugs such as chlorpromazine and haloperidol. Many other of these first generation antipsychotic drugs followed, and included thioridazine, trifluoperazine, fluphenazine and others. These drugs are sometimes referred to as conventional or typical antipsychotics, and many remain in use today, although other, newer drugs have largely superseded these agents in developed nations. Like all antipsychotics, the first generation agents reduce the positive symptoms of schizophrenia, but negative symptoms may be relatively refractory (and may be worsened). First generation antipsychotics are often sedating agents, especially drugs such as chlorpromazine and pericyazine. Alpha-adrenergic blockade causing a tendency to postural hypotension and falls is also a problem with these drugs. Anticholinergic effects may contribute to delirium, constipation, dry mouth (xerostomia), urinary hesitancy and blurred vision.

Newer antipsychotics such as olanzapine, risperidone, quetiapine and ziprasidone—as well as less commonly used agents such as amisulpride, aripiprazole, clozapine, paliperidone, quetiapine, risperidone, asenepine and sertindole—are collectively referred to as second-generation antipsychotics or atypical antipsychotics. The use of atypical antipsychotics is the usual standard of care for schizophrenia. Receptor interactions with these agents are complex, involving dopamine D2 receptor blockade but also additional blockade at different receptors including dopamine D1 and D4, and subtype of serotonin receptor (serotonin 5HT2A). The most effective atypical antipsychotic is clozapine, but the use of this drug is limited because of the possibility of life-threatening adverse effects. Potentially fatal agranulocytosis occurring in up to 4 per cent of all consumers has required a structured monitoring system to be implemented where this agent is used. Consumers must have regular and frequent complete blood tests to ensure that the white blood cell count remains normal. Serious cardiac effects such as myocarditis and cardiomyopathy resulting in death or the need for cardiac transplantation are also known side effects of the drug (also see Table 15.7). Clozapine is for this reason restricted to management of treatment-resistant cases. In comparison to the older drugs, atypical agents are as effective for the positive symptoms of schizophrenia, but generally more effective for negative symptoms. An additional characteristic shared by most of the atypical agents is a lesser likelihood of extrapyramidal side effects.

A new development in the treatment of psychosis has recently come about because it is now understood that the underlying pathophysiology of psychosis is more complicated than previously anticipated. The understanding of the molecular biology of psychosis has expanded, elucidating the contributory role of serotonin in the aetiology of psychosis. Pimavanserin, a selective inverse agonist with significant selectivity for the serotonin 5-HT2A receptor, has recently been approved for use in specific types of psychosis (most importantly, as a treatment for psychosis associated with Parkinson's disease), and as an adjuvant agent to be used in combination with other antipsychotic agents. Importantly, pimavanserin has no significant affinity for dopamine receptors, challenging the prevailing paradigm for antipsychotic drug action. It is anticipated that a new wave of drug therapy options for the management of psychosis will now follow the introduction of pimavanserin, perhaps offering new hope in cases where an individual has a psychotic illness that has been resistant to the treatment options that have been available to date.

All antipsychotic drugs have the potential to cause adverse effects, and these may cause serious drug-related harm in some cases. It is also important to understand that the occurrence of adverse effects can also have a significant adverse impact upon adherence to the medication regimen. Adverse effects associated with antipsychotics can be divided into extrapyramidal side effects and metabolic side effects.

Extrapyramidal side effects

Extrapyramidal side effects (EPSE) are much less common with atypical drugs. They arise through dopaminergic blockade and are dose-related, and may be very distressing for the consumer. EPSE are often manageable with anticholinergic drugs, although it is best to avoid these agents for long-term use. Various EPSE include the following:

- Dystonas (dystonia) may be described as muscle cramps or spasm in the face, neck, trunk and limbs. It can have a rapid, acute onset. Examples include torticollis, retrocollis, carpopedal spasm, trismus and perioral spasm. Serious dystonias include oculogyric crisis, laryngeal spasm and opisthotonos, and are medical emergencies.
- Akathisia is a subjective sensation of restlessness. It can be difficult to differentiate between akathisia and psychotic agitation. Akathisia will usually improve with dose reduction and deteriorate when the dose is increased. It is not usually responsive to anticholinergic drugs, but may respond to low dose propranolol.

TABLE 15.7 SELECTED PRESCRIBING CONSIDERATIONS FOR VARIOUS ANTIPSYCHOTIC DRUGS

Drug	Dosage and formulations*	Clinical characteristics*
Amisulpride	Tablet, oral liquid: acute dose 200–400 mg twice daily, decrease for maintenance	Thought to be more likely than other atypical agents to cause parkinsonian side effects. Dosage adjustment required in renal impairment.
Aripiprazole	Tablet: 15–30 mg daily	Partial dopamine agonist. May have a higher incidence of akathisia than other atypical agents.
Asenepine	Wafer: 5–10 mg twice daily	Consumer should not eat or drink for 10 minutes after administration.
Chlorpromazine	Tablet, oral liquid: variable, up to 1000 mg daily for acute psychosis Short-acting injection 25–50 mg every 6–8 hours by deep IM injection for management of acute psychiatric emergency	Associated with photosensitivity rash. Very sedating, significant anticholinergic effects, prominent orthostasis. Poorly tolerated by the elderly. IV injection can cause catastrophic hypotension; IM injection causes significant orthostasis and is associated with injection site pain and development of sterile abscess.
Clozapine	Tablet, oral liquid: slowly titrated to usual dose range of 200–600 mg daily, max 900 mg daily; response may correlate with serum concentrations	Significant adverse effects; although regarded as the most clinically effective antipsychotic, serious reactions such as agranulocytosis, myocarditis and seizures mean that this agent is not used for first-line treatment (reserved for severe/refractory causes and used with intensive monitoring). Weight gain and metabolic dysregulation with hyperglycaemia/diabetes/dyslipidaemia are frequently observed. Significant drug interactions occur including decrease in serum concentration with carbamazepine, increased serum concentration with fluvoxamine and also after smoking cessation.
Droperidol	Short-acting injection: IM/IV injection of 5–25 mg for extreme psychotic or manic agitation	Potential for QT prolongation and serious arrhythmias. Avoid concurrent use with other agents that prolong the QT interval.
Flupenthixol	Long-acting depot injection: usual dose 20–40 mg every two weeks by deep IM injection	Delayed onset of action—not suitable for management of acute psychotic agitation.
Fluphenazine	Long-acting depot injection: usual dose 12.5–50 mg every two weeks by deep IM injection	Delayed onset of action—not suitable for management of acute psychotic agitation.
Haloperidol	Tablet, oral liquid: up to 30 mg daily in two or three divided doses Short-acting injection: 2–10 mg IMI repeated as needed for psychotic agitation Long-acting depot injection: usual dose 50–100 mg every four weeks by deep IM injection	Prominently associated with parkinsonian side effects. High potential for tardive dyskinesia. Unlikely to cause orthostasis.

CHRIS ALDERMAN AND KAREN-LEIGH EDWARD

Drug	Dosage and formulations*	Clinical characteristics*
Olanzapine	Tablet, oral liquid: up to 20 mg daily in 2 or 3 divided doses Short-acting injection: 5–10 mg IM repeated as needed for psychotic agitation (max 30 mg/24 hours) Long-acting depot injection: usual dose 210–300 mg every two weeks by deep IM injection	Most sedating of the atypical agents. Weight gain and metabolic dysregulation with hyperglycaemia/diabetes/dyslipidaemia are frequently observed. Significant drug interactions occur including decrease in serum concentration with carbamazepine, increased serum concentration with fluvoxamine and also after smoking cessation. Oral wafers may be used to enhance likelihood of adherence in acute psychosis. Monitor for post-injection delirium for three hours after injection of long-acting depot product.
Paliperidone	Slow-release tablet: 3–12 mg daily Long-acting depot injection: titrate to maintenance dose of 25–150 mg monthly	Closely related to risperidone.
Pericyazine	Tablet: antipsychotic dose of 30 mg daily in divided doses	Often used at more moderate doses for sedative and anxiolytic effects.
Quetiapine	Tablet: 300–800 mg daily in divided doses	Sustained-release formulation may be administered once daily.
Risperidone	Tablet, wafer, oral liquid: titrate to 2–8 mg daily in divided doses Long-acting injection: 25–50 mg every two weeks	Associated with significant hyperprolactinaemia and metabolic disturbance. Long-acting injection must be stored in refrigeration.
Sertindole	Tablet: Initially 4 mg once daily titrated as needed to maximum of 12–20 mg daily	Potential for QT interval prolongation and serious arrhythmias. Avoid concurrent use with other agents that prolong the QT interval.
Trifluoperazine	Tablet, oral liquid: 2–15 mg twice daily	First generation agent associated with high incidence of parkinsonism, tardive dyskinesia, metabolic disturbance/weight gain.
Ziprasidone	Capsule: 40 mg twice, titrated to maximum of 80 mg twice daily if needed Short-acting injection: 10–20 mg every four hours to a maximum of 40 mg daily, duration no greater than two or three days	Evidence suggests least likelihood of weight gain or metabolic dysregulation. Take capsules with food.
Zuclopenthixol	Tablet: 10–15 mg daily in divided doses Intermediate-acting injection: 50–150 mg every two or three days Long-acting injection: 200–400 mg every 2–4 weeks	Caution is required to ensure that the correct dosage form is selected.

*Note that this is not a comprehensive guide—refer to reference texts and manufacturers' information.

- Parkinsonism (also referred to as pseudoparkinsonism or parkinsonian side effects) may resemble idiopathic Parkinson's disease. Features include tremor, rigidity or bradykinesia. It may necessitate treatment with an anticholinergic drug such as benztropine.
- Tardive dyskinesia (TD) is an abnormal involuntary movement syndrome commonly affecting the face, mouth or tongue, and occasionally the head, neck, trunk or limbs. It is most commonly observed after extended treatment, and more common with the older agents than atypicals. It is potentially irreversible.
- Neuroleptic malignant syndrome (NMS) is a potentially fatal condition with fulminant symptoms including fever, rigidity and autonomic instability. Plasma creatine kinase (CK) concentration may be elevated.

Metabolic side effects

Metabolic side effects such as weight gain associated with antipsychotic drug treatment are very common. Clozapine and olanzapine are the drugs most likely to be associated with weight gain, and in some cases the extent and rate of increased body mass index (BMI) can be rapid and extreme. Dietary advice and lifestyle assessment and assistance must be provided. Antipsychotic drugs increase the risk of hyperglycaemia and diabetes mellitus. Clozapine and olanzapine are prominently associated with abnormal glucose tolerance. Similarly, antipsychotic drug treatment confers additional risk of dyslipidaemia. With impaired glucose tolerance, elevated lipids and obesity—plus a sedentary lifestyle and a high prevalence of smoking—the risk for cardiovascular disease is significant.

There is now research examining pharmacological treatment options that may mitigate the metabolic impact of antipsychotic drug treatment. One agent that appears to be promising for this purpose is metformin (although this drug has been widely used for the treatment of type 2 diabetes for many years, it appears that the beneficial effects in protecting against the metabolic effects of antipsychotics can be achieved for people who do not have diabetes). Another agent showing promise as a preventative measure against the metabolic impact of antipsychotic treatment is the anticonvulsant drug topiramate, which was noted to be associated with weight loss during clinical trials.

Other metabolic effects such as hyperprolactinaemia are associated with antipsychotic drug treatment. Hyperprolactinaemia causes secondary complications such as gynaecomastia, galactorrhoea, abnormal menses and anovulation, as well as sexual dysfunction. Hyperprolactinaemia may also reduce bone mineral density and contribute to the development of osteopaenia or osteoporosis.

Drug treatment for affective disorders

'Mood disorders' and 'affective disorders' are terms that are sometimes used interchangeably, primarily because the terms 'mood' and 'affect' are closely related but describe slightly dissimilar occurrences. Mood is used to describe a person's main state of emotions or feelings (subjective experience), while affect is more suitably used to describe the external manifestation of the current internal emotional state of the person (objective observation). Mood disorders consist of depression and bipolar affective disorders.

■ TOPIC LINK

See Chapter 10 for more on mood disorders.

Depression

Non-drug treatments are useful for the management of major depression; however, drug therapy is the most commonly employed treatment modality. The drugs of use for this purpose are referred to as antidepressants or antidepressant agents/drugs. These agents/drugs are also used for anxiety disorders and some eating disorders. There are differences between individual agents (such as adverse effects, drug interactions, suitability for specific consumer populations and toxicity in overdose), but the overall safety, tolerability and effectiveness are broadly similar for most drugs and drug classes. Various factors may influence the selection of an antidepressant for an individual consumer, and are represented in Figure 15.3. For example, the presence of a specific medical condition may mean that a particular drug would not be effective or advisable—a man with prostatomegaly should not be treated with a highly anticholinergic tricyclic antidepressant (TCA) because of the risk of urinary hesitancy or retention. Drug interactions will need to be taken into account with respect to the other drug treatment a person might already be treated with.

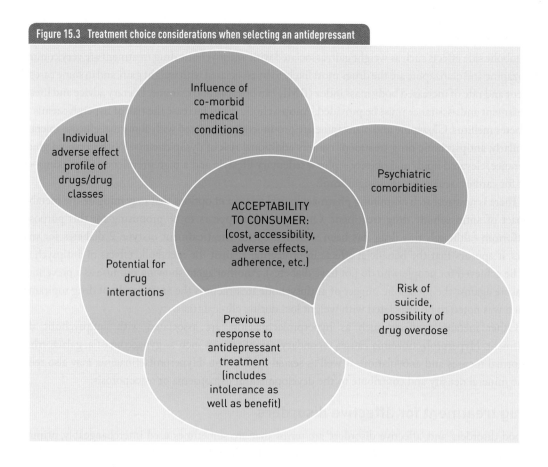

Figure 15.3 Treatment choice considerations when selecting an antidepressant

Influence of co-morbid medical conditions

Individual adverse effect profile of drugs/drug classes

Psychiatric comorbidities

ACCEPTABILITY TO CONSUMER: (cost, accessibility, adverse effects, adherence, etc.)

Potential for drug interactions

Risk of suicide, possibility of drug overdose

Previous response to antidepressant treatment (includes intolerance as well as benefit)

An important drug interaction that needs to be considered is serotonin toxicity, caused by an excess of serotonergic activity and reflected by symptoms of neuromuscular excitation, autonomic stimulation and mental status changes. Antidepressants that can cause serotonin toxicity include such medications as SSRIs, TCAs and MAOIs, as well as non-antidepressant agents such as pethidine, tramadol, the herbal supplement St John's Wort and illicit substances (for example, MDMA or 'ecstasy'). The term 'serotonin toxicity' has come to replace the previously used terminology, 'serotonin syndrome', largely because significantly dangerous/disabling symptoms can be present in some cases without the case satisfying a full suite of syndromal requirements.

Antidepressant interactions can also have a pharmacokinetic basis, where the effects of one drug alter the clearance of another. For instance, some anticonvulsants increase the rate of hepatic drug metabolism, compromising the effectiveness of many antidepressants. SSRIs can inhibit the hepatic metabolism of other drugs, producing unintended toxicity. Examples include pronounced methadone or clozapine toxicity after treatment with fluvoxamine, or enhanced beta blockade with metoprolol if combined with paroxetine or fluoxetine.

Some antidepressants are very toxic in overdose and should be avoided in cases where there is high risk of suicide, or a history of past drug overdose. The safest drugs to use under these circumstances are the SSRIs or moclobemide.

Treatment with antidepressants usually involves a standard dose for three or four weeks, after which there may be consideration of a dosage increase. If there is little response, or intolerable side effects, the usual approach would be to switch to a different drug or to add an augmentation agent (for example, lithium or an atypical antipsychotic).

Bipolar affective disorder

Pharmacotherapy for bipolar disorder is complex, and is often initiated and supervised by a specialist psychiatrist. Treatment goals include management of episodes of mood disturbance and ongoing prophylaxis against further episodes of depression or mania.

The primary aim when treating mania is to promptly control symptoms of abnormally elevated mood. This is usually undertaken using medications: if symptoms are severe or there are prominent psychotic features, antipsychotic drugs are the mainstay of the management approach. Commonly used agents are olanzapine (up to 20 mg daily), quetiapine (up to 800 mg daily in divided doses), risperidone (up to 6 mg daily) or ziprasidone (80 mg twice daily). Concurrent treatment with a benzodiazepine medication can be used to potentate sedation.

The other approach to the management of mania involves the use of mood stabiliser medications. It is common to combine mood stabiliser treatment with antipsychotics and benzodiazepines during an episode of acute mania, and later phase out treatment of antipsychotics after euthymia (or near euthymia) has been achieved. Mood stabiliser medications are usually left in place as part of the prophylactic approach to treatment. The mood stabiliser drugs used for acute mania are lithium, sodium valproate (also called valproic acid or divalproex sodium) and carbamazepine.

Bipolar disorder also involves episodes of major depression. Treatment of depression in bipolar disorder is the same as that used for major depressive disorder, with standard treatment approaches including antidepressants, electro-convulsive therapy and psychological treatments. Currently evidence suggests that maintenance of antidepressant therapy does not reduce the likelihood, severity, refractoriness or duration of depressive episodes in bipolar disorder. Also, treatment-emergent affective switch (sometimes referred to as 'manic switch') can cause a consumer to switch from depression to mania, hypomania or a mixed episode: antidepressants should be stopped and management of elevated mood implemented.

Prophylactic mood stabiliser treatment is used to reduce the frequency, duration and severity of episodes of mania and depression. Lithium, valproate, carbamazepine, lamotrigine, olanzapine and quetiapine are all effective for this purpose, although lithium continues to be regarded as the treatment of choice. Lamotrigine may be preferred where episodes of major depression are predominant. Combinations involving lithium with an anticonvulsant may be used for those with refractory illness. Lithium can cause serious toxicities if the serum concentration is not maintained within the reference range, and nurses can play an important role in educating consumers about the early signs of toxicity.

CHRIS ALDERMAN AND KAREN-LEIGH EDWARD

TABLE 15.8 STANDARD DAILY DOSES* FOR A RANGE OF ANTIDEPRESSANTS

	Starting dose (mg)	Maintenance (mg)	Maximum (mg)
SSRIs			
Citalopram	10	20	40
Escitalopram	5	10	20
Fluoxetine	10–20	20–30	60
Paroxetine	10–20	20–30	50
Sertraline	25–50	50–100	200
Fluvoxamine	50	50–100	200
TCAs			
Amitriptyline	25–50	50–150	300
Clomipramine	25–50	75–150	300
Dothiepin	25–50	75–150	300
Doxepin	25–50	75–150	300
Imipramine	25–50	75–150	300
Nortriptyline	25–50	75–150	150
Trimipramine	25–50	75–150	300
MAOIs			
Phenelzine**	15–30	30–60	90
Tranylcypromine**	10–20	20–40	60
Moclobemide**	300	600	600
Other			
Agomelatine	25	25–50	50
Bupropion	150	300**	300**
Desvenlafaxine	50	50–100	200
Duloxetine	30	30–60	90
Mirtazapine	15	30	45–60
Reboxetine**	8	10	12
Venlafaxine	75	75–225	375**

*Doses may require adjustment for renal or hepatic impairment. More conservative doses should be used for children and the elderly. Caution is needed in the presence of polypharmacy or multiple medical co-morbidities.

**Administered in divided doses.

Drug treatment for anxiety disorders

Non-pharmacological treatments are often the preferred first-line approach for the management of anxiety disorders, but pharmacotherapy can also prove to be very helpful, particularly where the symptoms are refractory to another therapy. The drugs used for anxiety disorders are also used for other mental and medical disorders, but dosage titration and duration of treatment need to be tailored to accommodate the specific issues to be addressed with anxiety disorders. It is also important to acknowledge that there is a high prevalence of associated substance disorders among people with anxiety disorders, creating a range of additional challenges in pharmacotherapy.

People with anxiety disorders will often present seeking treatment to address somatic complaints such as muscular tension headache, nausea, constipation or diarrhoea, tachycardia and insomnia. Partly because of this, people with severe anxiety disorders may use strong analgesic and hypnosedative drugs with considerable potential for drug abuse, dependence and withdrawal, which is especially dangerous if there is co-morbid alcohol use.

Drugs with potent anti-anxiety effects such as the benzodiazepines (for example, diazepam, oxazepam and alprozolam) produce rapid anxiolytic effects, but these agents have potential disadvantages. Benzodiazepines have potential for abuse, dependence, tolerance and withdrawal, producing potentially serious physiological and psychological adverse effects. Unpleasant withdrawal effects can make it difficult to discontinue treatment, and there may be serious medical complications such as withdrawal seizures if the discontinuation process is not appropriately managed. Sometimes people may visit a number of prescribers to obtain the drugs ('doctor shopping'). Benzodiazepines do not alter the underlying psychopathology associated with serious anxiety disorders, instead offering only temporary alleviation of anxious moods or symptoms such as sleep disturbance. When the effects of the benzodiazepines wear off, symptoms usually return and more benzodiazepine is required. Long-term treatment with benzodiazepines is often associated with tolerance and tachyphylaxis (greater doses needed to achieve the same effect), leading to dose escalation and the continuation of treatment for longer than initially intended. The hazards of injudicious use of benzodiazepines for symptomatic management of an anxiety disorder are represented in Figure 15.4.

An in-depth discussion of the detailed management of each of the different types of anxiety disorders is beyond the scope of a generalist text. Selected aspects for clinically important anxiety disorders include the following.

■ TOPIC LINK

See Chapter 10 for more on anxiety disorders.

Generalised anxiety disorder (GAD)

Excessive anxiety or worrying is present on more days than not, extending over a period of six months or more and concerning a range of specific events or activities. It is difficult or impossible to control, and features restlessness, easy fatigability, difficulty with concentration, irritability, muscle tension or sleep disturbance.

First-line treatment approaches include psychoeducation, relaxation techniques and positive coping skills, supplemented with ongoing supportive psychotherapy or CBT. During periods of severe or acute exacerbations, symptoms may be managed with long-acting benzodiazepine (for example, diazepam 5–15 mg daily). Short-acting, rapid onset drugs such as alprazolam should be avoided. Commonly used antidepressants for management of GAD are SSRIs and venlafaxine or duloxetine.

Panic disorder

This relatively common form of anxiety disorder is often accompanied by agoraphobia (fear of having a panic attack in a social place, which would be difficult and embarrassing to escape from, and leads

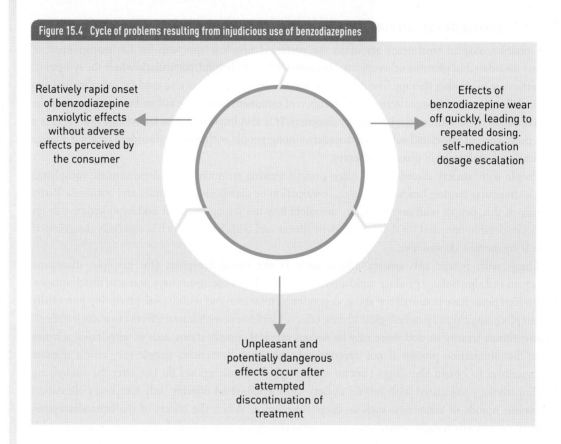

Figure 15.4 Cycle of problems resulting from injudicious use of benzodiazepines

Relatively rapid onset of benzodiazepine anxiolytic effects without adverse effects perceived by the consumer

Effects of benzodiazepine wear off quickly, leading to repeated dosing. self-medication dosage escalation

Unpleasant and potentially dangerous effects occur after attempted discontinuation of treatment

to avoidance). Symptoms include recurrent, unexpected panic attacks, at least one month of persistent apprehension about the possibility of further attacks, worry about implications of attacks and significant behavioural changes.

CBT is the first-line treatment. Drug therapy involves the use of SSRIs or venlafaxine, commencing at a modest dose with slow upward titration. Drug treatment for panic disorder will usually need to continue for up to a year, usually combined with non-drug treatment. If benzodiazepines have been prescribed for symptomatic treatment, it is very important to gradually decrease the dosage, if possible using a long-half-life agent.

Post-traumatic stress disorder (PTSD)

This is a serious anxiety disorder that occurs after exposure to extremely traumatic stressful events or circumstances, often involving actual or threatened death or serious injury, or witnessing a horrendous event that could involve death or injury. Responses involve intense fear, helplessness or horror. Key symptoms clusters include re-experiencing phenomena, avoidance and hyperarousal.

First-line therapy should be non-pharmacological with specialised CBT techniques, including strategies such as graded exposure therapy involving desensitisation. SSRIs are now accepted as first-line drug treatment for PTSD, and other antidepressants (mirtazapine and venlafaxine) may also be used. The addition of an anticonvulsant mood stabiliser drug may prove helpful where there is severe hyperarousal and angry outbursts. Topiramate, prazosin, propranolol and atypical antipsychotics (for example, quetiapine or olanzapine) may be used under specialist supervision.

Obsessive-compulsive disorder (OCD)

Symptoms include recurrent obsessions or compulsions that are time-consuming, distressing or cause significant impairment. People with OCD recognise that the obsessions and compulsions are excessive or unreasonable, and include persistent thoughts, impulses or images that the person perceives to be intrusive or inappropriate. Obsessional themes are commonly centred on contamination, repeated doubts (Is the door locked? Are the appliances turned off?) or the need for specific ordering of objects. In response to the obsessions, the person attempts to ignore or suppress such thoughts or impulses, or to neutralise them with a corresponding thought or action—a compulsion such as repetitive behaviours or mental acts.

Non-drug therapy may be used for OCD, but drug treatment is usually required. First-line pharmacotherapy is high-dose SSRIs. Alternatives include high-dose venlafaxine or the tricyclic antidepressant clomipramine.

Drug treatment for other mental disorders

Pharmacotherapy has proven efficacy in a range of other mental disorders, in some cases primarily for the purpose of symptom relief, but in others the treatment is directed at the underlying mental illness itself. A general textbook cannot provide in-depth coverage of the full range of situations in which psychotropic pharmacotherapy may prove to be helpful, but examples include the use of:

- SSRI drugs for some eating disorders such as bulimia nervosa
- abstinence-promoting agents such as naltrexone and acamprosate in the treatment of dependence upon alcohol and some other drugs
- cholinesterase inhibitors such as donepezil, rivastigmine and galantamine—as well as other agents such as memantine—to address cognitive dysfunction that might be seen in dementia illness such as Alzheimer's disease, Lewy body dementia and vascular dementia
- amphetamines and other stimulant medications for children with attention deficit hyperactivity disorder (ADHD)
- psychotropic drugs as a part of a broader composite approach to the management of chronic pain.

The exploration of the pharmacology of orexin modulators is expected to deliver significant new drug therapy options over the next decade. Sub-types of orexin receptors are through to govern various human functions such as sleep modulation and appetite. The first of the agents relating to clinical effects of orexin, suvorexant, has recently been approved by the US Food and Drug Administration for the management of insomnia.

Adherence and recovery

Adherence, compliance, and concordance are related terms. Compliance is the oldest of the terminologies and, put in simple terms, has been used to refer to the extent to which a person follows instructions with respect to medications or other treatment instructions. Having lost favour in modern practice because of paternalistic overtones not consistent with quality use of medicines principles (focused upon the primacy of consumer views) the term 'compliance' has eventually been replaced with other concepts. The World Health Organization (WHO) has ultimately adopted the term 'adherence' to refer to the extent to which a consumer follows medical instructions (WHO, 2003, p. 3), such as using medications or adopting a specific diet or other lifestyle principles recommended by health-care providers.

The idea of 'recovery' has been part of the terminology of health services for the last few decades. The recovery model adopted in such countries as the UK, Ireland, Australia, New Zealand, the USA and Canada puts the consumer at the centre of care. There has been a lack of consensus on the meaning of recovery, since the notion of recovery can be seen from many viewpoints, such as an individual and self-determined recovery, the absence of symptoms, a return to premorbid functioning, the ability to fulfil roles and obligations, or a stable sense of well-being and quality of life.

'Concordance' is a relatively modern term that is used to represent the extent of agreement between a consumer and clinician with respect to the plans for therapy. Implicit in the practice of concordance is working with the consumer's beliefs about their condition and treatment. The key elements of a concordance approach are working collaboratively and with flexibility, working with the beliefs that consumers have about medication and medication regimens, and working towards agreed goals towards addressing non-adherent medication behaviours the consumer may be experiencing. This is a shared decision-making approach and involves the consumer at the centre of care. Shared decision-making is suitable for long-term decisions, especially in the context of a chronic illness (Edward & Alderman, 2013).

In terms of adherence, there are many factors that have an impact upon medication adherence, and these have specific and considerable relevance in relation to the successful treatment of mental disorders. Evidence suggests that people in the general population, including those with mental illness, are at risk of non-adherence; and non-adherence can have profound negative impact upon treatment outcomes. The health belief model (Kasl, 1974) goes part of the way to elucidating some of the factors that may be influential with respect to psychotropic drug adherence. Briefly, factors that are positive influences upon adherence include experience of daily benefit, lack of adverse effects that have meaning for the consumer, maintenance of supportive relationships and infrastructure, and minimal exposure to illicit drug use. On the other hand, as might be expected, the absence of perceived benefits, severe adverse effects, loss of supportive relationships and infrastructure, and extensive exposure to illicit drugs will usually compromise adherence and negatively affect treatment outcomes for individuals. Overlaying these factors are many other issues that can adversely affect adherence. The characteristics of mental illness may lead to a lack of insight or impaired judgment that can reduce the likelihood that medications are taken as intended. Additionally, cultural and/or religious factors can affect belief systems. The simple matter of access to medications can be highly influential: if a person cannot get to a dispensary to have a prescription filled (perhaps because of disability or geographical isolation), or cannot afford to have a prescription filled, adherence will be compromised.

Adherence can present a special problem when dealing with a consumer affected by psychosis. Pharmacotherapy may be delivered in the context of a community treatment order (CTO) that compels a consumer to receive treatment at an approved place. Long-acting depot formulations of drugs such as risperidone, paliperidone, haloperidol, fluphenzaine, flupenthixol, olanzapine or zuclopenthixol are used for this purpose, and indeed may also be useful even if a CTO is not required.

If adherence is compromised, evidence suggests that response to treatment will also be compromised and outcomes will be poorer. Nurses and other health professionals such as pharmacists can provide crucial support in the form of psychoeducation and medication management services. These approaches have been proven to improve both adherence and treatment outcomes and recovery.

A relatively new term has recently entered the technical lexicon relating to adherence. The extent to which therapeutic success sensitive under imperfect adherence is driven by the property known as 'forgiveness'. Ultimately, it is possible that drug development will become more focused upon forgiveness, meaning that the reality of occasional missed doses of a drug may not be so critical to the success of treatment.

SUMMARY

Psychotropic drug therapy is a fundamental element of the range of treatment modalities used for the management of nearly all mental disorders. New treatments in psychiatry have developed rapidly and will continue to emerge. A multidisciplinary approach to the use of drug treatment is required, involving nurses, medical staff and other relevant people such as pharmacists. It is incumbent upon all nurses working in the mental health field to establish, maintain and expand a working understanding of the principles of psychotropic pharmacotherapy, and to be able to access appropriate resources to optimise the safe and effective use of medicines for therapy of people affected by serious mental disorders.

DISCUSSION QUESTIONS

1   What is meant by the term 'drug-related problem'?

2   Discuss examples whereby various health professionals may contribute specific expertise in designing and implementing pharmacotherapy for those with mental illness.

3   Which aspects of pharmacokinetics can be used in the nursing assessment and evaluation processes?

4   Describe two different types of adverse drug reactions.

5   What are the standard pharmacotherapy options that are used for the management of major depression?

TEST YOURSELF

1   Pharmacotherapy is:

   a   fundamental in the treatment of all cases of mental disorders

   b   unusual in the treatment of a large proportion of all cases of mental disorders

   c   fundamental in the treatment of a large proportion of all cases of mental disorders

   d   all of the above

2   What is medication-related harm?

   a   Any undesirable event experienced by the consumer that involves or is suspected to involve drug therapy, potentially interfering with desired outcomes

   b   Harm that focuses exclusively on adverse drug reactions at the organisational level

   c   Harm that is only actual medication-related harm

   d   All of the above

3   The medicines management pathway cycle:

   a   is related to medications for consumers that include such activities as consumer medication adherence, followed by prescribing, reviewing, issuing, administering, monitoring and communicating

   b   is the complex interplay related to medications for consumers including such activities as decision to treat, followed by prescribing, reviewing, issuing, administering, monitoring and communicating

   c   includes such activities as adverse drug reactions, side effects of medication, preference of administration for consumers and family shared decision making related to medication management

   d   is a pathway only available in New Zealand

CHRIS ALDERMAN AND KAREN-LEIGH EDWARD

4   Pharmacokinetics is the term that:

a   refers to blood vessels that form a part of the hepatic portal circulation system

b   describes drugs that only produce a therapeutic effect after entering the systemic circulation and accessing the site of action

c   describes reversible movements of drugs within the body, usually from one compartment to another

d   is used to refer to the science of the disposition of drugs and metabolites in the body

USEFUL WEBSITES

Beyondblue—Anxiety: https://www.beyondblue.org.au/the-facts/anxiety

Healthline—Drug interactions: www.healthline.com/druginteractions

Merck Manual—Overview of pharmacodynamics www.merckmanuals.com/professional/clinical_pharmacology/pharmacodynamics/overview_of_pharmacodynamics.html

National Institute of Mental Health: Anxiety disorders: www.nimh.nih.gov/health/topics/anxiety-disorders/index.shtml

Pharmaceutical Management Agency of New Zealand (PHARMAC): www.pharmac.health.nz

PubMed Health—Major depression: www.ncbi.nlm.nih.gov/pubmedhealth/PMH0001941

QUMMAP—Mapping quality medicine use initiatives: https://www.nps.org.au/australian-prescriber/articles/quality-use-of-medicines-are-we-nearly-there-yet

Sane Australia—Bipolar disorder: www.sane.org/information/factsheets-podcasts/199-bipolar-disorder

World Health Organization—Adverse drug reactions monitoring: www.who.int/medicines/areas/quality_safety/safety_efficacy/advdrugreactions/en

REFERENCES

Department of Health and Ageing (2002). *The national strategy for quality use of medicines.* Canberra: DoHA.

Department of Health and Ageing (2010). *National medicines policy.* Canberra: DoHA. Retrieved from www.health.gov.au/internet/main/publishing.nsf/Content/National+Medicines+Policy-1.

Edward, K., & Alderman, C. (2013). *Psychopharmacology: Contexts and current practices.* Melbourne: Oxford University Press.

Frances, A. (2013). Saving normal: An insider's revolt against out-of-control psychiatric diagnosis, DSM-5, big pharma and the medicalization of ordinary life. *Psychotherapy in Australia, 19*(3), 14.

Kasl, S. V. (1974). The health belief model and behavior related to chronic illness. *Health Education & Behavior, 2*(4), 433–454.

Krystal, J., Tolin, D., Sanacora, G., Castner, S., Williams, G., Aikins, D. E., Hoffman, R. E., & D'Souza, D. C. (2009). Neuroplasticity as a target for the pharmacotherapy of anxiety disorders, mood disorders, and schizophrenia. *Drug Discovery Today, 14*(13–14), 690–697. doi: 10.1016/j.drudis.2009.05.002.

Lenhardt, R., Marker, E., Goll, V., Tschernich, H., Kurz, A., Sessler, D. I., Lackner, F. (1997). Mild intraoperative hypothermia prolongs postanesthetic recovery. *Anesthesiology, 87*(6), 1318–1323.

Sessler, D. I. (2001). Complications and treatment of mild hypothermia. *Anesthesiology, 95*(2), 531–543.

Strand, L. M., Morley, P. C., Cipolle, R. J., Ramsey, R., & Lamsam, G. D. (1990). Drug-related problems: Their structure and function. *DICP, 24*(11), 1093–1097.

World Health Organization (2003). *Adherence to long-term therapies: Evidence for action.* Geneva: WHO.

CHAPTER 16

The Older Person

ROBYN GARLICK

Acknowledgment

The authors would like to acknowledge Susan Koch who co-wrote this chapter in the first edition of this text and Helen Rawson for co-writing in the second edition.

KEY OUTCOMES

AFTER READING THIS CHAPTER, YOU SHOULD BE ABLE TO:

- discuss the prevalence of depression, dementia and delirium in older adults

- describe the most appropriate methods for screening processes to differentiate clinical features of depression, dementia and delirium in the older adult

- identify delirium, dementia and depression and the overlapping clinical features that may coexist in the older adult

- describe the implications of medication, multiple co-morbidities and chronic illnesses on older persons with a mental illness

- identify differences caused by masking of symptoms in psychosis, anxiety, depression and dementia

- describe the risks, signs and symptoms and assessment of suicide in the older person.

KEY TERMS

- behavioural and psychological symptoms of dementia (BPSD)
- delirium
- dementia
- depression
- hoarding
- person-centred care
- pharmacological management

Introduction

In this chapter you will explore the ageing population of Australia and New Zealand, the causes of mental illness in this population and its impact upon health, mental health services provision and the main illnesses seen in older adults. Depression, delirium, dementia, anxiety and amnestic conditions are discussed. Medication issues specific to the older person and the interplay between physical health and mental illness is further explored. The key component of care provision is person-centred care: the treatment and care provided by health services that places the person at the centre of their own care and considers the needs of the older person's carers (Victorian Department of Human Services, 2006).

The ageing population

In Australia, between 1995 and 2015 the number of persons aged 65 years and over increased from 11.9 per cent to 15 per cent of the population; those aged 85 years and over increased by 148 per cent; and the number of centenarians increased by 254 per cent. These figures compare with a total population increase of 32.1 per cent over the same period, according to the Australian Bureau of Statistics (2015a). The country of birth is also changing, with more people born overseas moving into each of the age groups over 65 than those under 65 years (Australian Bureau of Statistics, 2012).

In New Zealand significant change in the age structure is also occurring, with the number of people over 65 doubling between 1984 and 2014, with the expectation that this demographic will double again by 2039, according to Statistics New Zealand (2016). The largest growth period began in 2011 and will continue to 2037 as baby boomers (people born immediately after the Second World War) move into the over-65 age group. This age group will account for up to 26 per cent of the New Zealand population by 2068 (Statistics New Zealand, 2016). By 2068, half the population could be older than 45 years.

Population ageing is a significant feature of most developed countries and is related to both sustained low fertility (fewer children) and increasing life expectancy (Gerland et al., 2014; Reckel et al., 2013). Patterns of ageing within Australia and New Zealand differ across states and regions, and are dependent on fertility, mortality and migration trends. Falling fertility, increasing life expectancy and the effect of baby boomers becoming older have all contributed to the increase in number and proportion of people aged over 65 years.

If disability rates, physical health and co-morbidities continue to increase in prevalence with the increase in older people, then this group will also be the highest consumers of health services. The most distinctive symptom of older adults over younger persons is the existence of multiple co-morbid disorders. There issues include the 'old old' (85 years and over) people who have a range of typical age-related health problems (for example, arthritis, dementia and cancer); and secondly, the '65 and over' age bracket with a larger burden of lifestyle-related diseases (for example, type 2 diabetes) than previous generations, according to the Australian Institute of Health and Welfare (2014).

CRITICAL THINKING OPPORTUNITY

1   If health is seen as one of the top growth areas of employment, how might the nursing workforce appear within a shrinking workforce and therefore fewer taxpayers available to fund it?

2   If there are more people born overseas who are aged over 65, 85 and 100 years, what are the implications of nursing people with poor English-langauge skills and different cultural expectations?

Older adults and mental health

The mental health of older people is impacted by whether they can live independently due to frailty, reduced mobility and/or disability, or a pre-existing or recent onset of a chronic physical condition worldwide (World Health Organization, 2013) and in Australia (Australian Institute of Health and Welfare, 2015). In addition, there is an impact of poor mental health on physical health and/or quality of life (World Health Organization, 2013). In 2012, 87 per cent of older Australians reported a long-term medical condition and 42 per cent needed assistance with at least one everyday activity (Australian Bureau of Statistics, 2012).

Older adults with a mental illness fall into two main groups: those who have longstanding mental health challenges, and those who develop a mental illness when they are older. Factors that place older individuals at risk for developing a mental illness include physical frailty, an ageing brain, chronic illnesses, threats to identity and self-esteem, bereavements, inadequate social supports and a low socioeconomic position. Older people are particularly at risk of anxiety and depression, especially where there are co-occurring physical health issues, dementia and disability; or, for those experiencing bereavement, loss of independence or social isolation (Arola et al., 2010; El-Gabalawy et al., 2011; World Health Organization, 2013). The Australian Institute of Health and Welfare (2013) estimates that 52 per cent of residential aged care residents display symptoms of a depression.

In the fifth edition of the *Diagnostic and Statistical Manual of Mental Disorders* (DSM 5; American Psychiatric Association, 2013), three groups of mental disorders—delirium, dementia and the amnestic disorders—form a broad category: neurocognitive disorders. These are characterised by the primary symptoms common to all the disorders: impairment in cognition (for example, memory, language or attention). Cognitive functioning can also be affected in depression and psychosis (Ohmuro et al., 2015). Acute and chronic illness (for example, pain or dementia) can mask depression, leading to misdiagnosis and inadequate treatment (Martin, Neighbors & Griffith, 2013; Scherrer et al., 2014).

※ CRITICAL THINKING OPPORTUNITY

1   What are some of the challenges of nursing an older person that has experienced bereavement, loss of independence or social isolation?

2   Why would having more than one mental illness at one time and/or a co-morbid physical illness increase the complexity of assessment and treatment?

Mental health services for older adults in Australia and New Zealand

Services for aged mental health consumers differ across Australia and New Zealand. Aged people's mental health services are primarily for people with a longstanding mental illness who are now over 65 years of age, or who have developed functional illnesses such as depression and psychosis in later life. Service provision may also include people with severe behavioural difficulties associated with organic disorders such as dementia (Department of Human Services, 2006). Major cities of Australia and New Zealand have specific services for older people due to population needs, but in smaller cities and rural areas, services for older people tend to be provided by adult mental health services or through a generic aged service. The implication is that older people requiring a psychiatric admission will enter an adult mental health unit or be assessed in a mainstream aged person's facility. The mainstream aged or adult psychiatric unit may not have the expertise or specific knowledge required for working with an older person. When there is an aged-specific service for mental health consumers, a current adult consumer who turns 65 may remain with the adult service (servicing 18–64 year olds) until an ageing process is implicated. The age for entry into older adult mental health services is likely to change as the population continues to age (Department of Human Services, 2009), but consideration of a person's health and well-being may also be taken into account considering the link between high mortality and poor physical health of people with a mental illness.

Brodaty, Draper and Low (2003) suggest a seven-tiered model of service delivery for those with behavioural and psychological symptoms of dementia (see Figure 16.1). Traditional mental health caters to the tiers higher in the pyramid, but mainstream residential care covers all tiers.

Coverage of services for older adults includes community, inpatient and residential.

■ TOPIC LINK
See Chapter 3 for more on physical health and mental illness

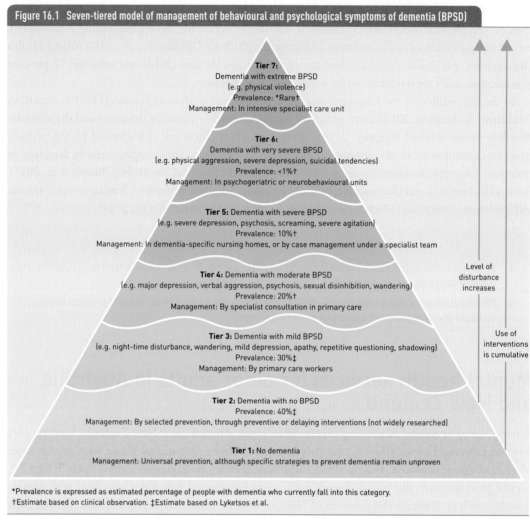

Figure 16.1   Seven-tiered model of management of behavioural and psychological symptoms of dementia (BPSD)

Tier 7:
Dementia with extreme BPSD
(e.g. physical violence)
Prevalence: *Rare†
Management: In intensive specialist care unit

Tier 6:
Dementia with very severe BPSD
(e.g. physical aggression, severe depression, suicidal tendencies)
Prevalence: <1%†
Management: In psychogeriatric or neurobehavioural units

Tier 5: Dementia with severe BPSD
(e.g. severe depression, psychosis, screaming, severe agitation)
Prevalence: 10%†
Management: In dementia-specific nursing homes, or by case management under a specialist team

Tier 4: Dementia with moderate BPSD
(e.g. major depression, verbal aggression, psychosis, sexual disinhibition, wandering)
Prevalence: 20%†
Management: By specialist consultation in primary care

Tier 3: Dementia with mild BPSD
(e.g. night-time disturbance, wandering, mild depression, apathy, repetitive questioning, shadowing)
Prevalence: 30%‡
Management: By primary care workers

Tier 2: Dementia with no BPSD
Prevalence: 40%‡
Management: By selected prevention, through preventive or delaying interventions (not widely researched)

Tier 1: No dementia
Management: Universal prevention, although specific strategies to prevent dementia remain unproven

Level of disturbance increases

Use of interventions is cumulative

*Prevalence is expressed as estimated percentage of people with dementia who currently fall into this category.
†Estimate based on clinical observation. ‡Estimate based on Lyketsos et al.

Brodaty, Draper & Low (2003)

Community services

Community services include aged persons assessment and treatment teams (APATTs) and psychogeriatric assessment and treatment teams (PGATs). These multidisciplinary teams provide community-based assessment, treatment, rehabilitation and case management for older people. The team offers specialist expertise in medical assessment and treatment, psychological, behavioural, social and functional assessments, and a corresponding range of therapeutic interventions. The focus of care in these teams is recovery and strength-based rehabilitation.

There are also community teams that focus on short-term intensive treatment at home (intensive community treatment team; ICT) and long-term recovery aspects and community teams that specialise in behavioural and psychiatric symptomatology of residents in residential care (behavioural assessment and specialist intervention consultations services; BASICs).

Services that may assist with diagnoses include Cognitive, Dementia and Memory Services (CDAMs) or memory clinics and neuropsychology services. CDAMs are specialist multidisciplinary services that

TOPIC LINK

See Chapter 6 for more on the recovery model.

provide diagnostic, referral and educational service for people experiencing memory loss or changes to their thinking, and their carers.

Aged acute inpatient care

These services provide short-term inpatient management and treatment during an acute phase of mental illness until sufficient recovery allows the person to be treated effectively in the community. They are usually located with other aged care facilities and/or general hospitals. Co-location occurs for a number of reasons:

- the ability to access a residential service for those who require assessment from aged care assessment services (ACAS)
- common co-morbidities in this age group
- the nature of physical illness and treatments that interplay with psychiatric symptoms.

The team is similar to those in adult mental health units and includes a consultant psychiatrist and nurse unit manager who manage the team, plus social workers, occupational therapists and clinical and neuropsychologists. The team of the acute care inpatient unit may also include geriatricians and other therapists, such as physiotherapists and art or music therapists.

Residential aged care services

Psychogeriatric (aged people's mental health) residential aged care facilities provide a range of specialist bed-based services to older people who cannot be cared for in mainstream aged care residential services. The level of persistent cognitive, emotional or behavioural disturbances the resident experiences determines the need for this admission. Mental health residential aged facilities, where available, offer longer-term accommodation, ongoing assessment, treatment and rehabilitation in units designed to have a familiar, home-like atmosphere, and residents are encouraged to participate in a range of quality of life activities. CADE (confused and demented elderly) units located in New South Wales were created for high levels of challenging behaviours. In rural units, these services may assist when neuropsychology or memory clinics are not available or accessible.

Clinical liaison and emergency crisis assessment and treatment

The general hospital is often where older adult psychiatry emerges. The role of clinical liaison and emergency crisis assessment and treatment (ECAT) may be a separate or dual role. Consultation–liaison mental health nursing is concerned with assisting non-mental health staff to care for people with psychiatric problems during their hospital admission. Such concerns may be a mental illness or a medically induced mental health concern, and include side effects from medication, shock and trauma, or effects of a physical illness that present with psychiatric symptomatology. The role of the consultation–liaison nurse includes education, knowledge and skills acquisition, strategy and intervention assistance, confidence development and cultural change towards mental illness. Much of the time is spent working with other nurses to identify strategies to deal with symptoms and develop documentation to measure changes. The consultation–liaison role may also include assistance with coping with grief and loss, debriefing and support groups.

■ TOPIC LINK

See Chapter 19 for more on crisis assessment and treatment teams, and the online chapter for more on consultation–liaison mental health nursing.

Recruitment and workforce

Australia has an ageing workforce and older adult mental health is no exception. The labour force in both Australia and New Zealand will age, reflected in a rising median age and an increasing proportion of the labour force in the older age brackets. In Australia, there are nineteen broad industries and 'registered nurse' is the second of the top ten occupations. Health care and social assistance is projected to make the largest contribution to employment growth over the next five years (Australian Bureau of Statistics, 2014). The growth in health-care employment will have an impact upon service provision within older adult mental health. Research exploring undergraduates' future career choices indicate mental health and aged have poorer preference outcomes (McCann, Clark & Lu, 2010; Happell, Byrne et al., 2014). The *Australia's Future Health Workforce* report (Health Workforce Australia, 2014) indicates that Australia's demand for nurses will exceed supply in the next decade and both mental health and ageing will experience shortages. More will need to be done to encourage nurses to move into these specialities.

CRITICAL THINKING OPPORTUNITY

1   How might the attitudes of undergraduate nursing students need to change for them to pursue older adult mental health as a career choice?

2   How can older adult mental health theory and clinical placement be improved to ensure change occurs in recruiting the future workforce?

ABOUT THE CONSUMER   Ruby's story

Ruby is a retired 69-year-old widowed woman who lives alone. She worked previously as school teacher. She has always been very independent and has lived alone for the past fifteen years since the death of her husband. She presents with her daughter for assessment for dementia at an emergency department.

Ruby presents with a long history of depressive symptoms that were treated by her general practitioner (GP). Currently, her signs and symptoms include not looking after herself properly (not showering, not eating at mealtimes, leaving the gas on the hotplates and cooking excessive amounts of food and leaving it in the oven for days at a time). She is also misplacing things: 'I think I had the car keys and placed them on the hook and now someone has taken them.' She describes being okay and says that there is nothing wrong with her. She has never been hospitalised for her depressive symptoms, but has had time away from work in the past. She has disturbed sleep, which has also been a problem in the past. Her sleep pattern is now erratic with daytime sleeping and night-time wakening occurring. In the past, she would sometimes either sleep excessively or have trouble getting to sleep, but only during periods that she was depressed and her sleep patterns would return to normal within weeks. According to her daughter, Ruby is also forgetting to pay bills, which is unusual as she has always been organised. Ruby does not seem concerned about her forgetfulness. She displays signs of agitation in the waiting area and her daughter states that this behaviour is new and it happens more outside the home.

TOPIC LINK   ■
See Chapter 10 for more on depression.

REFLECTION QUESTIONS

1   As Ruby's health-care worker, would you consider your role to include involvement in her activities of daily living?

2   What characteristic of Ruby's presentation would you consider in determining if there were more than one illness process involved or to differentiate between illnesses?

3   What specific signs, symptoms and behaviours would you monitor?

4   Would you consider bringing multidisciplinary input or external services into assessments to determine whether Ruby should stay living at home? If so, who and why?

Nursing practice reflection

Ruby presents with a long history of depression. Her signs and symptoms indicate that she may also have dementia, but it is difficult to differentiate between the illnesses and to determine whether she has both depression and dementia. She has no insight into her condition and is unconcerned by her symptoms, but this presentation may be signs of a dementia developing. As her nurse you will need to consider that she may no longer be able to live alone. In addition, the family may now have to be more involved in her care and her decision making, so you must consider how you can engage the family to facilitate this process in a formal way. The adjustment of becoming dependent on others may be difficult for Ruby and for her family. Ruby is likely to have concerns if her capacity for decision making is questioned and this is often a difficult conversation to have with older people. You will need to consider your role in the nursing care of Ruby through these discussions.

Assessment

A detailed history is essential when assessing any recent change in health or mental health status. The assessment should include a comprehensive history of past and current medical diagnoses, psychiatric history and treatment, and a full physical assessment. It is important to have all information validated by carers and relatives. The consumer is likely to have had some cognitive decline, and the decline is likely to have had an effect on memory and intelligence.

The *informant interview* (that is, an interview with someone who has known the consumer for some time) often provides information on changes that the consumer does not or cannot recognise. Carers and relatives can also provide insight into the needs assessment of the consumer. The informant interview will also give an indication of the carer's stress burden, and may identify the needs of the carer when keeping an older adult consumer at home and independent. Carers and relatives can comment on the functional aspects of their lives, and about their coping mechanisms and support networks.

■ TOPIC LINK

See Chapter 2 for more on mental health assessment.

Biopsychosocial older adult psychiatric nursing assessment

The *biopsychosocial older adult mental health nursing assessment* is based on the special needs and challenges of older people in relation to biological, psychological and social needs. As with all assessments, it is important to determine the older person's ability to participate. That is, language skills—reading, writing and comprehension—are assessed as a common initial sign of cognitive impairment and deterioration in dementia, and hearing is assessed to ensure correct interpretation of questions. It is also important to pace the interview to the consumer's ability to respond.

As well as past and present health status, physical examination results and physical functioning, a pharmacology review should be undertaken with nurses responsible for the ongoing physical health and behaviour monitoring. Behaviour may be the only indicator to a health issue due to communication difficulties. Pharmacokinetics and pharmacodynamics change with age, so even medication that a person may have been on for some time may cause new side effects and interactions because of changes in the ability to absorb, distribute, metabolise and excrete. Polypharmacy due to co-morbidities increases with age (Elliott & Booth, 2014; Vyas, Pan & Sambamoorthi, 2012), as does the potential for adverse medication effects (Salive, 2013).

The impact of physical problems on the long-term mentally ill and on mental well-being is of particular note. Mental health consumers have shorter life expectancies, poorer health outcomes and poorer health behaviours than the general population (De Hert et al., 2011; Happell, Stanton at al., 2014) and are more likely to have multiple illnesses (Barnett et al., 2012). Multiple illnesses increase polypharmacy, risk of interactions, pain and disability (Maher, Hanlon & Haijar, 2014). Suicide appears to occur more often in those with physical co-morbidities that are chronic, particularly if these have as a consequence a decrease in function and role leading to hopelessness (Podgorski et al., 2010). Polypharmacy, interactions, pain and chronic physical co-morbidities are risk factors for suicide in older people (Almeida et al., 2012). Coping skills/mechanisms, pain and hope in relation to their physical health should be explored in suicide assessment (see Suicide in this chapter).

While the below is not a definitive list, psychiatric symptoms that occur in the following medical conditions:

- Hypothyroidism, pneumonia, hepatitis, hyperthyroidism and mononucleosis can present as neurosis and depression.
- Hyperthyroidism, ulcerative colitis, hypothyroidism and paroxysmal atrial tachycardia can present as anxiety.
- Hypotension, neurosyphillis, cirrhosis, drug and alcohol withdrawal, diabetes (hyperglycaemia) and cerebral vascular accidents can present as psychosis.
- Antiretroviral drugs, antiparkinsonian drugs, antiepileptics, cardiovascular medications, antibiotics, antihistamines and respiratory medications may all cause psychiatric symptoms.

The initial assessment of the older person is more commonly carried out in the person's living environment/home. The home environment provides information on activities of living (such as bathing and hygiene, cooking, laundry, shopping, help and assistance), and adds to the information given by the mental status examination and other screening tools. The physical examination may indicate nutrition and hydration deficiencies, health issues, and signs of neglect, injury or abuse, and disability.

CRITICAL THINKING OPPORTUNITY ✳

1 How and why might you involve the family/carers in any assessment (for example, memory confirmation, baseline or collateral information, and cultural norms)?

2 Some medical illnesses are more common in some mental illnesses, and medical illnesses and their treatment can cause psychiatric symptoms. How might you assess the difference between symptomatology of a medical illness and signs and symptoms of depression or anxiety? How can the nursing care differ?

Screening tools

Screening tools are not used in isolation but as an addition to the history, mental status examination and physical assessment. The diagnoses for individuals are not made just as a result of a screening; a medical history should be taken before the application of any screening tool. It is important to note that language skills, education level and intelligence affect some assessment tools, such as the Mini-Mental Status Examination (MMSE). The MMSE (or Folstein test) is one of the most commonly used cognition screens (Stein et al., 2015) and has been translated and culturally validated in a number of community languages, including Spanish (Contador et al., 2016), Singapore Chinese (Feng et al., 2012) and Urdu (Venneri & Malik, 2014). The key features of the MMSE are the same for any age group.

The Psychogeriatric Assessment Scales (PAS) incorporate MMSE, Abbreviated Mental Test Scores (AMTS), Geriatric Depression Scale (GDS), and cognitive decline and behavioural change scales.

The PAS is a method of assessing psychogeriatric disorders, but will not inform nurses of what action is required. PAS gathers information in a systematic way and provides guidance on how this information should be interpreted by comparing the results to the normal range found in the community (Jorm & Mackinnon, 2016).

Nurses can screen for cognitive changes by using one or more tools to substantiate clinical observations. The AMTS is a simple and validated cognitive impairment test, initially used with older adults but now adapted for other settings including the emergency department (Jackson, Naqvi & Sheehan, 2013; Pendlebury et al., 2015). The test focuses on orientation and memory. Scores of 7 or less suggest cognitive impairment. The MMSE is the most widely used. The main strengths of this tool are that it covers cognitive function and orientation, memory, concentration, language (naming an everyday item followed by more unusual objects), praxis (pentagons intersecting) and gnosis (recognition of pictures and commands).

The Clifton Assessment Procedures for the Elderly (CAPE) and the Cambridge Examination for Mental Disorders of the Elderly (CAMDEX-R) include cognitive, information and orientation scales. The CAPE measures behavioural and functional ability in the areas of physical disability, apathy, communication difficulty and social disturbance (Chan et al., 2014; Wenborn et al., 2013) and can rate dependency, which is used to assess aged care residential funding. CAMDEX-R, devised by Roth and colleagues at Cambridge University, is a diagnostic assessment to identify dementia and differentiate between other diagnoses and normal processes of ageing (Roth et al., 1999) and includes executive function assessment by verbal fluency (Gale et al., 2014).

A common and simple test of clock drawing assists in supporting a diagnosis of dementia, or indicates areas of difficulty for that individual. Clock drawing can assess executive function, attention and visuospatial ability (Cosgrove et al., 2015). Trojano and Gainotti's 2016 study concluded that analysing the drawing errors rather that the overall accuracy of the drawing differentiates between dementias. Even if consumers can tell the time, it is often difficult for them to spatially design a clock. Some cannot space the twelve numbers, some start with the 3, 6, 9 and 12, and others line them up at the start of the dial. Many have difficulty with the minute and the hour hands.

Depression scales help to collate symptoms and screen for depression. They can also be used to monitor the course and response to treatment. The daily presence of five or more symptoms (including sleep, interest and appetite) indicate a major depression that requires pharmacotherapy in the treatment. See Table 16.1 for a summary of the leading assessment scales.

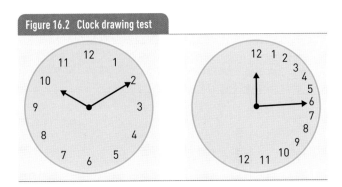

Figure 16.2 Clock drawing test

ROBYN GARLICK

TABLE 16.1 ASSESSMENT SCALES USED IN THE OLDER ADULT

Indicator	Assessment / Screening Tool	Comments
Depression	Geriatric Depression Scale (GDS)	The most widely used, it comes in a long and short version, and avoids somatic symptoms; the overall score indicates the possibility of depression. Not for significant cognitive impairment.
	Cornell Scale for Depression in Dementia (CSDD)	It screens for suspicion of dementia; includes information from the nurse, consumer and carer; and is recommended for use in moderate-to-severe cognitive impairment.
	Psychogeriatric Assessment Scales (PAS)	Designed to gather information on dementia and depression, it assesses an individual and an informant in areas of stroke, depression and cognitive impairment. It aims to assess, not decide what actions are to be taken.
Dementia	Mini-Mental Status Examination (MMSE)	Validated in many settings, it is commonly available, translated and validated in many languages. In the older person it is worth noting anxiety symptoms, masked depression, suicidal ideation and any cognitive impairment.
	Clifton Assessment Procedures for the Elderly (CAPE)	It includes cognitive, information and orientation scales.
	Psychogeriatric Assessment Scales (PAS)	It is designed to gather information on dementia and depression. It assesses an individual and an informant in areas of stroke, depression and cognitive impairment. Its aims are to assess, not to decide what actions are to be taken.
	Confusion Assessment Method Instrument (CAMI)	It assists in distinguishing between delirium and dementia, and discerns consciousness and attention and the clinical course with any fluctuations. This test has also been modified for the intensive care unit (ICU) setting.
	Behavioral Pathology in Alzheimer's Disease Rating Scale (BEHAVE-AD)	A behaviour rating scale for Alzheimer's disease, it is in two parts: symptomatology and a global rating of the symptoms' severity. It covers paranoid and delusional ideation, hallucinations, activity disturbances, aggression, diurnal variation, mood, and anxieties and phobias.
Agitation in older people	Cohen-Mansfield Agitation Inventory	A rating questionnaire consisting of twenty-nine agitated behaviours, each rated on a 7-point scale of frequency, assessing the frequency of agitated behaviours in elderly persons; originally used with caregivers in the long-term care setting.

Indicator	Assessment / Screening Tool	Comments
Life and living	Instrumental Activities Of Daily Living (IADL)	It assesses eight areas of daily living, including ability to use a telephone, shop, prepare food, do housekeeping, use the laundry, use transport, and manage medications and personal finances.
	Barthel scale	The Barthel scale, or Barthel ADL index, is used to measure performance in basic activities of daily living and mobility. It assesses independent living skills.
	Quality of Life (QoL)	This measures quality-of-life indicators in dementia. It is taken from the consumer and a carer.
Mental health	Cambridge Examination For Mental Disorders In The Older Adult (CAMDEX-DS)	It includes cognitive, information and orientation scales.
	Brief Psychiatric Rating Scale (BPRS)	This is used for global mental health assessment.
Delirium	Confusion Assessment Method Instrument (CAMI)	It assists in distinguishing between delirium and dementia and discerns consciousness and attention and the clinical course with any fluctuations. This test has also been modified for the intensive care unit (ICU) setting.
	Neecham Confusion Scale	It measures level of confusion in processing and alertness, behaviour, motor and physiological areas.
Suicide	Harmful Behaviours Scale	It is scored based upon observations of direct and indirect self-destructive behaviour among nursing home residents; it is reliant on the observer and their skills.
	Reasons for Living Scale: Older Adult Version (RFL–OA)	It is a longer version that rates reasons to live and is self-rating.
	Geriatric Suicide Ideation Scale (GSIS)	It measures suicidal ideation and is not for the cognitively impaired. Areas of investigation are suicide ideation, death ideation, loss of personal and social worth, and perceived meaning in life.

Note: Suicidality should always be assessed, and should include static (historical markers that are permanent and fixed) and dynamic (amenable to change, including skills and coping) risk factors. Suicide is screened using depression scales and the MMSE, and documented in a risk assessment.

ROBYN GARLICK

1   How could losses such as retirement, physical health deterioration, deafness and diminished eyesight have an impact on the Reasons for Living Scale and older adults' suicidality?

2   Why would poor physical health and polypharmacy make diagnoses difficult? (Hint: review the psychiatric symptoms list in the 'Biopsychosocial older adult psychiatric nursing assessment' section.)

Diagnostic tests

Appropriate diagnostic tests are the same as for younger adults, and include urine and blood specimens for vitamin B12; folate; venereal disease and chemical profile for urea and electrolytes; liver function tests and thyroid function; chest X-ray; brain MRIs; and toxicity screens. Vitamin B12 and venereal disease testing are considerations depending on the findings. These tests will rule out the most life-threatening causes of the health problem. It is also important, for treatment and care, that discrimination between organic and functional diseases is made.

Vitamin B12 deficiency, hypothyroidism, hyperparathyroidism, neurosyphilis and folate deficiency can cause reversible dementia. Delirium is investigated by identifying the underlying cause, and tests include full blood examination, calcium, urea and electrolyte levels, liver function tests, thyroid function tests, glucose levels, chest X-ray, electrocardiograph, blood cultures and urinalysis.

Delirium

Delirium is a medical emergency (Han, Wilson and Ely, 2010; Gareri et al., 2016) and not a normal part of ageing (Rosen et al., 2015). Delirium is a common accompaniment to physical illness in the older adult, and advanced age is a major risk factor for its development (Australian Commission on Safety and Quality in Health Care, 2016; Rosen et al., 2015). The presence of delirium in the older adult often has a poor prognosis.

Delirium is also known as acute confusional state, toxic psychosis, acute brain syndrome and acute organic brain syndrome. It is an acute organic disturbance of higher cerebral function associated with impaired ability to attend to the environment. Delirium is an acute decline in attention and cognition, according to Day, Higgins and Koch (2010).

It is important that clinicians are vigilant in their observation and monitoring to the possibility of delirium occurring after surgical procedures and acute medical conditions, and in exacerbations of chronic medical conditions. Delirium is often unrecognised, misdiagnosed and untreated (ACSQHC, 2016; Rosen et al., 2015; Traynor et al., 2016).

The blood–brain barrier may be impaired by ageing, and therefore it becomes more susceptible to toxins. Delirium is associated with an increased risk for the development of dementia and the highest risk factor for developing a delirium is a pre-existing dementia (ACSQHC, 2016; Fong et al., 2015). Delirium is often caused by potentially modifiable factors, such as medications, dehydration, malnutrition and sleep disturbances (Rosen et al., 2015). Delirium is also linked to functional decline (Fong et al., 2015). Overall, it appears prevention of delirium is more efficacious than early detection and treatment (ACSQHC, 2016).

Delirium is characterised by disturbances of consciousness, including reduced awareness and reduced ability to sustain concentration, often referred to as *clouding of consciousnesses*. Changes in cognition include perceptual disturbance (illusions and visual hallucinations are common); memory deficit, especially recent; disorientation, often with alteration in the sleep–wake cycle; and language disturbance. Always suspect delirium when there is a disturbance of behaviour, thinking, sleep or orientation, particularly if it is worse at night.

Delirium develops rapidly within hours or days. Signs and symptoms also fluctuate over the course of the day, and could be mistaken for 'sundowning' in someone who has a dementia. It is reversible when the underlying cause is addressed, but can be irreversible if not treated, and, if unable to be treated, can lead to coma and ultimately death.

Delirium risk factors include pre-existing dementia, presence of a serious medical condition (such as ischaemic heart disease and diabetes), increased age, depression, alcohol abuse, abnormal serum sodium, hearing and/or visual impairment, and disability. Over-the-counter medications are commonly used by older adults, with fewer herbal therapies being used (Maher, Hanlon & Haijar, 2014; Stone et al., 2017). The over-the-counter medication or herbal therapies such as St John's Wort can lower concentrations and thus not meet therapeutic ranges (for example, clopine) (Van Strater & Bogers, 2012). There is an increased risk of drug interactions, especially from pharmacokinetics, in the older adult (twice that of 30–40-year-olds). Alcohol, analgesics and benzodiazepine tend to be the drugs that older adults misuse at present, and these are also often implicated in the development of delirium (Airagnes et al., 2016; Gareri et al., 2016).

Delirium can be divided, according to level of arousal or psychomotor activity, into three 'subtypes': hyperactive, hypoactive and mixed form (Department of Health, 2012a). Hyperactive features include increased motor activity, restlessness, agitation, hallucinations and delusions, and inappropriate behaviour. Hypoactive or 'quiet' delirium features include reduced motor activity, lethargy, withdrawal, drowsiness and staring off into space. The 'mixed' subtype is characterised by alternating features of the two forms. Hypoactive delirium is the most common manifestation in older people and can be misdiagnosed as dementia, depression or negative symptoms of psychosis (such as de-motivation or lethargy) (O'Regan et al., 2016).

There are many screening tools available; the symptoms investigated should match the criteria of the *Diagnostic and Statistical Manual of Mental Disorders* (fifth edition; DSM 5). Neurocognitive measures are often taken, but they should be combined with clinical observation and clinical features before diagnosis or treatment is recommended. In complex cases, more in-depth neuropsychological testing may be required. The delirium symptom interview should be utilised to assist other confusion monitors. A MMSE should be repeated at least hourly, and increase or decrease depending on response and behaviour. Mental state may not fluctuate as much as mood and behaviour during a delirium.

ABOUT THE CONSUMER Ruby's story (continued)

When Ruby is admitted to the aged inpatient psychiatric unit, she is found to be malnourished. Investigations indicate Ruby has type 2 diabetes and had symptoms of metabolic syndrome over many years. Ruby is on medication for dyslipidaemia and hypertension, and from her history has shown symptoms of dysglycaemia. Ruby has abdominal obesity. These factors, plus the administration of a tricyclics antidepressant, increased Ruby's chances of insulin resistance and development of metabolic syndrome.

ROBYN GARLICK

Prior to admission Ruby had been taking four different medications. On admission she was administered a benzodiazepine at the emergency department as she was agitated and very restless. Ruby has had sleep deprivation, poor hydration and nutrition, and has a cognitive impairment. She has been inactive and unmotivated to be involved in any activity. She develops a delirium.

REFLECTION
QUESTIONS

1 How would you identify factors from Ruby's history that may have contributed to the risk of delirium developing?

2 What do you consider are other risk factors for the development of a delirium?

3 Reflect on the capacity for decision making in Ruby's story with reference to any legislation regarding electro-convulsive therapy (ECT).

Management and care for the older adult

The first principle of management is to investigate and treat the underlying medical cause. Nurses should monitor closely vital signs, oxygenation, and food and fluid intake.

Pharmacological management is the medical care that incorporates the use of medications with the aim of medication review is to reduce or rationalise as many medications as possible. Anticholinergic medications, including antiparkinsonians (for example, benztropine and biperiden), antidepressants (for example, amitriptyline), antihistamines (for example, promethazine) and antipsychotics (for example, chlorpromazine and thioridazine), need to be slowly altered as these medications can cause cognitive impairment. Small dosage increases usually occur so that any changes can be monitored by nursing care. The slow increase is related to polypharmacy, ageing changes in liver enzymes and other ageing processes affecting medication (absorption, distribution, metabolism and excretion) (Davies & O'Mahony, 2015).

Nursing care should include anticipated nocturnal deterioration; therefore, medication provided early in the evening rather than late (such as before sleep) can ensure the medication has an effect before behaviour changes. If a benzodiazepine must be utilised, it should be a specific medication for a known cause (for example, diazepam per alcohol withdrawal guidelines). Care must be taken with the use of benzodiazepines as they can cause paradoxical worsening of confusional states. A paradoxical reaction is the opposite effect to the expected outcome of appropriate treatment or a clinical deterioration that may be transient (Gryschek et al., 2010). Benzodiazepines may be prescribed for their calming effect, but in the elderly a paradoxical aggression may occur with nurses noting signs of anxiety and restlessness (Dell'osso & Lader, 2012; Nicholas, Lee & Roche, 2011). The outcome of the paradoxical aggression may be to increase the benzodiazepine or to introduce another medication, increasing the risk of delirium. Beware of exacerbating delirium with high doses of antipsychotics and benzodiazepines.

Behavioural interventions require frequent assessment. The nurse will need to assess agitation and intervene when it occurs. A gentle approach with regular reassurance—especially regarding safety—should be implemented. Anxiety is also common in older adults, so a non-threatening approach is recommended. Information and communication provided to the consumer should be short and simple due to their memory changes, confusional status, sensory impairment (such as hearing and hallucinations) or cognitive processing ability. Information may need frequent repeating by the nurse. Prompts for orientation and memory, such as familiar faces, especially of family and friends, are helpful.

The involvement of familiar staff also assists. Changing the lighting level over the day to simulate the day–night cycle is important as artificial lighting gives the false illusion of daytime for long periods. This may be important in areas such as the ICU where lighting is the same night and day. Use of a night-light can help reduce disorientation.

CRITICAL THINKING OPPORTUNITY

1   Consider an older adult admitted to a general ward with a delirium. What nursing challenges could occur?

2   How could delirium symptoms become confused with features of dementia, depression or negative symptoms of psychosis?

Depression

According to the DSM 5 (American Psychiatric Association, 2013) depression requires five criteria for diagnoses. The first criterion is five or more symptoms being present for at least two weeks and changing functioning, with symptoms that include depressed mood most of the day on most days, marked decrease in interest or pleasure in most activities, and significant weight, sleep, energy and concentration changes. The other criteria include exclusion of a mixed episode, due to substance or a medical condition; exclusion of a manic or hypomanic episode; or exclusion of a better explanation through alternative depression diagnoses. Older adults often deny feeling sad or depressed, but may still have major depression. Depression is expressed in mood, which is a subjective feeling state, and often shows in this age group as somatic symptoms. It is seen as a sustained state of low mood, unhappiness and sadness. Subtypes of depression are major clinical depression, dysthymic disorder and adjustment disorder with depressed mood, grief and bereavement.

Recognising depression in the older adult starts with knowing the signs and symptoms. Depression red flags include sadness, fatigue, abandoning or losing interest in hobbies or other pastimes that were pleasurable, social withdrawal and isolation (reluctance to be with friends, engage in activities or go out of the home), weight loss, loss of appetite, sleep disturbances (difficulty falling asleep or staying asleep, oversleeping or daytime sleepiness), loss of self-worth (worries about being a burden to carers or loved ones, and feelings of worthlessness or self-loathing), increased use of alcohol or other drugs (including benzodiazepines and painkillers), fixation on death and suicidal thoughts or attempts.

Older adults do not always fit a typical picture of depression. Many depressed older people do not claim to feel sad at all. They may complain, instead, of low motivation, a lack of energy or physical problems. In fact, physical complaints, such as arthritis pain or headaches, appear to have become more significant, and are often the predominant symptom of depression in an older person. Older adults with depression are also more likely to show symptoms of anxiety or irritability. They may constantly wring their hands, pace around the room or fret obsessively about money, their health or the state of the world.

The DSM 5 (American Psychiatric Association, 2013) is specific to diagnostic groups and includes four disorder types: anxiety, dissociative, mood and somatoform. Many presentations within these diagnoses may be associated with an underlying depression or have overlapping features of dementia (Rodrigues, Petersen & Perry, 2014; Tobe, 2012). Anxiety symptoms may dominate and mask depression. Behaviours may also point to an underlying depression; consider behavioural disorders (aggression or inappropriate micturition), shoplifting, alcohol dependence for a first time and an accentuation of premorbid personality traits (theatrical past behaviours) as warning signs.

Pseudodementia is an important reminder that severe depression can mimic dementia. Pseudodementia is described as a cognitive deficit secondary to a primary mood disorder (Kennedy, 2015; McCutcheon et al., 2016). Depressed older people may not perform well on dementia screening tools because of poor concentration and memory. Depressed people of all ages perform poorly on cognitive impairment tests. The distinction is that depressed older adults have a general impairment in effortless tasks, especially those concerned with memory, rather than cortical function impairment (language, construction and praxis). The older consumer may be perplexed and difficult to interview. The history, to indicate depression, involves months at most, and the poor memory can be dated or a rough time indicated. The dementia consumer is more likely to be inaccurate, but not aware or concerned by the deficit, while the pseudodementia consumer may become irritable and complain and be aware of the poor memory. People who experience pseudodementia can remember afterwards that they had a poor memory. Duration of illness, symptom severity, harm risk, functional impairment and history will determine treatment, as it is with all depressions, with antidepressants involvement occurring in persistent or severe depression (including pseudodementia) (Gutzman & Qazi, 2015; Symonds & Anderson, 2016). Pseudodementia responds well to electro-convulsive therapy (Waite & Easton, 2013).

There are different theories about pseudodementia and the link to dementia. As stated, depression can occur in dementia but the nature of a possible deterioration or pathway to dementia (Kobayashi & Kato, 2011) is developing. Research indicates that oxidative stress (lifetime of nitrogen–oxygen balance) in the brain at a molecular, cell and pathological level is linked to reduced cerebral metabolic rate for glucose (Roderigues, Petersen & Perry, 2014), changes in neural plaque and neurofibrillary (McCutcheon et al., 2016) and genetic causes with links to dementia (Bieniek et al., 2014).

All medications have side effects, but some can actually cause symptoms of depression or make a pre-existing depression worse. Harmful drug interactions or a failure to take a medication as prescribed can also contribute to depression. For older adult individuals with multiple prescriptions, the risk of medication-induced depression is particularly high (Thomas et al., 2014; Wu & Okusaga, 2014)). Medications that can induce depression include steroids, painkillers, hormones, arthritis medication, high blood pressure drugs, heart disease medication, tranquillisers and cancer drugs.

Assessment of depression in an older adult consumer is similar to that for a younger person, and screening tools have already been discussed. The main difference is in physical health. This interplays with mental health, and also how a person copes with physical health will have an impact on mental health. Physical health issues such as dehydration, falls, hip fractures, urine retention, constipation and heart arrhythmias are common in the older adult; all can be caused by medication and all can affect mental health. This is another reason why medication is introduced slowly with the older adult.

ABOUT THE CONSUMER   Ruby's story (continued)

Following a fall, Ruby's restriction of movement has exacerbated an existing depression, and she does not appear to be responding to her medication. Ruby is not eating or drinking and does not want to take her medication. It is becoming urgent that the depression respond to treatment. The decision from the multidisciplinary team and from the mental health tribunal is for Ruby to undergo a series of electroconvulsive treatments.

After three treatments in a week, Ruby reveals to her daughter that she is feeling more energetic and is looking forward to going home. She tells her daughter that she wants her own bedroom and her own space, and cannot imagine what life would be like in a retirement village or, worse, a nursing home. Ruby still has fleeting feelings of overwhelming sadness and feels she has nothing to offer in life. These feelings pass, but are intense when she experiences them. Ruby's injuries are improving and she is now able to move freely about.

REFLECTION QUESTIONS

1   What are some nursing care considerations to make when considering risk for Ruby?

2   Reflect on the signs and symptoms you may want to monitor when caring for Ruby. How would you document this in a nursing care plan?

3   How might you measure any change in behaviour?

Nursing care and management of depression

The goals of management are to reduce symptoms of depression, to improve social functioning and to develop support networks. Other goals may be to eliminate or reduce the risk of suicide and to improve physical health. Linkage to a general practitioner is essential. Supportive psychosocial interventions or psychotherapy should be considered, either alone or in combination with other treatments. Psychotic features often mean that an antidepressant and an antipsychotic medication may be required. If there are no contraindications, consumers with psychotic depression should be offered ECT, which should also be considered if medication is not tolerated or there is no improvement, and when there are severe physical complications (attempted suicide or metabolic distress) or response is too slow and is affecting physical health.

Serotonin reuptake inhibitors have limited use in older adults as side effects include agitation, sleep disturbance and anorexia (Edward & Alderman, 2013) so nurses need to monitor behaviour, sleep and nutrition. Selective serotonin reuptake inhibitors (SSRI) antidepressants including fluoxetine, citalopram and paroxetine are most commonly prescribed in older adults (Greenblatt & Greenblatt, 2016).

Psychotherapies are available to the older adult, but there is little supporting research, except in limited cognitive behavioural studies (Kishita & Laidlaw, 2017). Therapies include behaviour therapy, cognitive behaviour therapy (CBT), problem-solving therapy, brief dynamic therapy, interpersonal therapy and reminiscence therapy (Gaggiolo et al., 2015; Jayasekara et al., 2014; Kobayashi & Kato, 2011).

Older consumers give the same response as younger consumers do to antidepressants. Even when there are physical co-morbidities and physical illnesses, antidepressants should be used. Co-morbid psychiatric illnesses, such as anxiety and substance misuse, adversely affect the outcomes for depression. Benzodiazepines should be used sparingly, and gradually discontinued whenever possible.

When taking multiple medications, an antidepressant with the lowest risk of drug–drug interactions should be administered. It is not uncommon for the older adult to be taking more than nine medications, and these could include multiple benzodiazepines. Antidepressants that are safer for the older adult are those with the lowest anticholinergic properties. When commencing antidepressants, serotonin-related side effects should be monitored; these include agitation and also self-harm or attempted suicide, as symptoms may initially worsen. Sodium blood levels should be monitored, as they will affect tolerance and response rates. Tricyclic antidepressants (TCAs) should not be used with those who have a postural hypotension or cardiac abnormalities.

ROBYN GARLICK

Lithium carbonate has a narrow therapeutic range, and that is problematic in older people. Extreme care needs to be taken with older adults who have any fluctuation with their nutrition and hydration. Lithium may take four to six weeks to have a therapeutic effect, and consumers may need to remain on medication for a year or two. Maintenance therapy should be followed for at least a year. Maintenance treatment may also be required for ECT. All mood stabilisers require monitoring over time for adverse events. Sodium valproate is often used in the older adult and increased monitoring of serum levels and toxicity signs are recommended (Edward & Alderman, 2013). Lithium is a salt, so consider this with nursing care. Serum lithium levels and signs of toxicity need close monitoring especially in hot weather. Oedema, electrolyte imbalances, weight gain and toxicity are side effects, so increased serum levels and lower doses of lithium are required in older adults (Edward & Alderman, 2013).

Antidepressants should be tapered off when being ceased. Fluoxetine, despite its effects, is not recommended as the main antidepressant, because of its long half-life. An antidepressant is prescribed based on side-effect profile, past response and severity of the depression.

Herbal medications, such as St John's Wort and gingko, should be noted, as the herbs can effect drug metabolism, lower seizure threshold, increase blood pressure and heart rate, and interact with some medications (Tachjian, Maria & Jahangir, 2010).

Suicide

Suicide risk increases with age, and is highest for Caucasian men aged over 85 years. There is an association between physical illness and suicide with older persons (Conwell et al., 2010; De Leo et al., 2013). People with this risk factor who suicide usually have had contact with medical services (Conwell et al., 2010; Raue, Ghesquiere & Bruce, 2014; Webb et al., 2012). Depression is the greatest risk factor for suicide. Older people with depression and poor physical health have a sense of being a burden. Burdensomeness and functional impairment is associated with suicide ideation (Conwell et al., 2010; Cukrowicz et al., 2011; De Leo et al., 2013).

Characteristics associated with high risk for suicide include history of depression, attempted suicide in the past, family history of suicide, firearms in the home, abuse of alcohol or other substances, unusual stress, chronic medical condition and, importantly, social isolation. Suicide in the older adult is more likely with deterioration in physical health and with a depressive illness compared with younger people. Physical health problems were most common in the oldest age group (85 years and over); and for older adults, as age increases until 95 years old so does suicide risk (Shah et al., 2016). People with more severe illness, clinical deterioration and functional impairment compose the higher suicide risk (Conwell et al., 2010).

A thorough risk assessment should be completed. It should include any presence of suicidal or homicidal ideation or intent, new or increased confusion, persecutory or depressive psychotic symptoms, exhaustion in the carer, and whether any psychotropic medication has been prescribed.

Mania

Mania can occur in the older adult, although it is uncommon but not rare as a first presentation later in life—consumers commonly have mania episodes at a younger age (Dols et al., 2013; Forester et al., 2015). Sami, Khan and Nilforooshan (2015), in their review of case files, indicate a strong association between late onset mania and underlying organic illness. Sami and colleagues (2015) also discuss iatrogenic and vascular risk factors being involved.

1   Reflect on how you think mania in an older person could be a greater risk when compared to a younger person.

2   How would you care for and manage the behaviours of an older adult consumer presenting with promiscuous sexual behaviour?

Dementia

Dementia is a broad diagnostic term that includes a group of brain disorders characterised by gradual decline in cognitive abilities and changes in personality and behaviour (Hunter, 2012). Dementia is diagnosed when there is a development of multiple cognitive deficits that are manifested by memory impairment, and at least one of the following cognitive impairments: *aphasia* (affects language comprehension and production; for example, they can sing but are unable to speak, or can read but not write), *apraxia* (inability to execute purposeful movements, such as a command to make a motion like cleaning teeth or drawing), *agnosia* (inability to recognise known objects) and disturbance in *executive functioning* (the ability to plan to attain a goal and to make steps and to adapt to achieve a goal). A person's personality is also affected.

Dementia is inclusive of a variety of neurological disorders depicted by memory loss and cognitive impairment (Winblad et al., 2016). Dementia is a general term used to describe a form of cognitive impairment that is chronic and generally progressive, occurring over a period of months to years. More than 52 per cent of those living in residential aged care facilities have dementia (Australian Institute of Health and Welfare, 2012). Heart disease was the leading cause of death in 2015, but as death rates from dementia increase and heart disease and stroke decline, dementia is predicted to become the leading cause of death (Australian Bureau of Statistics, 2015b).

There are different forms of dementia, and each has its own causes. Some of the most common forms of dementia are Alzheimer's disease, vascular dementia, frontal lobe dementia, and dementia with Lewy body syndrome (Sheehan, 2012; Winblad et al., 2016). There are two types of dementia:

1   *primary dementia*—progressive and not reversible, and not secondary to any other disorder (examples include Alzheimer's disease and multi-infarct dementia)

2   *secondary dementia*—occurs as a result of some other pathological process, such as infections, trauma, toxicity, neoplasm or neurological diseases. Some can be treated, but are reversible only if the underlying cause is able to be eliminated.

At the initial stages of dementia, consumers show fatigue, difficulty in sustaining mental performance and a tendency to fail when the task is novel or complex or requires a shift in problem-solving strategy. The inability to perform tasks becomes increasingly severe, and spreads to everyday tasks such as grocery shopping and dressing as the dementia progresses.

Dementia is essentially a disease of older people but not a normal part of the ageing process (Edward & Alderman, 2013). The distribution of dementia is according to type, and includes Alzheimer's disease (50–60 per cent), which involves changes to the structure and chemical functioning of the brain; vascular dementia (20 per cent) (Rizzi, Rosset & Roriz-Cruz, 2014; Thompson et al., 2010), resulting from infarction or vascular disease; while the remaining diagnoses include dementia with Lewy bodies, mixed dementia, a combination of Alzheimer's and vascular dementia, and other dementias, especially acquired

ABOUT THE CONSUMER Ruby's story (continued)

Ruby has type 2 diabetes and metabolic syndrome. Review the evidence-based literature on high triglycerides, diabetes and vascular dementia, and consider the risk of Ruby developing vascular dementia.

Ruby has not been diagnosed with dementia, but it was an area of concern for Ruby and her daughter when Ruby was unwell. Difficulty concentrating, sleep disturbance, forgetting things on a regular basis and lack of engagement would have all given Ruby and her daughter some fodder for thoughts of dementia.

REFLECTION QUESTIONS

1 Consider how the picture of Ruby's presentation differs from that of dementia.
2 What supports would you consider for Ruby as her treating nurse?

immunodeficiency syndrome (AIDS), Parkinson's disease, Huntington's disease, Korsokoff's syndrome, Creutzfeldt-Jakob disease and head trauma. Alzheimer's disease, vascular demenetia and Lewy body dementia make up 90 per cent of all dementias (Sheehan, 2012).

Worldwide distribution of dementia varies according to cultural and socioeconomics differences, with Japan having the lowest prevalence (Rizzi, Rosset & Roriz-Cruz, 2014). The distribution of dementia is expected to change because of a change in vascular dementia numbers. There are now new medications that treat and manage some dementias. There is far more screening before birth for illnesses such as Huntington's disease. Vascular dementia, because of lifestyle changes and psychotropic medication that cause insulin resistance and lipid changes, is expected to increase more than others.

The classic course of dementia is an onset in a consumer's fifties or sixties, with gradual deterioration over five to ten years, leading eventually to death. The exception to this is sudden onset resulting from head trauma, infection or cerebral hypoxia. The word 'dementia' is used widely to describe a group of diseases that affect the brain and cause progressive decline in a person's abilities to remember, think and learn. The main abilities affected are judgment, orientation, emotions, memory and thinking. Cognitive impairment of dementia modifies the clinical presentation of other mental disorders. It can be difficult to tease out the specific target symptoms; for example, depression can be masked by cognitive slowing. It is always wise to monitor for depression signs if a consumer with vascular dementia becomes irritable or aggressive.

Approximately 6 per cent of people over 75 years of age have dementia, and the risk of developing dementia increases with age. The onset is usually but not always gradual. One in four of the population aged over 85 years will develop dementia (Edward & Alderman, 2013). Dementia incidence and as a consequence costs will increase extraordinarily in the next 40 years (Brodaty & Cumming, 2010). Alzheimer's dementia is more common in people with Down syndrome than in the general population, and it can occur at an earlier age (Wiseman et al., 2015).

When a person has dementia, one or more areas of the brain are damaged, with the areas of damage different for each person. The person cannot control the behaviour resulting from this brain damage. People with dementia are individual, both in the way they are affected (their behaviour) and the nature and extent of the underlying brain damage.

Behavioural and psychological symptoms of dementia

Behavioural and psychological symptoms of dementia (BPSD) are defined as:

- *behaviour symptoms*—including restlessness, physical aggression, screaming, agitation, wandering, culturally inappropriate behaviours, sexual disinhibition, hoarding, cursing and shadowing
- *psychological symptoms*—including anxiety, depressed mood, hallucinations and delusions.

Causes of BPSD include physical causes (medically unwell, especially delirium, medication effects, visual or hearing difficulties, fatigue, pain, constipation or urinary tract infection), environmental causes (a new environment or a change in environment, over- and under-stimulation, lack of orientation cues, lighting, including dimness and glare, and over-restriction, such as lack of places to wander) and communication difficulties, both *from* the consumer (inability to communicate needs, and communication problem as a result of cardiovascular accidents or sensory deficits in hearing or sight) and *to* the consumer (over-complication of the message, or the communication is too confronting). Because of communication difficulties, acute health issues can be difficult to identify. Sensory deficits may also be an issue. (Burns et al., 2012; New South Wales Ministry of Health, 2013).

Treatment for agitation often involves sensory input at multiple levels. Observation of individual responses should guide person-centred treatment.

Management of dementia medications

Cognitive enhancers used to reduce symptoms and disease progression have limited effectiveness—a significant amount of people do not respond at all (Cappell et al., 2010; Tricco et al., 2013). Acetyl cholinesterase inhibitors are used against the effects of Alzheimer's disease and delay the onset of some symptoms, and may lessen the severity and impact of behavioural and psychological symptoms of dementia (NSW Ministry of Health, 2013).

The most common cholinesterase inhibitors used are donepezil, rivastigmine and galantamine (Edward & Alderman, 2013). Nurses should monitor nutrition, weight and gastro effects, as gastrointenstinal side effects are common. Another drug, Memantine, works on neurotransmitters and can be used alone or in conjunction with cholinesterase inhibitors (Edward & Alderman, 2013). Cholinesterase inhibitors seem to slow progression at early stages of dementia, but the research evidence is limited.

Management is also focused on person-centred care that takes into account the person's past history. This management dependent of diagnoses may include interventions such as attendance at men's sheds, mock bus stops, activity baskets, memory corners, raised garden beds for resident participation, cars that have been disabled for simulation activities, chook runs or pet therapy, etc. Treatments include sensory modulations; for example, light-based sensory input can have an effect on mood. Behavioural issues can also be treated with multisensory input, with all senses stimulated at the same time. Response to treatments is essential to monitor as it can affect consumers in different ways, with some consumers becoming more agitated.

CRITICAL THINKING OPPORTUNITY

1 How could orientation cues (reminders to who they are, who others are, where they are, and what time/season/weather it is) be used in a home or an inpatient or residential service?

2 How could the signs and symptoms of the diagnoses of late onset psychosis and anxiety be confused?

ROBYN GARLICK

Psychotic disorders

Schizophrenia and delusional disorders in old age can be longstanding or of recent onset, and affect 17–23 per 100,000 people (Hall & Hassett, 1998). These conditions usually occur when the consumer is isolated. The presentation is normally one of harassment or feeling harassed, and usually comes to attention after a dispute. Late-life psychotic symptoms often occur as a result of a medical illness. The illness may be undiagnosed or drug induced. Other co-morbid mental illnesses should also be ruled out. There are also high rates of visual and auditory impairments in psychotic consumers. Nursing care management will include psychosocial interventions. Cognitive behaviour therapy (CBT), medication and group therapy are beneficial in the older age group (Goncalves & Byrne, 2012). Antipsychotics are likely to be administered to assist with psychotic symptoms.

Anxiety disorders

It is unusual for primary anxiety disorders to develop for the first time in old age. If they develop, be alert to the possibility of underlying depression, or hidden physical illness such as cardiac or thyroid disease. Like dementia and post-traumatic stress, anxiety may be longstanding but unrecognised. Anxiety may be triggered by the death of a spouse or sudden discontinuation of prescribed or non-prescribed medication. The Geriatric Anxiety Inventory (GAI), which is adapted from the Geriatric Depression Scales (GDS), is specific for assessing older adult anxiety.

CRITICAL THINKING OPPORTUNITY

How could anxiety be hidden or a longstanding issue and only become a problem when a spouse dies?

Hoarding disorder

The term 'hoarding' is of limited use because it can be a symptom of multiple organic and mental disorders, and cannot be utilised as a single entity for diagnoses (Mataix-Cols et al., 2010). Compulsive hoarding has been described as the acquisition of and failure to discard a large number of possessions that appear to be useless or of limited value (Timpano et al., 2011), living spaces cluttered to the point they cannot be used for activities they were designed for, and significant distress or impairment in functioning caused by the hoarding (Ayers et al., 2013).

A separate hoarding disorder has been included in the DSM 5 (American Psychiatric Association, 2013). Hoarding beliefs and behaviours will assist to classify the severity of hoarding (American Psychiatric Association, 2013). Hoarding was until 2013 listed in DSM-IV as a symptom of obsessive-compulsive personality disorder (OCPD) (Steketee, 2011). Hoarding disorder has a link with obsessive-compulsive disorder (OCD), other anxiety and mood disorders, and impulse control disorders (Mataix-Cols et al., 2010). Indecisiveness, perfectionism, and difficulty in planning and organising tasks are other common features of hoarding disorder (American Psychiatric Association, 2013). Research by Tolin and colleagues (2012) suggests differences in neural functioning, with hoarding disorder related to problems in identifying the emotional significance of belongings and the appropriate emotional response to these belongings. Tolin and colleagues' study (2012) proposed that the regulation of affect during decision-making was impaired.

Risk management is a priority and includes falls, fires, hygiene and health review (Department of Health, 2012b). The treatment of hoarding is complex and may not respond well to medical or psychological treatments. (CBT and combination therapy are often employed, and CBT has been tested and found to be beneficial in individual and group settings (Tolin et al., 2015.) The Hoarding Scale and self-reports of the Saving Inventory Scale and the Clutter Image Rating Scale are validated instruments for evaluation of the severity of the problem (Tolin, Frost & Steketee, 2010).

Older adults' medication contemplations for nurses

There are biological changes that occur in an older adult. There is typically a decrease in renal clearance; a decreased blood flow to the liver; central and peripheral neuronal cell loss; and slowed transmission. Declining organ function, increased brain and central nervous system sensitivity to medication, multiple disease and polypharmacy are special considerations due to the physical effects of ageing (Edward & Alderman, 2013) and should be considered when monitoring medication side effects. All five senses decline with age, but sexuality is maintained. There are major changes occurring in organ systems. There is a slowing of the neurological system with brain changes (shrinking brain weight after 30 years of age). Neuroplasticity of the brain may be challenged. All of these implications need to be considered when administering and managing medications in older adults.

Consider polypharmacy when reviewing medication. When listing all the medications that the consumer is taking, include over-the-counter medications, vitamins and herbal supplements. Assessment should include the consumption of grapefruit juice (this interacts with liver enzymes, affecting many medications, including hypertension and cholesterol medications). Polypharmacy increases risks to the older adult consumer by increasing the likelihood of falls (an increased likelihood of suffering blood pressure changes early), increasing the difficulty in properly diagnosing mental illness, and increasing the likelihood of adverse medication reactions, especially if not properly dosed, and interactions (Bennett et al., 2014; Kojima et al., 2012; Maher, Hanlon & Haijar, 2014; Richardson, Bennett & Kenny, 2015). Neuroleptic malignant syndrome (NMS) can occur in the older adult, and is more common in those with Parkinson's disease or Lewy body dementia. NMS from antipsychotics risk increases with the dose and duration of treatment and abrupt withdrawal; even short-term use of antipsychotics can lead to death in the older adult (Inouye, Marcantonio & Metzger, 2014; Oruch et al., 2017).

Start slowly and always go slowly when medicating older adults. Monitor closely for signs of improvement, and report signs and symptoms so changes can be made to the dose. Few studies have been undertaken on depot medication and outcomes in older adults. Low dose risperidone can be given for BPSD, but the preferred view is to remain as drug-free as possible (Edward & Alderman, 2013).

Other factors

Other care considerations and assessments should be considered when caring for older adults. Prevention of falls and assessing clinical symptoms and the environment for the potential for falls are essential. Home visiting is an issue, as it is in any area of psychiatry. A risk assessment should be completed before and after visits, considering who else is in the home, whether there are obvious risk factors such as firearms and medications, and what animals are on the property. The property itself should also be noted for safety, including any holes in floors, roads that are in disrepair and obstacles to be aware of within the property. 'No lifting' is a policy in all older adult units, and should be considered and monitored from the outset. Increasing numbers of bariatric consumers may be admitted because of vast weight gains with some antipsychotic medications.

Pain in the older person

Due to natural ageing, bodily changes and the vulnerability of risks of accidents leading to chronic pain (for example, falls), the older adult is likely to experience pain more than younger adults. If pain is expressed or identified, a pain assessment should be undertaken. Special attention should be paid to those cognitively impaired consumers who may not be able to express their pain. The Abbey scale is an example of a pain instrument that can be used on consumers not able to express themselves.

CRITICAL THINKING OPPORTUNITY

1   How could 'pain' play a part in someone's mental health?
2   How could language or speech difficulties affect the ability to measure pain?

SUMMARY

The proportion of people aged over 65 is increasing in Australia and New Zealand, while the proportion of people under 15 is declining. Population ageing will have an impact on health and health care, family composition and living arrangements. The dependency burden on future workers for support for providing pensions, housing and health care is rising. The main increase is in the over 85s and in centenarians, and these are also the age groups that have increased levels of dementia and increasing disability, more complex physical conditions and an increasing sense of hopelessness and uselessness. These conditions also link to suicide risk which is at significant levels. Misuse of alcohol and other substances is also on the increase. Good health promotion, prevention interventions and interventions targeting loneliness assist in maintaining good mental health for people of an older age.

Mental health for older people is complex. Delirium can be misinterpreted as depression or dementia. Physical health interplays with delirium, dementia and depression. The risk assessment needs to broader and are more complex. Falls, cognitive impairment, dysphagia and physical health assessments contribute to risk assessments and care.

Medication needs to be monitored closely as side effects increase due to ageing body and body systems. The ageing body causes an increase in numbers and types of medication required. Doses need to be increased slowly and need closer titration, and medication routes may have to be reviewed (crushed tablets or wafers) with dysphagia assessed.

DISCUSSION QUESTIONS

1   What might be some of the reasons that mental health problems in older adults remain undetected?
2   What types of diagnostic tools can be used to aid health professionals in diagnosing mental illness in older adults?
3   What are some of the challenges of diagnosing mental illness in older people?
4   Why must health professionals be vigilant in recognising signs of delirium and accurately treating it in older adults?
5   What factors should a health professional consider when monitoring medication effects and in consumer/carer education with an older person experiencing mental illness?

TEST YOURSELF

1. Older adults with a mental illness fall into two main groups:
   a. Those who have longstanding mental health symptoms and those who develop a mental illness when they are older.
   b. Those who are responsive to medications and those that are treatment resistant to all medications
   c. Those who have no symptoms of their mental illness and those that get minor symptoms and need their medication altered
   d. Those who have suicidal ideation and those that do not have any suicide risk.

2. Pharmacokinetics and pharmacodynamics change with age resulting in:
   a. Larger doses of all medication being required
   b. Fewer medications as often the one drug can be used for multiple reasons
   c. Even medication that a person may have been on for some time may cause new side effects and interactions because of changes in the ability to absorb, distribute, metabolise and excrete
   d. Fewer side effects as organs begin to deteriorate and have less effects from the medication

3. An example of a screening or assessment tool for delirium includes:
   a. Mini-mental status examination
   b. Cornell Scale for Depression in Dementia
   c. Confusion Assessment Method Instrument (CAMI)
   d. Psychogeriatric assessment scales (PAS)

4. The risk of developing dementia
   a. Decreases with age
   b. Increases with age
   c. Remains constant throughout life
   d. Increases with delirium

USEFUL WEBSITES

Alzheimer's Australia: www.alzheimers.org.au

Canadian Coalition for Seniors' Mental Health: www.ccsmh.ca

HealthInsite https://www.healthdirect.gov.au/older-people-and-mental-health

International Psychogeriatric Association: www.ipa-online.org

Registered Nurses' Association of Ontario—Screening for delirium, dementia and depression in older adults: http://rnao.ca/bpg/guidelines/screening-delirium-dementia-and-depression-older-adult

Victorian Government Health Information—Dementia: www.health.vic.gov.au/older/toolkit/06Cognition/02Dementia/index.htm

REFERENCES

Airagnes, G., Pelissolo, A., Lavallée, M. Flament, M., & Limosin, F. (2016). Benzodiazepine misuse in the elderly: Risk factors, consequences and management. *Current Psychiatry Reports, 18*, 89. doi:10.1007/s11920-016-0727-9.

Almeida, O. P., Draper, B., Snowdon, J., Lautenschlager, N. T., Pirkis, J., Byrne, G., Pfaff, J. J. (2012). Factors associated with suicidal thoughts in a large community study of older adults. *British Journal of Psychiatry, 201*, 466–472. doi: 10.1192/bjp.bp.112.110130.

American Psychiatric Association (2013). *Diagnostic and statistical manual of mental disorders* (5th ed.; DSM 5). Arlington: American Psychiatric Publishing.

Arola, H. M., Nicholls, E., Mallen, C., & Thomas, E. (2010). Self-reported pain interference

ROBYN GARLICK

and symptoms of anxiety and depression in community-dwelling older adults: Can a temporal relationship be determined? *European Journal of Pain, 14*(9), 966–971.

Australian Bureau of Statistics (2012). *Reflecting a nation: Stories from the 2011 Census.* ABS cat. no. 2071.0. Canberra: ABS.

Australian Bureau of Statistics (2014). *Employment projections.* ABS cat. no. 6291.0.55.003, Canberra: ABS.

Australian Bureau of Statistics (2015a). *Australian demographic statistics.* ABS cat. no. 3101.0, Canberra: ABS.

Australian Bureau of Statistics (2015b). *Disability, ageing and carers, Australia: Summary of findings.* ABS cat no. 4430.0. Canberra: Australian Bureau of Statistics.

Australian Commission on Safety and Quality in Health Care (2016). *Delirium Clinical Care Standard.* Sydney: ACSQHC.

Australian Institute of Health and Welfare (2012). *Residential aged care and home care 2013–14.*

Australian Institute of Health and Welfare (2013). *Depression in residential aged care 2008–2012.* Aged care statistics series No. 39. Cat. No AGE 73. Canberra: AIHW.

Australian Institute of Health and Welfare (2014). *Australia's welfare 2014.* Australia's welfare series no. 12. Cat. no. AUS 198. Canberra: AIHW.

Australian Institute of Health and Welfare (2015). *Australia's health 2014.* Australia's health series no. 14. Cat. no. AUS 178. Canberra: AIHW.

Ayers, C. R., Wetherall, J. L., Schiehser, D., Almklov, E., Golshan, S., & Saxena, S. (2013). Executive functioning in older adults with hoarding disorder. *International Journal of Geriatric Psychiatry, 28*(11), 1175–1181.

Barnett, K., Mercer, S. W., Norbury, M., Watt, G., Wyke, S., & Guthrie, B. (2012). Epidemiology of multimorbidity and implications for health care, research, and medical education: a cross-sectional study. *The Lancet, 380*(9836), 37–43 doi: http://dx.doi.org/10.1016/S0140-6736(12)60240-2.

Bennett, A., Gnidic, D., Gillett, M., & Carroll, P. (2014). Prevalence and Impact of Fall-risk increasing drugs, polypharmacy, and drug-drug interactions. *Drugs and Aging, 31*(3), 225–232 doi: 10.1007/s40266-013-0151-3.

Bieniek, K. F., van Blitterswijk, M., Baker, M. C., Petrucelli, L., Rademakers, R., & Dickson, D. W. (2014). Expanded C9ORF72 hexanucleotiderepeat in depressive pseudodementia. *JAMA Neurology, 71*(6), 775–781 doi: 10.1001/jamaneurol.2013.6368.

Brodaty, H., & Cumming, A. (2010). Dementia services in Australia. *International Journal of Geriatric Psychiatry, 25,* 887–895 doi:10.1002/gps.2587.

Brodaty, H., Draper, B. M., & Low, L. F. (2003). Behavioural and psychological symptoms of

dementia: A seven-tiered model of service delivery. *Medical Journal of Australia, 178*(5), 231–235.

Burns, K., Jayasinha, R., Tsang, R., & Brodaty, H. (2012). *Behaviour management. A guide to good practice: Managing Behavioural and Psyychological Symptoms of Dementia.* Sydney, Dementia Collaborative Research Centre, University of New South Wales.

Cappell, J., Herrmann, N., Cornish, S., Lanctot, K. L. (2010). The pharmacoeconomics of cognitive enhancers in moderate to severe Alzheimer's disease. *CNS Drugs, 24*(11), 909–927 doi: 10.2165/11539530-000000000-00000.

Chan, G. Z. P., Chin, C. K. L., McKitrick, D. J., & Warne, R. W. (2014). *Australasian Journal on Ageing, 33*(2), 121–123.

Contador, I, Bermejo-Pareja, F., Fernandez-Calvo, B., Boycheva, E., Tapias, E., Llamas, S., & Benito-Leon, J. (2016). The 37 item version of the Mini-Mental State Examination: Normative data in a population-based cohort of older Spanish adults (NEDICES). *Archives of Clinical Neuropsychology, 31*(3), 263–272.

Conwell, Y., Duberstein, P. R., Hirsch, J. K., Conner, K. R., Eberly, S., & Caine, E. D. (2010). Health status and suicide in the second half of life. *International Journal of Geriatric Psychiatry, 25*(4), 371–379 doi: 10.1002/gps.2348.

Cosgrove, J., Jamieson, S., Smith, & Alty, J. (2015). The relationship between clock drawing and cognition in Parkinson's. *Journal of Neurology Neurosurgery and Psychiatry, 86*(11), 82–84, doi:10.1136/jnnp-2015-312379.172.

Cukrowicz, K. C., Cheavens, J. S., van Orden, K. A., Ragain, R. M., & Cook, R. L. (2011). Perceived burdensomeness and suicide ideation in older adults. *Psychological Aging, 26*(2), 331–338 doi: 10.1037/a0021836.

Davies, E. A., & O'Mahony, M. S. (2015). Adverse drug reactions in special populations: The elderly. *British Journal of Clinical Pharmacology, 80*(4), 796–87, doi: 10.1111/bcp.12596.

Day, J., Higgins, I., & Koch, T. (2010). Delirium and older people in acute care. In R. Nay & S. Garratt (Eds.), *Older people: Issues and innovations in care.* Sydney: Elsevier.

De Hert, M., Correll, C. U., Bobes, J., Cetkovich-Bakmas, M., Cohen, D., Asai, I., Leucht, S. (2011). Physical illness in patients with severe mental disorders. 1. Prevalence, impact of medications and disparities in health care. *World Psychiatry, 10*(1), 52–77.

De Leo, D., Draper, B. M., Snowdon, J., & Kolves, K. (2013). Suicides in older adults: a case control psychological autopsy study in Australia. *Journal of Psychiatric Research, 47,* 980–988 doi: http://dx.doi.org/10.1016/j.psychires.2013.009.

Dell'osso, B., & Lader, M. (2012). Do benzodiazepines still deserve a major role in the treatment of psychiatric disorders?

A Critical reappraisal. *European Psychiatry, 28*(1), 7–20, doi: http://dx.doi.org/10.1016/j.eurpsy.2011.11.003.

Department of Health. (2012a). *Best care for older people everywhere: The toolkit.* Melbourne: Victorian Government.

Department of Health. (2012b). *Discussion paper: Hoarding and squalor.* Melbourne: Ageing and Aged Care Branch, State of Victoria.

Department of Human Services (2006). *An introduction to Victoria's public clinical mental health services.* Melbourne: Government of Victoria.

Department of Human Services (2009). *Because mental health matters—Victorian mental health reform strategy 2009–2019.* Melbourne: Department of Human Services.

Dols, A., Kupka, R. W., van Lammeren, A., Beekman, A. T., Sajatovic, M., & Stek, M. L. (2013). The prevalence of late-life mania: a review. *Bipolar disorders, 16*(2), 113–118 doi:10.1111/bdi.12104.

Edward, K. L.& Alderman,C. (2013). *Psychopharmacology: Practice and Contexts.* Melbourne: Oxford University Press.

El-Gabalawy, R., Mackenzie, C. S., Shooshtari, S., & Sareen, J. (2011). Comorbid physical health conditions and anxiety disorders: a population-based exploration of prevalence and health outcomes among older adults. *General Hospital Psychiatry, 33*(6), 556–564.

Elliott, R. A., & Booth, J. C. (2014). Problems with medicine use in older Australians: a review of the recent literature. *Journal of Pharmacy Practice and Research, 44*(4), 258–271.

Feng, L., Chong, M. S., Lim, W. S., & Ng, T. P. (2012). The modified Mini-Mental State Examination test: normative data for Singapore Chinese older adults and its performance in detecting early cognitive impairment. *Singapore Medical Journal, 53*(7), 458–462.

Fong, T. G., Davis, D. D., Growdon, M. E., Albuquerque, A., & Inouye, S. K. (2015). The interface between delirium and dementia in elderly adults. *The Lancet Neurology, 14*(8), 823–832.

Forester, B. P., Ajilore, O., Spino, C., & Lehmann, S. (2015). Clinical Characteristics of Patients with Late Life Bipolar Disorder in the Community: Data from the NNDC Registry. *American Journal of Geriatric Psychiatry, 23*(9), 977–984 doi:10.1016/j.jagp.2015.01.001.

Gaggiolo, A., Scaratti, C., Morganti, L., Stramba-Badiale, M., Agostoni, M., Spatola, C. A. M. Riva, G. (2014). Effectiveness of group reminiscence for improving wellbeing of institutionalized elderly adults: study protocol for a randomized controlled trial. BioMed Central, 15, 408, doi: 10.1186/1745-6215-15-408.

Gale, C. R., Cooper, C., Deary, I. J., & Sayer, A. A. (2014). Psychological wellbeing and incident frailty in men and women: The English

Longitudinal Study of Ageing. *Psychological Medicine, 44*(4), 697–76, doi: 10.1017/S0033291713001384.

Gareri, P., Castagna, A., Ruotolo, G., Merante, A., Russo, G., & De Sarro, G. (2016). Drug-induced delirium: A frequent and important matter for geriatricians. *Journal of Pharmaceutical and Biomedical Science, 6*(1), 70–74.

Gerland, P., Raftery, A. E., Sevcikova, H., Li, N., Gu, D., Spoorenberg, T., Wilmoth, J. (2014). World population stabilization unlikely this century. *Science, 346*(6206), 234–237.

Goncalves, D. C., & Byrne, G. J. (2012). Interventions for generalized anxiety disorder in older adults: Systematic review and meta-analysis. *Journal of Anxiety Disorders, 26*(1), 1–11.

Greenblatt, H. K., & Greenblatt, D. J. (2016). Antidepressant associated hyponatremia in the elderly. *Journal of Clinical Psychopharmacology, 36*(6), 545–549 doi:10.1097/JCP.0000000000000608.

Gryschek, R. C. B., Pereira, R. M., Kono, A., Patzina, R. A., Tresoldi, A. T., Shikanai-Yasuda, M. A., & Benard, G. (2010). Paradoxical reaction to treatment in 2 patients with severe acute paracoccidiodomycosis. *Clinical Infectious Disease, 50*(10), 56–58, doi: https://doi.org/10.1086/652290.

Gutzman, H., & Qazi, A. (2015). Depression associated with dementia. *Gerontologic Geriatrics, 48*(4), 305–311 doi: 10.1007/s00391-015-0898-8.

Hall, K. A., & Hassett, A. M. (1998). Assessing and managing old age psychiatric disorders in the community. *Medical Journal of Australia, 168*(6), 299–305.

Han, J. H., Wilson, A., & Ely, E. W. (2010). Delirium in the older emergency department patient: A quiet epidemic. *Emergency Medicine Clinics of North America, 28*(3), 611–631.

Happell, B., Byrne, L., Platiana-Phung, C., Harris, S., Bradshaw, J., & Davies, J. (2014). Lived-experience participation in nurse education: Reducing stigma and enhancing popularity. *International Journal of Mental Health Nursing, 23*(5), 427–434.

Happell, B., Stanton, R., Hoey, W., & Scott, D. (2014). Cardiometabolic health nursing to improve health and primary care access in community mental health consumers: Baseline physical health outcomes from a randomised controlled trial. *Issues in mental health nursing, 35*(2), 114–121.

Health Workforce Australia (2014). *Australia's Future Health Workforce.* Canberra, Department of Health.

Hunter, S. (2012). *Miller's nursing for wellness in older adults. First Australian and New Zealand edition.* Sydney, Lippincott, Williams & Wilkins.

Inouye, S. K., Marcantonio, E. R., & Metzger, E. D. (2014). Doing damage in delirium: the hazards of antipsychotic treatment in elderly persons. *The Lancet Psychiatry, 1*(4), 312–315 doi: 10.1016/S2215-0366(14)70263-9.

Jackson, T. A., Naqvi, S. H., & Sheehan, B. (2013). Screening for dementia in general hospital inpatients: a systematic review and meta-analysis of available instruments. *Age and Ageing, 42,* 689–695 doi: 10.1093/ageing/aft145.

Jayasekara, R., Procter, N., Harrison, J., Skelton, K., Hampel, S., Draper, R., & Deuter, K. (2015). Cognitive behavioural therapy for older adults with depression: a review. *Journal of Mental Health, 24*(3), 168–171 doi: 10.3109/09638237.2014.971143.

Jorm, A. F., & Mackinnon, A. J. (2016). *Psychogeriatric assessment scale: 4th Edition.* Melbourne, Mental Health Research Institute.

Kennedy, J. (2015). Depressive pseudodementia— how 'pseudo' is it really? *Old Age Psychiatrists, 62,* 30–37.

Kishita, N., & Laidlaw, K. (2017). Cognitive behaviour therapy for generalized anxiety disorder: Is CBT equally efficacious in adults of working age and older adults? *Clinical Psychology Review, 52,* 124–136.

Kobayashi, T. Kato, S. (2011). *Depression–dementia medius: Between depression and the manifestation of dementia symptoms.* Psychogeriatrics, 11 (3), 177–182.

Kojima, T., Akishita, M., Nakamura, T., Nomura, K., Ogawa, S., Iijima, K., Ouchi, Y. (2012). Polypharmacy as a risk for fall occurrence in geriatric outpatients. *Geriatric Gerontologist International, 12,* 425–430 doi: 10.1111/j.1447-0594.2011.00783.

Maher, R. L., Hanlon, J. T., & Haijar, E. R. (2014). Clinical consequences of polypharmacy in elderly. *Expert Opinion Drug Safety, 13*(1), doi: 10.1517/14740338.2013.827660.

Martin, L. A., Neighbors, H. W., & Griffith, D. M. (2013). The experience of symptoms of depression in men versus women: Analysis of the National Comorbidity Survey Replication. *Journal of American Medical Association Psychiatry, 70*(10), 1100–1106.

Mataix-Cols, D., Frost, R. O., Pertusa, A., Clark, L. A., Saxena, S., Leckman, J. F., Wilhelm, S. (2010). Hoarding disorder: A new diagnosis for DSM-V? *Depression and Anxiety, 27*(6), 556–572.

McCann, T. V., Clark, E., & Lu, S. (2010). Bachelor of Nursing students career choices: A three – year longitudinal study. *Nurse Education Today, 30*(1), 31–36.

McCutcheon, S. T., Han, D., Troncoso, J., Koliatso, V. E., Albert, M., Lyketsos, C. G., & Leoutsakos, J. M. S. (2016). Clinicopathological correlates of depression in early Alzheimer's disease in the NACC. *International Journal of Geriatric Psychiatry, 31*(12), 1301–1312.

New South Wales Ministry of Health (2013). *Assessment and Management of People with Behavioural and Psychological Symptoms of Dementia (BPSD).Handbook for NSW Health Clinicians.* North Sydney, Royal Australian and New Zealand College of Psychiatrists.

Nicholas, R., Lee, N., & Roche, A. (2011). *Pharmaceutical Drug Misuse in Australia: Complex Problems, Balanced Responses.* National Centre for Education and Training on Addiction (NCETA), Flinders University, Adelaide.

O'Regan, N., Fitzgerald, J., Adamis, D., Molloy, D. W., Meagher, D., & Timmons, S. (2016). Frequency and stability of motor subtypes in older medical inpatients with incident delirium. *Age Ageing, 45*(supp. 2), ii1–ii12, doi: https://doi.org/10.1093/ageing/afw159.04.

Ohmuro, N., Matsumoto, K., Katsura, M., Obara, C., Kikuchi, T., Hamaie, Y., Matsuoka, H. (2015). The association between cognitive deficits and depressive symptoms in at-risk mental state: A comparison with fist-episode psychosis. *Schizophrenia Research, 1-3*(162), 67–73.

Oruch, R., Pryme, I. F., Engelsen, B. A., & Lund, A. (2017). Neuroleptic malignant syndrome: an easily overlooked neurologic emergency. *Neuropsychiatric Disorder Treatments, 13,* 161–175 doi: 10.2147/NDT.S118438.

Pendlebury, S. T., Klaus, S. P., de Brito, M., & Wharton, R. M. (2015). Routine cognitive screening in older patients admitted to acute medicine: abbreviated mental test score (AMTS) and subjective memory complaint versus Montreal Cognitive Assessment and IQCODE. *Age Ageing, 44*(6), 1000–1005.

Podgorski, C. A., Langford, L., Pearson, J. L., & Conwell, Y. (2010). Suicide prevention for older adults in residential communities: Implications for policy and practice. *PLoS Medicine, 7*(5), doi: 10.1371/journal.pmed.1000254.

Raue, P. J., Ghesquiere, A. R., & Bruce, M. L. (2014). Suicide risk in primary care: identification and management in older adults. *Current Psychiatric Reports, 16*(9), 466–470 doi: 10.1007/s11920-014-0466-8.

Reckel, B., Grundy, E., Cylus, J., Mackenbach, J. P., Knai, C., & McKee, M. (2013). Aging in the European Union. *The Lancet, 381*(9874), 1312–22.

Richardson, K., Bennett, K., & Kenny, R. A. (2015). Polypharmacy including falls risk-increasing medications and subsequent falls in community-dwelling middle-aged and older adults. *Age and Ageing, 44,* 90–96 doi: 10.1093/ageing/afu141.

Rizzi, L., Rosset, I., & Roriz-Cruz, M. (2014). Global epidemiology of dementia: Alzheimer's and vascular types. *BioMed Research*

International, 908915, 8 pages, http://dx.doi. org/10.1155/2014/908915.

Rodrigues, R., Petersen, R. B., & Perry, G. (2014). Parallels between major depressive disorder and alzheimer's disease: Role of oxidative stress and genetic vulnerability. *Cell Molecular Neurobiology, 34*(7), 925–949 doi:10.1007/s10571-014-0074-5.

Rosen, T., Connors, S., Clark, S., Halpem, A., Stern, M. E., deWald, J., Flomenbaum, N. (2015). Assessment and management of delirium in older adults in the emergency department: Literature review to inform development of a novel clinical protocol. *Advanced Emergency Nursing Journal, 37*(3), 183–E3 doi: 10.1097/TME.0000000000000066.

Roth, M., Huppert, F. A., Mountjoy, C. Q., & Tym, E. (1999). *CAMDEX-R boxed set: the revised Cambridge examination for mental disorders of the elderly* 3rd Edition. Cambridge, Cambridge University Press.

Salive, M. E. (2013). Multimorbidity in older adults. *Epidemiologic Reviews, 35*(1), 75–83.

Sami, M., Khan, H., & Nilforooshan, R. (2015). Late onset mania as an organic syndrome: a review of case reports in the literature. *Journal of Affective Disorders, 188*, 226–231 doi: http:// dx.doi.org/10.1016/j.jad.2015.08.027.

Scherrer, J. F., Lustman, P. J., Loveland Cook, C. A., Salas, J., Burge, S., & Schneider, F. D. (2014). Factors that influence the association between severity of pain and severity of depression in primary care patients. *Journal of Pain Management, 7*(2), 117–128.

Shah, A., Bhat, R., Zarate-Escudero, S., De Leo, D., & Erlangsen, A. (2016). Suicide rates in five-year age-bands after the age of 60 years: the international landscape. *Aging & Mental Health, 20*(2), 131–138 doi: http://dx.doi.org/10.1080/13 607863.2015.1055552.

Sheehan, B. (2012). Assessment scales in dementia. *Therapeutic Advances in Neurological Disorders, 5*(6), 349–358 doi: 10.1177/1756285612455733.

Statistics New Zealand (2016). *Population Projections Overview*. Wellington, New Zealand Government.

Stein, J., Luppa, M., Kaduszkiewicz, H., Eisele, M., Weyerer, S., Werle, J., Maier, W. (2015). Is the Short Form of the Mini-Mental State Examination (MMSE) a better screening instrument for dementia in older primary care patients than the original MMSE? Results of the German study on ageing, cognition, and dementia in primary care patients (AgeCoDe). *Psychological Assessment, 27*(3), 895-904.

Steketee, G. (2011). *The Oxford handbook of obsessive compulsive and spectrum disorders*. Oxford, Oxford University Press.

Stone, J. A., Lester, C. A., Aboneh, E. A., Phelan, C. H., Welch, L. L., & Chui, M. A. (2017).

A preliminary examination of over-the counter medication misuse in older adults. *Research in Social and Administrative Pharmacy, 13*(1), 187–192, doi: http://dx.doi.org/10.1016/j. sapharm.2016.01.004.

Symonds, C., & Anderson, I. M. (2016). Unipolar depressive disorders. *Psychiatric Disorders, 44*(11), 654–660 doi: http://dx.doi.org/10.1016/j. mpmed.2016.08.013.

Tachjian, A., Maria, V., & Jahangir, A. (2010). Use of herbal products and potential interactions in patients with cardiovascular diseases. *Journal of the American College of Cardiology, 56*(11), 515–525 doi: http://dx.doi.org/10.1016/jacc.2009.07.074.

Thomas, K. H. Martin, R. M. Potokar, J. Pirmohamed, M., & Gunnell, D. (2014). Reporting of drug induced depression and fatal and non-fatal suicidal behaviour in the UK from 1998 to 2011. *BMC Pharmacology and Toxicology, 15*: 54 doi: 10.1186/2050-6511-15-54.

Thompson, C., Brodaty, H., Trollor, J., & Sachdev, P. (2010). Behavioural and psychological symptoms associated with dementia subtype and severity. *International Psychogeriatrics, 22*(2), 300–305 doi: 10.1017/S1041610209991220.

Timpano, K. R., Exner, C., Glaesmer, H., Rief, W., Keshaviah, A., Brähler, E., & Wilhelm S. (2011). The epidemiology of the proposed DSM 5 hoarding disorder: Exploration of the acquisition specifier, associated features, and distress. *Journal Clinical Psychiatry, 72*(6), 780–786, doi: 10.4088/ JCP.10m06380.

Tobe, E. (2012). Pseudodementia caused by severe depression. *BMJ Case Reports* doi:10.1136/ bcr-2012-007156.

Tolin, D. F., Frost, R. O., & Steketee, G. (2010). A brief interview for assessing compulsive hoarding: The hoarding rating scale—interview. *Psychiatry Research, 178*(1), 147–152.

Tolin, D. F., Frost, R. O., Steketee, G., & Muroff, J. (2015). Cognitive behavioural therapy for hoarding disorder: a meta-analysis. *Depression and Anxiety, 32*(3), 158–166 doi: 10.1002/da.22327.

Tolin, D. F., Stevens, M. C., Villavicencio, A. L., Norberg, M. N., Calhoun, V. D., Frost, R. O., … Pearlson, G. D. (2012). Neural mechanisms of decision making in hoarding disorder. *Archives of General Psychiatry, 69*(8), 832–841, doi:10.1001/ archgenpsychiatry.2011.1980.

Traynor, V., Cordato, N., Burns, P., Britten, N., Duncan, K., deVries, L., & McKinnon, C. (2016). Is delirium being detected in emergency? *Australasian Journal on Ageing, 35*(1), 54 -57.

Tricco, A. C., Sooiah, C., Berliner, S., Ho, J. M., Ng, C. H., Ashoor, H. M. Straus, S. E. (2013). Efficacy and safety of cognitive enhancers for patients with mild cognitive impairment: a

systematic review and meta-analysis. *Canadian Medical Association Journal, 185*(16), 1393–1401 doi: 10.1503/cmaj.130451.

Trojano, L., & Gainotti, G., (2016). Drawing disorders in Alzheimer's disease and other forms of dementia. *Journal of Alzheimer's Disease, 53*(1), 31 -52 doi:10.3233/JAD-160009.

Van Strater, A. C. P., & Bogers, J. P. A. M., (2012). Interaction of St John's Wort (Hypericum perforatum) with clozapine. *International Clinical Psychopharmacology, 27*(2), 121–124.

Venneri, A., & Malik, B. (2014). Assessing mental status in Pakistanis living in the UK: A comparison of two different Urdu versions of the MMSE. *Alzheimer's & Dementia: Journal of the Alzheimer's Association, 10*(4), 433–434.

Victorian Department of Human Services (2006). *What is person-centred health care?* Melbourne, Victorian Department of Human Services.

Vyas, A., Pan, X. & Sambamoorthi, U. (2012). Chronic condition clusters and polypharmacy. *International Journal of Family Medicine*, 1–8, doi:10.1155/2012/193168.

Waite, J., & Easton, A. (Eds.) (2013). *The ECT Handbook. 3rd Edition.* London, Central Policy Committee, Royal College Psychiatrists.

Webb, R. T., Kontopantelis, E., Doran, T., Qin, P., Creed, F., & Kapur, N. (2012). Suicide risk in primary care patients with major physical diseases: a case control study. *Archives of General Psychiatry, 69*(3), 256–264.

Wenborn, W., Challis, D., Head, J., Miranda-Castillo, C., Popham, C., Thakur, R., Illes, J., & Orrell, M. (2013). Providing activity for people with dementia in care homes: A cluster randomised controlled trial. *International Journal of Geriatric Psychiatry, 28*(12), 1296–1304.

Winblad, B., Amouyel, P., Andrieu, S., Ballard, C., Brayne, C., Brodaty, H., Wimo, A. (2016). Defeating Alzheimer's disease and other dementia: a priority for European science and society. *The Lancet Neurology, 15*, 455–532.

Wiseman, F. K., Al-Janabi, T., Hardy, J., Karmiloff-Smith, A., Nizetic, D., Tybulewicz, V. L. J. Strydom, A. (2015). A genetic cause of Alzheimer disease: mechanistic insights from Down Syndrome. *Nature Review Neuroscience, 16*(9), 564–574 doi: 10.1038/nrn3983.

World Health Organization (2013). *Mental health and older adults*. Factsheet no. 381, Geneva, WHO.

Wu, H. E., & Okusaga, O. O. (2014). Antipsychotic Medication-Induced Dysphoria: Its Meaning, Association with Typical vs. Atypical Medications and Impact on Adherence. *Psychiatric Quarterly, 86*(2), 199–205 doi:10.1007/ s11126-014-9319-1.

CHAPTER 17

Young People's Mental Health

KRISTY YOUNG AND
CHRISTINE POOLE

KEY OUTCOMES

AFTER READING THIS CHAPTER, YOU SHOULD BE ABLE TO:

- define infancy, childhood, adolescence and parenting
- identify factors affecting development, including skills deficits
- describe attachment theory and the impact of attachment disturbance
- describe trauma theory and the impact of trauma on the developing brain
- describe the processes involved in psychosocial assessment of infants, children, adolescents and families
- describe therapeutic interventions

KEY TERMS

- adolescence
- attachment
- childhood
- development
- infancy
- parenting
- trauma

Introduction

In this chapter you will explore early developmental stages and family relationships as well as infant, child and adolescent mental health, and the factors that contribute to the development of mental health disorders.

Stages of development

The early years of development are fundamentally important for neurological development. This has a direct impact on how the child learns new skills, including social and emotional skills throughout their life. Having a developmental perspective allows us to understand how humans continually grow and learn new skills throughout their life in physical, cognitive (intellectual), social, emotional and language realms. Human development generally follows a predictable pattern, making it possible for us to identify potential problems and intervene early. It also allows us to better understand how our consumers might behave, think, learn and feel, allowing us, as nurses, to better able to engage and communicate with them.

These stages form a continuum along which development proceeds.

- prenatal and neonatal
- infancy: newborn, baby and toddler
- childhood: preschool and school age
- adolescence: the period between puberty and maturity
- adulthood: young, middle age and old age.

Infancy

The period of infancy ranges from newborn to three to four years of age. Within this period there are three phases: newborn, baby and toddler. Social interactions and relationships that infants have with their parents or carers influence their emotional development (Mares, Newman & Warren with Cornish, 2011). The term 'infancy' is applied to the first year of life at which time the baby begins to learn about their immediate environment. Their learning is helped by the baby having the ability to focus their vision. Cognitively the baby is already learning about language and making sounds. It is also at this stage that the baby is able to develop secure attachments if they receive responsive, consistent and sensitive parenting.

The toddler period extends from 15 months to two and a half years. During this phase toddlers are becoming more independent and mobile, leading them to have a desire to explore their surroundings. They are also learning to manage frustration and strong emotions; and may show defiant behaviour leading to tantrums when they are thwarted. The toddler begins to understand right from wrong, and by two years of age shows some self-awareness. Language is also increasing and by two years of age they should be able to form simple phrases and sentences.

Childhood

According to the Centre for Community Child Health (2006), childhood includes the following periods:

- The preschool period (two and a half to six years) is a time of growing independence. Children at this age want to be considered more responsible; for example, they may want to choose their clothes. They develop a greater sense of empathy, and past experiences with others are remembered and can become part of the self-concept. During this period children develop an understanding of social rules, and therefore there is a systematic increase in pro-social behaviour and a decrease in aggressive behaviour. Children prefer to play with specific peers, and they develop friendships.
- In the school-age period (six to twelve years; also known as the middle or latency years), personality traits are developing. The school-age child is becoming more social, and is gaining more autonomy by exploring relationships outside of the family while maintaining good relationships with family members. The main tasks are friendships, self-control (of body and emotions) and mastery of the environment. They understand the clear distinction between public and private life (secrets), understand that they have an external and internal life (fantasy) and engage in hobbies.

Adolescence

Martin and Volkmar (2007) define adolescence as a period of rapid growth and development from puberty to maturity, generally occurring between the ages of 13 and 18 years, but sometimes continuing until the age of 20. This period of growth varies from person to person. Physical, social, cognitive and psychological changes occur simultaneously. The general magnitude of change in adolescence makes this a period of upheaval, ambivalence and turmoil for young people and their families. Physical and sexual growth and maturation are intertwined with the development of a clearer sense of personal, sexual and vocational identity; individuation from family; firmer personality characteristics; expectation or assumption of greater responsibility; development of an appropriate set of values; and a heightened capacity for peer relationships and intimacy.

Adulthood and parenting

The importance of assessing and treating the parent–child relationship when working within the infant, child and adolescent mental health setting is critical. The quality of parenting that people receive is

---

BOX 17.1 **KEY CONSIDERATIONS FOR NURSES: INCLUDING PARENTS**

■ Parents are *usually* doing the best they can. Therefore, support them, coach them and teach them—but don't blame them.

■ The nurse should consider how the young person's family can become an asset to

therapy. More often than not, they know the young person better than you do. The parents will also have significantly more contact with the young person than you will and hence more opportunity for encouraging and promoting change.

---

probably the most influential factor in their physical, psychological, social and economic development and well-being (Martin & Volkmar, 2007). Factors affecting parenting behaviour include a parent's own personal experiences and trauma, mental health, family experiences, cultural background, parents' temperaments, domestic violence, marital discord and the child's characteristics and temperament.

The development of parenting roles and tasks is critical for meeting children's needs for safety, care, control, intellectual stimulation and emotional literacy (that is, understanding feelings in self and others). The parents must establish routines in order to meet these needs, which is a complex process. Specific types of problems can arise if parents have difficulty with routines, including emotional and conduct problems.

Sensitive responsiveness in relation to a child's developmental needs is a key aspect of the parenting task. It refers to the emotional relationship with the child, and involves how parents respond and attune to their child's demands, behaviours and distress, and how they deal with the resolution of interpersonal conflicts. Protectiveness, emotional regulation, disciplining and play are key areas associated with sensitive responsiveness (Martin & Volkmar, 2007).

Nurses can fall into the trap of 'parent blaming' in their attempts to advocate for the infant, child or adolescent. This should be avoided, as it can further result in feelings of inadequacy, helplessness, hopelessness and self-doubt in the parent, adding to the disharmony in parentz–child relationships and causing ongoing difficulties for the family. Nurses instead are encouraged to take a position of neutrality, understanding, empathy, curiosity, warmth and respect, while being able to reflect on themselves and what they bring to each and every interaction with a consumer and their family, for example, their own family of origin experience (Flaskas, 2011).

1   What are the important developmental tasks of infancy, childhood and adolescence?

2   Complete the following table:

CRITICAL THINKING OPPORTUNITY

Stage	Age range	Physical	Cognitive	Social	Emotional	Language
Infancy						
Toddler						
Pre-school						
School age						
Adolescence						

KRISTY YOUNG AND CHRISTINE POOLE

Factors affecting development

Normal development may be affected by biological, psychological and environmental factors:

- *biological factors*—genetic makeup, internal factors, and temperament and biological vulnerability
- *psychological factors*—experience, reinforcement, motivation, attachment, nurturance, protection and support
- *environmental factors*—prenatal (a critical time for rapid growth), trauma, infection, nutrition, social and cultural factors (for example, gender and expectations of children), family stress and parenting style.

CRITICAL THINKING OPPORTUNITY

Why is it important to have a developmental framework when working in the field of infant, child and adolescent mental health?

Theories of development

There are a number of theories associated with early childhood development. Table 17.1 summarises the major theories.

TABLE 17.1 MAJOR THEORIES IN EARLY CHILDHOOD DEVELOPMENT		
Theoretical framework	**Theorists**	**Theory**
Psychodynamic	Sigmund Freud	Unconscious urges control behaviour
Emotional and psychological development	Erik Erikson	Built upon Freud's work; described eight stages of development
	John Bowlby	Explored attachment and recognised four aspects
	Mary Ainsworth	Built on Bowlby's work and devised a procedure to test the quality of attachment between carers and their child
Cognitive development	Jean Piaget	Children go through four stages of thinking in their cognitive development
Behavioural and learning theories	Albert Bandura	Social and observational learning
	B. F. Skinner	Operant conditioning
Language development	Lev Vygotsky	Four stages of speech development
	Noam Chomsky	All children are born with an innate ability to learn language
Moral development	Lawrence Kohlberg	Morality starts in early childhood and development can be affected by many factors

BOX 17.2 KEY CONSIDERATIONS FOR NURSES: DEVELOPMENT

- Children and adolescents with mental health problems 'do well if they can'. According to Greene (2005), if a child *could* do well, they *would* do well. Children and adolescents who don't do well may not have the *internal skills* to behave adaptively (Greene, 2005).

- Children and adolescents also may have *developmental delays*—their chronological age may not match their developmental progress. Consult with your colleagues if you are unsure: paediatricians, psychologists, occupational therapists and speech therapists regularly perform developmental assessments.

- Understanding whether a child or adolescent has skills deficits helps us to understand the context of their behaviour. For nurses and parents, understanding the context and meaning behind the young person's behaviour and interpreting it is critical to ensure a fair, flexible and appropriate (fitting) response to the behaviour. Nurses have a role in assessing and identifying skills deficits and implementing strategies to teach new skills. Nurses also need to work with parents to better understand their child and their behaviour (Regan, 2006).

- Skills deficits can be understood as a form of developmental delay according to Greene (2005). Children with skills deficits may have a history of trauma and disrupted attachment. Children and adolescents with social, emotional or behavioural problems may not have the internal skills to manage emotions, behave appropriately and get on with others. Problems can occur in any of the following domains:

- Executive functioning—the cognitive processes required to organise, plan, initiate, prioritise, monitor, reflect, self-evaluate and change.

- Social competency—includes the ability to process and make sense of social information as well as the development of appropriate social skills and conflict resolution skills.

SKILLS DEFICITS

- Emotional regulation and processing— includes the ability to identify and understand one's own emotions, use emotions during social interactions, use emotional awareness to guide problem-solving, deal with frustration, keep distress from overwhelming the ability to think, and be in control of how and when feelings are expressed (Havighurst, Harley & Prior, 2004).

- Language and communication—includes the ability to express oneself (verbally and written) and to understand what is being said by others. It also includes understanding social communication (pragmatics) such as body language, facial cues, conversation (staying on and changing topics, checking and clarifying), jokes, slang and colloquialisms, and adapting language according to the setting and people.

- Auditory processing—the ability to make sense of what is heard.

- Arousal and sensory processing—how physically and mentally alert one feels (arousal) and the ability to organise and interpret information received through the senses (sensory processing). Senses include visual, auditory, tactile, oral, olfactory, vestibular (gravity and balance) and proprioception (position and movement) (Ayres, 2005).

Bowlby's attachment theory

John Bowlby's attachment theory is utilised widely and in many different forms in the field of infant, child and adolescent mental health, and we turn to it now.

Healthy attachment is a reciprocal, enduring emotional connection between a child and his primary caregiver that is sensitive, consistent and responsive, resulting in the child's emotional and physical needs being met and the formation of a secure attachment with the carer. This then becomes the core template for all future relationships later in life. Attachment is necessary for the development of closeness and the satisfaction of the human need for love and belonging (Sameroff, McDonough & Rosenblum, 2004). Bowlby, who is considered to be the father of attachment theory, believed that there are four distinguishing characteristics of attachment:

1 *proximity*—the desire to be near the people we are attached to
2 *safe haven*—returning to the attachment figure for comfort and safety in the face of distress
3 *secure base*—the attachment figure acts as a base of security from which the child can explore the surrounding environment
4 *separation distress*—anxiety that occurs in the absence of the attachment figure (Siegel & Hartzell, 2004).

Attachment behaviour is expected to appear in infants at around seven to nine months of age. It is through the experience of a secure attachment relationship that children have greater ability to master and/or solve problems, are more creative and complex in their symbolic play, are more attractive to other children as playmates, learn to regulate their emotional state (learning to self-sooth or self-regulate) and come to feel safe and build resilience and trusting relationships with others.

Children who experience disrupted attachment may suffer damage to all developmental systems, including the brain, and may exhibit increased social and emotional withdrawal and indiscriminate sociability; that is, the child will become friendly very quickly with strangers, develop clingy behaviour towards parents, become hypervigilant (believing the world is unsafe and dangerous), exhibit dysregulation of emotions such as sleep disturbance and an inability to sooth self, and have difficulty in communication as a result of language delays.

Factors that may affect attachment include parental mental illness, parental neglect, lack of responsive and consistent parenting, physical or sexual abuse, absence of parent (either physically or emotionally), unplanned pregnancy, witnessing domestic violence, substance use and abuse by parents, and parents suffering financial hardship and trauma (Mares, Newman & Warren, 2005).

Attachment disturbance is an important risk factor for various clinical disorders, but attachment may also be compromised by other risk factors that give rise to symptom presentation and mental health disorders (such as trauma) (AACAP, 2005).

ABOUT THE CONSUMER Ella's story

Ella is a 6-month-old unplanned baby whose mother, Rachel, is a 28-year-old teacher. Ella's father works long hours and her extended family live interstate so the family are quite isolated with no supports. Ella and her mother were referred by the child health nurse to the local Infant Mental Health Service, where it was noted that Ella was rarely making eye contact, gave very few smiles and made no verbal noises; she was also not rolling over. Whenever the child health nurse visited, Ella was either in her cot or in the baby swing, and was receiving little stimulation from toys or mobiles. Rachel looked tired and admitted to being depressed since the birth of Ella, but had not sought help from the GP as she felt that because she was a teacher, who was used to managing a class of 25 seven-year-olds, she should be able to cope with her own baby. Rachel also stated that she was only meeting the basic care needs for Ella, such as feeding and bathing, and added that she had no energy and had no desire to cuddle or play with Ella when she was awake.

REFLECTION
QUESTIONS

1   Do you think that Ella and Rachel have a positive attachment relationship?

2   If not, what do you think are the factors preventing Rachel from having a positive relationship with Ella?

3   Is Ella on track developmentally?

4   What are the signs that Ella's development is delayed?

5   What other signs are there that suggest Ella's attachment to her mother is disrupted?

Trauma

Trauma can be broadly defined as an experience that threatens the individual's psychological or physical well-being or physical existence, and that overwhelms the individual's coping mechanisms (Mares, Newman & Warren, 2005, p. 173). According to Downey (2007), 80 per cent of trauma occurs within the family home. The most difficult trauma for children is that experienced in the parent–child relationship, as the person who you depend on to love you and keep you safe is also the person who is hurting you.

Trauma exposure is associated with antisocial behaviour and mental health disorders, which can lead to social disruption for the victim (Paz, Jones & Byrne, 2005). According to Caffo, Forresi and Lievers (2005), high-risk populations, such as homeless adolescents and juvenile offenders, have been shown to experience particularly high rates of trauma, including physical and sexual abuse, and being victims of violent crime. Exposure to domestic violence and physical maltreatment is a predictor of later antisocial behaviour. The majority of young people admitted to mental health units have histories of trauma and have experienced significant loss and grief in their lives. Most have experienced cumulative complex trauma (for example, chronic abuse, chaotic households and neglect) rather than a one-off trauma (for example, a car accident or bushfire).

Research has found that trauma affects neurological development as a result of alterations to the structures and functions of the brain. This therefore affects learning and day-to-day functioning, including abstract thought, concrete thought, memory, concentration, social skills, affiliation, attachment, sexual behaviour, emotional reactivity, motor regulation, arousal, appetite, sleep, blood pressure, heart rate and body temperature (National Executive Training Institute, 2005).

Our brains are built to cope with stress using the fight–flight–freeze response, which is a normal and protective response when confronted with a potentially dangerous and life-threatening situation. This response is heightened and overdeveloped in those who have experienced trauma. This can mean that they are often operating in a state of physiological arousal and are therefore rarely calm. Their body responds to perceived threats and possibly non-threatening situations as if they are under threat and at risk (Downey, 2007).

All children respond differently to trauma, depending on their temperament and their level of resilience. Trauma may disrupt attachment and can impede child development. Children are more vulnerable to trauma than adults because trauma has a detrimental impact on the developing brain. Younger children who experience trauma are more likely to have long-term problems such as anger and anxiety. (Downey, 2007).

KRISTY YOUNG AND CHRISTINE POOLE

Children and adolescents with trauma histories may develop maladaptive and challenging behaviours, such as problems with self-regulation, and may try to self-regulate using self-harming behaviours such as cutting, developing eating disorders and/or engaging in substance abuse behaviours (van der Kolk et al., 1996). It is important to remember that the behaviours that children and adolescents demonstrate—for example, dissociation (National Executive Training Institute, 2005)—have been adaptive and have been helpful in surviving in difficult and abusive environments.

Children who have been traumatised often do not discuss their fears and traumas freely. These children have little insight into the connection between their actions and feelings and the events that have happened to them (van der Kolk, 2005, p. 405). However, if clinicians fail to look through a trauma lens and conceptualise consumer problems as related possibly to current or past trauma, they may fail to see that trauma victims, young and old, organise much of their lives around repetitive patterns of reliving and warding off traumatic memories, reminders and affects (van der Kolk, cited in Moroz, 2005, p. 12).

Secure attachment has a role in protecting people against the impact of trauma, and supportive parenting may help children recover (Caffo, Forresi & Lievers, 2005). However, attachment disturbance and trauma can coexist—each may be the originating event giving rise to the other.

BOX 17.3   KEY CONSIDERATIONS FOR NURSES: ATTACHMENT AND TRAUMA

- Mandatory reporting—nurses have legal obligation to report suspected cases of child abuse and neglect. This may vary across different states and territories in Australia.

- Given the trauma usually occurs within relationships, the healing usually needs to occur in the child's or adolescent's day-to-day supportive and nurturing relationships; hence it is critical to involve parents or carers in our interventions.

- Inpatient units should be calm and nurturing environments, and nursing staff should be caring and compassionate.

- Nurses should help children identify their triggers and recognise when young people are moving from calm to heighted states.

- Tips to help people calm down when they are heighted: a drink of water, taking deep breaths or going for a walk.

- Keep calm—manage your own emotions and manage the way you react and respond.

Working with children who have experienced trauma can be really hard work and self-care is important.

- These children do not have a solid, secure experience of a relationship and so have difficulty forming such relationships. Just because you and your colleagues are caring does not mean the child will be able to perceive this and trust you.

- Evidence suggests that the more severe an attachment disorder experienced by the child, the less likely they are able to respond to usual forms of behaviour management. Children with reactive attachment disorder never respond to this type of intervention because reward and consequence rely on an attachment relationship where the child ultimately wants the approval of the parent (or nurse within the inpatient setting) (Downey, 2007).

Think about a time when you experienced a strong and possibly overwhelming emotion.

1 What was the event prompting the emotion?

2 What were the physical manifestations?

3 How did you express the emotion?

4 What was helpful in regulating and managing the emotion?

5 What did you need from your loved ones or the people who were caring for you?

6 How can your own experiences help to inform your practice with consumers who have experienced trauma?

Psychosocial assessment of infants, children and adolescents

Psychosocial assessment is usually conducted in three or four sessions of 45–60 minutes' duration and should include:

- one interview with the whole family
- one interview with the child or adolescent (infants and toddlers are always seen with their parents)
- one interview with the parents
- a feedback session, generally with the whole family but at least with the parents and identified client.

The assessment can occur on an outpatient or inpatient basis. The nurse should be aware of the developmental status of the child or adolescent in order to conduct the interview appropriately, for example, children may be better able to express themselves through play and drawing. Children may struggle to separate from parents, and so should be seen with their parents in the first instance, while adolescents may prefer to be seen alone at first. The primary goal of the assessment process is to understand the inner world of the child or adolescent through the development of a therapeutic relationship (which will be discussed later in this chapter) and by gathering information using a clear, structured interview and a variety of therapeutic questioning styles.

Following the assessment, the clinician makes a formulation that examines the factors contributing to the presenting problem in biological, social and psychological domains, under each of the following headings:

- *Precipitating factors*—what started the problem?
- *Predisposing factors*—what predisposed the child to the problem?
- *Perpetuating factors*—what is maintaining the problem?
- *Protective factors*—what are the personal resources of the child or adolescent and the family? For example premorbid stability, strengths, psychosocial factors such as education (Rhodes & Wallis, 2011).

Risk factors for suicide include sociodemographic factors (being male, social and geographical isolation), significant life events and family adversity (experiencing family difficulties or violence, or family history of suicide, loss of a friend or family member) and psychiatric and psychological factors (mental health disorders such as depression, anxiety, bipolar disorder and substance misuse; having a mental illness is the strongest risk factor for suicide).

Self-harm

It is believed that the number of young people who self-harm is very high. Self-harm refers to deliberately hurting or injuring oneself without trying to end life. Examples of self-harming behaviours include cutting, burning and head banging. True prevalence rates are hard to assess as many young people do not disclose their self-harming behaviour or present to health-care professionals.

BOX 17.4 PRESENTING DISORDERS DURING CHILDHOOD AND ADOLESCENCE

For those nurses that would like to read further on presenting disorders during childhood and adolescence please research the terms below:

- Neurodevelopmental disorder
- Communication disorder
- Autistic Spectrum disorder
- Attention deficit hyperactivity disorder (ADHD)
- Depressive disorders
- Anxiety disorders
- Conduct disorders

Therapeutic interventions

When deciding on a particular therapeutic intervention, developmental, family and social issues—as well as the young person's strengths and weaknesses—should be taken into account. The psychotherapeutic approach should be chosen to address individual needs. Young people should be evaluated in the context of their family, school, community and culture. Treatment must be multifaceted, and include education for the young person, family and teachers, and consultation with the young person's general practitioner. However, evidence-based practice is also relevant in choosing a therapeutic modality; for example, research tells us that cognitive behavioural therapy and antidepressant medication are the most effective means of alleviating symptoms of depression.

The importance of the therapeutic relationship or alliance

The importance of a good therapeutic relationship and the use of self has been widely documented and is a critical component of successful outcome for the young person and their family (Flaskas, 2011; McClellan & Werry, 2003). A therapeutic alliance, which supports the young person's best functioning, is a prerequisite for successful intervention, regardless of the specific aims. Successful therapy goes far beyond mere technique or conceptual framework, and involves providing the consumer with hope and creating a corrective emotional experience (Hartman & Zimberoff, 2004).

Care planning

The following is an example care plan for Ella. This plan addresses what can be done for Ella—her mother is mentioned, but in a child and youth mental health setting the mother would be encouraged to seek help for her depression elsewhere. The areas of daily living that are considered include biopsychosocial factors and the plan is mapped out using the nursing process (assessment; plan; implementation; evaluation). Remember, the success is in the detail, so be specific about who, when and what in the collaborative plan; and never include someone in the plan if they were not consulted in the planning process.

Date: [Today's date]						
Consumer name: Ella			**Case manager: Mental health nurse**			
Areas of daily living	Assessment of current situation	Goal	Plan (undertaken with consumer)	Implementation	Who is responsible (include only those who have been consulted in the planning process)	Evaluation/ review date
Ella's delayed milestones	Ella's lack of positive attachment to Rachel presents as a delayed milestone.	Ella to have positive attachment to her mother and achieve appropriate milestones.	Rachel to work with the mental health nurse on attachment based parenting strategies using a theoretical framework of John Bowlby.	Offer Rachel weekly appointments with baby Ella present.	Case manager and Rachel	Ongoing
Rachel's depression	Rachel is unable to form a positive bond with Ella due to depression.	Rachel to have a positive bond with Ella.	Encourage Rachel to seek help through her GP for her depression and possible referral to a psychologist.	Liaise with GP and psychologist so Ella and mother receive holistic care.	Rachel, GP and psychologist	Ongoing

SUMMARY

Many factors and situations contribute to the development of psychiatric disorders. Clinicians must recognise that developmental stage, environmental and social stressors and family relationships are an integral part of the overall picture of a child or adolescent and therefore interventions must incorporate these elements. Inpatient care is relational, empathetic and strengths based.

Working in the area of infant, child and youth mental health is challenging, complex and very rewarding. In this chapter, the factors and situations that contribute to the development of mental health disorders in children and young people have been explored, including developmental, environmental and social stressors and family relationships. Treatment approaches therefore must be multifaceted and must include involvement of the wider systems that support the child or young person in their daily lives. Viewing parents and families as resources is critical and we should support them, coach them and teach them.

KRISTY YOUNG AND CHRISTINE POOLE

DISCUSSION QUESTIONS

1 Why is it important to have a 'developmental perspective' when treating an infant, child or young person?

2 Name the common skills deficits that may be observed in children or young people suffering behavioural or emotional problems. Why is it important to consider a child or young person's possible skills deficits?

3 What is attachment theory? Why is attachment important for healthy development?

4 What are the factors and situations that may contribute to the development of mental health disorders in children and adolescents?

TEST YOURSELF

1 Factors that affect development are:

a Biological

b Psychological

c Environmental

d All of the above

2 Adolescence can be defined by which ages

a 13–18 years

b 6–12 years

c 11–20 years

d 21–23 years

3 A major developmental theorist in cognitive development is

a Sigmund Freud

b John Bowlby

c Jean Piaget

d Albert Bandura

USEFUL WEBSITES

Child Trauma Academy: http://childtrauma.org

Daniel Hughes: www.danielhughes.org

Dr Dan Siegel: http://drdansiegel.com

Lives in the Balance: www.livesinthebalance.org

Nursing and Midwifery Board of Australia—Professional Standards: www.nursingmidwiferyboard.gov.au/Codes-Guidelines-Statements/Professional-standards.aspx

Zero to Three: www.zerotothree.org

REFERENCES

AACAP, see American Academy of Child and Adolescent Psychiatry.

American Academy of Child and Adolescent Psychiatry (2005). Practice parameter for the assessment and treatment of children and adolescents with reactive attachment disorder of infancy and early childhood. *Journal of the American Academy of Child and Adolescent Psychiatry, 44*(11).

Ayres, J. A. (2005). *Sensory integration and the child: 25th anniversary edition.* Western Psychological Services.

Caffo, E., Forresi, B. & Lievers, L. S. (2005). Impact, psychological sequelae and management of trauma affecting children and adolescents. *Current Opinion in Psychiatry, 18*(4), 422–428.

Centre for Community Child Health (2006). *Behaviour problems: Practice resource.* Retrieved from http://raisingchildren.net.au/verve/_resources/Behaviour_problems.pdf.

Downey, L. (2007). *Calmer classrooms: A guide to working with traumatised children.* Melbourne: Child Safety Commissioner.

Flaskas, C. (2011). The therapeutic use of self. In P. Rhodes & A. Wallis (Eds.), *A practical guide to family therapy: Structured guidelines and key skills* (pp. 1–15). Melbourne: IP Communications.

Greene, R. W. (2005). *The explosive child.* New York: HarperCollins.

Havighurst, S. S., Harley, A. & Prior, M. (2004). Building preschool children's emotional competence: A parenting program. *Early Education and Development, 15*(4): 423–446.

Hartman, D. & Zimberoff, D. (2004). *Corrective Emotional Experience in the Therapeutic Process.* Journal of Heart-Centered Therapies, Vol. 7, No. 2, pp. 3-84.

Mares, S., Newman, L., Warren, B., with Cornish, K. (2005). *Clinical skills in infant mental health, first 3 years.* Victoria: Acer Press

Mares, S., Newman, L., Warren, B., with Cornish, K. (2011). *Clinical skills in infant mental health, first 3 years* (2nd ed.). Victoria: Acer Press.

Martin, A. & Volkmar, F. (Eds.) (2007) *Lewis's child and adolescent psychiatry: A comprehensive textbook* (4th ed.). Philadelphia: Lippincott Williams & Wilkins.

McClellan, J. M. & Werry, J. S. (2003). Evidence based treatments in child and adolescent psychiatry: An inventory. *Journal of the American Academy of Child and Adolescent Psychiatry, 42*(12), 1388–1400.

Moroz, K. (2005). *The effects of psychological trauma on children and adolescents.* Vermont: Department of Health.

National Executive Training Institute (2005). *Training curriculum for reduction of seclusion and restraint. Draft Curriculum Manual.* Alexandria: National Association of State Mental Health Program Directors (NASMHPD), National Technical Assistance Center for State Mental Health Planning (NTAC).

Paz, I., Jones, D. & Byrne, G. (2005). Child maltreatment, child protection and mental health. *Current Opinion in Psychiatry, 18*(4), 411–421.

Regan, K. (2006). *Opening our arms: Helping troubled kids do well.* Colorado: Bull.

Rhodes, P. & Wallis, A. (2011). *A practical guide to family therapy.* Melbourne: IP Communications.

Sameroff, A. J., McDonough, S. C. & Rosenblum, K. L. (2004). *Treating parent–infant relationship problems.* New York: Guilford Press.

Siegel, D. & Hartzell, M. (2004). *Parenting from the inside out: How a deeper self- understanding can help you raise children who thrive.* New York: Jeremy P. Tarcher Inc.

van der Kolk, B. (2005). Developmental trauma disorder: Toward a rational diagnosis for children with complex trauma histories. *Psychiatric Annals, 35*(5), 401–408.

van der Kolk, B., McFarlane, A. & Weisaeth, L. (Eds.) (1996). *Traumatic stress: The effects of overwhelming experience on mind, body, and society.* New York: Guilford Press.

PART 3
Praxis of Mental Health Nursing

Praxis in healthcare relates to informed reasoning and practice. That is, putting a theory into action. In mental health nursing, interventions such as psychotherapy and case management are informed by theories. It is the theoretical framework that helps us to organise ideas about things and can assist in making ideas easier to remember and apply to real world situations.

This next part of the book is where you will learn about the concepts of psychotherapy and case management and the role of mental health nurses. The theoretical framework for these interventions will be discussed further assisting you in comprehending these topics. This part of the book also cover the topics of culture and diversity as seen in Australia and New Zealand. Finally, you will examine the theoretical background and application of care of people who have a criminal history and who have mental illness.

CHAPTER 18

Psychotherapy Essentials in Mental Health Nursing

ROBERT TRETT AND
HALEY PECKHAM

KEY OUTCOMES

AFTER READING THIS CHAPTER, YOU SHOULD BE ABLE TO

- place psychotherapeutic practice in nursing within a brief history of psychotherapy and nursing theory development
- link psychotherapeutic practice to interpersonal and humanistic approaches in mental health nursing
- situate psychotherapeutic practice in the context of attachment theory, therapeutic alliance neuroscience and consumer focused nursing
- demonstrate an understanding of the common factors approach to psychotherapeutic practice in mental health nursing
- appreciate the value of psychotherapeutic practice in relation to both neurological and social learning perspectives.

KEY TERMS

- attachment
- coping
- epistemic trust
- humanism
- neuroplasticity
- not knowing stance
- psychotherapy
- recovery alliance theory of mental health nursing
- therapeutic alliance

Introduction

This chapter presents a perspective on nursing drawing on the work of both nurses and others whose core practice is based in psychotherapeutic knowledge and principles.

Psychotherapeutic essentials for nursing practice house a range of ideas, knowledge and practices that attend to processes of the mind. By this we mean mental states such as thoughts, feelings, memories, beliefs, ideas and desires. Nurses whose practice is informed by psychotherapeutic essentials assist consumers to reflect, integrate and gain perspective on their mental processes. This serves the purpose of finding meaning in their experiences and improvement in their relationships with others.

Psychotherapy's founders began to publish in the nineteenth century. Figures such as William James (1842–1910), Sigmund Freud (1856–1939), Carl Jung (1875–1961), Ivan Pavlov (1849–1936) and Jacob Moreno (1889–1974) founded theoretical lineages; broadly speaking these are the psychoanalytic, behavioural and humanistic/existential schools of twentieth century psychology (Clarkson, 1992; Meares, 2004). Arguably the first half of the twentieth century was dominated by psychoanalysis, but this was contested by behavioural psychology, which brought a culture of empiricism and criticised the psychoanalytic hegemony from the position of natural and social science (Magnavita, 2006). Some would say that by the late twentieth century both had given way to cognitive science and psychopharmacology in terms of the major influences on clinical mental health professions (Burston, 2003). Countering this view, the value of psychopharmacology, cognitive science and empiricism as sole informants to practice has been challenged by those seeing the need for deeper ethical and philosophical underpinnings to inform both nursing and medical practice (Allen, 2016; Bracken et al., 2012; Watson, 2009). Arguably, nursing sits most comfortably within a humanistic framework; we demonstrate this further in the next section.

Humanistic perspective

Humanistic approaches have their primary concern with subjective present moment experiences. Relief of suffering occurs not through expunging unwanted symptoms of illness, nor prompting insight into unconscious processes through analytic interpretation (Clarkson, 1992). Rather, humanistic clinicians work more collaboratively, focusing on finding meanings that may have been in some way obscured by adverse life experiences (Burston, 2003).

Adversity in the field of mental illness includes suffering associated with mental ill-health, hospitalisation, social alienation and marginalisation, as well as earlier (and possibly traumatic) experiences that may have shaped beliefs, perspectives and interpersonal relating styles in ways less adapted to the demands of citizenship, self-determination and social inclusion. Humanistic approaches are active in seeking engagement on the clinician's part, and oriented to curiosity about people's subjective experiences. Mental health nursing focuses ever more fully on recovery principles, including identifying people's strengths, supporting decision-making and valuing learning from experience (over nurses controlling and limiting experience). We return to the fit that humanistic psychotherapy has to nursing practice later, but for now draw attention to a 2013 study of nurses working in acute care settings (Cleary et al., 2013) where the theme of humanism was prominent in nurses' perceptions of their contribution to mental health recovery. Humanistic care included categories such as therapeutic relating, kindness, encouragement, listening, discussing options, hope, optimism and future focus. The qualities inherent in these categories speak to processes of interpersonal relating; this is the heart of nursing's contributions to mental health care.

Interpersonal relating

Aligned to developments in psychotherapeutic thought outlined above, some quintessential contributors to the discipline of mental health nursing emerged from the mid-twentieth century. Hildegard Peplau's (1909–1999) work foreshadowed the role of the nurse-therapist and generated the term 'psychodynamic nursing' (Peplau, 1952). She was forerunner for subsequent nurse theories and approaches (Barker, 2001; Barker, Jackson & Stevenson, 1999; Cameron, Kapur & Campbell, 2005; Moyle, 2003; Shanley & Jubb-Shanley, 2007, 2012; Shanley, Jubb & Latter, 2003; Wheeler, 2005; Wheeler & Delaney, 2008). In bringing focus to the interpersonal, Peplau and others speak to a quality of relationship that mental health nurses develop with consumers. We believe that this relationship is ubiquitous to psychotherapeutic practice within nursing. It requires us to focus on creating alliances with consumers that in turn contribute to strengthening a sense of self.

Therapeutic alliance and development of self

Relationships have their foundations in human attachment theory. Both contemporary nursing and psychotherapy have been re-examining the primacy of human attachment and the effects of insecure attachment, as a part explanation for the troubled times that mental health consumers experience. We discuss this further below. Therapeutic relating based in attachment theory develops a shared understanding achieved through an alliance between two people, rather than an act performed by a clinician on or about the person (Blum, 2016). Nursing literature is vocal on the issues of relationship and alliance (Brimblecombe, Tingle & Murrells, 2007; Cameron, Kapur & Campbell, 2005; Cardell & Pitula, 1999; Carlsson et al., 2006; Cleary et al., 2013; Cutcliffe & Grant, 2001; Cutcliffe & Barker, 2002; Cutcliffe & Stevenson, 2008; Delaney & Handrup, 2011; Shanley, Jubb & Latter, 2003). In addition, empirically supported psychotherapies emphasise attachment/loss and the importance of stimulating strong attachment relationships in psychotherapy as a way of developing the alliance required between clinicians and consumers, to stimulate change (Bateman, 2012; Bateman & Fonagy, 2006b).

We contend that this relationship focus is not an incidental factor that nurses use to help people feel better. Rather it reflects something essential to the recovery process. Nurses and psychotherapists point to therapeutic relating as a mechanism for developing a sense of self (Meares, 2004; Paley et al., 2003). Domains of self, such as continuity, coherence, embodiment and agency (Ramachandran, 2003), can inform nurses' psychotherapeutic practice by centring attention on supporting coping in relation to each discrete area.

While we accept that early attachment losses impact severely on the development of self, authenticity of relationship goes beyond ideas of repairing earlier attachment failures. Therapeutic relating represents the healing power of validation and acceptance that can occur between people (Elliott et al., 2013). A strong boundaried therapeutic relationship is the vehicle that conveys these benefits. We now explore the importance of this to psychotherapeutic nursing.

Evidence supporting therapeutic relating in nursing

Therapeutic alliance is achieved through therapeutic relationship. While much is yet to be discovered in this field, we can be confident that nurses' use of therapeutic relating does achieve general positive outcomes for consumers. While gold standard evidence is yet to be published, three studies support this. The first is a model for working with consumers facing suicidal crises (Cutcliffe et al., 2007); the second, a study into violent encounters in psychiatric settings that investigated the consumers' perspectives (Carlsson et al., 2006), and the third, a study of psychodynamic interpersonal psychotherapy delivered by nurses (Cahill, Paley & Hardy, 2013). These studies explored very different consumer groups in a range of mental health settings including inpatient units. The results confirm strong consumer desire for relationships and clear benefits from therapeutic relating. Nurse qualities such as listening, non-judgment, interpersonal warmth, authenticity, truthfulness of connection to the consumer's suffering, consumer involvement and reassurance were all highly rated. In the first two studies, these qualities provided the vehicle for harm reduction (suicide in one case and violence in the other). In the third study, consumers rated issues of reassurance and involvement more highly than nurses having a solution focus.

Another way to consider the question of benefits derived from therapeutic relating can be found in the results of mental health systems where such relating seems absent. A recent review of inpatient mental health care across six countries, including Australia, paints a sorry picture (Cutcliffe et al., 2015).

It points to lack of warmth in relationship and a general absence of formal or informal talk-based therapy as standout issues. More grimly, it paints a picture of 'coercion, disinterest, inhumane practices, custodial and controlling practitioners and a gross overuse of pharmacological "treatments" in inpatient settings' (Cutcliffe et al., 2015, p. 381–2). They note that formal and informal talk-based therapy is largely absent in inpatient units covered in the reports they reviewed and that consumer satisfaction is understandably low. While results such as these are inconsistent with Cleary and colleagues' (2013) findings, they are shocking. We believe that a psychotherapeutically equipped nursing workforce oriented to providing humanistic talk-based therapy within inpatient settings would improve outcomes. Sixty-five years have passed since Peplau (1952) anticipated the role of nurse-therapist. In our view this role, with its emphasis on self-awareness and positive therapeutic use of nurses' personalities (Vandemark, 2006), is crucial to recovery oriented care.

Further validation for the primacy of interpersonal relating can be extracted in the emerging science of neuroplasticity. We use this science to examine the neurobiological effects of early childhood traumatic experiences in relation to brain adaptation. Neuroplasticity explains certain behaviours we observe clinically in those who have suffered adverse experiences. It also provides support to the proposition that people continue to change and adapt according to new social experiences. Nurses' efforts to create benign interpersonal experiences with those suffering past trauma are thus supported by this science.

What does 'humanistic' nursing practice mean for you?

CRITICAL THINKING OPPORTUNITY

Neuroplasticity and psychotherapeutic nursing

Neuroplasticity is the capacity that our brain has that allows adaption to experiences. It offers a way of understanding how abuse and neglect in childhood leave a biological trace in the brain that predispose to apparent adult psychopathology.

Our early environment shapes our brains so that we can learn how to survive or thrive and can anticipate what we are likely to face in the future based on what we have experienced so far. Nature wants us to survive long enough to procreate, ensuring the survival of our genetic line. The plastic adaptations made to our brain and brain–body systems through early adverse experiences, such as abuse and neglect, steer us along a developmental pathway that is more threat-focused. This increases our chances of survival, and possibly orients us to early sexual behaviour to increase the chances of survival of our genetic line (Hillis et al., 2004; Teicher, 2002). So while these behaviours are often thought of as psychopathological, they are in fact nature's way of prompting survival.

Experiences in childhood profoundly impact on our mental and physical well-being as adults (Shonkoff, Boyce & McEwen, 2009). The Adverse Childhood Experiences study of 9500 respondents found that if children experienced four or more of psychological, physical or sexual abuse; domestic violence; or living with substance abusers, and those who were mentally ill or suicidal, or ever imprisoned, then as adults they were between four and twelve times more likely to develop substance abuse problems or depression, or to attempt suicide (Felitti, 1998). Experiences of trauma and abuse in childhood are consistently associated with an increased risk for what the literature describes as psychopathology (Chapman et al., 2004; Chen et al., 2010; Herman, Perry & van der Kolk, 1989; MacMillan, 2001).

ROBERT TRETT AND HALEY PECKHAM

Contemporary research indicates that child abuse leads to enduring structural and functional changes in the brain (Teicher, 2002; Teicher & Samson, 2016), as well as in brain–body systems, such as the hypothalamic pituitary adrenal axis and the autonomic nervous system (McEwen et al., 2015), all of which are calibrated by early experience.

Social and emotional factors have a profound influence on our survival and for this reason they can induce powerful neuroplastic change. Neglect, abuse and maltreatment, especially when they are clear acts of commission or omission by our caregivers, elicit powerful emotional experiences such as fear, helplessness, shame and rage, and impact dramatically on the relational bond between the child and caregiver. Thus maltreatment is a powerful influence on the developing brain and importantly on what that developing brain learns to anticipate in terms of safety and relationships.

Neuroplasticity occurs at every level of the brain, from the genes through to the connections between gross brain regions. Genes may be marked with chemical groups following significant experiences that result in the expression of that gene being increased or decreased. This is epigenetics, which allows nurture (experiences) to be written into nature (the genes) providing a mechanism for adapting gene expression to experience. Epigenetic changes may be brief or enduring, and may be inherited. Studies in rodents indicate that gene expression is affected by early social and emotional experiences (Peckham, 2013; Roth, 2009; Suri et al., 2013; Turecki & Meaney, 2016; Weaver, 2005). These changes are thought to be adaptive (Suri et al., 2013). Studies in humans are limited, but indicate that adults who have suffered early abuse or trauma exhibit a different epigenome from adults without abuse histories (Labonte et al., 2012; Suderman et al., 2014). The increased incidence/prevalence of PTSD in children whose mothers survived the holocaust may be due to transmission through epigenetic mechanisms (Yehuda, 2008).

Nature's assumption is that the child will be born into life-threatening danger and the inherited epigenetic tendency towards high anxiety and hypervigilance creates difficulties in present day life, but is protective and survival positive from an evolutionary–biological standpoint.

Similar to epigenetics, neurogenesis, the birth of new neurons, is also affected by experience of the environment (Egeland, Zunszain & Pariante, 2015; Kempermann, Kuhn & Gage, 1997; Lieberwirth & Wang, 2012; Opendak & Gould, 2015). Once generated, new neurons must integrate into the pre-existing neural network where they contribute to the formation of new memories or the moderation of existing memories (Deng, Aimone & Gage, 2010). As experience promotes adaptive change in the brain, our ability to learn and remember is itself malleable. Exercise and new experiences enhance neurogenesis and facilitate our capacity for change, presenting a clear therapeutic opportunity for mental health nurses (Shaffer, 2016).

Neurons communicate through synapses, which increase in strength with increased activity (Sweatt, 2016). Similarly, highly active neural pathways acquire increased levels of myelin, which makes the impulse transmission down a pathway faster and more efficient (Fields, 2015). These forms of plasticity are known as synaptic and white matter plasticity, respectively, and together form the basis of learning and memory (Fields, 2015; Sweatt, 2016). Practice, in the form of repeated experience, builds up neural pathways, which are then myelinated. With this they become more efficient, and more automatic. The brain cannot discriminate between healthy and unhealthy experiences and learns through repetition, so the cumulative impact of a childhood consisting of days, months and years of experiences of neglect, shaming, hostility, criticism and physical or sexual violence cannot be underestimated. The brain learns from past experiences and is shaped by them to anticipate a future of similar experiences, and at this level of neuroplasticity it is clear that common symptoms experienced by mental health consumers such as generalised anxiety, despair, fear of abandonment, low self-worth and emotional dysregulation may be outcomes of repeated childhood experiences of fear, helplessness, neglect, lack of attunement and having no safe person to help regulate one's emotional state.

Connections between the limbic system, where we experience emotions such as fear and the pleasure associated with reward, and the prefrontal cortex where we reflect, plan and make decisions, are also forged through experience. Ideally, as infants and children we would have parents that could help us identify, name and soothe our emotions and reflect on how they shape our behaviour. Without such experiences this emotional regulatory circuit cannot develop, leaving individuals unable to self-soothe, as the prefrontal cortex is not sufficiently connected to lower brain regions to modulate them. Consequently, these individuals are at risk of chronic anxiety and for acting with impulsive aggression towards the self or others. Nurses' roles in actively soothing consumers as well as supporting new self-soothing coping is critical for consumers who experience emotion regulatory problems.

At every level the brain is shaped by experience. Abuse and neglect in childhood shape us to anticipate a harsh and dangerous world, one in which we may be impotent and helpless. We adapt to these experiences and adopt the best strategy for our survival, which may be defensive, aggressive, dissociative or passive, and this can give rise to symptoms of distress and control associated with mental illness. Some view these difficulties as signs of psychopathology; however, we do not view it this way. A healthy brain is one that can adapt to experience and environments. Neuroplasticity – the brain's capacity to adapt – suggests that symptoms of distress and control reflect an adaptation to support survival. However, survival priorities assume the worst and act defensively, which can in turn create interpersonal difficulties for the consumer who has had these experiences. New benign and benevolent experiences – particularly of safety and relationships that contradict the expectations and anticipations of the world that were established in childhood by abuse or neglect – allow us to anticipate a safer world and safer relationships. The intrinsically relational nature of nurse-led psychotherapeutic approaches offer respect, empathy, emotional attunement, attention and physical, sexual, psychological and emotional safety. These qualities contradict negative expectations and set up new anticipations of safety and autonomy. These in turn may ameliorate symptoms of control, aggression and passivity that stem from fear, isolation and helplessness.

In summary, a reparative present moment relationship between nurses and consumers allows for something new to happen within an attachment context.

Attachment and its implications for psychotherapeutic nursing

The development of an attachment pattern can be thought of as an example of a functional neuroplastic adaptation to experiences with a caregiver. Just as all human babies are biologically primed to learn a language, they are also biologically primed to form attachment bonds that are critical for healthy development in early life and important for our well-being 'from the cradle to the grave' (Bowlby, 1979). Continuing with the language metaphor, the language the infant encounters in their environment becomes the language they speak and the same applies to the emotional language of attachment theory. The baby adapts and, through repeated experiences with the caregiver, learns how to optimally relate to that caregiver.

The purpose of attachment first put forward by John Bowlby was to promote infant survival through a psycho-biological mechanism that motivates infants to seek proximity from their caregivers (Bowlby, 1988). Smiling, clinging, crying and exploring are attachment-related behaviours that have evolved to

ROBERT TRETT AND HALEY PECKHAM

build and maintain the attachment bond. Seeking proximity to the caregiver through the formation of an attachment bond is critical for the survival of the infant, but caregivers differ greatly in terms of:

- the quality of care they can give
- their physical and emotional availability
- their attitude towards neediness in their baby.

It is survival that is positive for the baby to be able to adapt to the caregiver's attachment style by achieving and maintaining the life-serving proximity of that caregiver. This is the premise on which secure and insecure patterns of attachment are based.

Mary Ainsworth observed that attachment patterns fall into classifications of secure and insecure with the insecure group being further subdivided into insecure avoidant and insecure anxious or preoccupied (Ainsworth et al., 1978). An infant receiving care from a parent who is physically and emotionally available to them, and who correctly interprets their needs and responds to them swiftly and sensitively, will come through repeated experiences to anticipate more of that attuned care. This is a neuroplastic adaptation: learning that comes about through repeated experience. Confident that they will be promptly responded to and that their needs will be accepted and met by their caregiver, the infant becomes *securely attached* and from this secure position can confidently explore the world. In this scenario the infant has to minimally adapt to his or her caregiver as the caregiver is open and available to the needs of the child.

If caregivers are perhaps more preoccupied with their own needs and available to their child sometimes but not consistently, the infant may adapt to this by anxiously or fretfully trying to ensure the availability of the caregiver. This presents as an infant who seems to want attention but isn't able to be soothed by it. This is behaviour typically seen in an infant with an insecure *anxious or preoccupied attachment*.

An infant developing an *avoidant attachment* may have repeated experiences of not being favourably responded to when they are overtly distressed and needy, but are more favourably responded to and can maintain proximity to their caregiver if they are less vocal and appear more self-contained and less needy.

Each of these attachment patterns—secure and insecure—is a functional adaptation to caregiver, providing a means for the infant to maintain proximity to the caregiver, thus ensuring their protection and their survival.

Further study into attachment patterns led to the introduction of a fourth classification, that of 'disorganised/disorientated' (Main & Solomon, 1989). The attachment bond is an evolutionarily successful strategy to promote the survival of the infant by ensuring proximity to the caregiver and their protection. For some infants the threat to their survival *is* their caregiver. This catches the infants in a biological paradox. They are biologically motivated to seek the proximity of their caregiver who is both the protector and the greatest threat to them. This paradox is manifest in the behaviours of these attachment traumatised children. They may turn in circles, walk backwards to their caregivers or display other contradictory behaviours, literally acting out their paradoxical experience. Imaging studies exploring brain activity and attachment reveal a consistent picture on the effects of maltreatment in childhood. Maltreatment and a disorganised/disorientated attachment classification predict a stronger limbic activity and reduced prefrontal cortex activity (Lenzi et al., 2015; Teicher & Samson, 2016). The adult outcomes for maltreated children parallel those of children with a disorganised/disorientated attachment classification. The consequences of a lack of relational safety and emotional regulation in childhood manifest as disrupted, dysregulated and unsafe relating in adulthood. Impulsive and extreme forms of emotional regulation, such as self-harm and substance use, are often to the fore.

Attachment patterns can be gradually changed through gaining a new relational experience and thus in principle could be provided by an ongoing therapeutic relationship with a nurse. However, many hospital and community settings are not structured to provide or allow for the development of enduring therapeutic relationships with individual practitioners.

Psychotherapeutic practice in nursing calls health services to think through their structural processes so that enhanced therapeutic relating between nurses and consumers can take centre stage. We also ask nurses to think through the improvements they can make in their day-to-day, hour-to-hour, minute-by-minute interactions with consumers (particularly those with trauma and neglect histories) that would improve therapeutic relating, even when service systems emphasise other priorities. Nurses' roles as therapists need to form the comfortable centre to practice, rather than a secret art practised on the margins of a biomedical mental health system.

CRITICAL THINKING OPPORTUNITY

1 How might Bowlby's attachment theory and the sciences of neuroplasticity inform psychotherapeutic practice?

2 What might nurses do practically to ensure more focus is placed on therapeutic relating in the context of busy mental health settings?

Conceptualising the role of the mental health nurse-therapist

So far we've looked at psychotherapeutic practice within mental health nursing through the lens of a humanistic relationship oriented approach and referenced growing evidence for this perspective from both social and neuro-sciences. But what framework might best support a humanistic psychotherapeutic approach to nursing?

In the light of poor consumer satisfaction, we feel some urgency to craft approaches as useful to nurses working in inpatient units as they are to community settings. Advancing practice ideas in the remainder of this chapter, we complement the findings in other parts of this textbook, in particular Chapter 20, which covers therapeutic methodologies that can be used in case management and Chapter 12, which looks at nursing in the field of personality disorders.

To distinguish the work of nurse-therapists, we suggest psychotherapeutic ideas must be conceptualised within nursing frameworks. The recovery alliance theory (RAT; Shanley & Jubb-Shanley, 2007) has particular applicability. Developed in Australia, their theory references care delivered in this part of the world. Arguably, more than the other models, it reflects contemporary consumer–nurse co-production values. The model, based on recovery partnerships, consumer strengths and ideas of common humanity occurring between nurses and consumers, inform the authors' companion work describing a nursing specific therapeutic approach called coping focused counselling (Shanley & Jubb-Shanley, 2012).

RAT's fit to a nurse-specific approach for psychotherapeutic practice is attractive in that the theory captures something of the culture and practice of nursing. These are evident in three core constructs: coping, working alliance and self responsibility/control.

The idea of working alliance is a core construct in psychotherapeutic nursing. Its origins, dating back to Freud, are advanced as a pan-theoretical factor in psychotherapeutic literature (Horvath & Luborsky,

■ TOPIC LINK

TOPIC LINK See Chapter 20 for therapeutic methodologies.

See Chapter 12 for nursing in the field of personality disorders.

1993). Working alliance has been validated in psychotherapeutic practice (Taylor et al., 2015) and beautifully illustrated in a clinical vignette of her own practice in psychoanalytically influenced nursing by Alicia Evans (2005). In our view, working alliance offers a heuristic bridge between psychotherapy and nursing approaches.

BOX 18.1 **TAXONOMY OF PSYCHOTHERAPEUTIC NURSING PRACTICES**

TRUST IN RELATIONSHIP

1 Create an emotionally bonded healing setting where distress is soothed, allowing mutual communication to be established.

2 Discover with the person a shared language representing their experiences, which is understandable and usable *between* nurse and consumer.

3 Using this language, discover together how subjective aloneness, emptiness and related life struggles might be best accepted/ validated (trust through emotional knowing).

4 Support person struggles to encounter, defuse from and accept feared situations, in the service of meaning making and new or novel learning.

5 Teach a present moment focus, taking the perspective that memories help inform current feelings, thoughts, ideas and desires, while change occurs in the present moment (not the past). Prompt by asking *what does this mean for your life now, or what does this mean for you and me now?*

KNOWLEDGE OF MIND

1 In the parlance of the person's language, support exploration and linking between feelings, emotions, memories, ideas, thoughts and desires.

2 Puzzle together on the meanings and linkages between these various states of mind and real-world experiences.

3 Support reflection and perspective taking, through observing mental processes in conversation or through contemplative activity such as mindfulness practices.

4 Consider how these ideas and insights might support coping.

CONNECTION BETWEEN PEOPLE

1 Support strengths evident in the person's current coping and explore how these might inform social connections.

2 Considering the meaning of others' expressions, behaviours and possible mental processes.

3 Together, generate ways to test out ideas and observations of self and other through engaging in social, occupational and/ or treatment settings (social experiential learning).

4 Support the process by offering safe role plays between nurse and person (benign exposure).

In RAT, the working alliance is seen as the vehicle for therapeutic approaches. Specific characteristics in the working alliance are described that distinguish nurse-led therapeutic approaches from other professions. These are the use of everyday speech, variable context and times, self-disclosure to enhance therapeutic relationship and shared humanity, unscripted dialogue and holistic perspectives encompassing wide ranging consumer life experiences. RAT advances that the primary value of therapeutic practice in nursing is to support a person's coping. In this, RAT distinguishes nursing practice as support oriented, and differentiates nurse-led psychotherapeutic practice from approaches that may emphasise insight or behavioural change. This is not to say that supporting coping precludes consumers developing new perspectives or insights, nor would it suggest that change in behaviour does not occur in the context of nurse-supported coping. Rather, it suggests that the author of new insights or behavioural changes is the consumer not the clinician. This viewpoint is a core construct for psychotherapeutic nursing.

BOX 18.2 PSYCHODYNAMIC INTEPERSONAL THERAPY

Psychodynamic intepersonal therapy (PIT) emphasises the linking of emotions, memories and patterns of relating through everyday language between clinician and consumer (Guthrie & Moghavemi, 2013). It has been empirically tested in relation to nursing by Paley and colleagues (2008) and emphasises personal relationship between nurse and consumer. The approach focuses on mutuality, careful attention to the content of conversation offered by consumers, and tentative attempts by the nurse to understand the emotional meanings as of past interpersonal problems become present between the nurse and consumer in current situations—the here and now. If the significance of the presentation of problems is sufficiently understood, it becomes the moment where the nurse can work collaboratively with the consumer to link emotions, memories and social relating. The aim is for the person to experience something new in the context of the present conversation.

RAT emphasises the person's language as central to conceptualising their mental health concerns. This is contrasted to professional-led language found in diagnosis–pharmacotherapy–symptom reduction approaches. RAT purposefully veers away from conceptual jargon that can sometimes creep into psychologically led formulations.

RAT's privileging of ordinary language is considered to empower consumer responsibility and control, and sits comfortably with consumer-led approaches such as those developed for hearing voices (Corstens, Longden & May, 2012; Romme & Escher, 1989), living with difficult emotions (Daya, 2013) and/or working with unusual experiences (Knight, 2009).

BOX 18.3 MENTALISATION BASED TREATMENT

Mentalisation based treatment (MBT) skill sets, which are part of a broader mentalising orientation, have been found to be useful to nurses working with consumers diagnosed with borderline personality disorder (Warrender, 2015). While this study relates to a specific diagnosis, MBT's approaches (such as understanding people in the context of their mental processes), alongside broad clinician contributions (such as empathy, an active here and now orientation and a not knowing curious stance) reveal the common factors approaches embedded within MBT. Furthermore, mentalising has a broad application in that it is linked to the reduction in vigilance and rigidity, prompting a style of trust that underpins social learning (Fonagy & Allison, 2014).

Life concerns, being formulated strictly from their own descriptions, place the consumer (not the professional) in the power seat. Possible solutions are considered to be located internally within the person's language and expression, rather than in the professional's external wisdom and knowledge. Nurses' therapeutic endeavours are therefore firmly focused on supporting consumer subjective coping during periods of mental health disruption, rather than offering clinician-led solutions. We will now examine how common therapeutic practices support this.

1   How is supporting coping different from a behaviour change orientation?

2   Which of these models appeals more to my approach to nursing?

Common therapeutic factors

RAT assists us to formulate and differentiate a nurse-specific approach to psychotherapy. What, however, do we know of the common factors that nurses may call upon to shape and inform a coping focused psychotherapeutic nursing? What methodologies are consistent to this orientation, and what might we reasonably predict as an outcome to such endeavour?

Recent years have seen the ascendency of evidence-based practice in mental health. This has focused resources and effort on generating empirical evidence for all mental health interventions, based on randomised control trials (RCTs). One claim for this approach is that this evidence focus allows us to scientifically specify both psychopharmacological and psychological interventions applicable to classified disorders.

It is certainly hard to argue against the role of medication in limiting the neurological damage associated with repeated psychotic episodes. Yet cogent positions are advanced within psychiatry, quoting meta-analyses that show the effectiveness of both medication and specific psychological interventions is far lower than originally thought (Bateman, 2012; Bracken et al., 2012).

Interestingly, what is ever clearer from meta-studies into the effectiveness of psychological treatments is that they all seem to work about as effectively as each other. This raises a question as to why different therapies, each claiming that their effectiveness relies on mechanisms specific to their approach, work as effectively as rival approaches, despite large variations in their theory and interventions strategies.

Additionally, consumer perspectives (Corstens, Longden & May, 2012; Daya, 2013; Knight, 2009; Romme & Escher, 1989), advance complementary approaches to mental health problems that are growing in popularity among those who might meet criteria for disorders, but who choose a different way to conceptualise, explore and integrate experience.

In 1936 (Rosenzweig, 2002/1936) proposed that a set of *common factors* must exist with regard to different psychological approaches. This idea is now resurfacing (Paley & Shapiro, 2001; Wampold et al., 1997). Restricting the combination of factors under consideration to those located within evidence-based approaches avoids the pitfalls of an ill-disciplined eclecticism that focuses investigators' efforts onto elements that empirically supported therapies have in common. This contrasts with the specific factors that each claim as the mechanisms for their brand's success (Bracken et al., 2012; Budd & Hughes, 2009; DeFife & Hilsenroth, 2011). These efforts have revealed a combined perspective of what works (Bateman, 2012; Shanley & Jubb-Shanley, 2012; Weinberger, 2014).

To think through what common factors may be present in psychotherapeutic nursing practice, we return to humanism. As mentioned above, humanism is a core element in RAT (Shanley & Jubb-Shanley, 2007). In research into nurses' work with suicidal people, Cutcliffe et-al identified reconnection with humanity as a core variable to successful outcome (Cutcliffe et al., 2006; Cutcliffe et al., 2007). In addition, humanistic and experiential approaches have been shown to be as effective as cognitive-behavioural approaches (Elliott et al., 2013)

Bruce Wampold (2012) identifies that distinctively human characteristics—such as making sense of the world, influencing things by social means, connecting to others, expecting things and mastering obstacles—as core common factors in therapy. He makes the case that all therapy is humanistic; that is, 'psychotherapy evolved as a culturally embedded healing practice because of human traits' (Wampold, 2012, p. 445).

BOX 18.4 ACCEPTANCE AND COMITTMENT THERAPY

In his recent essay aligning Jean Watson's theory to acceptance and comittment therapy (ACT) clinical practice, Houghton (2016) brings attention to practices such as:

- mindfulness—a process of contemplative attending to self and environment in the present moment
- cognitive defusion—a process of observing mental processes as an alternative to being convinced that the content is literally true
- acceptance—validation for things as they are, as a precondition to growth and change

- values orientation—a process of systematically recognising the essential ideals held paramount by the individual
- committed action—action aligned to personal values that direct behaviour towards what truly matters to that individual.

These interventions have been empirically validated in the context of ACT treatment across a number of diagnostic categories (Hayes, 2004). We contend they contribute well to a common psychotherapeutic practice for mental health nurses.

Similar factors such as an emotionally charged bond, a confiding healing setting, ways of understanding emotional distress and consumer-centred options for overcoming troubled times emerge across the common factors literature (Laska, Gurman & Wampold, 2014).

Reconciling common and specific factors, Weinberger reviews features that he considers to have either empirical support or strong argument (Weinberger, 2014). Similar to RAT, he finds that therapeutic alliance is a prominent factor; this includes items such as cohesion between clinician and consumer, fostered through empathy, goal consensus and collaboration.

Weinberger's second factor is a person's expectancy. He makes the point that if the person expects something good to occur then this will increase successful outcome. Third, a sense of control and mastery is identified. Weinberger identifies clinician activities that support control and mastery and, in so doing, anticipates a methodology for a common factors psychotherapeutic practice. These concur with a coping-focused model for mental health nursing (specified above).

CRITICAL THINKING OPPORTUNITY

1   If specific approaches are endorsed by randomised control trials, why focus on common approaches/ factors?

2   What are the three factors Weinberger (2014) suggests that reconcile specific and common approaches to psychotherapeutic practice?

3   What do you need to be aware of when attempting to engage an involuntary consumer using a common factors approach?

The common factors approach is a developing empirically supported method that can inform psychotherapeutic nursing. These factors are also harnessed in specific empirically supported psychotherapies such as psychodynamic interpersonal therapy (Guthrie & Moghavemi, 2013; Paley et al., 2008), mentalisation based treatment (Allen, Bateman & Fonagy, 2008; Bateman & Fonagy, 2004), and third wave behavioural approaches such as acceptance and commitment therapy (Dimidjian et al., 2016; Hayes, 2004) (see Boxes 18.2, 18.3 and 18.4).

From all these approaches, we suggest a taxonomy for psychotherapeutic nursing practice:

- trust in relationship
- knowledge of mind
- connection between people.

Each of these three areas has accompanying sets of therapeutic capabilities that relate to empirically supported common factors. We propose these as a nonspecific psychotherapeutic nursing approach that should alleviate the real-world mental suffering encountered by people who utilise nursing supports. While empirical support sufficient to fully evidencing our position is yet to be developed, we propose that a key mechanism for reduction in long-term suffering will be found in the linkages proposed between natural pedagogy and psychotherapeutic practice (see the following 'Future directions' section). This advancing field of inquiry points to trust as the basic building block for social participation and lifelong learning. Our intention in promoting the style of psychotherapeutic nursing proposed here is to pivot practice to three primary tasks:

1 Establishing trust between nurses and consumers as a basic social template;
2 Supporting consumer self-trust through linking subjective processes of mind to a cohesive self-narrative;
3 Supporting capacity for social trust within communities of peers.

Future directions

ABOUT THE CONSUMER Lucy's story

Lucy is a 32-year-old woman with a history of bipolar disorder that was diagnosed in her late teens. She had a number of hypomanic and depressed episodes throughout her twenties, but these seemed to settle and she hadn't been seen by the mental health service for two years. She is the youngest of three siblings. Their mother was a single parent and she died six months ago. Lucy recently suffered a breakdown in an important relationship and over the past three weeks has had intrusive thoughts about her ex-boyfriend's shortcomings. She began feeling increasingly invincible, as if she could control her ex-boyfriend's life and activities, and began leaving aggressive messages on his voicemail.

This was reported to police, resulting in Lucy became abusive and threatening to police officers. She eventually agreed to a brief hospital admission as an alternative to being charged. On the ward she has been irritable, but she remembers positive relationships with the ward nurses and agreed to a medication review, period of observation and 'psycho-social support'. She is thought by some to 'lack insight', but despite her doubts Lucy has opted for hospital and you notice that when not over-stimulated she responds to your curiosity about her and says she would like to develop perspective on her current situation. In one of these quieter moments Lucy confided that she feels embarrassed by some of the messages she left on her former boyfriend's voicemail and very alone after her mother died. On the other hand, she finds hospital irritating and doesn't really see the point of it. She is particularly irritated when she hears some staff think she lacks insight and, when irritated she closes herself off from any perspective taking.

REFLECTION QUESTIONS

1   How would you prioritise Lucy's needs from a psychotherapeutic practice perspective?

2   What common factors might be useful when Lucy is irritated by staff thinking that she lacks insight?

3   What factors might indicate Lucy is progressing in relation to her desire to 'develop perspective'?

4   From the psychotherapeutic perspective, what do you consider the most important qualities for you to bring to the therapeutic alliance with Lucy?

Implicit to all we say here is the primacy of interpersonal relating in nursing practice. This field is not static and future considerations are turning to social pedagogy to further explain and support the sort of psychotherapeutic practices that we have described. To close, we briefly outline these ideas as a way of continuing our gaze into the future of psychotherapeutic practice.

From the mentalisation field, Peter Fonagy, George Gergely, Elizabeth Allison and Jon Allen (Allen, 2016; Fonagy & Allison, 2014; Fonagy, Gergely & Target, 2007) have introduced ideas of epistemic trust and epistemic vigilance. This is knowledge that integrates the field of natural pedagogy to psychotherapeutic practice.

Epistemic vigilance is associated with closing off to learning, a state of being unable to be reached: 'the self-protective suspicion towards information coming from others that may be potentially damaging, deceptive, or inaccurate' (Fonagy & Allison, 2014, p. 373).

Vigilance is naturally occurring, but in infancy it is moderated by caregivers providing ostentatious cues to a child of their intention to communicate. The result is epistemic trust, proposed as a biological effect that opens the infant to social learning, which is then perpetuated through an ongoing secure attachment. Epistemic trust is the precondition for social learning. The attached child 'will believe his/ her caregiver to be a reliable source of knowledge' (Fonagy & Allison, 2014), thus secure attachment becomes instrumental in paving the way to knowledge acquisition.

Consumers who encounter mental health services may for a variety of reasons suffer from low levels of trust. This constrains their ability to make sense of and take in information, as well as inhibiting the natural ability we humans have to create knowledge through social means.

Mentalising, in the psychotherapeutic use of the word, is the process of the clinician holding in their mind, *the mind of the person they are working with*. This involves connecting in a way that attends to the subjective experiences of the other person. It requires an unmistakeable and ostentatious willingness to hear what is on the mind of the other and help make sense of that. It is, we propose, the essential thing that occurs when nurses connect using the common factor approaches we outline above.

This process requires us to step outside of our *knowing*, and enter a *not knowing stance*, (something that can be difficult for nurses who are trained to know things, ask about signs and symptoms and impart their knowledge). A *not knowing* nurse gives the person the chance to speak about what is on their mind. In return, this provides the nurse with an opportunity to discover that person's subjective experiences. This enhances empathy, connection and then a dialogue where a process of linking various experiences that inform meaning and social learning becomes possible. This process reduces vigilance and rigidity, increases trust and opens natural pathways to knowledge:

> [T]he very experience of having our subjectivity understood—of being mentalized—is a necessary trigger for us to be able to receive and learn from the social knowledge that has the potential to change our perception of ourselves and our social world.

Fonagy and Allison (2014, p. 372)

It is the *social world* that people return to from their ventures in mental health-care systems. In opening the pathways to epistemic trust, the psychotherapeutic practice of mental health nurses assists people (re)acquire a level of openness to experience that allows participation in sharing, learning and developing their own knowledge *in that world*.

Care planning

The following is an example care plan for Lucy informed by the recovery alliance theory and a common psychotherapeutic factors approach.

	Lucy's viewpoint	Lucy's desires	Mutual goals/plan	Agreed approach	Review
Working alliance	What alliance? When I'm told I have 'no insight' I say f*ck your alliance; but some of you are okay. Actually when you listen you're okay—it's just when you don't I get pissed off.	I need to understand stuff. It's like I've been through the wringer and I put (former boyfriend) through hell when my mum died. What happened to us? (He's a right pr*ck too. Everything's all about him, his mates and his f*cking football club. Sometimes I want to kill him!) I want you to help me with that not all the other crap.	Have quiet space each day for a half-hour chat to try to figure out what's happened and what to do next. Main aim is to get some perspective and see what happens next, rather than feel as if everything needs to be solved immediately; it's okay to take time. No interrogation about symptoms or medication compliance in this space (that will be in sessions with the doctor). This space is for trying to put my ideas together.	Find a language that makes sense to us both so we can talk about what's been going on and what is meant by certain statements (such as 'I want to kill him'). No taboos on what feelings get talked about, but care when talking about angry feelings so these don't overwhelm things. It's okay to talk about the past, but we'll try to figure out what is most relevant to my present and immediate plans. If/when things feel out of control we slow down and focus on breathing, rather than mind stuff.	Lucy will review each day in her diary with the help of pm shift nurse before bed. Overall review of progress at end of the week with further goals to be discussed at that point.
Coping focus	I cope best when I can get a moment to settle down. Sometimes there is just too much noise in this place. The quiet room helps but sometimes it's hard being alone.	I think there is too much going on emotionally. I've got to pace myself; I need help with that sometimes. Being alone isn't good as sometimes my mind races and I need someone to help slow it down.	When feeling alone it's okay to approach the contact nurse to seek some company. We need to learn more about why being alone feels like sh*t and why I hate my ex boyfriend! Just accept me when I feel like crap (or when I feel bubbly). Reassurance about my feelings helps, but I need to understand why I feel certain things.	Time allocation as above. Ask questions about what helps, what doesn't and when things are worse or better.	Review approaches in sessions to keep track of what is helping build coping.
Self-responsibility/control	I feel out of control sometimes, but I know far more than you think I do.	Listen to me and help me figure things out, then I have more control.	Nurses to help link different parts of Lucy's ideas, thoughts, memories and feelings but more as questions, not conclusions—as that feels too much like our insight not hers.	As above.	As above.

1 How would you prioritise Lucy's needs from a psychotherapeutic practice perspective?

2 What common factors might be useful when Lucy is irritated by staff thinking that she lacks insight?

3 What factors might indicate Lucy is progressing in relation to her desire to 'develop perspective'?

4 From the psychotherapeutic perspective what do you consider the most important qualities for you to bring to the therapeutic alliance with Lucy?

SUMMARY

We have located our approach to psychotherapeutic practice in mental health nursing within a long tradition of psychotherapeutic thought. This originated in the nineteenth century in separate traditions influenced by founding figures whose approaches were largely disconnected. Psychoanalytic/psychodynamic, behavioural and humanistic frameworks competed for the high ground over much of the twentieth century with mental health nursing approaches aligned to both psychodynamic and humanistic frameworks. While cognitive and psychopharmacological perspectives seemed to dominate by the end of the twentieth century, the twenty-first century has seen the growth of common psychotherapy factors, consumer-led perspectives and a revolution in neurobiological understandings based in neuroplasticity science.

In nursing, our practice theories are concerned with supporting consumer self-determination beyond diagnosis, treatment and remission paradigms. The recovery alliance theory of mental health nursing focuses nurses on interpersonal practices that support coping. We believe that such coping happens when, within securely attached therapeutic relationships where aloneness is reduced, arousal lowers and new neural pathways develop to sustain change. In this, linkages between a wide range of mental processes and real-world relationships support consumer meaning making. While this is what nurses may be aiming for, it should be said that the nature of what coping fits best to what person is ultimately determined by that person, as citizen rather than passive recipient of nursing care.

DISCUSSION
QUESTIONS

1 From an attachment theory perspective, what is your understanding of the relationship between creating alliances with consumers and strengthening of a sense of self?

2 In what way/s is a therapeutic alliance achieved through the development of a therapeutic relationship?

3 In what way/s does the use of neuroplasticity theory held us understand apparent adult psychopathology?

4 What are the key foci of psychodynamic interpersonal therapy and does it relate to your practice?

5 What are the common therapeutic factors underpinning psychodynamic nursing practice?

TEST YOURSELF

1 Humanistic frameworks for psychotherapeutic nursing are concerned with:

a creating high levels of collaboration that, in turn, assist consumers discover personal meaning in their experiences

ROBERT TRETT AND HALEY PECKHAM

b making lemonade out of lemons

c helping nurses make meaning of their professional experiences by developing self-compassion

d competing with and ultimately replacing cognitive science and psychopharmacology

e supporting consumer rights and self-determination

2 The importance of therapeutic relationships is upheld by:

a customer surveys that show that both consumers and carers place high value on nurses showing kindness to them

b relationships being generally thought to help consumers to better cope with their illnesses

c review data showing that clinical remission from mental illnesses requires high-quality therapeutic relationships be established with both consumers and carers

d nursing studies showing high correlation between therapeutic relationship and harm reduction and consumer satisfaction

e nurses' experiences of higher job satisfaction when given adequate time to relate therapeutically with consumers

3 Neuroplasticity science is important in psychotherapeutic nursing because:

a it is a way of understanding why some consumers habitually repeat behaviours and patterns that do not serve them

b it keeps consumers and nurses positive about change

c psychotherapy needs some science to validate it

d it is an alternative rationale to diagnosis and pharmacotherapy

e it is a way of understanding behaviours and patterns as attempts to adapt to past experiences, as well as a hopeful stance that new experiences will lead to change

4 The taxonomy of psychotherapeutic nursing practices is derived from:

a an analysis of specific evidence-based psychological techniques

b common therapeutic factors established across a range of empirically validated psychotherapies

c mental health nurse focus groups comprising nurses who practise psychotherapy

d an eclectic approach to psychotherapy

e a lively debate between consumers, carers and senior nurses

USEFUL WEBSITES

Organisations

International Society for Psychological and Social Approaches to Psychosis: www.isps.org

New Zealand Association of Psychotherapists/Te Rōpū Whakaora Hinengaro: http://nzap.org.nz

Psychotherapy and Counselling Federation of Australia: www.pacfa.org.au

Psychodynamic interpersonal and psychoanalytic therapy

Psychodynamic Interpersonal Therapy (PIT) Special Interest Group: www.psychodynamic-interpersonal-therapy.uk/index2.html

Acceptance and commitment therapy

ACT Mindfully: https://www.actmindfully.com.au/

Mentalisation based therapy

YouTube—Mentalizing and MBT: https://www.youtube.com/watch?v=kxUHILbZNaY

Integrative psychotherapy

YouTube—Integrative Psychotherapy—Its Roots, History and Methods: https://www.youtube.com/watch?v=Xxq79TMdKNs

Common empirically validated factors and epistemic trust in psychotherapy

YouTube—David H. Barlow on Evidence-Based Treatments, Common Factors and Recent Psychotherapy Research: https://www.youtube.com/watch?v=GWNo6y2gU0g

Voice hearing

YouTube—Compassion for Voices: A Tale of Courage and Hope: https://www.youtube.com/watch?v=VRqI4lxuXAw

REFERENCES

Ainsworth M., Blehar M., Waters E., & Wall S. (1978). *Patterns of attachment: a psychological study of the strange situation.* New Jersey: Lawrence Erlbaum Associates.

Allen, J. G. (2016). Should the century-old practice of psychotherapy defer to science and ignore its foundations in two millennia of ethical thought? *Bulletin of the Menninger Clinic, 80*(1), 1–20.

Allen, J. G., Bateman, A. W., & Fonagy, P. (2008). *Mentalizing in Clinical Pracice.* Washington D. C.: American Psychiatric Publishing.

Barker, P. (2001). The Tidal Model: Developing a Person-Centered Approach to Psychiatric and Mental Health Nursing. *Perspectives in Psychiatric Care, 37*(3), 79–87.

Barker, P., Jackson, S., & Stevenson, C. (1999). What are psychiatric nurses needed for? Developing a theory of essential nursing practice. *Journal of Psychiatric and Mental Health Nursing, 6,* 273–281.

Bateman, A. (2012). Treating Borderline Personality Disorder in Clinical Practice. *American Journal of Psychiatry, 169*(6), 560–563.

Bateman, A., & Fonagy, P. (2004). *Psychotherapy for Borderline Personality Disorder: Mentalization-based treatment.* New York: Oxford University Press.

Bateman, A., & Fonagy, P. (2006b). Progress in the treatment of borderline personality disorder. *British Journal of Psychiatry, 188,* 1–3.

Blum, H. P. (2016). Interpretation and Contemporary Reinterpretation. *Psychoanalytic Inquiry, 36,* 40–51.

Bowlby, J. (1979). *The making & breaking of affectional bonds*: London: Tavistock Publications, 1979.

Bowlby, J. (1988). *A secure base: parent-child attachment and healthy human development / John Bowlby*: New York: Basic Books, 1988.

Bracken, P., Thomas, P., Timimi, S., Asen, E., Behr, G., Beuster, C., Yeomans, D. (2012). Psychiatry beyond the current paradigm. *British journal of psychiatry 201*(6).

Brimblecombe, N., Tingle, A., & Murrells, T. (2007). How mental health nursing can best improve service users' experiences and outcomes in inpatient settings: responses to a national

consultation. *Journal of Psychiatric and Mental Health Nursing, 14,* 503–509.

Budd, R., & Hughes, I. (2009). The dodo bird verdict—controversial, inevitable and important: a commentary on 30 years of meta-analyses. *Clinical Psychology & Psychotherapy, 16*(6), 510–522.

Burston, D. (2003). Existentialism, Humanism and Psychotherapy. *Existential Analysis 14*(2), 309–319.

Cahill, J., Paley, G., & Hardy, G. (2013). What do patients find helpful in psychotherapy? Implications for the therapeutic relationship in mental health nursing. *Journal of Psychiatric and Mental Health Nursing, 20,* 782–791.

Cameron, D., Kapur, R., & Campbell, P. (2005). Releasing the therapeutic potential of the psychiatric nurse: a human relations perspective of the nurse–patient relationship. *Journal of Psychiatric and Mental Health Nursing, 12,* 64–74.

Cardell, R., & Pitula, C. R. (1999). Suicidal Inpatients' Perceptions of Therapeutic and Nontherapeutic Aspects of Constant Observation. *Psychiatric Services, 50*(8).

Carlsson, G., Dahlberg, K., Ekebergh, M., & Dahlberg, H. (2006). Patients Longing For Authentic Personal Care: A Phenomenological Study of Violent Encounters In Psychiatric Settings. *Issues in Mental Health Nursing, 27,* 287–305.

Chapman D., Whitfield C. V. F., Dube S., Edwards V., & Anda R. (2004). Adverse childhood experiences and the risk of depressive disorders in adulthood. *Journal of Affective Disorders, 82*(2), 217–225.

Chen, L., Murad, M., Paras, M., Colbenson, K., Sattler, A., Goranson, E., Zirakzadeh, A. (2010). Sexual Abuse and Lifetime Diagnosis of Psychiatric Disorders: Systematic Review and Meta-analysis. *Mayo Clinic Proceedings, 85*(7), 618–629.

Clarkson, P. (1992). *Transactional analysis Psychotherapy an integrated approach.* London: Tavistock/Routledge.

Cleary, M., Horsfall, J., O'Hara-Aarons, M., & Hunt, G. E. (2013). Mental health nurses' views

of recovery within an acute setting. *International Journal of Mental Health Nursing, 22,* 205–212.

Corstens, D., Longden, E., & May, R. (2012). Talking with voices: exploring what is expressed by the voices people hear. *Psychosis, 4*(2), 95–104.

Cutcliffe, J., Stevenson, C., Jackson, S., & Smith, P. (2006). A modified grounded theory study of how psychiatric nurses work with suicidal people. *International Journal of Nursing Studies, 43,* 791–802.

Cutcliffe, J., & Grant, G. (2001). What are the principles and processes of inspiring hope in cognitively impaired older adults within a continuing care environment? *Journal of Psychiatric and Mental Health Nursing, 8,* 427–436.

Cutcliffe, J. R., & Barker, P. (2002). Considering the care of the suicidal client and the case for 'engagement and inspiring hope' or 'observations'. *Journal of Psychiatric and Mental Health Nursing, 9,* 611–621.

Cutcliffe, J. R., Santos, J. C., Kozel, B., Taylor, P., & Lees, D. (2015). Raiders of the Lost Art: A review of published evaluations of inpatient mental health care experiences emanating from the United Kingdom, Portugal, Canada, Switzerland, Germany and Australia. *International Journal of Mental Health Nursing, 24,* 375–385.

Cutcliffe, J. R., & Stevenson, C. (2008). Feeling our way in the dark: The psychiatric nursing care of suicidal people—A literature review. *International Journal of Nursing Studies, 45,* 942–953.

Cutcliffe, J. R., Stevenson, C., Jackson, S., & Smith, P. (2007). Reconnecting the Person with Humanity: How Psychiatric Nurses Work with Suicidal People. *Crisis, 28*(4), 207–210.

Daya, I. (2013). Living With Difficult Emotions. Retrieved from www.indigodaya.com/wp-content/uploads/2013/05/Difficult-Emotions-Self-Help-Booklet-Indigo-Daya.pdf.

DeFife, J., & Hilsenroth, M. (2011). Some Implicit Common Factors in Diverse Methods of Psychotherapy. *Journal of Psychotherapy Integration, 21*(2), 172–191.

Delaney, K. R., & Handrup, C. T. (2011). Psychiatric Mental Health Nursing's

Psychotherapy Role: Are We Letting It Slip Away? *Archives of Psychiatric Nursing,, 25*(4), 303–305.

Deng, W., Aimone, J. B., & Gage, F. H. (2010). New neurons and new memories: how does adult hippocampal neurogenesis affect learning and memory? *Nature Reviews Neuroscience, 11*(5), 339–350.

Dimidjian, S., Arch, J., Schneider, R., Desormeau, P., Felder, J., & Z. S. (2016). Considering Meta-Analysis, Meaning, and Metaphor: A Systematic Review and Critical Examination of 'Third Wave' Cognitive and Behavioral Therapies. *Behaviour Therapy* Retrieved from http://dx.doi.org/10.1016/j.beth.2016.07.002.

Egeland M., Zunszain P., & Pariante, C. (2015). Molecular mechanisms in the regulation of adult neurogenesis during stress. *Nature Reviews Neuroscience, 16*(4).

Elliott, R., Greenberg, L. S., Watson, J. C., Timulak, L., & Freire, E. (2013). Research on humanistic-experiential psychotherapies. In M. J. Lambert (Ed.), *Bergin & Garfield's Handbook of psychotherapy and behavior change* (6th ed.) (pp. 495–538). New York: Wiley.

Evans, A. M. (2005). Patient or consumer? The colonization of the psychiatric clinic. *International Journal of Mental Health Nursing, 14*, 285–289.

Felitti, V. (1998). Relationship of childhood abuse and household dysfunction to many of the leading causes of death in adults: the Adverse Childhood Experiences (ACE) Study. *American Journal of Preventive Medicine, 14*(4), 245–258.

Fields, R. D. (2015). A new mechanism of nervous system plasticity: activity-dependent myelination. *Nature Reviews Neuroscience, 16*(12), 756–767.

Fonagy, P., & Allison, E. (2014). The Role of Mentalizing and Epistemic Trust in the Therapeutic Relationship. *Psychotherapy, 51*(3), 372–380.

Fonagy, P., Gergely, G., & Target, M. (2007). The parent–infant dyad and the construction of the subjective self. *Journal of Child Psychology and Psychiatry, 43*(3/4), 288–328.

Guthrie, E., & Moghavemi, A. (2013). Psychodynamic-Interpersonal Therapy: An Overview of the Treatment Approach and Evidence Base. *Psychodynamic Psychiatry, 41*(4), 619–636.

Hayes, S. (2004). Acceptance and Commitment Therapy, Relational Frame Theory, and the Third Wave of Behavioral and Cognitive Therapies. *Behaviour Therapy, 35*, 639–665.

Herman, J., Perry, J., & van der Kolk, B. (1989). Childhood Trauma in Borderline Personality Disorder. *American Journal of Psychiatry, 146*(4), 490–496.

Hillis, S., Anda, R., Dube, S. V. F., Marchbanks, P. & Marks, J. (2004). The association between adverse childhood experiences and adolescent pregnancy, long-term psychosocial consequences, and fetal death. *Pediatrics, 113*(2), 320–328.

Horvath, A., & Luborsky, L. (1993). The role of the therapeutic alliance in psychotherapy. *Journal of Consulting and Clinical Psychology, 6*(4), 561–573.

Houghton, J. (2016). *The influence of Watson's world in the psychotherapeutic interventions of acceptance and commitment therapy (act) and mindfulness.* Essay. Royal Melbourne Hopsital.

Kempermann, G., Kuhn, G., & Gage, F. (1997). More hippocampal neurons in adult mice living in an enriched environment. *Nature, 386*(6624).

Knight, T. (2009). *Beyond Belief, alternative ways of working with delusion, obsessions and unusual experiences*. Shrewsbury: Peter Lehmann Publishing.

Labonte, B., Suderman, M., Maussion, G., Navaro, L., Yerko, V., Mahar, I., Turecki, G. (2012). Genome-wide epigenetic regulation by early-life trauma. *Archives of General Psychiatry, 69*(7).

Laska, K., Gurman, A., & Wampold, B. (2014). Expanding the Lens of Evidence-Based Practice in Psychotherapy: A Common Factors Perspective. *Psychotherapy, 51*(4), 467–481.

Lenzi, D., Trentini, C., Tambelli, R. & Pantano, P. (2015). Neural basis of attachment-caregiving systems interaction: insights from neuroimaging studies. *Frontiers in Psychology, 24*(6).

Lieberwirth, C., & Wang, Z. (2012). The social environment and neurogenesis in the adult Mammalian brain. *Frontiers In Human Neuroscience, 6*.

MacMillan, H. (2001). Childhood Abuse and Lifetime Psychopathology in a Community Sample. *The American Journal of Psychiatry, 158*(11), 1878 -1883.

Magnavita, J. J. (2006). In Search of the Unifying Principles of Psychotherapy: Conceptual, Empirical, and Clinical Convergence. *American Psychologist*, 882–892.

Main, M., & Solomon, J. (1989). Procedures for identifying infants as disorganized/disoriented during the Ainsworth Strange Situation. In M. T. Greenberg, D. Cicchetti, & E. M. Cummings (Eds.), *Attachment in the preschool years: Theory, research, and intervention* (pp. 121–160.). University of Chicago Press: Chicago.

McEwen, B. N. B., Gray, J., Hill, M., Hunter, R., Karatsoreos, I., & Nasca, C. (2015). Mechanisms of stress in the brain. *Nature Neuroscience, 18*(10), 1353–1311.

Meares, R. (2004). The Conversational Model: an outline. *American Journal of Psychotherapy, 58*(1), 51–66.

Moyle, W. (2003). Nurse–patient relationship: A dichotomy of expectations. *International Journal of Mental Health Nursing, 12*, 103–109.

Opendak, M., & Gould, E. (2015). Adult neurogenesis: a substrate for experience-dependent change. *Trends in Cognitive Sciences, 19*(3), 151–161.

Paley, G., Cahill, J., Barkham, M., Shapiro, D., Jones, J., Patrick, S., & Reid, E. (2008). The effectiveness of psychodynamic-interpersonal therapy (PIT) in routine clinical practice: A benchmarking comparison. *Psychology and Psychotherapy: Theory, Research and Practice, 81*, 157–175.

Paley, G., Myers, J., Patrick, S., Reid, E., & Shapiro, D. A. (2003). Practice development in psychological interventions: mental health nurse involvement in the Conversational Model of psychotherapy. *Journal of Psychiatric and Mental Health Nursing,, 10*, 494–498.

Paley, G., & Shapiro, D. (2001). Evidence-based psychological interventions in mental health nursing. *Nursing Times, 97*(03).

Peckham, H. (2013). Epigenetics: The Dogma-defying Discovery That Genes Learn From Experience. *International Journal of Neuropsychotherapy, 1*(1), 9–20. doi:10.12744/ijnpt.2013.

Peplau, H. E. (1952). *Interpersonal relations in nursing.* New York: Putnam.

Ramachandran, V. (Writer) (2003). Neuroscience—the New Philosophy *Reith Lectures The Emerging Mind Lecture 5*. www.bbc.co.uk/radio4/reith2003/lecture5.shtml: BBC.

Romme, M. A., & Escher, A. D. (1989). Hearing voices. *Schizophrenia bulletin, 15*(2), 209.

Rosenzweig, S. (1936). Some Implicit Common Factors in Diverse Methods of Psychotherapy. *Journal of Psychotherapy Integration*, (published in 2002), *12*(1), 5–9.

Roth T. (2009). Lasting Epigenetic Influence of Early-Life Adversity on the BDNF Gene. *Biological psychiatry, 65*(9), 760 -769.

Shaffer J. (2016). Neuroplasticity and Clinical Practice: Building Brain Power for Health. *Frontiers in Psychology*.

Shanley, E., & Jubb-Shanley, M. (2007). The recovery alliance theory of mental health nursing. *Journal of Psychiatric and Mental Health Nursing,, 14*, 734–743.

Shanley, E., & Jubb-Shanley, M. (2012). Coping focus counselling in mental health nursing. *International Journal of Mental Health Nursing, 21*, 504–512.

Shanley, E., Jubb, M., & Latter, P. (2003). Partnership in Coping: an Australian system of mental health nursing. *Journal of Psychiatric and Mental Health Nursing, 10*, 431–441.

Shonkoff, J., Boyce, W., & McEwen, B. (2009). Neuroscience, molecular biology, and the childhood roots of health disparities: building a new framework for health promotion and disease prevention. *Journal of the American Medical Association, 301*(21), 2252–2259.

Suderman, M., Borghol, N., Pappas, J., Pereira, S., Pembrey, M., Hertzman, C., Szyf, M. (2014).

Childhood abuse is associated with methylation of multiple loci in adult DNA. *BMC Medical Genomics, 7*(13), 12.

Suri, D., Veenit, V., Sarkar, A., Thiagarajan, D., Kumar, A., Nestler, E., Vaidya, V. (2013). Early Stress Evokes Age-Dependent Biphasic Changes in Hippocampal Neurogenesis, Bdnf Expression, and Cognition. *Biological psychiatry, 73*(7), 658–666.

Sweatt, J. D. (2016). Neural plasticity and behavior: Sixty years of conceptual advances. *Journal of Neurochemistry, 139*(2), 179–199.

Taylor, P. J., Rietzschel, J., Danquah, A., & Berry, K. (2015). The role of attachment style, attachment to therapist, and working alliance in response to psychological therapy. *Psychology and Psychotherapy: Theory, Research and Practice, 88*, 240–253.

Teicher, M. (2002). Scars that won't heal: the neurobiology of child abuse. *Scientific American, 286*(3), 54–61.

Teicher M, & Samson J. (2016). Annual Research Review: Enduring neurobiological effects of childhood abuse and neglect. *Journal Of Child Psychology And Psychiatry, And Allied Disciplines, 57*(3), 241–266.

Turecki G, & Meaney M. (2016). Effects of the Social Environment and Stress on Glucocorticoid Receptor Gene Methylation: A Systematic Review. *Biological Psychiatry, 79*(2), 87–96.

Vandemark, L. (2006). Awareness of self and expanding consciousness: using nursing theories to prepare nurse-therapist. *Issues in Mental Health Nursing, 27*, 605–615.

Wampold, B. (2012). Humanism as a Common Factor in Psychotherapy. *Psychotherapy, 49*(4), 445–449.

Wampold, B., Mondin, G., Moody, M., Stich, F., Benson, K., & Ahn, H. (1997). A meta-analysis of outcome studies comparing bona fide psychotherapies: Empirically, 'All must have prizes'. *Psychological Bulletin, 122*(3), 203–215.

Warrender, D. (2015). Staff nurse perceptions of the impact of mentalization-based therapy skills training when working with borderline personality disorder in acute mental health: a qualitative study. *Journal of Psychiatric and Mental Health Nursing, 22*, 623–633.

Watson, J. (2009). Caring science and human caring theory: transforming personal and professional practices of nursing and health care. *Journal of Health & Human Services Administration 31*(4), 466–482.

Weaver I. (2005). *Epigenetic programming by maternal behavior.* (Electronic Thesis or Dissertation), McGill University.

Weinberger, J. (2014). Common Factors are not so common and specific factors are not so specified: Toward an inclusive integration of psychotherapy research. *Psychotherapy, 51*(4), 514–518.

Wheeler, K. (2005). The Primacy of Psychotherapy. *Perspectives in Psychiatric Care, 41*(4), 151.

Wheeler, K., & Delaney, K. (2008). Challenges and Realities of Teaching Psychotherapy: A Survey of Psychiatric-Mental Health Nursing Graduate Programs. *Perspectives in Psychiatric Care, 44*(2), 72–80.

Yehuda R. (2008). Maternal, not paternal, PTSD is related to increased risk for PTSD in offspring of Holocaust survivors. *Journal of psychiatric research, 42*(13), 1104–1111.

CHAPTER 19

Case management

KAREN-LEIGH EDWARD

Acknowledgment

The authors would like to acknowledge Gilles Terrière and Di Hawthorne who co-wrote this chapter in the second edition.

KEY OUTCOMES

AFTER READING THIS CHAPTER, YOU SHOULD BE ABLE TO:

- define case management
- distinguish between assertive case management and the 'standard' model of case management
- understand the central tasks of a case manager and the disciplines a case manager can come from
- identify the professional skills a nurse will bring to case management
- demonstrate an understanding of the recovery model and how this is used in the case management framework.

KEY TERMS

- assertive case management
- brokerage model
- case management
- cognitive behaviour therapy (CBT)
- clinical case management model
- narrative therapy
- recovery model
- self-efficacy
- strengths model

Introduction

In this chapter you will discover the role of case management for consumers within the community mental health setting. Case management is the central model for providing care and coordination of care in community mental health services. There are many definitions of case management that can be located within the literature, and varying models of application of the case management model. However, the overarching focus of case management is to provide holistic care aimed at improving the overall biopsychosocial needs of the individual at the centre of care. The purpose of case management is to work collaboratively with consumers and their carers or families in order to maximise the potential to live independently in the community. It is important to highlight that case management refers to management of service provision, not management of people.

Case management: an international outlook

Central to contemporary mental health services is an effort to ensure that people who experience mental disorders spend fewer days as a hospital inpatient and are discharged to home with follow-up as soon as possible. Unnecessary mental health hospital care can be stigmatising and expensive, and can cause significant interruption to the individual's roles at home and at work. Case management was introduced into mental health service provision to reduce hospital length of stay while still enhancing the continuum of care that people require as they move through the health system. It is important to look to local and international trends related to case management, and the implications of those trends with regard to nursing in Australia and New Zealand, as this can ensure care management is provided in a contemporary and evidence-based manner. For instance, a systematic review with meta-analysis of the efficacy of case management undertaken in the late 1990s established clear benefits for consumers receiving care under the case management framework. Mueser and colleagues (1998) established that a reduction in length of hospital stay and symptomatology existed for those in case management. This has been supported in subsequent research related to the benefits of case management versus standard care, revealing case management can reduce the length of hospital stay and prevent clients being lost to follow-up in mental health-care services; there is also some suggestion that consumers receiving case management are more adherent with their treatment and medication regimes compared to standard care (Dieterich et al., 2010).

Although case management has been established and used as a key factor of mental health service delivery in many countries, it has not been practised in a similar way globally. For example, some Asian countries are embarking on variations of case management to address the issues of inflexibility and fragmentation found in their systems (Wong, Yeung & Ching, 2009). In particular, the Hong Kong government has dedicated additional funding for the development of community-based mental health services for their mental health consumers. These services are named Community Link (Com-Link), which is a supportive social and prevocational service for people with severe mental illness and their carers; and Community Care (Com-Care), an active outreach and support service that includes crisis intervention for those more prone to relapse (Wong, Yeung & Ching, 2009). More recently, personal care plans and an integrated approach to individualised and engaged care for people with severe mental illness have been trialled in Hong Kong, with positive results seen through an audit of outcomes in 2011 (Cheng et al., 2012). Also in China, the Chinese University of Hong Kong, Asia-Australia Mental Health and the Institute of Mental Health Peking University are currently collaborating to develop and deliver a culturally sensitive, tripartite training program in case management for mental health workers across China (Lui et al., 2011).

A nationwide survey in Australia highlighted that the odds of hospitalisation for individuals with severe mental illnesses was higher for those without a case manager (Morgan et al., 2012). In addition, results of the survey indicate service integration was needed to meet the considerable and varied mental and physical health needs of individuals with severe mental illness. The Australian Government's establishment of the Partners in Recovery (PIR) initiative provides an opportunity for the development of more effective and efficient models of coordinated care for identified people with severe mental illness and their families and carers (Brophy et al., 2014). In the USA, assertive community treatment teams utilise case management as a mode of treatment intervention, and it has become one of the most researched interventions in mental health-care delivery (Marshall & Lockwood, 2011). Several studies exploring proactive community treatment have stressed that keeping true to the model—that is, fidelity— leads to better consumer outcomes for those experiencing mental disorders. In the USA, the philosophy of mental health case management is to focus on each person's strengths, interests and abilities and to decrease, if not to avoid, hospitalisations. A systematic review, with meta-regression techniques applied to data from randomised controlled trials, demonstrates that when hospital use is high, case management can reduce it. However, case management is less successful when hospital use is already low for the consumer. In the UK, case management teams are mainly resourced by nurses, and these nurses have access to other multidisciplinary members, especially allied health and medical (Killaspy et al., 2009).

In most examples of case management care for those who experience mental disorders, nurses are the linchpin in the continuum of care for the mental health consumer. This is an important point, and one to reflect upon in terms of your own contribution and the impact you and your nurse colleagues can have upon the care interventions and care continuum for those in your care, including the consumer's carers.

Rapp and Goscha (2004) describe nine principles of effective case management:

1 Case managers ought to deliver as much of the service as possible, rather than making referrals to multiple formal services.
2 Work is in the community.
3 Case management consists of both individual and team case management.
4 Case managers have primary responsibility for a person's required services.
5 Case managers can be para-professionals (from different fields such as nursing, social work, psychology, medicine, occupational therapy and community work). Supervisors of case managers should be experienced and fully credentialed.
6 Caseload size should be small enough to allow for a relative high frequency of contact (if possible no more than 20:1).
7 Case management service should be time-unlimited, if appropriate. However, individuals in receipt of case management services should be able to exit case management (called case closure) and then re-enter case management if needed.
8 People need access to familiar people.
9 Case managers should foster choice.

There are many different models of case management; however, they typically involve a single case manager working with a mental health consumer.

Models of case management

Case management is a system for assisting people to overcome the complex issues that can be a consequence of a serious and longstanding mental or developmental problem. These issues may result from an interruption to developmental stages; for example, if the normal progress through adolescence to adulthood is interrupted by early onset psychosis, or if the previous achievements in functioning are lost to later onset serious illness. Areas affected can include social relationships, learning and further education, skills of independent living, ability to earn an income and, for many, the questioning of the very meaning of their life. In such circumstances, the reduction or elimination of the symptoms of illness is insufficient as an intervention outcome as the consumer requires a holistic approach to assisting their recovery.

Case management is not unique to mental health services and is offered by disability, housing, welfare and physical health organisations. Each sector has a particular approach to case management. In the Australian mental health field, when case management emerged on the mental health-care landscape in the 1990s the most common models of delivering case management were the assertive model and the 'clinical' model (Ziguras & Stuart, 2000; Dieterich et al., 2010).

Assertive case management is quite intensive (Rosen, Meuser & Teesson, 2007); the consumer may be seen several times a week and is more likely to be seen at home or in community settings. Practical assistance is given, as consumers may need to be guided in developing budgets, shopping, cooking and learning to manage other everyday tasks. Significant family support or reconciliation may be required if the consumer's illness has impacted on family relationships. The consumers often need assistance in developing the appropriate social skills and self-confidence that will allow them to successfully interact with their families and the broader community. Staff working in assertive type teams will have a caseload of fewer than twenty consumers and work closely with their colleagues and with consumers of other case managers, helping them to achieve their daily tasks and goals (Dieterich et al., 2010; Issakidis et al., 1999). Considering the available evidence, assertive community treatment case management is one of the most effective interventions in mental health service provision today. Assertive community treatment (ACT) case managers provide health-care services to people with severe and persistent mental illness, and often this type of approach is used by teams such as mobile support and treatment teams. ACT consumers have shown significant reduction in symptom severity and better outcomes in their global assessment of functioning (GAF) (Jeong, Lee & Jon, 2016).

Case managers working with the clinical case management model will have a larger caseload of about twenty-five to thirty consumers that have less complex needs, and will see each consumer fortnightly or monthly. Less practical assistance will be provided and the work of the team will be more focused on the treatment of the mental illness. The case manager or another treating clinician will work with the consumer to develop both an understanding of their illness and an increased ability to moderate the effects of symptoms that may be ongoing despite medication. The case manager may use one of the psychotherapeutic intervention approaches covered later in this chapter. Clinical case management is more likely to be office-based with less community outreach visiting (Wong, Rosenburg & Wessman, 2006) than in assertive case management.

In Australia, the clinical model is more common and often used by Continuing Care, Clinical Consultancy teams. The early community mental health clinics were established in the 1970s and 1980s, and subsequently adopted the clinical model when community care became the preferred treatment option in mental health (Lewis, 2003). However, assertive case management teams were implemented to address the needs of the more severely ill consumers who had persistent symptoms and very limited community living skills. Many mental health services in Australia are either integrating their clinical and assertive case management teams or replacing the clinical model with an assertive model (Castle, Mander & Gomes, 2002) showing improved clinical outcomes for consumers similar to that seen in other countries such as the USA and the UK (Harvey et al., 2012).

In the *Fourth National Mental Health Plan* (Commonwealth of Australia, 2009), the Australian Government established priority areas for the period 2009–2014 that were directly applicable to outcomes for case management. These priorities were the promotion of social inclusion and recovery, prevention and early intervention, access, coordination and continuity of care. This means that the consumer's quality of life should improve via case management—they should be able to enjoy mainstream recreational and vocational activities, and develop and maintain rewarding social relationships. Relapses should be prevented if possible; if not, intervention should take place very early in the relapse to minimise disruption to the person's social and personal life. The *Fifth National Mental Health Plan* (Commonwealth of Australia, 2016) shapes care dependent upon the level of need as determined by a health professional and care will be integrated dependent upon the person's needs. Mental health services reform is high on the agenda for Australia, where care will have a stepped care model (depending on level of need determined by a health professional), integrated care packages, national coordinated services for children and youth, and a greater use of mental health technologies (Council of Australian Governments, 2012).

Recovery, strengths and self-efficacy

As well as models of the system of case management (defining the staff–consumer ratio and the tasks of the case manager), there are therapeutic models of care. Older models of care often emphasised 'doing to' the consumer, which in mental health gave rise to the large institutions. However, newer models emphasise 'doing with' and empowering consumers, which fits well with community-based care and other changes within the health system.

Nationally, mental health in Australia and New Zealand has adopted a particular model of care—the recovery model—as a pathway to improve consumer outcomes. The principles of the model are outlined in the *National Standards for Mental Health Services* (Commonwealth of Australia, 2010) and supported by all mental health services. The standards quote Jacobson and Greenley (2001, p. 42):

> Recovery refers to both internal conditions experienced by persons who describe themselves as being in recovery—hope, healing, empowerment and connection—and external conditions that facilitate recovery—implementation of human rights, a positive culture of healing and recovery oriented services.

This is a very different approach from only treating the symptoms of the illness. In contemporary mental health-care service provision there are new approaches to empowering consumers, fostering hope and encouraging the development of self-management skills that will assist in implementing a recovery model (such as therapeutic optimism and fostering resilience).

One of these is the strengths approach. The strengths approach is underpinned by the belief that the person has strengths and abilities that they might not be applying to the current situation or that they do not realise they possess. Often consumers become so overwhelmed by their problems that they cannot view their abilities realistically. The traditional medical approach of focusing on problems or symptoms often compounds this, and both the consumer and the case manager can feel helpless. A case manager working from a strengths model is optimistic about change and the consumer's abilities, and will place high importance on the consumer's aspirations and values as significant motivators for moving forward (McCashan, 2005; Rapp & Goscha, 2011).

Underlying the strengths approach is self-efficacy theory (Bandura, 1977). This theory of motivation proposes that a person is more likely to attempt a task if they believe that they will succeed. There are three factors that influence self-efficacy: behaviour, environment and cognitive factors. Bandura's theory underpins the development of cognitive therapy (discussed later in this chapter). Recent research in Australia has shown that a community-based self-efficacy approach has significantly reduced hospitalisation for consumers in the Australian Capital Territory (Gilbert et al., 2012).

Who is a case manager and what do they do?

In mental health in Australia and New Zealand, the case manager is usually a clinician. Their role is to work with the consumer and the consumer's family or significant other, and coordinate the completion of a comprehensive and holistic assessment to identify the consumer's psychosocial and medical needs. Several clinicians may contribute to the assessment if their clinical expertise is relevant; for example, the nurse can complete the physical assessment and the occupational therapist can complete a functional assessment to determine the consumer's capacities and needs in carrying out activities of daily living. The case manager will also draft a plan in collaboration with the consumer and the consumer's family or significant other. The plan will identify and prioritise needs, interventions, responsibilities and timelines. Typically, there is no discriminatory funding attached to providing interventions for the consumer. For example, if the consumer needs a support worker, then the case manager liaises and negotiates with a service that is funded to provide the required service to the consumer. In this case, the consumer may be restricted to using services that are free of charge and only available to people living in a certain area. The treatment or care plans will be reviewed by the multidisciplinary team and are often presented to legal review boards or panels if the consumer is on an involuntary community order. A relapse prevention plan should also be developed with the consumer as part of the individual treatment plan. In Victoria this is recommended by the Chief Psychiatrist (Victorian Government, 2004).

The case manager has an ongoing role in the consumer's recovery process, working actively to coordinate care, liaise with other services providing resources to the consumer (for example, housing), evaluate outcomes and engage the consumer in treatment. The quality of the relationship between the consumer and the case manager is a potential predictor of good consumer outcomes. A case manager with a good supportive and understanding relationship with a consumer is able to motivate her to achieve goals and to engage with treatment (Howgego et al., 2003; Rosen, Meuser & Teesson, 2007).

In some instances, the case manager is not a clinician and may not work in a public health service but in an organisation (such as a disability support or primary health service) that is also funded to provide services to people with mental illness. In such organisations, it is not essential that staff have a clinical qualification. In Victoria, several projects have been funded where 'care coordination'—a process similar to case management—is provided by organisations that are not public mental health services but still target consumers of mental health services with complex needs. In this case, the care coordinator would liaise with the mental health service and request particular services on behalf of the consumer. These projects are funded by the Australian Government as part of the *Fourth National Mental Health Plan* (Commonwealth of Australia, 2009). Internationally there are programs with peer case managers that have had some success (Sells et al., 2006).

Less common in Australia is the brokerage model of case management in mental health. In this model, funding is available to purchase services that the consumer requires. Generally, the case manager purchases services for the consumer; however, they may not work directly with the consumer. In extended brokerage services, the case manager may also provide direct support via a clinical service to the consumer (Willis, Reynolds & Keleher, 2008). Although brokerage is not the overarching funding model in Australia, many small brokerage programs assist in the provision of community treatment and rehabilitation. A comprehensive evaluation of some of the recent initiatives funded by the Australian Government is detailed in the *Evaluation of the FaHCSIA Targeted Community Care Mental Health Initiatives* (Commonwealth of Australia, 2012).

Case management skills can be developed through postgraduate education, peer support and professional organisations such as the Case Management Society of Australia & New Zealand & Affiliates (CMSA). The CMSA has also developed Standards for Case Management to assist the novice case manager. Most commonly, though, the case manager in Australian mental health services will develop skills in the clinical setting with assistance from policy and procedures, mentoring and ongoing clinical supervision.

1 How could you engage an involuntary consumer in community-based treatment of their illness?

2 Why is community mental health so important in the Australian setting?

3 What skills, knowledge and attitudes prepare the nurse for the role of case manager?

CRITICAL
THINKING
OPPORTUNITY

KAREN-LEIGH EDWARD

Therapeutic interactions used in case management

Case managers work in a close therapeutic relationship with consumers with the central focus on such activities as assessment, planning, linking the consumer to services they require, advocating on their behalf, brokering (purchasing services needed by the consumer) and monitoring consumer progress. The key function and focus for the case manager is relapse prevention while working in a recovery framework. In this context, the case manager will require therapeutic treatment skills. The most commonly used therapeutic treatment skills include cognitive behaviour therapy (colloquially referred to as 'talking therapy'), dialectical behaviour therapy and narrative therapy.

Cognitive behaviour therapy

Cognitive behaviour therapy (CBT) is well established as an effective treatment for a range of disorders (such as anxiety and affective disorders). CBT utilises a combination of behavioural and cognitive techniques to target a consumer's symptoms. CBT is a type of psychological therapy that assists people to change unhelpful or unhealthy thoughts, behaviours and feelings.

The focus of CBT is on teaching consumers how to control and correct faulty thinking patterns in order to manage their own disorder. Beck and colleagues (1979, p. 3) describe cognitive therapy as 'an active, directive, time-limited, structured approach used to treat a variety of mental health disorders (for example, depression, anxiety, phobias, pain problems, etc.)'. CBT works on the principle that negative, unhelpful beliefs need to be 'tested' to determine whether they are accurate, realistic and truthful. In most cases, the thoughts are actually irrational misconceptions, commonly known as 'cognitive distortions'. Cognitive distortions serve to maintain a negatively skewed and unhelpful belief system, leading to distress and increased difficulty coping in situations.

Some common cognitive distortions include:

- *All or nothing thinking*—some people see things in black or white categories.
- *Overgeneralisation*—people who engage in this style of thinking tend to draw conclusions on the basis of one or more isolated events.
- *Selective abstraction (filtering)*—sometimes a person focuses on a specific detail of an event and takes it out of context.
- *Discounting or disqualifying the positive*—some people tend to reject a successful experience or a positive event by generating a reason why it does not count.
- *Jumping to conclusions*—sometimes people tend to draw a conclusion even when there are no facts to support it.
- *Magnification or minimisation*—sometimes a person assigns too much or too little importance to an event.
- *Personalisation*—some people blame things on themselves when there is no reason for taking part or any of the blame.

Additional strategies used in conjunction with CBT include:

- relaxation techniques
- breathing techniques
- distraction
- coping statements

- thought stopping
- problem solving
- social skills training:
  - assertion
  - conflict management
  - conversation skills
  - vocational and employment skills
  - relationship and interpersonal skills.

Dialectical behavioural therapy

Dialectical behavioural therapy (DBT) has been used successfully as a therapeutic approach with people who have a diagnosis of borderline personality disorder and parasuicidal behaviour. DBT is eclectic and draws on supportive, cognitive and behavioural therapies. It is a form of psychological therapy developed by Marsha Linehan and has been shown to be a very effective intervention for people with significant emotional and relationship problems. Linehan (1993) pioneered this treatment, based on the idea that psychosocial treatment of those with borderline personality disorder was as important in controlling the condition as traditional psychotherapy and pharmacotherapy. Basically, DBT maintains that some people, due to invalidating environments during upbringing and biological factors as yet unknown, react abnormally to emotional stimulation. There are four primary modes of treatment in DBT:

1 individual therapy
2 group skills training (family)
3 telephone contact
4 therapist consultation.

Before a consumer will be taken on for DBT, they will be required to give a number of undertakings:

1 to work in therapy for a specified period of time and, within reason, to attend all scheduled therapy sessions
2 if suicidal or parasuicidal behaviours are present, to work on reducing these
3 to work on any behaviours that interfere with the course of therapy ('therapy interfering behaviours')
4 to attend skills training.

Narrative therapy

Narrative therapy centres on people as the experts in their own lives and views problems as separate from people. Narrative therapy assumes that people have many skills, competencies, beliefs, values, commitments and abilities that will assist them to reduce the influence of problems in their lives. It is a form of psychological therapy using narrative. Initially developed in the 1970s, the approach uses a collaborative and non-blaming approach

Narrative therapy differs from many therapies in that it puts a major emphasis on identifying people's strengths—particularly as they have mastered situations in the past—and therefore seeks to build on their resilience rather than focus on their failures or negatives. Narrative therapy is sometimes known as 're-authoring' or 're-storying' conversations. Stories consist of events, linked in sequence, across time, according to a plot. A narrative is like a thread that weaves the events in our lives together, forming a story.

What narrative therapy is not

Narrative therapy is not about 'looking at the positives' and 'ignoring the negatives'. Nor is about saying: 'Just get over it. Look at these other things—you should be happy.' Narrative therapy is centred on examining the whole picture, selecting stories that have been missed or lost and bringing them to the forefront of the therapeutic moment in discussion.

ABOUT THE CONSUMER   Tony's story

Tony is a 29-year-old single man who has been referred for case management following a recent relapse that necessitated an acute admission. The cause of the relapse was thought to be due to increased substance misuse (cannabis and methamphetamine). In light of Tony's tendency for non-adherence to prescribed antipsychotic medication since being diagnosed with schizophrenia at 21 years of age, the psychiatrist has replaced Tony's oral medication with a fortnightly antipsychotic depot injection.

Tony lives with his parents and younger brother. The parents report that he blames them for his hospitalisations and often argues with them and his brother. Tony does not have many friends and spends most of his days sleeping or playing computer games; he has not worked since dropping out of university at the age of 21.

Tony has a BMI of 29.4 and his waist to hip ratio is 1:2. He is overweight and blames this on his medications, which is one of the likely reasons for his non-adherent behaviour. During the initial assessment and using the Basis-32 questionnaire (Eisen, Dill & Grob, 1994; Department of Health and Ageing, 2003), Tony identified that he would like to address the following issues:

- He wants to lose weight in order to find a girlfriend.
- He wants to do more than sit at home, but does not know what that might be.
- He wants to stop being anxious when in public (because of his weight and his voices).
- Although he does not see the use of cannabis a being a problem, he wants to stop using methamphetamine. He also wants to stop smoking cigarettes due to increasing prices, but does not agree that it has a bad effect on his health.

Tony says: I sleep all the time for two to three days after receiving [the depot medication] and even after that I still have trouble getting up. I don't have any energy or money to go to the gym to lose this weight. No girl will have me because of this and because of my schizophrenia. I'm happy though that I've now got a case manager as he listens to me and doesn't talk down to me like the doctors. The one good thing I have about the illness is the voices and the psychiatrists always try to take them away from me by giving me medications. My case manager asked me what I wanted from this experience and explained to me what this Basis-32 was about. I feel good that someone is listening to me and helping me. Things have already been better at home after he spoke with my parents. My old man has not been bugging me about getting a job. That's one reason I've been using cannabis—to de-stress from them. I need to give up ice though because this last experience scared me, as it made my voices turn bad, like bad spirits trying to take me with them to hell.

REFLECTION QUESTIONS

1 How would you prioritise Tony's needs?
2 How would you address the concept of personal recovery versus medical recovery?
3 How would you address the needs of Tony's family in planning his care?
4 As well as motivational interviewing, what other approaches could you use?
5 When would you review these plans and why?

Care planning

The following is an example care plan for Tony. The recovery framework is a central consideration for the development of this care plan with Tony. The areas of daily living that are considered include biopsychosocial factors and the plan is mapped out using the nursing process (assessment, planning, implementation and evaluation). Remember, the success is in the detail, so be specific about who, when and what in the collaborative plan; and never include someone in the plan if they were not consulted in the planning process.

Date: [Today's date]						
Consumer's name: Tony			**Case Manager: Gary**			
Areas of daily living	**Assessment of current situation**	**Goal**	**Plan** (undertaken with consumer)	**Implementation**	**Who is responsible** (include only those who have been consulted in the planning process)	**Evaluation/ review date**
Mental health	Tony wants to keep his good voices and not suffer from the evil ones.	For Tony to feel comfortable with his symptoms	Tony has agreed to a referral to a voices clinic to meet other people with voices and learn how to live with them.	Tony will attend the weekly meetings with help from his father.	Tony and his father	Review in three months
Social	Tony is single and wants to have a girlfriend. He is afraid that his weight and his illness (both his voices and side effects of medication) will prevent him from achieving that goal. As a result he gets anxious when going out.	For Tony to have opportunities to socialise	Provide with anxiety management strategies.	Tony to practise anxiety management techniques.	Tony and Gary	Review in three months
			Tony will engage his brother in exploring local activities and hobbies.	Tony and his brother will explore and attend local activities.	Tony and his brother	
	Tony and his parents argue regularly. He believes that they do not like him as much as his brother. They would like him to stop smoking, stop using drugs and to get a job.	For Tony and his parents to have better relationship	Tony and his family have agreed to family sessions.	Monthly family sessions to focus on communication and better understanding of problems as well as being solution focused. Parents to attend Well Ways sessions.	Tony, Gary and parents	Review every three months
			The parents have agreed to referral to carer support organisations as well as carer education sessions (for example, Well Ways)	Parents to contact carer support as needed.	Tony, Gary and parents	

KAREN-LEIGH EDWARD

Date: [Today's date]

Biological	Tony does not like his body image due to his weight. He is also at risk of developing diabetes and/or heart-related diseases due to the weight and smoking.	For Tony to lose weight	Tony has agreed to see a dietician to help with his diet.	Tony is keeping a diary of his food intake. He is also adhering to recommendations from his meeting with the dietician.	Tony	Review every four weeks
			Tony will use money saved from smoking to buy a Wii for exercise games.	Tony is saving money in a jar towards purchase of the Wii.	Tony	
			Tony's has agreed to walk with his mother for 30 minutes each day.	Tony and his mother are walking the dogs each evening.	Tony and his mother	
	Tony has disclosed that he has trouble getting an erection since he started medication.	For Tony to feel comfortable with his sexual functions	Tony will see his GP to discuss and rule out biological problems. Explore role of anxiety, substance use and possible co-morbid depression in sexual dysfunction.	Liaise with the GP regarding findings. Review with psychiatrist to address role of medication, substance use and co-morbid illnesses.	Tony, GP and psychiatrist	Review in three months
Environmental	Tony does not want to sit in the house any more but is not sure what he wants to do.	For Tony to find his niche in the community	Tony will accept his brother's offer to explore opportunities in the neighbourhood regarding activities based on previous and ongoing hobbies. Tony will explore returning to education or employment.	Tony and his brother will research local activities online and attend meetings together. Tony will discuss and work with the case manager to identify his goals regarding education or employment.	Tony, his brother and Gary	Review in three months
Substance using behaviours	Tony does not believe that cannabis is bad for his mental health.	To increase Tony's knowledge of the role of cannabis	Using motivational interviewing techniques, explore Tony's perceptions and beliefs of cannabis use and the role of cannabis in mental health, and promote harm minimisation until he moves from a precontemplative stage.	Discuss these issues during review sessions and ongoing assessment of his stage of change. Discuss harm-minimisation techniques as regards his use of cannabis.	Tony and Gary	Review in three months

Date: [Today's date]						
	Tony has decided to cease using amphetamine.	Tony to remain abstinent	Tony has referred himself to a drug and alcohol service for support and started seeing an AoD counsellor.	Liaise with AoD counsellor in order to better support Tony during review sessions and ensure case manager and AoD counsellor are working together.	Gary and AoD counsellor	Review in three months
	Tony has decided to stop smoking.	For Tony to stop smoking	Identify with Tony if he has had previous attempts at giving up to help him plan for a more successful quit attempt.	Refer Tony to his GP for nicotine replacement therapy and to Quitline to assist his quit attempt. Liaise with his parents so they can support his quit attempt.	Tony, GP, Gary, Quitline and parents	Review in three months
			Explore his beliefs about effects of smoking on his health to promote his decision to quit for financial gains.	Tony will save the money he uses to buy cigarettes in a jar. He can use the savings for treats such as the purchase of a Wii.	Tony	
Risk behaviours	Tony stops adherence to his medication, increasing the potential for relapse.	For Tony to adhere to prescribed medication	Explore with Tony and his doctors, using motivational interviewing, his beliefs about medication and his views of his illness.	Conduct regular reviews with the doctors to discuss effects and side effects of medication. Advocate on Tony's behalf if he is unable to verbalise his needs. Provide education as required on the role of medication in relapse prevention.	Tony, Gary and doctors	Review every three months

SUMMARY

Case management is not unique to mental health services and is offered by disability, housing, welfare and physical health organisations. In the mental health field, the most common models of delivering case management are the assertive model and the 'clinical' model. Case management is a model of care used for the provision and coordination of care in community mental health. Considering the available evidence, assertive community treatment case management is one of the most successful interventions in mental health service provision today. There are many different models of case management; however, they typically involve a single case manager working with a mental health consumer. A case manager works from a strengths approach and within a recovery framework, and is hopeful about change, including the consumer's abilities for change. Case managers place high importance on the consumer's goals, aspirations and values as significant motivators for the consumer. Case managers also work in a close therapeutic relationship with consumers with the central focus of the case management role, including assessment, planning, linking the consumer to services they require, advocating on their behalf, brokering (purchasing services needed by the consumer) and monitoring consumer progress.

Q
**DISCUSSION
QUESTIONS**

1   Why do case mangers place high importance on the consumer's goals, aspirations and values?

2   What clinical skills or educational background do you need to be a case manger within the assertive case management approach?

3   Many frameworks and models are used to understand the mental illness–health continuum. Using the recovery framework as a guide, what model of care approach would the case manager be most likely to use and why?

4   Think about the therapeutic skills identified that case managers use with consumers and families. Which of these appeal to you? Why?

TEST YOURSELF

1   Case managers:

a   have secondary responsibility for a person's required services

b   work within the community

c   only work in team case management

d   are only drawn from the nursing profession

2   The strengths approach:

a   is underpinned by the belief that person has strengths and abilities that they might not be applying to the current situation

b   has been used in mental health for many decades

c   is underpinned by the belief that person has strengths and abilities that they do not realise they possess

d   all of the above

3 Dialectical behavioural therapy (DBT):

 a is eclectic and draws on supportive, cognitive and behavioural therapies

 b is based upon story-telling principles

 c can only be used with families

 d guides the consumer towards recovery using the consumer-dependent person model

4 CBT is described as the following by Beck and colleagues

 a an inactive, indirective, time-limited, unstructured approach used to treat a variety of psychiatric disorders

 b an active, directive, time-limited, semi-structured approach used to treat a variety of physical and mental disorders

 c a non-verbal, directive, time-limited, structured approach used to treat a variety of psychiatric disorders

 d an active, directive, time-limited, structured approach used to treat a variety of psychiatric disorders

USEFUL WEBSITES

Assertive Community Treatment Association: www.actassociation.org

Case Management Society of Australia & New Zealand & Affiliates: www.cmsa.org.au

Department of Health—The role of case management: http://health.gov.au/internet/publications/publishing. nsf/Content/mental-pubs-p-mono-toc~mental-pubs-p-mono-bas~mental-pubs-p-mono-bas-acc~mental-pubs-p-mono-bas-acc-cas

Health & Disability Commissioner—Mental health services: www.hdc.org.nz/about-us/mental-health-and-addictions/mental-health-services

REFERENCES

Bandura, A. (1977). Self-efficacy: Toward a unifying theory of behavioural change. *Psychological Review, 84*(2), 191–215.

Beck, A. T., Rush, A. J., Shaw, B. F., & Emery, G. (1979). *Cognitive therapy of depression.* New York: Guilford Press.

Brophy, L., Hodges, C., Halloran, K., Grigg, M., & Swift, M. (2014). Impact of care coordination on Australia's mental health service delivery system. *Australian Health Review, 38*(4), 396–400.

Castle, D., Mander, A., & Gomes, A. (2002). The management of change in a community mental health team. *Australian Health Review, 25*(2), 115–121.

Cheng, K. M., Chan, C., Wong, R., Leung, K. T., Mui, J., Chui, W., & Cheung, E. (2012). Integrated care pathway for the personalized care programme for patients with severe mental illness in Hong Kong. *International Journal of Care Pathways, 16*(3), 72–75.

Commonwealth of Australia (2009). *Fourth national mental health plan: An agenda for collaborative government action in mental health 2009–2014.* Barton.

Commonwealth of Australia (2010). *National standards for mental health services.* Barton.

Commonwealth of Australia (2012). *Evaluation of the FaHCSIA targeted community care mental health initiatives.* Barton: Department of Families, Housing, Community Services and Indigenous Affairs.

Commonwealth of Australia (2016). *Fifth National Mental Health Plan: Draft for consultation.* Retrieved from from http://www.health.gov.au /internet/main/publishing.nsf/content /8F54F3C4F313E0B1CA258052000ED5C5 /$File/Fifth%20National%20Mental %20Health%20Plan.pdf.

Council of Australian Governments (2012). *The roadmap for national mental health reform 2012–2022.* Council of Australian Governments. Retrieved from www.coag.gov.au/sites/default/ files/The%20Roadmap%20for%20National%20 Mental%20Health%20Reform%202012–2022. pdf.pdf.

Dieterich, M., Irving, C. B., Park, B., & Marshall, M. (2010). Intensive case management for severe mental illness. *The Cochrane Database of Systematic Reviews,* (10), CD007906. Advance online publication. http://doi.org/10.1002/14651858. CD007906.pub2.

Department of Health and Ageing (2003). *Mental health national outcomes and casemix collection: Overview of clinician-rated and consumer self-report measures,* Version 1.50. Canberra: DHA.

Eisen, S. V., Dill, D. L., & Grob, M. C. (1994). Reliability and validity of a brief patient-report instrument for psychiatric patient outcome evaluation. *Hospital and Community Psychiatry, 45,* 242–247.

Gilbert, M. M., Chamberlain, J., White, C., Mayers, P., Pawsey, B., Liew, D., Musgrave, M., Crawford, K., & Castle, D. (2012). Controlled trial of a self-management program for people with mental illness in an adult mental health service—the Optimal Health Program (OHP). *Australian Health Review, 36*(1), 1–7.

Harvey, C., Killaspy, H., Martino, S., & Johnson, S. (2012). Implementation of assertive community treatment in Australia: Model fidelity, patient characteristics and staff experiences. *Community Mental Health Journal, 48*(5), 652–661.

Howgego, I., Yellowlees, P., Owen, C., Meldrum, L., & Dark, F. (2003). The therapeutic alliance: the key to effective patient outcomes? A descriptive review of the evidence in community mental health case management. *Australian and New Zealand Journal of Psychiatry, 37*(2), 169–183.

KAREN-LEIGH EDWARD

Issakidis, C., Sanderson, K., Teesson, M., Johnston, S., & Buhrich, N. (1999). Intensive case management in Australia: A randomized controlled trial. *Acta Psychiatric Scandinavia, 99*(5), 360–367.

Jacobson, N., & Greenley, D. (2001). What is recovery? A conceptual model and explication. *Psychiatric Services, 52*(4), 482–485.

Jeong, J. H., Lee, K. H., & Jon, D. I. (2016). Fifteen-month follow-up of an assertive community treatment program for chronic patients with mental illness. *European Psychiatry, 33,* S480–S481.

Killaspy, H., Johnson, S., Pierce, B., Bebbington, P., Pilling, S., Nolan, F., & King, M. (2009). Successful engagement: A mixed methods study of the approaches of assertive community treatment and community mental health teams in the REACT trial. *Social Psychiatry and Psychiatric Epidemiology, 44*(7), 532–540.

Lewis, M. (2003). *The people's health: Public health in Australia, 1950 to the present.* Oxford: Greenwood Press.

Linehan, M. (1993). Cognitive behavioral treatment of borderline personality disorder. Guilford Press, NY, USA.

Liu, J., Ma, H., He, Y. L., Xie, B., Xu, Y. F., Tang, H. Y., Yu, X. (2011). Mental health system in China: history, recent service reform and future challenges. World Psychiatry, 10(3), 210–216.

Marshall, M., & Lockwood, A. (2011). Assertive community treatment for people with severe mental disorders. *The Cochrane Library.*

McCashan, D. (2005). *The strengths approach.* Bendigo: St Luke's Innovative Resources.

Morgan, V. A., Waterreus, A., Jablensky, A., Mackinnon, A., McGrath, J. J., Carr, V., … & Galletly, C. (2012). People living with psychotic illness in 2010: the second Australian national survey of psychosis. *Australian and New Zealand Journal of Psychiatry, 46*(8), 735–752.

Mueser, K. T., Bond, G. R., Drake, R. E., & Resnick, S. G. (1998). Models of community care for severe mental illness: A review of research on case management. *Schizophrenia Bulletin, 24*(1), 37–74.

Rapp, C. A., & Goscha, R. J. (2004). The principles of effective case management of mental health services. *Psychiatric Rehabilitation Journal, 27*(4), 319–333.

Rapp, C. A., & Goscha, R. J. (2011). The strengths model: a recovery-oriented approach to mental health services. Oxford University Press, NY.

Rosen, A., Meuser, K., & Teesson, M. (2007). Assertive community treatment: Issues from scientific and clinical literature with implications for practice. *Journal of Rehabilitation, Research and Development, 44*(6), 1–13.

Sells, D., Davidson, L., Jewell, C., Falzer, P., & Rowe, M. (2006). The treatment relationship in peer-based and regular case management for clients with severe mental illness. *Psychiatric Services, 57*(8), 1179–1184.

Victorian Government (2004). *Treatment plans under the Mental Health Act.* Melbourne: Department of Health.

Willis, E., Reynolds. L., & Keleher, H. (2008). *Australian health care.* Churchill Livingstone.

Wong, D. F., Rosenburg, G., & Wessman, A. (2006). *Clinical case management for people with mental illness: A biopsychosocial vulnerablity stress model.* Pennsylvania: Haworth Press.

Wong, D., Yeung, M., & Ching, C. (2009). Evaluating a case management model for people with severe mental illness in Hong Kong: A preliminary study. *Hong Kong Journal of Psychiatry, 19,* 11–17.

Ziguras, S., & Stuart, G. (2000). A meta-analysis of the effectiveness of mental health case management over 20 years. *Psychiatric Services, 51*(11), 1410–1421.

CHAPTER 20

Prevention and Management of Aggression

GERALD A. FARRELL

Acknowledgment

The author would like to acknowledge the contribution of Rod Mann who co-wrote this chapter in the second edition.

KEY OUTCOMES

AFTER READING THIS CHAPTER, YOU SHOULD BE ABLE TO:

- appreciate the factors that lead to consumers' aggression, including the influence of the environment
- understand the concepts of advanced statements and safety plans
- appreciate the importance of skilled communication training for staff
- understand best practice principles in risk assessment
- consider the influence of culture in managing aggression
- highlight the importance of health-care organisations having a culture of safety in helping to establish effective reporting of incidents.

KEY TERMS

- aggression
- assault
- culture
- staff training
- risk assessment
- violence

Introduction

In this chapter you will explore the concept of aggression, including violence and assault. You will learn that these are contestable terms and are not easily defined because of their subjectivity. While definitions remain elusive, our understanding of the causes and steps to manage the problem are advancing, including the critical role that staff play in the prevention and management of aggression. Aggression should not be seen simply as arising from 'within' the consumer; rather, we need to understand the contributions of the environment in triggering and maintaining it, which includes mental health nurses and other clinical staff. A large section is devoted to staff training, and the need for staff to act in a partnership arrangement with their consumers. A final section looks at how we can best manage risks associated with consumers who are deemed to be aggressive. Risk management is now firmly embedded in occupational health and safety legislation.

The concept of aggression

Aggression at work is a serious worldwide problem: 'Crossing borders, cultures, work settings and occupational groups, violence in the health-care workplace is an epidemic in all societies, including the developing world' (World Health Organization, 2002, p. 1). In nursing, aggression from consumers or their relatives remains a major concern. Traditionally, mental health settings, along with aged care and emergency departments, have been designated hot spots for consumer aggression; however, staff in all health-care settings are vulnerable to threats of violence and assault (Farrell & Shafiei, 2012). To put the extent of the problem in context in Australia, from 1 July 2001 to 30 June 2002, 42,338 incidents related to consumer safety were reported to the Australian Client Safety Foundation. Of these, 3621 (9 per cent) involved physical violence or abuse and threats by consumers, with staff injury reported in 5 per cent of cases. The proportion of incidents was higher in emergency departments and higher still in mental health settings (Benveniste, Hibbert & Runciman, 2005).

At the level of individual staff, Australian survey research indicates that across health-care settings about one-third of nurses experience verbal and/or physical aggression, with nearly half indicating three or more instances over their last four working weeks. Consumers and their visitors were mainly responsible for the aggression. For staff who had reported being aggressed against, verbal abuse, physical abuse and threat of harm were experienced by 90 per cent, 45 per cent and 27 per cent, respectively (Farrell, Shafiei & Chen, 2012). In the mental health context, aggression is a common experience of many nurses, although much of it is described as non-threatening (Maguire & Ryan, 2007). It should be noted that comparing findings between studies is highly problematic due to difference in definitions of aggression used and study design. Also, relying on official statistics is problematic as aggressive incidents are underreported by staff.

While health service staff, and particularly nurses, are the main targets of consumer 'aggression', other consumers can be victims, too. For example, some years ago an entire ward was closed after an elderly consumer died following an attack from another consumer (Benveniste, et al. 2005). A more recent event, with tragic outcomes, was reported in *The Age* newspaper in December 2012, where an inpatient in a forensic mental health facility was allegedly strangled by another consumer (Cook & Silvester, 2012).

Despite physical injury to health-care staff being low, most staff involved in aggressive incidents report feeling angry and emotionally upset, and complain about feeling unsafe at work (Needham et al., 2005; Rose & Cleary, 2007). There are also consequences for service providers due to staff going off sick (O'Connell et al., 2000), leaving their job or permanently leaving the nursing field (Farrell, Bobrowski & Bobrowski, 2006).

Definition of aggression

Despite the surge in articles and reports on the subject, we are still a long way off agreeing on a definition of aggression or violence. It is a contestable term. While most people might agree that a person wielding a shotgun and threatening to shoot people is behaving aggressively, the vast majority of incidents at work are not so overtly obvious.

BOX 20.1 AGGRESSION, VIOLENCE AND ASSAULT

Aggression, violence and assault are largely subjective notions and thus open to interpretation. For instance, at what point does assertive behaviour or 'letting off steam' cross over into aggression? Is the confused elderly consumer behaving aggressively when she lashes out, or is she simply trying to protect herself? If I knock someone over without intending to hurt them, is that an accident or an act of 'violence'? When does a 'pat' become an assault? Further, where a person agrees to participate in an activity, and then remains silent throughout the activity, is that 'passive aggression' or simply a rebellious act?

The concern around finding an acceptable definition of aggression is not to be taken lightly. Where organisations use different definitions of aggression, it is impossible for researchers to reach a consensus on the nature and extent of the problem. It is also impossible to meaningfully compare findings from different studies. Consumers can suffer, too. What might be tolerable consumer behaviour in one setting may be penalised in a different one. Even where 'acceptable' behaviour is spelled out for consumers, they may not be able to fully appreciate the gravity of their actions, especially when they are unwell. But it is not just consumers who may be confused—staff may be, too. Where staff are uncertain as to what is acceptable consumer behaviour, their interventions to prevent and manage 'aggression' can be compromised or, alternatively, they may manage consumers' aggression and other challenging behaviours in a more restrictive fashion than is necessary.

While it may be fanciful to arrive at a definition applicable in all situations and acceptable to everyone, we should strive for consistency in how we use terms, at least within jurisdictions. In this chapter, the Victorian Government's definition of occupational violence is used (Department of Human Services, 2007, p. 10), which has been adopted across that state's public health settings, and provides a comprehensive, although not watertight, definition. It states:

> Occupational violence is defined as:
>
> Any incident where an employee is abused, threatened or assaulted in the circumstances arising out of, or in the course of their employment (Adapted from WorkSafe guidance note, 2003).
>
> With this definition of occupational violence:
>
> - 'threat' means a statement or behaviour that causes a person to believe that they are in danger of being physically attacked, and may involve an actual or implied threat to safety, health or wellbeing.
> - 'physical attack' means a direct or indirect application of force by a person to the body of, or clothing or equipment worn by, another person, where the application creates a risk to health and safety.
> - Neither intent nor ability to carry out the treatment is relevant, the key issue is that the behaviour creates a risk to health and safety.
> - Examples of occupational violence include, but are not limited to, verbal, physical or psychological abuse, threats, throwing objects, sexual harassment.

The definition is broad enough to encompass aspects of behaviour such as bullying and harassment.

CRITICAL THINKING OPPORTUNITY

1 What do you see as both the positives and negatives in the definition of occupational violence?

2 Can you suggest how it might be improved?

3 Do you think a definition can cover all aspects of aggression?

Causes of consumer aggression

Much has been written on the causes of consumer aggression. Some relate it to properties originating from 'inside' the person, such as the commonly held view that men are more likely to be perpetrators of violence (Turnbull, 1999, p. 25). Other examples of 'inside' causes include consumers with delusional paranoia (Whittington & Richter, 2006) or severe psychopathology (Nijman, 2002), and especially those with substance abuse disorders (Stuart, 2003). Many causes of verbal abuse towards health-care staff are related to drug or alcohol intoxication (Wondrak, 1999).

Other causes of consumer aggression highlight 'outside' influences, such as the quality of staff–consumer relationships, ward regime and consumers' access to privacy (Daffern, Mayer & Martin, 2004). Whittington and Richter (2006, p. 51) note that the average ward can be a source of unpleasant emotional and/or physiological arousal for consumers. Other consumers and staff may either intentionally engage in ways that are upsetting for some consumers, such as through unsolicited touch, invasion of personal space, use of gestures and tone of voice. More generally, adverse staff working conditions (Camerino et al., 2008) and even poorly illuminated interior environments (Gerberich et al., 2005) have been cited as associated with increased risk of assault towards staff.

A third focus is 'interactional'; that is, where aggression is seen as a product of 'inside' and 'outside' factors. This emphasises the role of environmental factors in both triggering and maintaining consumer aggression. For instance, Henderson (2011) notes that consumers in a manic state can be easily angered and become aggressive if limits are set on their behaviour. Sometimes the interplay between 'inside' and 'outside' factors and consumer aggression is not immediately obvious. Interestingly, when staff were asked to account for consumer aggression, they cited consumer-related 'inside' causes, whereas consumers thought that situational or 'outside' factors triggered incidents (Duxbury, 2002). The contribution of 'inside' and 'outside' factors and their interaction is examined in more detail when we look at staff training later in the chapter.

Thus, it is rarely sensible to take at face value a consumer's aggression as a product of herself or her mental illness without carrying out a careful examination of root causes, which should include both 'inside' and 'outside' factors and their interactional effects. The fact that someone has a mental illness diagnosis does not mean that they will be 'aggressive'. Indeed, people with mental health problems are more likely to be victims of aggression (Stuart, 2003). We need to move away from the general public's exaggerated view that associates mental illness, aggression and their personal risk (Stuart, 2003).

That said, of course it is sensible to be cautious (and at the same time be warm and friendly) where you have little information about past behaviour, or the best 'approach' of engagement, especially when meeting consumers for the first time. On admission, consumers can be highly aroused and fearful; their mental disorder is often at its most severe (Whittington & Richter, 2006, p. 50); and they may resent the fact that they are there in the first place, seeing their admission as a violation of their liberty. They may also have substance abuse problems, which, as noted above, are major determinants for aggression.

Strategies for the prevention and management of aggression

Health-care employers have a responsibility to ensure staff, consumers and others are protected against aggression, and that occupational health and safety risks are effectively managed (*Prevention and Management of Aggression in Health Services*, 2009). There is a plethora of policies and directives available at state and national levels, both here and overseas, on the prevention and management of aggression. While many of these directives provide detailed information, it is left up to individual settings to decide what is best for their organisation and situation. Most address three main strategies, which we have termed 'active', 'passive' and 'administrative'.

Active strategies

One major 'active' strategy is staff training. Many organisations emphasise the need for a stepped approach to training; that is, fitting training to staff needs. In this way, front-line staff get more intensive hands-on training than, say, office staff. An example of the different training foci suggested for different levels of staff is provided in Table 20.1. Level 1 training is focused mainly on awareness raising around what is to count as aggression, and the policies and reporting mechanisms in place in the organisation. Level 2 training includes additional information on the identification of triggers of aggression, how to recognise signs of escalating aggression, awareness of environmental hazards and negotiation skills to try to defuse incidents. Level 3 training is designed for staff who are in close contact with consumers and addresses such issues as self-defence and use of restraints. Level 4, the most comprehensive training, is reserved for managers and includes levels 1–3 as well as how to organise an incident management team response, how to provide support for staff involved in incidents and how to conduct a post incident investigation.

Mental health services, particularly those with inpatient units, have for a long time focused considerable effort and attention on aggression management and prevention training programs for staff. These programs range from tiered approaches (as described above) offered in online training formats to multi-day intensive courses, including train-the-trainer programs. Such programs typically focus on medico-legal aspects of aggression management, underlying reasons for aggression, strategies to prevent and minimise violence, restraint techniques and personal safety techniques, such as breakaway manoeuvres.

TABLE 20.1　EXAMPLE OF A TIERED TRAINING MODEL

Content	Level 1 (for all new staff)	Level 2 (for non-clinical staff)	Level 3 (for clinicians)	Level 4 (for managers)
OHS policy framework—responsibilities of employees and employers, consumer and staff rights and responsibilities	+	+	+	+
Reporting mechanisms	+	+	+	+
Definition of consumer-initiated aggression and violence, and emergency codes	+	+	+	+
Identification of triggers to aggression and violence		+	+	+
Recognition of signs of escalating aggression		+	+	+
Awareness of environmental hazards and exit points		+	+	+
Negotiation skills		+	+	+
Self-defence			+	+
Use of restraints—awareness of their risks			+	+
Incident management and team response				+
Support for staff following incidents				+
Post-incident investigation				+

Adapted from *Prevention and Management of Aggression in Health Services* (2009)

GERALD A. FARRELL

Content varies across programs and is dependent to a large extent on the training provider and their background experience. For example, some programs will include restraint techniques, while others will not. Some are designed and delivered by mental health clinical staff, while others are contracted out to training organisations, whose trainers may have a police or security background.

Passive strategies

A major focus of the 'passive' strategy is the work setting. The environment in which consumers are cared for includes the physical surroundings, which requires an understanding of the principles of safe design for work (*Prevention and Management of Aggression in Health Services*, 2009). Areas of interest here include building security, including access and egress; space and privacy for consumers; fixtures and fittings; lighting; noise; colour (of buildings and staff uniforms); duress alarms; car park safety; and signage. Communication by way of signage can range from assistance with way-finding—minimising frustration in being able to locate services—to information in the form of posters about the role of health-care staff and expected behaviours while visiting friends or relatives, or when receiving health-care services.

Administrative strategies

Administrative strategies focus on policies, procedures and practices, and are mainly concerned with the provision of a safe and healthy workplace—where workers are not subjected to aggression, and where there is a commitment to workers who are exposed to, or have witnessed, aggression. They also focus on risk control, which may include any or all of the following:

- file flagging and care planning for consumers who are or are thought to be likely 'aggressors'
- restriction of visiting rights
- alternative treatment arrangements
- limit-setting
- contracts of acceptable behaviour
- conditional treatment agreements
- use of restraints
- refusal of service.

A recent study highlights the importance of paying attention to 'passive' and 'administrative' factors in reducing consumer aggression. Farrell, Shafiei and Chen (2012) found that most protection for staff from consumer aggression was afforded in settings when there was sufficient staff to provide safe care; when managers effectively enforced policies/sanctions; where personal protective equipment, such as mobile phones and personal duress alarms, were provided to staff; and where consumer facilities were of a high order.

Despite the emergence of numerous policies and guidelines around the control of consumer 'aggression', its management remains problematic. A major impediment to its successful regulation is that our responses to aggression have been limited and, in many respects, counterproductive. They are limited in that aggression is principally seen as a product of the consumer, while ignoring the contributions of the environment in triggering and maintaining it, which includes mental health nurses themselves. Thus such policies and guidelines decontextualise and oversimplify the problem of consumer aggression. They are counterproductive in that they limit therapeutic avenues for its prevention and management.

In the next section, we concentrate on staff training, as this is an area in which many organisations expend considerable resources. Staff training is time-consuming and expensive, and guidelines are now readily available regarding program content (see, for example, *Prevention and Management of Aggression in Health Services,* 2009). However, there is little in the way of decent advice on teaching methods, how long programs should last for or how often staff should attend refresher courses. Also, the advice on program evaluation appears weak. More worryingly, the evidence for the effectiveness of training programs is patchy (Farrell, Shafiei & Chen, 2012; Nachreiner et al., 2005). Few programs have been the subject of robust evaluation (Farrell & Cubit, 2005), and those that have suggest that they do not help reduce the frequency of assaults on staff (Richter, Needham & Kunz, 2006).

Staff training

A comprehensive training program to prevent, reduce and manage aggression in mental health settings requires, first and foremost, a change in attitude among some service providers. We need to move away from a 'zero tolerance' approach to its management, which sees the problem as originating mainly from within the consumer and presses consumers to be responsible for their actions. We also need to reassess the value of how we assert that aggression against nurses is unacceptable; that is, it is not to be tolerated (Australian Nursing Federation, 2010; Department of Health, 1999) and must be stamped out (Cameron, 2011).

Granted, some people may be 'naturally' aggressive; however, there are dangers in thinking about people in general terms, such as 'aggressive'. Labels are 'sticky' and can blind us to an individual's positive attributes, as well as distract us from looking for other causes for a person's anger; for example, how we, as nurses, are behaving towards them. So berating consumers to 'behave' neglects the consideration of factors 'outside' the individual. It should be remembered that aggression rarely occurs in a vacuum and consideration of factors both 'inside' and 'outside' the individual, and their interaction, is necessary (Farrell & Gray, 1992, p. 40).

Further, we argue that therapeutic management of consumer aggression in mental health settings is part of the job of a nurse. It comes with the territory. If mental health nurses believe that they should not have to put up with consumers' aggression—that it is an unacceptable aspect of their work—then they are likely to miss important opportunities for therapeutic engagement with these consumers. Indeed, some experienced nurses do abdicate any responsibility for dealing with incidents and instead call in non-clinical staff or hospital security personnel whenever an 'issue' arises. This can lead to strident managerial and coercive approaches, which are unlikely to serve the consumer's best interests.

We are advocating for nurses to take the lead in recognising the inevitability that consumers (and their relatives) will, from time to time, get worried, upset or angry, or misinterpret circumstances around them. Accepting this reality is not to say that we should stop trying to prevent or minimise the occurrence of consumer aggression, or to discourage reporting of incidents. However, by being open to what might be producing and maintaining a consumer's aggression, including our own behaviour and organisational 'irritants', we will be in a better position to reduce it, now and in the future.

CRITICAL THINKING OPPORTUNITY

1 If you accept that aggression and other challenging behaviours by consumers or their relatives are an inevitable aspect of mental health care, why then do you think that some mental health nurses may not see the management of aggression from consumers as a legitimate and an important aspect of their work?

2 What are some likely long-term consequences if nurses do not take the lead in aggression management training and research?

GERALD A. FARRELL

Developing a training program: the SOS model

The solution to understanding and reducing consumer aggression is through focusing on the consumer's predicament, which includes the environment and care staff behaviour. Farrell, Shafiei and Salmon (2010) use the SOS acronym (Self, Other, Situation) when they discuss a training model for nurses in respect to consumers' 'challenging behaviour', which includes aggression. 'Self' refers to nurses' values—the worth they attach to others, their emotional responses towards others, and their communication skills; 'Other' includes the factors influencing consumers' reactions to illness and care; and 'Situation' denotes the ways that the cultural and physical environment influences staff–consumer interaction. Each of these domains is expanded upon below.

Self

The most obvious way in which staff influences consumer aggression is by perceiving—that is, labelling—consumer behaviour as aggressive. As we touched on above, the same behaviour can be interpreted differently by different people: what one person may see as aggression, another may perceive as assertion. For instance, in the mental health setting, consumers with a diagnosis of borderline personality are often viewed less sympathetically than consumers with depression or schizophrenia (Markham & Trower, 2003).

Other

As we have seen, the association between mental illness and aggression is equivocal; therefore, it may be more helpful to look at 'everyday' factors to explain why an individual is 'aggressive' (Farrell & Gray, 1992, p. 40). These authors note that being admitted to hospital is stressful for most people, which can lower their tolerance and interfere with judgment and perception. This can be exacerbated for people with mental illness, who may be admitted against their will, may be experiencing highly intrusive thoughts, may have experienced past trauma and may be under the influence of alcohol or drugs. It is little wonder, then, that some may get defensive, annoyed, angry and 'aggressive'.

Situation

Dissatisfaction with services (Zampieron et al., 2010), a lack of facilities (Lyneham, 2000) and locked doors (Bowers, 2007) have been associated with increases in consumer 'aggression'. Understaffing, too, can be a factor. Lack of staff can lead to increases in consumer waiting times, which, in turn, can lead to consumer frustration and 'aggression' (Lanza et al., 1994; Nabb, 2000; Royal College of Nursing, 1998).

In the SOS training model, trainees need to be informed—using evidence-based knowledge—about consumer aggression and problems of interactions. They need to understand the factors influencing their own behaviours, including their emotional responses and values. With this understanding, they can begin to apply this knowledge to real-life situations. In this way, trainees can be mindful in responding to situations on the basis of a conscious assessment, rather than unthinkingly. Also, they need to be streetwise enough to respond immediately to protect themselves or others should a consumer's anger turn physical (Farrell & Salmon, 2009).

De-escalation skills and beyond

Today, a major focus of many training programs centres on the attainment of de-escalation skills (that is, diffusing aggressive situations by talking). While perhaps important when incidents begin to arise or aggression occurs—although there is little evidence to back up this view (Richter, et al. 2006)—they do not help staff avoid aggressive encounters occurring.

A certainty of practice is that front-line nurses will often have to interact with consumers around situations that are potentially aversive; for example, getting consumers to do something they would prefer not to do; stopping consumers from doing something they want to continue doing; and/or saying no to consumers' requests (Newbill et al., 2010). Common examples include asking consumers to take medications that they would rather avoid because of their unwanted effects (some undesirable effects of the commonly used major antipsychotic medications include weight gain and sexual dysfunction), asking a consumer to refrain from swearing, and refusing a consumer's request to be discharged immediately.

Newbill and colleagues (2010) suggest that rather than teaching staff de-escalation skills, a better approach is to alert them to how to navigate potentially aversive interactions with consumers. These authors suggest that by becoming aware of or sensitised to these occasions, staff will come to monitor both the consumer's and their own response more carefully, and to act with greater intentionality, thereby helping to avoid agitating consumers to begin with. They go on to suggest that 'validation' of the consumer's emotional response to aversive interactions should occur first, followed by engaging the consumer in adaptive problem-solving skills—skills that are exportable to community living. An example of 'validation' in use for a consumer who is unwilling to take his medication might be: 'I know you are concerned about the medication's unwanted effects. Would you like to discuss what might be done towards minimising their effects?' The nurse could also enquire if there is anything else worrying the consumer.

Farrell and Gray (1992) illustrate a number of ways of coping with consumers' aggression that minimise the threat to carers, using verbal and non-verbal means. They recommend that nurses should:

- *Be supportive and avoid defensiveness*—this requires good listening skills, empathy and an 'open' attitude.
- *Be reassuring in what is said and done*—a warm and friendly approach, coupled with an air of confidence and control, will help the other person feel safe. Try to match the 'aggressor's friendly behaviour and meet the aggressive behaviour not with anger but with concern, gradually bringing the level down to calmness'.
- *Avoid situations where the other person fears 'loss of face' from backing down*—not wanting to look like a loser can turn encounters into fights. Avoid power struggles.
- *Ask themselves what is going on in the immediate environment that might be prolonging the incident*—are the nurse or consumer being stirred up by onlookers?
- *Avoid 'pat' responses*—too much reliance on one or two communication techniques may irritate the 'aggressor'.
- *At all times be respectful and courteous*—do not judge until you have heard the full story. While the customer is not always right, she should not feel that when she complains she is starting off on the wrong foot (Sieff, 1990).

The above suggestions are in line with the tenets of validation. Both Farrell and Gray (1992) and Newbill and colleagues (2010) acknowledge that consumers need to feel understood, and, as Newbill and colleagues (2010) indicate, they should not be left to feel they are at the mercy of an uncaring system. These authors advise that if a particular institutional 'rule' appears to generate conflict, then administrators should review the rule and see if the reason for it is appropriate and if it is being implemented as intended.

In respect to responding to consumers' verbal abuse, Wondrak (1999) outlines five assertiveness techniques that he has adapted from Smith (1975) to teach student nurses how to deal more effectively with verbal abuse (see Box 20.2).

BOX 20.2 ASSERTIVENESS TECHNIQUES FOR VERBAL ABUSE

1   Side-stepping. This is where the nurse responds totally non-defensively or non-aggressively to neutralise the possibility of the situation escalating further. Wondrak gives the example of a consumer who suddenly says, 'Call yourself a nurse? You are b***** useless'. The nurse could reply with, 'Yes, I agree. I have a lot to learn.'

2   Self-disclosure. Rather than being trapped by their professional image, Wondrak suggests that, used sensibly, self-disclosure can help de-escalate a situation; for example, if you admit that you are hurt by what the consumer said or did, or even that you are frightened.

3   Partial agreement. This is similar to side-stepping, where the nurse responds to criticism without arguing with the consumer.

4   Gentle confrontation. Used when the consumer is calmer, it follows from a 'partial agreement'. In the example provided in 'Side-stepping' above, the nurse then might say, 'You seem very upset with me. Is there something I have done, or is there something else that is worrying you?'

5   Being specific. This means deciding what it is you want to say to the consumer, and doing so as clearly as possible. Wondrak cautions that this is a difficult skill to master.

Wondrak (1999)

Staff training and creativity

All communication skills and techniques should be seen for what they are—simply suggestions for how nurses might respond. They cannot prescribe how nurses should respond in a given situation. By its nature, each consumer interaction is a unique event, and negotiating a successful consumer outcome requires imagination in how particular communication skills are deployed (Salmon & Young, 2011). For example, showing empathy and making eye contact may be appropriate in some situations, but in other circumstances these same skills may be interpreted by consumers as intrusive and hostile.

In the context of medical communication skills training, Salmon and Young (2011) note that consumers' demands on practitioners are more complex, context-dependent and inconsistent than can be captured by general principles for deploying communication skills. These authors provide the following example to illustrate this point. Ensuring consumers are informed and involved about their care requires practitioners to exercise considerable ingenuity. In a survey of cancer consumers, 100 per cent of respondents wanted practitioners to be honest, but 91 per cent also wanted them to be optimistic (Kutner et al., 1999). They go on to note that while consumers may want to feel involved in their care and for practitioners not to be paternalistic, some often need practitioners to take responsibility for treatment decisions (Mendick et al., 2010).

Trevor Lowe (1990, in Farrell & Gray, 1992, p. 71) provides a fine example of a creative staff response in a mental health context, when 'police and dogs were brought on to the ward because of the disturbance caused by a consumer. The situation remained extremely tense and frightening until a nurse suggested to the man that if he got into bed, she would see about getting rid of all the people, the dogs and associated pressure and unpleasantness'. Farrell and Gray suggest that the nurse's action offered a compromise that 'saved face' for all concerned. Also, by being in bed, the nurse strengthens her 'control' of the consumer—being in bed is incompatible with aggressiveness, and provides an opportunity for the consumer to 'cool down'.

Gaynor (2009), too, provides insightful comments around the complexities of caring, discussing a consumer with substance intoxication who was admitted to an accident and emergency department. On arrival, the consumer required 'all available resources' to restrain her because of her aggression; nevertheless, Gaynor managed to provide a care environment that was sensitive to the consumer's many clinical and dignity needs, while minimising disruption to the rest of the emergency department.

1 Can you think of examples from your own experience in nursing or elsewhere that involved creative approaches (including what may have been said or done) to help reduce another's anger, aggression or distress?

2 How do you 'feel' when faced with another's anger or distress?

Skilled communication

Skilled communication, whether it is breaking bad news to consumers or responding therapeutically to angry relatives, is both an art and a science; that is, it is how nurses adapt and imaginatively shape their own communication skills and styles to best fit the situation in hand (Salmon & Young, 2011). It is also about feeling comfortable with uncertainty. Sometimes incidents can arise spontaneously, leaving the unprepared practitioner fearful and apprehensive, and having to think on his feet. Consequently, teaching programs need to provide learners with the opportunity to 'experiment' in real situations in the company of effective role models. Learners will also need the opportunity to reflect on their practice, and trainers will need the appropriate expertise to help guide trainees in developing approaches that are evidence-based. In this way learners can continue to hone their 'skills' on their way to becoming effective practitioners. The following insights are apt here:

> In skilful, helpful action, when our awareness remains quiet and clear, there's breadth to our perspective. It's aerial, wide-screen, panoramic and yet able to focus quickly. With all this we are not only thinker-participants but observers of our thinking and participation as well … so the quiet mind makes possible an overall awareness of the total situation, including ourselves.

Dass and Gorman (1985, in Farrell & Gray, 1992, p. 72)

Effective training in clinical communication skills takes time; and one-off, class-based training programs are unlikely to be a helpful vehicle for practitioners to transfer classroom learning to the clinical context (van den Eertwegh et al., 2013). Training in clinical communication skills needs to be integrated into an organisational-wide response that encourages pro-social behaviour. For example, where there are good nurse–consumer relationships, and where staff work in supportive teams, there is a greater potential for protection from aggression (Alexander & Fraser, 2004; Camerino et al., 2008). Without nurturing, learners are likely to flounder in the face of workload pressures, time issues, inappropriate modelling and lack of valuing of such skills (Silverman, 2011).

Consequently, training staff in the prevention and management of consumer aggression requires a careful exploration of a number of interrelated factors, including those that concern the nurse, the consumer, their family and carers, and the health-care environment. Trainees will need time to acquire their understanding of these issues in order to be able to apply that understanding to effect skilled professional care for all consumers—even for those consumers for whom staff may not feel immediate empathy!

GERALD A. FARRELL

Partnering with consumers

Developing 'advanced statements' and 'safety plans' can help both the nurse and the consumer understand what is important for consumers in terms of their preference for ongoing care, including when their mental status deteriorates and when they are at their most vulnerable in terms of their safety needs. Box 20.3 outlines the scope of these plans.

BOX 20.3 ADVANCED CARE PLANNING, ADVANCE STATEMENTS AND SAFETY PLANNING

Advanced care planning is a process whereby a consumer—in consultation with health-care providers, family members and important others—makes decisions about his future health care, should he become incapable of participating in treatment decisions (Mental Health Bill—Austin Health Submission, 2011). Care planning processes or psychiatric advanced directives (PADs) have been developed and introduced in other countries (Srebnik, Applebaum & Russo, 2004; Elbogen et al., 2007). While competent and able to do so, the consumer can articulate and communicate their preferences for ongoing mental health treatment and care if they are no longer able to make decisions for themselves; for example, during a period of acute psychosis. The 2013 review of the *Mental Health Act 1986* (Vic) includes a proposal to enable a person to make an advance statement to record their treatment preferences in the event that they become unwell and require compulsory treatment:

> Advance statements facilitate a collaborative treatment approach at times where a client is so unwell that they are unable to communicate their treatment preferences. They will assist the authorised psychiatrist to understand the client's treatment preferences and enable the authorised psychiatrist to make substitute treatment decisions that better align with the client's wishes. Advance statements will improve communication, give clients greater control over their treatment when

> they are subject to a compulsory treatment order and promote an improved client experience.

Department of Health (2012)

Safety planning also involves a collaborative discussion about specific circumstances that may compromise the person or another person's safety; for example, where there is a risk of self-harm, suicidal impulses, or aggression or violence towards other people. A safety plan is an individualised, proactive intervention plan developed collaboratively between clinical staff and the consumer to help the consumer with their safety needs and preferences for care. According to the National Technical Assistance Centre (2006), a safety plan will help to inform and educate consumers about their safety needs and assist clinical staff in working with consumers to maintain their safety and the safety of others. Such plans can be developed at any point during the episode of care or at any point throughout the continuum of care, such as community-based care. Where possible, a safety plan is developed with consumers during their community episode of care (either with a community case manager, referring clinician or primary nurse) and where an inpatient admission is a possibility. It is during this phase of care that a consumer is more likely to be engaged in the process and can reflect on the circumstances that might lead to their and others' safety being compromised.

At times, developing a safety plan may be difficult to achieve, given the level of collaboration required to develop the plan; however, every effort should be made to discuss with the consumer triggers, warning signs and preferred coping and defusing strategies as soon as the consumer is able to participate. Wherever appropriate, and possible, next of kin and/or carers should be consulted with due regard to confidentiality, privacy and the provisions of mental health and privacy legislation. A safety plan does not replace an overarching care or recovery plan, but rather complements it.

REFLECTION QUESTIONS

1 Why are safety plans sometimes difficult to achieve?

2 When should the nurse think about initiating the development of a safety plan?

More generally, partnering with consumers also implies that we take regular soundings of what consumers see as relevant for their care, and act on them as appropriate. Respect for personal privacy, gender-related preferences for space and interactions, and experience of past trauma may also be factors in managing relationships and interactions. In the context of mental health nursing, men and women appear to have different needs. Women in particular, have voiced significant safety concerns about the inpatient environment. In 2006, the Victorian Women and Mental Health Network (VWMHN) surveyed female consumers and mental health staff about their experience of mixed-sex wards. This showed that nearly 60 per cent of women surveyed identified felt unsafe or very unsafe in the inpatient setting. Feeling unsafe was mainly due to issues related to the behaviours of male consumers, such as verbal and physical aggression, intimidation, and threatened and actual assault, including sexual assault. The issue is compounded by the high numbers of women consumers (50–60 per cent) who are victims of past sexual abuse, including child sexual assault. There is also a need to ensure that the needs of men are met in relation to safety within the inpatient unit. Men can also be vulnerable and at risk of bullying, intimidation, violence and sexual assault (Department of Health, 2011).

Risk management

To be an effective clinician, it is vital to be aware of consumers' health-care needs, which includes an awareness of the aggression risk they might pose to themselves or to others. According to the National Risk Management Programme (2007, p. 57), 'Risk [refers to] the nature, severity, imminence, frequency/ duration and likelihood of harm to self or others. A hazard that is to be identified, measured and ultimately, prevented.' While serious risk of harm to themselves, or to others, by people with a mental illness is small, the situation is rendered much more serious where consumers have a substance abuse problem. Further, despite the small risk, the consequences for consumers and victims can be catastrophic. So it is in everyone's interest that predictions of the likelihood that a consumer might be aggressive are as accurate as possible.

The management of consumer risk is now firmly embedded in occupational health and safety legislation. As well as having a duty to provide safe working conditions for staff, health-care employers are also obliged to provide safe environments for consumers and others in the workplace, which ideally includes an integrated approach to risk management in 'which risks are systematically identified, managed and reduced through building a safe culture; leading and supporting staff; promoting reporting; involving and communicating with service users; learning from and sharing safety lessons; and implementing solutions to prevent harm' (National Client Safety Agency, 2004 p. 1). It is also every clinician's responsibility to assess the likelihood of their consumers becoming a risk to themselves or to others, as well as to report real or likely environmental hazards; for example, poor or ineffective staff car park lighting.

The great majority of health-care settings have detailed policies and procedures in respect to occupational health and safety. For example, the *Prevention and Management of Aggression in Health Services* (2009) provides extensive information around the management of risk for the prevention of consumer aggression, through workplace design, violence hazard identification, support for those involved in incidents, consumer alerts and so forth; it also includes assessment tools and checklists for such areas as high-risk screening, violence hazard identification and risk assessment, aggression risk and behaviour assessment.

Clinical risk assessment for aggression or dangerousness

When conducting a clinical risk assessment of the likelihood of a consumer's future aggression or dangerousness, Scott and Resnick (2006) suggest that clinicians can divide the concept into five components:

1 *The magnitude of potential harm that is threatened*—this includes physical harm to property or others, as well as psychological harm to others.
2 *The likelihood that an aggressive act will take place*—these authors note that a person's past history of acting out on violent thoughts best predicts that an act of aggression will be carried out.
3 *The imminence of harm*—for example, is the person threatening harm in the next few hours?
4 *The frequency of the aggressive act*—the greater the frequency of the aggressive behaviour, the higher is the risk of its recurrence in the period of time.
5 *The situation that the person finds themselves in*—situational factors that increase the likelihood of aggression include association with peers who have a criminal record of offending, lack of financial resources and housing, easy access to weapons, and exposure to alcohol or drugs.

Scott and Resnick (2006) further distinguish between affective and predatory aggression. Affective aggression is when a person reacts to a perceived threat, either from 'inside' factors (such as delusional thoughts) or 'outside' factors (such as provocation from others). On the other hand, predatory aggression is planned, purposeful and goal directed towards a particular target or person. The person has no remorse and is acting independent of situational factors, the goal being to retaliate against others, to gain a sense of control or to obtain a desired outcome or goal.

In assessing the likelihood of a person becoming aggressive, it is vital that all relevant information is collected through both direct and indirect interaction with the person. Importantly, this information should be analysed to formulate a management plan, which must be communicated to all relevant staff through clinical handovers, nursing handovers and the medical record. Ideally, this should be done with the involvement of the consumer, her family and carers, and staff.

In practice, most assessments of consumer risk for aggression, whether in inpatient or community settings, are based on professional judgments, which may have some validity in predicting consumers' short-term aggression potential (Scott & Resnick, 2006); or on criteria or checklists that have not been subject to evaluation as to their usefulness. See Box 20.4 for an example of a clinical assessment framework used in practice.

To help improve the accuracy of prediction, there are now a number of validated risk-assessment tools. For example, the Violence Screening Checklist (VSC; McNeil & Binder, 1994) is thought to provide an efficient assessment of risk for violence on admission, whereas the Broset Violence Checklist (BVC; Almvik, Woods & Rasmussen, 2000) and Dynamic Appraisal of Situational Aggression: Inpatient Version (DASA IV; Ogloff & Daffern, 2003) can provide an efficient and accurate assessment of risk on a day-to-day basis (Ogloff & Daffern, 2006).

These tools address negative 'inside' factors, such as consumers' impulse control, their willingness to follow directions, their sensitivity to perceived provocation or to denial of requests, and whether they have violent thoughts and fantasies, issues with substance use and active positive psychotic symptoms. Factors external to or 'outside' the consumer that have an association with risk of aggression are also examined. They include staff experience and working conditions and their relationships with colleagues and managers (Johnson, 2004). Positive factors are also considered as these can be 'protective' against the development of aggression. Examples include strong supportive structures, stable employment and accommodation, prolonged abstinence from alcohol or drugs, and old age (Allnutt et al., 2010).

BOX 20.4 AN EXTRACT OF A CLINICAL RISK ASSESSMENT TOOL

Overall aggression risk summary	Details/comments
Aggression/harm to others (including sexual violence) Static factors ❏ History of violence ❏ Offending/forensic history ❏ Victimisation ❏ Conduct disorder/antisocial traits Dynamic factors ❏ Impulsivity ❏ Anger ❏ Intoxication/withdrawal ❏ Carries weapon/access to firearm ❏ Recent threats or other aggressive actions/thoughts ❏ Psychotic symptoms	
Interim risk management plan	
Significant past history and issues to be considered in managing longer-term risks: _____ _____ Plan to manage current risks: _____ _____	

Interventions required for inpatient services	Observation levels
• **Imminent** risk requires immediate intervention to ensure safety. This may include the need for **one-to-one nursing care**, PRN medication, use of high support area, medical review. • **High** risk rating for at least risk items 1, 2, 3, 4 and 5 may indicate **constant visual engagement**. • **Moderate** risk ratings for at least risk items 1, 2, 3, 4 and 5 may indicate **close engagement** with frequency of sighting specified between 15- to 60-minute visual observations. • **Low** risk ratings indicate **mealtime/handover** visual observations. NB. In instances where risk ratings are variable, always maintain a higher level of engagement. If for any reason there is variance to these interventions, **document** reasons in the medical record.	• **Level 1** (One-to-one nursing) • **Level 2** (Constant engagement) • **Level 3** (Close engagement) • **Level 4** (Standard engagement)

Austin Health, extract *Clinical Risk Assessment Screen* (2013)

It is beyond the scope of this chapter to detail specific risk-assessment methods and tools or to unpick risk-management plans. The reader is encouraged to view the handbook *Clinical Risk Assessment and Management*, produced for Justice Health, New South Wales (Allnutt et al., 2010), which provides mental health clinicians with practical guidance in relation to the assessment process and how to go about developing a risk-management plan, in both the inpatient and outpatient setting. The handbook *Best Practice in Managing Risk*, produced by the Department of Health, UK (National Risk Management Programme, 2007), also provides a framework to guide mental health professionals working with consumers to assess risk, where sixteen best practice points for effective risk management are discussed (see Box 20.5).

Despite the advances in risk prediction, Scott and Resnick (2006) acknowledge that the prediction of consumer aggression remains an imprecise science, akin to forecasting the weather where it is not possible to state with certainty that a future weather event will occur. However, they go on to say that gathering detailed consumer histories and using appropriate risk-assessment tools will help make risk assessments as accurate as possible.

BOX 20.5 BEST PRACTICE TIPS FOR EFFECTIVE RISK MANAGEMENT

INTRODUCTION

1. Best practice involves making decisions based on knowledge of the research evidence, knowledge of the individual service user and their social context, knowledge of the service user's own experience, and clinical judgment.

FUNDAMENTALS

2. Positive risk management as part of a carefully constructed plan is a required competence for all mental health practitioners.

3. Risk management should be conducted in a spirit of collaboration and based on a relationship between the service user and their carers that is as trusting as possible.

4. Risk management must be built on recognition of the service user's strengths and should emphasise recovery.

5. Risk management requires an organisational strategy as well as efforts by the individual practitioner.

BASIC IDEAS IN RISK MANAGEMENT

6. Risk management involves developing flexible strategies aimed at preventing any negative event from occurring or, if this is not possible, minimising the harm caused.

7. Risk management should take into account that risk can be both general and specific, and that good management can reduce and prevent harm.

8. Knowledge and understanding of mental health legislation is an important component of risk management.

9. The risk management plan should include a summary of all risks identified, formulations of the situations in which identified risks may occur, and actions to be taken by practitioners and the service user in response to crisis.

10. Where suitable tools are available, risk management should be based on assessment using the structured clinical judgment approach.

11. Risk assessment is integral to deciding on the most appropriate level of risk management and the right kind of intervention for a service user.

WORKING
WITH SERVICE
USERS
AND CARERS

12   All staff involved in risk management must be capable of demonstrating sensitivity and competence in relation to diversity in race, faith, age, gender, disability and sexual orientation.

13   Risk management must always be based on awareness of the capacity for the service user's risk level to change over time, and a recognition that each service user requires a consistent and individualised approach.

INDIVIDUAL
PRACTICE
AND TEAM
WORKING

14   Risk management plans should be developed by multidisciplinary and multi-agency teams operating in an open, democratic and transparent culture that embraces reflective practice.

15   All staff involved in risk management should receive relevant training, which should be updated at least every three years.

16   A risk management plan is only as good as the time and effort put into communicating its findings to others.

National Risk Management Programme (2007)

Further, as noted above, aggressive behaviour is not an objective phenomenon. Therefore, risk assessment must be made in consideration of consumers' total situations, and must be made on a regular basis, using validated risk-assessment methods; otherwise, we may unnecessarily attach a pejorative and potentially lifelong 'dangerousness' label to consumers, which can have disastrous consequences for them and for their care. Alternatively, we may fail to acknowledge the seriousness of consumers' propensity for aggression, which can have catastrophic outcomes for consumers themselves and their victims, including health-care staff.

CRITICAL THINKING OPPORTUNITY

1   What are some of the potential positive and negative consequences for the consumer labelled as 'dangerous'?

2   Why do you think staff sometimes do not take seriously a consumer's risk for aggression?

3   Conversely, why do you think some staff might overreact when a consumer is considered 'risky' or 'dangerous'?

Cultural considerations

As readers will no doubt appreciate, the concept of mental illness invites a certain degree of ambiguity and uncertainty. This situation is compounded by the diversity of Australia's culture. About one-fifth of the population was born overseas. More than 200 languages, including Indigenous Australian languages, are spoken in Australia, and about two million of the population (about 14 per cent) aged five years and over speak a language other than English at home. Over 60 per cent of Australians have at least two different ethnic origins, and 20 per cent have four or more. Around 2 per cent of the population is Aboriginal or Torres Strait Islander (Department of Immigration and Citizenship, n.d.). Therefore, there is the potential for bias, with clinicians making unfounded assumptions in estimating risk because of cultural and language barriers. To help clinicians overcome communication challenges to help make their assessment as accurate as possible, they should utilise transcultural mental health services when conducting risk assessments (Allnutt et al., 2010).

Reporting incidents of aggression

It is important that incidents of aggression are reported; otherwise, organisations will be in the dark as to the extent of the problem, and their management of risk compromised. In addition, staff and consumers may be left without recourse to appropriate support when incidents arise, learning opportunities will be lost, and it will be impossible to know if interventions to reduce the problem are working.

Incident reports need to be accurate, and relevant to the task in hand. If we want only a count of incidents, say, by type—verbal and physical—then a simple reporting method can be used. If more detail is required—for example, a description of possible antecedents to the incident—then a more nuanced report is needed. However, the reality is that staff do not always report incidents (Kowalenko et al., 2013). Nurses, it seems, weigh the benefits and risks of reporting incidents. Where staff perceive negative consequences of reporting, this negates their obligation to report (Gifford & Anderson, 2010). These authors found that cultural influences that discourage reporting were found to operate at all levels of the organisation they studied. Of particular importance were lack of follow-up after incidents, the cultural normalisation of assaults and the fear of blame.

Other factors that impacted on reporting were:

- *team relationships*—for example, when a staff member has done something wrong, peer pressure and/ or support can encourage or discourage reporting
- *consumer factors*—whether or not staff liked a consumer can influence both reporting and non-reporting
- *staffing*—for example, incidents occurring on a weekend when there are fewer and less experienced staff around can result in fewer reports, although reporting was likely to increase when staff thought it might potentially result in more appropriate staffing
- *the reporting process itself*—including the accessibility and ease of use of the reporting process.

Even when incidents are reported, there is the potential for partiality. In Gifford and Anderson's (2010) study, staff thought that the responsibility for incidents lay with consumer. Nurses weighted the pros and cons of reporting on their assessments as to the degree of culpability of consumers for incidents; that is, the extent to which they thought consumers were able to control their behaviour. There was little consideration of the contextual factors that result in incidents, with little or no reflection on how their own behaviour may have prompted or maintained the incident. Yet, it is through gaining an understanding of the surrounding landscape of triggers and mediators that is crucial for staff in learning how to reduce and manage incidents.

BOX 20.6 BIAS IN REPORTING

We should never lose sight of the fact that even in the best-run health-care organisations—where all incidents, however defined, are reported—bias in staff's observational reports is likely. As we have seen, incidents of aggression are difficult to define and influenced by numerous factors, including observers' judgments, which can be affected by their subconscious opinions and attitudes. What do you understand by the saying: I never have any difficulty finding evidence to back up my pet prejudices?

Nevertheless, health-care organisations have to press ahead with addressing these issues. All health-care organisations have to identify barriers to reporting and develop policies and procedures to assist staff report incidents. Gifford and Anderson (2010) highlight the crucial role of health-care organisations having a culture of safety in establishing effective reporting procedures. It is vital that organisational system factors as well as individual factors are included in this endeavour. Reporting is more likely where there are clear reporting policies; well designed and easy accessible reporting systems; protected time for staff to complete their reports; and where incidents are seen as opportunities for deep learning. For deep learning to occur, staff will need encouragement to provide an introspective account. They will need to think critically and creatively to develop a wide perspective on incidents and their management. This process can be a particularly sensitive issue for staff to navigate, so organisations need to pay particular attention to their reporting processes and how incident follow-up is managed. When sympathetically managed, review of incidents can offer another dynamic insight for staff (and consumers) to learn how best to help prevent and manage aggressive incidents.

Care planning

The following is an example of a clinical incident between a male consumer and a male nurse, and a care plan that was subsequently devised. The example is taken from a real-life incident. The consumer, Hamish (not his real name), was admitted to an acute care inpatient unit, following deterioration in his mental state. He had had two previous admissions to the unit in the past year. He was admitted as a voluntary consumer, following an assessment by the crisis team in his home, where he lives with his ageing parents. Hamish is 36 years old and has a history of psychotic episodes associated with amphetamine use. On admission, he was assessed as being a low risk for aggression. After three days in the unit, an incident occurred, as recorded in the following report.

Case notes entries

Date: [Today's date]
Consumer's name: Hamish Edwards Case Manager: T Walsh

Incident report:

In the morning Hamish seemed happy and responded appropriately to staff interactions. By mid-afternoon, however, he appeared to be distracted and refused to participate in ward activities. At about 4 pm, he said angrily, 'I have a mental problem,' and said he was 'depressed'.

He turned to me and said I was a 'nut case as well'. He then began to chest bump me. And without warning, he punched me in the chest. He said he wanted to provoke me to hit him in return, so that, in his words, 'I can go crazy'.

Hamish was then approached by another staff member, who offered him PRN medication (Olanzapine, 10 mg). By this time he was pacing, shouting and generally intimidating in his behaviour towards myself and other consumer and staff. After many attempts to give him the opportunity to take the medication orally, he became quite forceful and said to the staff member: 'Go on, give me an injection.'

He was intrusive of personal space and when the staff member attempted to open the double doors leading to the medication room, Hamish pushed his way through the doors (it seems he thought he could get out of the unit this way).

Eventually, after negotiation, he agreed to walk back into the lounge area. I immediately phoned the psychiatric registrar to apprise him of the situation with Hamish, and to request an intramuscular order of medication, which was obtained (IMI Olanzapine 10 mg @ 2255 hrs).

Hamish escalated (sic). He became physically aggressive again by punching a staff member in the arm. He was physically restrained and taken to his bed in his own bedroom and given IMI 10 Olanzapine at 2300 hrs. The physical restraint was released and he was reassured that he could remain in his room until the medication had effect and that staff would support him.

Within 10 minutes, he again became physically aggressive towards staff during a check on his progress. He was then escorted towards seclusion room 1. While in the seclusion area another consumer came in and started swinging punches and kicking at staff. A Code Grey was called and security staff arrived within 10 minutes. Despite the interaction, the second consumer was not secluded, as she quickly settled. Staff were able to discuss with her issues about acceptable behaviour and how, on discussion, it seemed her psychotic symptoms and her misinterpretation of events led to her outburst. She returned to her room.

Date: [Today's date]
Consumer's name: Hamish Edwards Case Manager: T Walsh

Hamish's seclusion lasted 30 minutes, following which he said he was willing to return to his room. In all other respects he was cooperative with staff. Shortly after, within 10 minutes, I received a phone call from staff in the next door unit indicating that one of their consumers had reported she had heard glass breaking and thought someone was breaking into their unit. Together with other staff members we did a search, including checking the courtyard. There was no obvious sign of damage viewing from the courtyard. However, due to the location of the consumer's bedroom the damage was not visible as it was behind a dividing wall.

Upon opening of the bedroom door the damage was extensive. The large and very heavy ensuite bathroom door had been removed from its hinges and used, along with a chair, to break the window and gain access to the walkway behind the courtyard. Staff noticed that the gate behind the large wall was opened and not locked, with the chain/padlock hanging off one side of the gate. Immediately I notified campus security—and a further Code Grey was called.

Phone call received from the site manager @ 0015 hrs offering support and organising for hospital maintenance to secure the broken window until it could be replaced. Security conducted a search behind the unit. The consumer had probably obtained access by using wall furniture to get up and over the fence. There was no sighting of the consumer on the hospital grounds.

I notified police/000 @ 0030 hrs, due to concerns for the consumer's safety and members of the public, as it was unknown if he had taken broken glass as a potential weapon, along with his unpredictable mental state. Police reported that they would conduct a search. Hamish's next of kin (father) was contacted and notified of the incident. He was asked to contact police and the ward if Hamish returned to the family home.

A phone call was made to the on-call nurse unit manager (NUM) to inform him of incident and photos sent to his mobile phone of the damage to the bedroom. NUM phoned back and informed staff that he had notified consultant psychiatrist at 0045 hrs.

Phone call from Police Communications @ 0110 hrs that the consumer had been located and was in the process of being transported back to the unit. I updated the on-call NUM of the incident/progress. The on call consultant psychiatrist was also notified of the incident.

Hamish was returned to the unit with police x 4 and transferred into the High Needs Area for his own personal safety/safety of others/potential for absconding/OHS. His own room still needed to be fixed. The patient was reviewed by the on-call psychiatric registrar and given PRN Olanzapine 10 mg @ 0205 hrs, while police remained present due to his reluctance to have the mediation and his level of agitation. Complied, although reluctantly.

Hamish was recommended as an Involuntary Consumer under the MHA and to be reviewed by the consultant psychiatrist in the morning. His father was notified of his return and reassurance provided. A carer consultant is to follow up with family.

The care plan below developed for Hamish concentrates on what the nurses might do to assist Hamish better manage his own anger and aggression and to minimise risks to themselves and others.

Note: The above care plan is a very truncated account and is for illustration only. The reality is that implementing aggression management programs (AMPs) for consumers is complex. Consumers may at first deny there is a problem and refuse to cooperate with staff. They may feel embarrassed to admit they have a problem, or they may be too ill to recognise the gravity of their situation. Therefore, patience and a careful assessment of the consumer's insight and readiness to participate are called for, as are good 'diplomatic skills'. Even where consumers are motivated to participate in a treatment program, treatment goals are unlikely to follow a linear process. Expect setbacks, especially where the consumer's problem behaviours s are long-standing or where their mental state fluctuates. Further, most AMPs for consumers occur mainly in inpatient settings and it is not clear how well skills and techniques learnt in the hospital environment carry over into the community setting. Staff involved in AMPs need to be specially trained to carry them out, and we are still some way off in determining the evidence-base for such programs.

Nevertheless, AMPs are a major step forward in assisting nurses' practice professionally and in a spirit of consumer collaboration to proactively intervene to prevent/reduce consumers' aggressiveness. For consumers involved in AMPs, there is the promise that their aggression and other challenging behaviours can be managed through non-restrictive means.

Care Plan

Areas of daily living	Assessment of current situation	Goal	Plan (undertaken with consumer)	Implementation	Who is responsible (including only those who have been consulted in the planning process)	Evaluation/ review date
Safety needs	Hamish is angry at having to stay in hospital. At times he is intimidating and threatening.	Immediate goal: Provide a safe and supportive environment for Hamish and minimise the risk of harm to himself or to others.	Hamish is helped to recognise the triggers for his anger/aggressive behaviour and resultant threats to his/others' personal safety. Hamish is assisted to communicate proactively how he feels in a constructive way.	Conduct a consumer risk assessment. This should be done in a spirit of collaboration with Hamish. Reduce stimulation and interactions that lead to arousal. Increase use of quieter areas and distraction techniques.	His 'key' nurse (with Hamish)	Ongoing
		Intermediate goal: Develop a treatment program to assist Hamish manage his aggression.	Compile a comprehensive list of early warning signs for Hamish's aggression, including precursors for aggression. Develop a Safety Plan as soon as Hamish can reasonably discuss.	Determine how best to detect early recognition of impending aggression and its precursors, prior to developing realistic strategies to diffuse them. Use a diary/ workbook to record progress.	Hamish and his 'key' nurse	Weekly chart review
		Long-term/ optimal goal: Consumer implements strategies to cope with aggression on his own; that is, without the assistance of nursing staff.	Hamish is taught to monitor his environment together with how he is thinking, feeling and behaving; and how to respond to lessen the risk for aggression.	Refine the aggression management plan, *prior* to Hamish taking responsibility for the plan's implementation.	Hamish and his 'key' nurse	Monthly follow-up with nurse

Incidents such as the one above are not unusual in inpatient units, but it should be noted that no serious injury to staff or others eventuated.

1   Why do you think Hamish behaved as he did?

2   What were the 'inside' factors at play? Were there 'outside' factors contributing to the incident?

3   Would a pre-existing safety plan have assisted nursing staff in managing Hamish's care?

4   What might Hamish be thinking and feeling about the situation he finds himself in? How might staff feel?

5   Can you think of other strategies that could be adopted to minimise aggressive behaviour? Would the SOS model be of assistance in a training program to manage this type of incident?

6   Does the care plan adequately address Hamish's aggressive tendencies? How could it be improved? Compare your ideas with those of your colleagues.

SUMMARY

Aggression is unfortunately a fact of life in health care, and mental health settings remain high on the 'at risk' list. However, it would be wrong to equate aggression solely with mental illness, despite the media hype and consequent irrational public concern around the association of mental illness, aggression and personal risk. Interestingly, research and practical experience inform us that the concept of consumer aggression is not straightforward—different staff can see and respond to the same behaviour differently. The cause of consumer aggression is not always obvious either. It frequently occurs due to a combination of interrelated 'inside' and 'outside' factors, including how staff interact and communicate with consumers. The organisational culture is important too. Staff need to feel supported and consumers need to feel wanted.

Front-line staff need to understand OHS policies and procedures; for example, incident reporting, risk control measures, and how to support colleagues involved in incidents. However, a major emphasis of training should be on the 'interactional 'nature of aggressive incidents. In the same way as the consumers they care for, staff will differ in their attitudes, values, emotional responses to illness or to stressful situations, and possess varying knowledge bases and communication skills. Therefore, aggression management training programs need to encourage trainees to explore these areas, as well as their habitual ways of responding to 'challenging' situations, including aggression. Training in communication skills is essential too, but training needs to be taught in context and in light of what seems to work for individual trainees. Trainees need time to experiment as each nurse–consumer interaction is a novel event. They will also need guidance by expert staff.

Mental health nurses are at the interface of direct consumer care, which puts them in a prime position to advance practice innovation, research and training around the prevention and management of consumer aggression. This should be a central part of nurses' clinical responsibility—and not left to non-clinicians. This view will need support at an organisational level if it is to be realised.

1   Why is the definition of consumer aggression difficult to pin down?

2   Why is it that the general public associates mental illness with aggression?

3   Discuss as many 'inside' and 'outside' factors as you can that may lead to a consumer becoming aggressive.

4   What do you understand by interactional effects when discussing causes of consumer aggression?

5   What type of organisation culture is required to successfully prevent and manage consumer aggression?

TEST YOURSELF

1   When thinking about the causes of aggression, which three factors do the authors say should be considered?

   a   Inside factors, outside factors and peripheral factors

   b   Interactional factors, transitional factors and inside factors

   c   Interactional factors, outside factors and intermediate factors

   d   Inside factors outside factors and interactional factors

2   File flagging, restriction of visiting rights, contracts of acceptable behaviour, limit setting, staff training, and attention to environmental design relate to:

   a   active and passive strategies

   b   active and administrative strategies

   c   administrative and passive strategies

   d   all of the above

3   Which is the best answer to the following statement? In the prevention and management of another's aggression, communication skills and techniques are:

   a   vital in showing staff how to deescalate incidents

   b   simply suggestions for how we should respond in a given situation

   c   vital in showing staff how to act assertively

   d   simply ideas for what to say to consumers when they are aggressive

4   Which of the following suggestions do you think will help staff best capture the likely risk for aggression posed by the consumer?

   a   Having policies and procedures in respect to occupational health and safety

   b   Using validated assessment forms

   c   Taking detailed consumer histories

   d   Using professional judgments

   e   All of the above

GERALD A. FARRELL

USEFUL WEBSITES

New Zealand Department of Labour—Managing the risk of workplace violence to healthcare and community service providers: Good practice guide: http://www.worksafe.govt.nz/worksafe/information-guidance/all-guidance-items/managing-the-risk-of-workplace-violence-to-healthcare-and-community-service-providers/preventing-violence.pdf

NICE—Violence and aggression (update): www.nice.org.uk/guidance/ng10/documents/violence-and-aggression-update-draft-full-guideline2

Victorian Auditor-General—Occupational violence against healthcare workers: https://www.audit.vic.gov.au/report/occupational-violence-against-healthcare-workers

Victorian Department of Health—Progress on occupational violence prevention in Victorian health services: www.health.vic.gov.au/__data/assets/pdf_file/0007/757105/1111008_Violence-in-Nursing_WEB_FA.pdf

Victorian Department of Health—Violence in healthcare taskforce report—Taking action to reduce violence in Victorian hospitals: https://www2.health.vic.gov.au/about/publications/researchandreports/violence-in-healthcare-taskforce-report

Victorian Department of Human Services—Preventing occupational violence in Victorian health services: www.health.vic.gov.au/__data/assets/pdf_file/0015/101643/nurse_safe_policy-Final.pdf

WorkSafe Victoria—Work-related

violence: www.worksafe.vic.gov.au/safety-and-prevention/health-and-safety-topics/occupational-violence

REFERENCES

Alexander, C., & Fraser, J. (2004). Occupational violence in an Australian healthcare setting: Implications for managers. *Journal of Health Care Information Management, 49*(6), 377–392.

Allnutt, S. H., O'Driscoll, C., Ogloff, J. R. P., Daffern, M., & Adams, J. (2010). *Clinical risk assessment and management: A practical manual for mental health clinicians.* Retrieved from www.justicehealth.nsw.gov.au.

Almvik, R., Woods, P., & Rasmussen, K. (2000). The Broset violence checklist: Sensitivity, specificity and interrater reliability. *Journal of Interpersonal Violence, 15*(12), 1284–1296.

Australian Nursing Federation (2010). *Zero tolerance: Occupational violence and aggression policy.* Retrieved from www.anfvic.asn.au/multiversions/3734/FileName/Zero_Tolerance.pdf.

Benveniste, K. A., Hibbert, P., & Runciman, W. B. (2005). Violence in health care: The contribution of the Australian Client Safety Foundation to incident monitoring and analysis. *Medical Journal of Australia, 183*(7), 348–351.

Bowers, L. (2007). *The City-128 study of observation and outcomes.* Retrieved from www.biomedcentral.com/1471–244X/7/S1/S122.

Camerino, D., Estryn-Behar, M., Conway, P. M., van Der Heijden, B. I. J. M., & Hasselhorn,

H. M. (2008). Work-related factors and violence among nursing staff in the European NEXT study: A longitudinal cohort study. *International Journal of Nursing Studies, 45*(1), 35–50.

Cameron, D. (2011). Speech to the Royal College of Nursing. In Design Council and Department of Health, *Reducing violence and aggression in A&E: Through a better experience* (p. 16). Retrieved from www.designcouncil.org.uk/Documents/Documents/OurWork/AandE/ReducingViolenceAndAggressionInAandE.pdf

Clinical Risk Assessment Screen (2013). Melbourne: Austin Health.

Cook, H., & Silvester, J. (2012). Patient 'strangled' in mental hospital. *The Age*, 28 December. Retrieved from www.theage.com.au/victoria/client-strangled-in-mental-hospital-20121227–2bxwi.html.

Daffern, M., Mayer, M. M., & Martin, T. (2004). Environment contributors to aggression in two forensic psychiatric hospitals. *International Journal of Forensic Mental Health, 3*(1), 105–114.

Dass, R., & Gorman, P. (1985). *How can I help?* London: Rider.

Department of Health (1999). *NHS zero tolerance zone: We don't have to take this.* Resource pack. London: Stationery Office.

Department of Health (2011). *Service guidelines on gender sensitivity and safety: Promoting a holistic*

approach to wellbeing. Melbourne: Victorian Government.

Department of Health (2012). *A New Mental Health Act for Victoria: Summary of proposed reforms.* Melbourne: Victorian Government.

Department of Human Services (2007). *Preventing occupational violence in Victorian health services: A policy framework and resource kit.* Melbourne: DHS.

Department of Immigration and Citizenship (n.d.). *National agenda for a multicultural Australia.* Retrieved from www.immi.gov.au/media/publications/multicultural/agenda/agenda89/australi.htm.

Duxbury, J. (2002). An evaluation of staff and patient views of strategies employed to manage inpatient aggression and violence on one mental health unit: A pluralistic design. *Journal of Psychiatric and Mental Health Nursing, 9*(3), 325–337.

Elbogen, E., Swanson, J., Applebaum, P., Swartz, M., Ferron, J., Van Dorn, R., & Wagner, H. (2007). Competence to complete psychiatric advance directives: Effects of facilitated decision making. *Law and Human Behaviour, 31*(3), 275–289.

Farrell, G., & Cubit, K. (2005). Nurses under threat: A comparison of content of 28 aggression management programs. *International Journal of Mental Health Nursing, 14*(1), 44–53.

Farrell, G., & Gray, C. (1992). *Aggression: A nurses' guide to therapeutic management*. London: Scutari Press.

Farrell, G., & Salmon, P. (2009). Challenging behaviour: An action plan for education and training. *Contemporary Nurse, 34*(1), 110–118.

Farrell, G., & Shafiei, T. (2012). Workplace aggression, including bullying in nursing and midwifery: A descriptive survey (the SWAB study). *International Journal of Nursing Studies, 49*(11), 1423–1431.

Farrell, G., Bobrowski, C., & Bobrowski, P. (2006). Scoping workplace aggression in nursing: Findings from an Australian study. *Journal of Advanced Nursing, 55*(6), 778–787.

Farrell, G., Shafiei, T., & Chen, S. P. (2012). Client and visitor assault on nurses and midwives: An exploratory study of employer 'protective' factors. *International Journal of Mental Health Nursing, 23*(1), 88–96. doi: 10.1111/inm.12002.

Farrell, G., Shafiei, T., & Salmon, P. (2012). Facing up to 'challenging behaviour': A model for training in staff-client interaction. *Journal of Advanced Nursing, 66*(7), 1644–1655.

Gaynor, N. (2009). Clinical management of acute behavioural disturbance associated with volatile intoxication. *Australian Emergency Nursing, 12*, 55–58.

Gerberich, S. G., Church, T. R., McGovern, P. M., Hansen, H., Nachreiner, N. M., Geisser, M. S., & Jurek, A. (2005). Risk factors for work-related assaults on nurses. *Epidemiology, 16*(5), 704–709.

Gifford, M. L., & Anderson, J. E. (2010). Barriers and motivating factors in reporting incidents of assault in mental health care. *Journal of the American Psychiatric Nurses Association, 16*(5), 288–298.

Henderson, S. (2011). Mood and anxiety disorders. In K. L. Edward, I. Munro, A. Robins & A. Welch (Eds.), *Mental health nursing: Dimensions of praxis* (pp 167–185). Melbourne: Oxford University Press.

Johnson, M. E. (2004). Violence on inpatient psychiatric units: State of the science. *Journal of the American Psychiatric Nurses Association, 10*(3), 113–21.

Kowalenko, T., Gates, D., Gillespie, G. L., Succop, P., & Mentzel, T. K. (2013). Prospective study of violence against ED workers. *American Journal of Emergency Medicine, 31*(1), 197–205.

Kutner, J. S., Steiner, J. F., Corbett, K. K., Jahnigen, D. W., & Barton, P. L. (1999). Information needs in terminal illness. *Social Science and Medicine, 48*, 1341–1352.

Lanza, M., Kayne, H. L., Pattison, I., Hicks, C., & Islam, S. (1994). Predicting violence: Nursing diagnosis versus psychiatric diagnosis. *Nursing Diagnosis, 5*(4), 151–157.

Lyneham, J. (2000). Violence in New South Wales emergency departments. *Australian Emergency Nursing Journal, 4*(1), 5–9.

Maguire, J., & Ryan, D. (2007). Aggression and violence in mental health services: Categorizing the experiences of Irish nurses. *Journal of Psychiatric and Mental Health Nursing, 14*(2), 120–127.

Markham, D., & Trower, P. (2003). The effects of the psychiatric label 'borderline personality disorder' on nursing staff's perceptions and causal attributions for challenging behaviours. *British Journal of Clinical Psychology, 42*(3), 243–256.

McNiel, D. E., & Binder, R. L. (1994). Screening for risk of inpatient violence: *Validation of an actuarial tool*. Law and Human Behavior, *18*(5), 579.

Mendick, N., Young, B., Holcombe, C., & Salmon, P. (2010). The ethics of responsibility and ownership in decision making about treatment for breast cancer: Triangulation of consultation with patient and surgeon perspectives. *Social Science and Medicine, 70*, 1904–2011.

Mental Health Bill—Austin Health Submission (2011). Mental Health Bill Exposure Draft, Submission by the Respecting Client Choices Program in collaboration with the Mental Health Clinical Service Unit, Austin Health. Retrieved from www.health.vic.gov.au/mentalhealth/archive/mhactreview/ed_submissions/submissions-2011/health-service-providers/eds207-silvester-professor-william-newton-professor-richard-fullam-dr-rachael.pdf.

Nabb, D. (2000). Visitors' violence: The serious effects of aggression on nurses and others. *Nursing Standard, 14*(23), 36–38.

Nachreiner, N. M., Gerberich, S. G., McGovern, P. M., Church, T. M., Hanson, H. E., Geisser, M. S., & Ryan, A. D. (2005). Impact of training on work-related assault. *Research in Nursing and Health, 28*(1), 67–78.

National Client Safety Agency (2004). *Seven steps to client safety: An overview guide for NHS staff.* London: NPSA. Retrieved from www.npsa.nhs.uk/health/resources/7steps.

National Risk Management Programme (2007). *Best practice in managing risk.* London: Department of Health.

National Technical Assistance Centre (2006). *Training curriculum for the reduction of seclusion and restraint.* National Association of State Mental Health Program Directors.

Needham, I., Abderhalden, C., Halfens, R. J., Fischer, J. E., & Dassen, T. (2005). Non-somatic effects of client aggression on nurses: a systematic review. *Journal of Advanced Nursing, 49*(3), 283–296.

Newbill, W. A., Marth, D., Coleman, J. C., Menditto, A. A., Carson, S. J., & Beck, N. C. (2010). Direct observational coding of staff who are the victims of assault. *Psychological Services, 7*(3), 177–189.

Nijman, H. L. I. (2002). A model of aggression in psychiatric hospitals. *Acta Psychiatrica Scandinavica, 106*(s412), 142–143.

O'Connell, B., Young, J., Brooks, J., & Lofthouse, J. (2000). Nurses' perceptions of the nature and frequency of aggression in general ward settings and high dependency areas. *Journal of Clinical Nursing, 9*(4), 602–610.

Ogloff, J. R. P., & Daffern, M. (2003). The assessment of inpatient aggression at the Thomas Embling Hospital: Toward the dynamic appraisal of inpatient aggression. *Forensicare: Victorian Institute of Forensic Mental Health Fourth Annual Research Report to Council, I July 2002–30 June 2003.*

Ogloff, J. R. P., & Daffern, M. (2006). The dynamic appraisal of situational aggression: An instrument to assess risk for imminent aggression in psychiatric clients. *Behavioural Sciences and the Law, 24*(6), 799–813.

Prevention and management of aggression in health services (2009). Retrieved from www.commerce.wa.gov.au/worksafe/pdf/guides/aggression_in_health_web.pdf.

Richter, D., Needham, I., & Kunz, S. (2006). The effects of aggression management training for mental health care and disability staff: A systematic review. In D. Richter & R. Whittington (Eds.), *Violence in mental health settings: Causes, consequences, management* (pp. 211–230). New York: Springer.

Rose, J. L., & Cleary, A. (2007). Care staff perceptions of challenging behaviour and fear of assault. *Journal of Intellectual & Developmental Disability, 32*(2), 153–161.

Royal College of Nursing (1998). *Dealing with violence against nursing staff: An RCN Guide for nurses and managers.* London: RCN.

Salmon, P., & Young, B. (2011). Creativity in clinical communication: From communication skills to skilled helper. *Medical Education, 45*, 217–226.

Scott, C. L., & Resnick, P. J. (2006). Violence risk assessment in persons with mental illness. *Aggression and Violent Behavior, 11*(6), 598–611.

Sieff, M. (1990). *On Management.* London: Weidenfeld & Nicolson.

Silverman, J. (2011). Clinical communication training in continuing medical education: Possible, do-able and done? *Client Education and Counselling, 84*(2), 141–142.

Srebnik, D., Applebaum, P., & Russo, J. (2004). Assessing competence to complete psychiatric advance directives with the competence assessment tool for psychiatric advance directives. *Comprehensive Psychiatry, 45*(4), 239–245.

Stuart, H. (2003). Mental health policy paper: Violence and mental illness: An overview. *World Psychiatry, 2*(2).

Turnbull, J. (1999). Violence to staff: Who is at risk? In J. Turnbull & B. Paterson (Eds.). *Aggression and violence: Approaches to effective management* (pp. 8–30). London: Macmillan.

van den Eertwegh, V., van Dulman, S., van Dalen, J., Scherpbier, A. J., & van der Vleuten, C. P. (2013). Learning in context: Identifying gaps in research on the transfer of medical communication skills to the clinical workplace. *Client Education and Counselling, 90,* 184–192.

Whittington, R., & Richter, D. (2006). From the individual to the environment and interaction in the escalation of violence in mental health settings. In D. Richter & R. Whittington (Eds.). *Violence in mental health settings. Causes, consequences, management* (pp. 47–68). New York: Springer.

Wondrak, R. (1999). Verbal abuse. In J. Turnbull & B. Paterson (Eds.). *Aggression and violence: Approaches to effective management* (pp. 79–94). London: Macmillan.

World Health Organization (2002). *New research shows workplace violence threatens health services.* Retrieved from www.who.int/mediacentre/news/releases/release37/en/— accessed.

Zampieron, Al. Galeazzo, M. Turra, S., & Buja, A. (2010). Perceived aggression towards nurses: Study in two Italian health institutions. *Journal of Clinical Nursing, 19,* 2329–2341.

CHAPTER 21

Aboriginal and Torres Strait Islander, New Zealand Māori and Remote Area Mental Health

VERENA TINNING AND
GRAEME THOMPSON

Acknowledgment

The authors would like to acknowledge the contribution of Kim Usher, Roianne West and Deb Spurgeon who co-wrote this chapter in the second edition.

KEY OUTCOMES

AFTER READING THIS CHAPTER, YOU SHOULD BE ABLE TO:

- identify the relevant health and mental health issues facing Māori, Aboriginal and Torres Strait Islander peoples
- identify changes that have occurred in providing mental health services for Māori, Aboriginal and Torres Strait Islander peoples.
- outline some of the culturally different presentations of mental illness that might be presented by Māori, Aboriginal and Torres Strait Islander consumers.
- understand the remote Aboriginal community setting
- understand the importance of family relationships
- understand the impact that Te Tiriti o Waitangi has in providing services for Māori.

KEY TERMS

- community and family relationships
- cultural assessment
- Kaiwhakaruruhau
- Māori models of health care
- mental status examination (MSE)
- remote Aboriginal communities
- social and emotional well-being
- social determinants
- Te Tiriti o Waitangi

Introduction

This chapter is divided into three sections. The first provides the reader with a historical perspective of Australian Aboriginal and Torres Strait islander peoples, the impact of colonisation and contemporary access to mental health care. The second section is written from a remote rural mental health nurse perspective, providing insight into some of the concerns and challenges of working in often far distant places, away from acute care services, to provide mental health care to Indigenous people within Australia. The last section comes from our colleagues in New Zealand, exploring the bi-cultural nature of mental health care in that country. This section offers insights into how care can be provided within a culturally safe and inclusive manner.

SECTION 1   THE MENTAL HEALTH OF AUSTRALIA'S ABORIGINAL AND TORRES STRAIT ISLANDER PEOPLES

ROIANNE WEST AND KIM USHER

There are approximately 669,881 Aboriginal and Torres Strait Islander people residing in Australia. This represents 3 per cent of the total Australian population (ABS, 2012). When compared with non-Indigenous Australians, Aboriginal and Torres Strait Islander people are less likely to be employed, are less likely to own a home and are overrepresented in supported accommodation for the homeless and those at risk of becoming homeless. While Australians enjoy relatively good health overall, Aboriginal and Torres Strait Islander people experience higher death rates than non-Indigenous Australians across all age groups (Australian Institute of Health and Welfare, 2008). Aboriginal and Torres Strait Islander people also experience higher rates of some mental disorders and social and emotional well-being problems than others (Australian Health Ministers' Advisory Council, 2004a). Prevalence estimates of mental illness in Aboriginal and Torres Strait Islander people are not well researched or documented in Australia (Henderson, Andrews & Hall, 2000).

As a way to understand the issues currently facing the Aboriginal and Torres Strait Islander people of Australia, and as a context for reflecting on these facts and figures, it is important to have some insight into the history of Indigenous peoples in Australia. For example, years of 'colonisation, welfare, the trauma of dispossession, removal of children, abuse and violence' have all taken their toll on the Aboriginal and Torres Strait islander peoples of Australia, and have triggered feelings of powerlessness (Cooperative Research Centre for Aboriginal Health, 2008, p. 35), as well as feelings of shame, loss, uncertainty and low self-esteem (Raphael & Swan, 1997). Other socio-historical-political factors involved in the development of illness among Aboriginal and Torres Strait Islander people include grief, separation from family and children, loss of cultural identity and the impact of social inequity, stigma and racism. This often results in Indigenous people externalising the cause of an illness to some past 'wrongdoing' (Vicary & Westerman, 2004). As a result, when dealing with the mental health needs of Aboriginal and Torres Strait Islander people, it is important to remember that individualised mental health care will always fall short unless it takes account of the broader social and structural improvements necessary to strengthen the entire community (Haswell et al., 2009).

Closing the life expectancy gap between Aboriginal and Torres Strait Islander people and non-Indigenous Australians within a generation is a critical priority of the Australian Government. Improving the mental health of Indigenous Australians is a key component in achieving this objective. The next section provides an overview of the issues facing Indigenous people in Australia, with particular emphasis on mental health problems and needs, and outlines a number of culturally appropriate nursing interventions.

Mental health and Aboriginal and Torres Strait Islander Australians

Aboriginal and Torres Strait Islander people often experience higher rates of mental health problems than non-Indigenous Australians. The rate of hospitalisations—one way of measuring use of mental health services—supports this observation. The most recent data available on hospitalisations indicate there were more hospitalisations of Indigenous males and females than expected, when based on the rates for non-Indigenous Australians (Australian Institute of Health and Welfare, 2008). In particular, hospitalisations related to psychoactive substance use were almost five times higher for Indigenous males and three times higher for Indigenous females. Those related to self-harm were also higher—three times as high for males and twice as high for females—when compared with non-Indigenous Australians (Australian Institute of Health and Welfare, 2008). Social and emotional responses experienced by Aboriginal and Torres Strait lslander people result from problems such as loss, grief, trauma, abuse, violence, substance misuse, physical health issues, child development problems, child removals, incarceration and family breakdown. Mental health problems include crisis reactions, anxiety states, depression, post-traumatic stress, self-harm and psychosis (Australian Health Ministers' Advisory Council, 2004a). Higher rates of psychiatric morbidity occur in other areas as well, especially depression, post-traumatic disorders and co-morbid disorders such as a physical condition or substance misuse. However, the rates for schizophrenia and bipolar disorder are similar to the rest of the population (Indigenous Health Infonet, 2009). Suicide rates are much higher for Aboriginal and Torres Strait Islander people (3.7 per cent in 2007) compared with non-Indigenous Australians (1.3 per cent in 2007; Australian Bureau of Statistics, 2009). In fact, from 2001 to 2005, the suicide rate was almost three times that of non-Indigenous males, making it the leading cause of death from external causes for Aboriginal and Torres Strait Islander males (Australian Institute of Health and Welfare, 2008).

The issue is further exacerbated where Aboriginal and Torres Strait Islander consumers reside in rural or remote areas and require transfer to larger regional areas for treatment. Consumers in this situation often find themselves without family members or support people nearby, current service providers are often not informed of their transfer, and feedback to usual service providers is generally protracted (De Crespigny et al., 2006). For Aboriginal and Torres Strait Islander consumers, being separated from family can be very stressful.

Aboriginal and Torres Strait Islander conceptualisations of mental health

Social and emotional well-being and mental health are similar concepts. The use of the term 'social and emotional well-being' by Aboriginal and Torres Strait Islander people is an attempt to move away from the biomedical perspective of mental health (especially mental illness). It also has a more positive and holistic connotation, which is in keeping with Indigenous beliefs about health. Principles of this approach are outlined in Table 21.1. Aboriginal and Torres Strait Islander mental health concepts also incorporate the holistic nature of health and well-being, and advocate the inclusion of mind, body, spirituality, and environmental and spiritual constructs (Vicary & Westerman, 2004). In addition, the concept of health includes not only the well-being of the individual but also that of the family and the community in which they live (Australian Institute of Health and Welfare, 2008). In the past, mental health services for Aboriginal and Torres Strait Islander people have been organised around a Western model of psychiatry, focusing on the individual, which has been found unsuitable. As a result, movement has begun towards creating a model that adopts the principles of Indigenous community-controlled services, which build capacity, strengthen and foster relationships, and retain flexibility in addressing needs and Aboriginal and Torres Strait Islander understandings of mental health. A similar philosophy of collaborative and consumer-oriented care is also occurring within mainstream mental health services across Australia.

TABLE 21.1 THE FIVE PRINCIPLES FOR DELIVERY OF SOCIAL AND EMOTIONAL WELL-BEING SERVICES	
Consumer and carer focus	Recognise that consumers, family members and carers all have experience of mental health problems, and their experience and role in recovery must be recognised and supported.
Context and community	Maximise engagement and involvement of people from the local community, understand kinship structures and promote the importance of family and appropriate cultural and linguistic assessments.
Continuity of care	Understand early warning signs, look for risk factors and triggers, and engage consumers in continual planning and regular review.
Checking for change	Identify Indigeneity, consult family and/or carer in assessment ratings, and provide feedback to consumers and carers in a way that supports communication about change and promotes hope.
Considered clinical care	Take into account the experience and knowledge of the individual and their family, and the knowledge of the broader relationship between consumer and community.

Adapted from Haswell et al. (2009)

These new services are urgently needed to address the current disparities in Aboriginal and Torres Strait Islander mental health (Haswell et al., 2009).

Therefore, understanding Aboriginal and Torres Strait Islander mental health and ill health requires consideration of not only the cause of the problems, but also the extent to which past influences have had an impact on Aboriginal and Torres Strait Islander people. To take this into account requires the nurse to reflect these differences in the treatment approach, while also taking into account existing frameworks and approaches for healing that are being used in the communities (Vicary & Westerman, 2004).

BOX 21.1 BELIEFS ABOUT MENTAL HEALTH AND ILLNESS

The following are some beliefs held by various Australian Aboriginal and Torres Strait Islander groups across Australia.

1 Thoughts and feelings can be shared telepathically between closely related individuals.

2 Magic spells can be cast, such as 'bone pointing' and 'being sung', and used to cause ill health and even death.

3 Dangerous spirits can make people ill.

4 Traditional healers are thought to have powers capable of restoring health.

Adapted from Haswell et al. (2009)

Policies and how they have an impact on service delivery

There are a number of important policies that have a direct impact on the provision of mental health care to Aboriginal and Torres Strait Islander people. Generic mental health policies such as the *National Action Plan on Mental Health 2006–2011* (Council of Australian Governments, 2008) are also relevant to

Aboriginal and Torres Strait Islander people. There are, however, some policies that relate directly to the delivery of mental health services to Indigenous people. The main ones are outlined below.

The Social and Emotional Well-being Framework 2004–2009 was designed to respond to the high levels of social and emotional well-being problems and mental ill health among Aboriginal and Torres Strait Islander people by providing a framework for national action. Within the framework, the importance of the delivery of culturally appropriate care is recognised, and the need for all services to work together for the best outcomes for Indigenous people is supported (Australian Health Ministers' Advisory Council, 2004a). An outcome of this framework is the *Protocols for the Delivery of Social and Emotional Well-being and Mental Health Services in Indigenous Communities*, which is designed to guide service delivery (Haswell et al., 2009).

Guidelines for Health Workers, Clinicians, Consumers and Carers were developed from the framework, and can be used by nurses and other health professionals when working with Aboriginal and Torres Strait Islander people. They offer background information as well as details of specific interventions (Haswell et al., 2009).

The *Cultural Respect Framework for Aboriginal and Torres Strait Islander Health 2004–2009* was developed as a guiding principle in policy construction and service delivery, as a means to strengthen relationships between the health-care system and Aboriginal and Torres Strait Islander people. In particular, it outlines a process for embedding cultural respect within health services and recognises important principles, such as a holistic approach, health sector responsibility, community control of primary health-care services, working together, localised decision-making, promoting good health, building the capacity of health services and communities, and accountability for health outcomes (Australian Health Ministers' Advisory Council, 2004b). These are therefore important principles to be used when developing and assessing health services in the future.

Current strategies to improve Indigenous mental health

There have been a number of strategies implemented as a way to improve the mental health of Australian Indigenous people. These include the following:

- *National Action Plan on Mental Health 2006–2011*—With the aim of improving the capacity of workers in Aboriginal and Torres Strait Islander communities, health practitioners are being trained to identify and address mental illness and associated substance use issues in Aboriginal and Torres Strait Islander communities and make referrals for treatment (Council of Australian Governments, 2008).
- *Bringing Them Home*—In response to the report of the 1997 National Inquiry into the Separation of Aboriginal and Torres Strait Islander Children from Their Families (Department of Health and Ageing, 2009), the Australian Government funded a number of programs for the social and emotional well-being of Aboriginal and Torres Strait Islander people, including the Bringing Them Home, Link Up, and Social and Emotional Well-being Regional Centre Programs.
- Beyondblue—Aboriginal and Torres Strait Islander mental health is a priority for the organisation Beyondblue, which has developed a range of culturally appropriate information sources, education and support strategies in consultation with communities and Indigenous organisations (Beyondblue, 2009).

- Living Is for Everyone (LIFE)—This is a national suicide prevention strategy that aims to improve access to suicide and self-harm prevention activities in Australia, and has a section devoted to reducing the high suicide rates among Australia's Aboriginal and Torres Strait Islander population (National Public Health Partnership, 2004).
- Headspace—The Headspace mission is to deliver improvements in the mental health, social well-being and economic participation of young Australians aged 12–25 years. It is in the process of developing an Aboriginal and Torres Strait Islander youth mental health strategic plan (Headspace).
- Australian Integrated Mental Health Initiative (AIM HI)—The AIM HI program was set up to improve outcomes for Aboriginal consumers of mental health services in remote Top End communities from 2003 to 2008. It developed two-way mental health promotion resources (for health professionals, consumers and carers), a story-telling project and new approaches to service delivery, including pictorial assessment and treatment tools (Cooperative Research Centre for Aboriginal Health, 2008).
- The Empowerment Program—As empowerment is a key to improving Aboriginal and Torres Strait Islander health and well-being, the Empowerment Program aims to encourage people to take control of their own lives and includes a family well-being program and men's groups (Cooperative Research Centre for Aboriginal Health, 2008).

Nursing interventions for working with Aboriginal and Torres Strait Islander people

We know that mental disorders do exist within Aboriginal and Torres Strait Islander communities (Haswell et al., 2009, p. 27; Westerman, 2003); however, their expression and treatment is different from those of the mainstream population, and Aboriginal and Torres Strait Islander people are often misdiagnosed or over-diagnosed as a result. Working with Aboriginal and Torres Strait Islander people requires respect for cultural difference. It is important to begin by finding out about the cultural norms of the community before making any assumptions about individual behaviour (Hart et al., 2009). In most cases, Aboriginal and Torres Strait Islander people are wary of mainstream health services. Therefore, it is essential that the nurse approaches people in a situation where they feel comfortable, such as in their own community. This may mean that the nurse or other health worker needs to travel to the community to see the consumer, rather than the other way around. Failure to take account of this important issue may lead to people presenting as more severely distressed than is actually the case (Westerman, 2004). It is also essential to make use of Aboriginal and Torres Strait Islander mental health workers who have knowledge of cultural issues and can assist with entry to the community. They must be considered as important members of the multidisciplinary team, and consulted on all issues of relevance to the Indigenous consumer. Consumers should be allowed to seek out help from a professional experienced in working with Indigenous people (Hart et al., 2009).

It is important to be aware that Aboriginal and Torres Strait Islander people will often be shy when first contact is made, and often reluctant to express their feelings and concerns. It might take time before the person will open up to you. To avoid being too confronting, it is helpful to avoid leading questions, but let people tell you their story at their own pace (Haswell et al., 2009). The use of culturally appropriate counselling techniques is therefore recommended (Westerman, 2004). The nurse also needs to be aware of gender issues. There are certain cultural requirements that mean there are things that a man cannot discuss with a woman and vice versa (Haswell et al., 2009). To do so would result in 'shame' for all concerned (Westerman, 2004).

The presentations of mental illness in Aboriginal and Torres Strait Islander people vary from the Western model, which often leaves nurses and other health workers unsure of the problem. Aboriginal people may talk about becoming unwell because of what they term 'longing for' or 'crying for' country—this may present in a similar way to depression. Furthermore, in a study of Indigenous people's perceptions of mental illness (Vicary & Westerman, 2004), the majority of Aboriginal and Torres Strait Islander people did not recognise depression as treatable, but rather conceived of it as 'just the way he is', which indicated a reference to a characteristic of the individual versus an illness. Aboriginal people are also known to grieve differently and for longer periods of time than non-Indigenous people. The death of an Aboriginal person signifies the beginning of an extended period of time when all relatives will engage in lengthy activities and rituals. Some Aboriginal people express their grief through acts of self-harm, called 'sorry cuts' (Haswell et al., 2009). Caution must also be taken when discussing bereavement, as it is often unacceptable to mention the name of the deceased (Haswell et al., 2009).

Family is extremely important in Aboriginal and Torres Strait Islander cultures. It is imperative that the consumer's family is encouraged to be involved in treatment, where the individual gives consent and the individual's right to confidentiality is respected. In addition, positive family relationships should be fostered as a way of ensuring support for the person during and after treatment (Hart et al., 2009).

CRITICAL THINKING OPPORTUNITY

1   Describe the steps you would take to ensure you acted in a culturally appropriate way when working with an Aboriginal or Torres Strait Islander consumer.

2   What do you perceive as the main differences necessary when approaching an Aboriginal or Torres Strait Islander mental health consumer compared with a non-Indigenous mental health consumer?

Assessment of Aboriginal and Torres Strait Islander people must also be adapted to include culturally relevant protocols and questions. Thus, when undertaking a mental status examination (MSE), the process must be adapted to include appropriate cultural considerations, as outlined in Table 21.2.

Aboriginal and Torres Strait Islander people have their own healers for all health issues, including mental health. There are many differences between the mainstream approach to treating mental illness and the approaches used by Indigenous healers. While both traditional healer approaches and mainstream approaches to mental health can be used together, when an Aboriginal or Torres Strait Islander consumer prefers to follow the advice of a traditional healer, this view must be respected (Haswell et al., 2009). Offering Aboriginal and Torres Strait Islander consumers the opportunity to incorporate traditional healers into their treatment plan is an important consideration. Likewise, the nurse should be prepared to consult traditional healers and cultural consultants when planning care (Westerman, 2004).

Medications may be conceived of in various ways by Aboriginal and Torres Strait Islander people. Psychotropic medications, used as one of the main treatments for mental illnesses, are often viewed with scepticism by Aboriginal and Torres Strait Islander people, who may prefer instead to use bush remedies as part of the traditional healing process (Haswell et al., 2009). In addition, as with many other

TABLE 21.2 CULTURAL ASSESSMENT AND AWARENESS AS PART OF THE MENTAL STATUS EXAMINATION (MSE)

Mental state examination (MSE)	Nursing cultural considerations	Nursing strategy
Spirituality	• Spiritual considerations are paramount when completing a MSE on an Indigenous consumer. • The greatest risk for the consumer and nurse is for an individual's spiritual experiences to be misinterpreted as a symptom. • To understand the cultural relevance of these experiences, specific strategies are required.	• Respectfully consult with family, Aboriginal and Torres Strait Islander health workers and other cultural informants in the community.
Appearance	• What might be an 'acceptable' standard of appearance for the general population might not necessarily be the same for the individual and/or community from which the consumer comes.	• Information can be sought from the consumer, family members, carers and Indigenous mental health and generalist health workers. • Identify what are acceptable standards of appearance in the community from which the individual comes.
Behaviour	• What might be an 'acceptable' standard of behaviour for the general population might not necessarily be the same for the individual and or community from which the consumer comes.	• Mental health providers need to be open-minded and observant about this area. • Be careful to separate signs of illness from culturally appropriate behaviours. • Avoid making assumptions.
Thought form	• There may be factors that prevented the consumer from getting an adequate education. Consequently, the consumer may exhibit problems with pronunciation, comprehension and grammatical structure. • For many Indigenous consumers, English will not be their first language.	• Determine how well the consumer knows English. • Ensure that a family member, Indigenous mental health worker and/or a generalist health worker is included in the assessment process as a support person and to interpret or translate as necessary.
Thought content	• Not all reported cases signify that there is a mental health problem.	• Caution must be exercised where cultural experiences and ideas are concerned. • Staff should explore whether such experiences and ideas make sense in cultural terms and are consistent with values and beliefs expressed by the consumer's family or community.
Affect	• For many Indigenous peoples across the world, revealing or showing emotion is a sign of weakness. Consequently, individuals might present as being reserved, even when discussing traumatic or happy experiences.	• This should be considered when determining flat affect. • Caution should also be used so as not to confuse the shyness of shame with sadness.
Attention and concentration	• Bear in mind that many Indigenous consumers might have vastly different concepts of what is considered to be general knowledge in comparison with the general population. Therefore, it is best to ensure that whatever topic is used to test this aspect is one that the consumer is familiar and comfortable with.	• Check with the local health worker or other specialists to determine appropriate levels of knowledge.

Mental state examination (MSE)	Nursing cultural considerations	Nursing strategy
Orientation	• Most people might not know the exact date, because of a different understanding of the concept of time.	• Assessment might include asking the day of the week, month and/or year. • Obvious disturbances could indicate a serious problem.
Memory		• Ensure that the topics used to test these areas are familiar to the consumer. Assessment in long-term memory might include recalling the names of family members instead of the last five prime ministers of Australia.
Intelligence	• Evaluating intelligence is a very complicated and controversial subject. This is because of the cultural and educational differences between Indigenous Australians and mainstream society.	• Establish the level of education of the consumer. • Establish how proficient the consumer is with English and its usage, and whether it is their first language. • Ensure that general knowledge questions are appropriate, considering that many Indigenous people have a different concept of general knowledge. • Ensure that how consumers present and communicate is not mistaken for slow or impaired functioning; for example, a consumer might be shy or generally sit back and contemplate a question before answering. • Actively engage Indigenous staff and support people for background information and assistance in the assessment process. • Be aware that the skills mainstream society values are not necessarily the same as those many Indigenous peoples view as important, such as values essential to survival, irrespective of how much schooling they have completed.
Insight	• As the understanding of mental health for some Indigenous people is different from that of mainstream understanding, this area can be difficult to assess.	• Ensure that a family member, Indigenous mental health worker or a generalist health worker is included in the assessment process as a support person, and to interpret or translate as necessary.
Judgment		• Mental health providers should consult Indigenous staff, families and community members to ensure that an accurate assessment is made.

Adapted from Haswell et al. (2009)

Aboriginal and Torres Strait Islander cultural groups, the concepts of time and time-related events, and issues of storage and sharing of prescriptions and medications, all have implications for medication management, and must be taken into account when planning care and selecting appropriate treatments. Furthermore, adherence to therapeutic regimens may also be problematic for Aboriginal and Torres Strait Islander consumers for many reasons (Usher, Foster & Bullock, 2009).

BOX 21.2 SUMMARY OF IMPORTANT FACTORS WHEN ASSESSING
AN ABORIGINAL AND TORRES STRAIT ISLANDER PERSON

When assessing Aboriginal and Torres Strait Islander consumers, the following issues need to be considered:

- Hallucinations, delusions or pathological thinking may be diagnosed incorrectly, when these may be the result of spiritual beliefs.
- Distress, even from what appear to be spiritual beliefs, must be taken seriously and treated in a considered way.
- Appearance may differ from what is expected, so there is a need to assess in relation to the community.
- Mental health providers need to be open-minded and observant when assessing behaviour and emotion and avoid making assumptions.
- Shyness or shame may be easily confused with sadness, or a reserved response with flat affect.

- It is important to establish whether English is the consumer's first language, and also determine the level of confidence with English.
- There is a danger of assuming that a delayed answer is a sign or slow or impaired functioning.
- The level of education of consumers should be determined.
- Many Aboriginal and Torres Strait Islander consumers will have a vastly different concept of what is considered general knowledge, so adjust general knowledge questions accordingly.
- Remain respectful of gender issues.

Adapted from Haswell et al., 2009

ABOUT THE CONSUMER   John's story

You are a registered nurse working in a primary health-care centre that services a number of remote Aboriginal communities. Concerned relatives ask you to go to their house to see John, a 19-year-old Aboriginal male, because he is acting strangely and refusing to attend the clinic. The family states that he has been acting strangely since his mother passed away. John was unable to attend the funeral, as he was out of town and could not get back. John has told the family that he sees and talks regularly to his mother and a cousin who committed suicide when he was the same age as John. He is blaming family members for his mother's death, and is threatening to 'kill them'. He finished school in Year 9, and has had a disrupted employment history. John has superficial cuts to his forearm and chest, and has a history of suicide attempts. He is the youngest of four siblings, the only male, and a family representative on a multi-family land claim—along with his father, who is a respected elder in the community. Although John's first language is English, he can speak his traditional language as well.

REFLECTION QUESTIONS

1   Using the information in this chapter, complete a MSE for John.
2   Identify which cues allow for the possibility of the misinterpretation of cultural experiences as symptoms.
3   Identify the strategies you would use to assist you to differentiate between a symptom and a cultural experience.
4   Complete a nursing care plan identifying the nursing intervention required for John.

SECTION 2 THE WORK OF A MENTAL HEALTH NURSE IN REMOTE ABORIGINAL COMMUNITIES

VERENA TINNING

The author acknowledges the Indigenous peoples of the Top End, especially those of the Larrakia and Thamarrurr Regions who have contributed their knowledge to the writing of this section.

This section of the chapter aims to enlighten readers about the unique work setting remote Aboriginal communities poses for mental health nursing. It discusses the many challenges affecting residents of remote communities, but also the opportunities to make a positive difference for an Aboriginal person experiencing a mental illness or disorder. The role entails facilitating both formal Western medicine-influenced treatments as well as engaging in activities that enhance the social and emotional well-being of individuals, families and the greater community.

The section is written from a mental health nurse practitioner's view and discusses how the role fits well into the remote context not only from a comprehensive Western treatment perspective but also from the nursing model view; that is, providing holistic care.

Setting the scene: the remote Aboriginal community context

Living in remote or very remote Australia is quite tough. Accessing services such as health, employment, telecommunications, Centrelink, banks and disability services or family assistance is more complicated than in the city—and in smaller communities may be non-existent or sporadic. Respondents to a general social survey in 2006 reported difficulties in accessing resources for reasons such as transport and distance, cost or inadequate services in the area (Baxter, Hayes & Gray, 2011); consequently, many miss out on such services.

Three per cent of Australians are Aboriginal and Torres Strait Islander people, or almost 670,000 people (Australian Bureau of Statistics, 2013b). In the Northern Territory, almost 30 per cent of the population identifies as Aboriginal and Torres Strait Islander, compared with much lower percentages in other jurisdictions in Australia, ranging from 0.9 per cent in Victoria to 4.7 per cent in Tasmania. Just over 21 per cent of Aboriginal and Torres Strait Islander people live in remote or very remote areas.

In the Top End of Australia, geographical distances between regional centres, rural and remote communities are vast. The territory occupies one sixth of Australia's land area. This frequently results in costly and delayed access to mental health care. The aero-medical service transports people to the regional hospitals in acute situations. Mental health consumers in crisis often meet the criteria to warrant air-ambulance rather than transfer to hospital via commercial flight, to manage potential or apparent risk factors safely.

Death by intentional self-harm ranked thirteenth in Australia in 2014 of all 'causes of death', compared with fourteenth in 2009 (Australian Bureau of Statistics, 2014). Of much more concern is that death by intentional self-harm is the leading cause of death in potential years of life lost.

In the Northern Territory, rates of death from suicide are almost three times higher in the Indigenous versus the non-Indigenous population. About a quarter of these occur in remote regions (Mental Health Directorate, 2015). The statistics show that there has been a recent decrease in this cause of death in the Northern Territory, especially in young Indigenous males. Other consequences of suicide on significant others—such as children, partners, parents and friends—is not included in this data, although they would add to the weighty adverse effects resulting from suicide; for example, complicated grief, blaming self and anger. In remote communities where suicide tends to occur in clusters, this only amplifies and prolongs the detrimental outcomes of suicide; grief is often 'never-ending' when coupled with dealing with death from premature natural deaths in family.

Problems resulting from violent behaviours within remote communities is unfortunately well documented and has been subject to extensive public discussion in recent years (Dudgeon et al., 2014). Statistics for incidents of aggression are three to five times higher among the Aboriginal and Torres Strait Islander population compared with non-Indigenous Australian residents, both as victims and perpetrators. The causes are believed to originate in events of the past such as colonisation, removal from families and country, marginalisation, welfare dependency, unemployment, lived experience of violence, substance abuse and mental health issues. It is quite obvious that addressing the problem of violence is an ongoing, complex and difficult task.

In the author's experience, it is not uncommon for violence to occur, but it is under-reported for fear of retaliation by the perpetrator and/or their families towards the person themselves or their family. For example, a 16-year-old girl was the victim of rape, which was reported under mandatory requirements. This led to inter-family conflict after the perpetrator's family pressured the victim's family to drop the charges. The victim and her family eventually moved to another community to escape the relentless stress from this situation. Blame was also pointed towards the girl's boyfriend for leaving her alone (in a house in the middle of the day). This example highlights some of the complexities of remote community living. Passive acceptance of violence seems to attract a response of 'It's always been like this'. Inevitably, this contributes to higher incidences of mental health issues and decreased resilience and functioning of individuals and families, and perpetuates inter-generational maladaptation.

Furthermore the social and emotional well-being and mental health of Aboriginal and Torres Strait Islander people is negatively influenced by the problematic use of alcohol and other drugs, at all age levels (Australian Bureau of Statistics, 2013a). There are, however, improvements reported in substance use as well as other health outcomes, including smoking and drinking alcohol during pregnancy. Nevertheless, there is still a statistically significant difference between Indigenous and non-Indigenous populations, with the former trailing behind.

A study in 2007 identified that almost a quarter of Australians had a lifetime substance-use disorder (Slade et al., 2009). Given that the numbers are increased among the Indigenous population, this has significant implications for the care of those who experience mental disorders, as it is well established that dual diagnosis in mental and substance-use disorders are high, which in turn calls for increased development of treatments that address both.

Ongoing and significant efforts are being made to improve social determinants such as education, housing and health (Meadows et al., 2012; Mental Health Directorate, 2015). Community visits by mental health clinicians are now more flexible in frequency, allowing mental health care to be better tailored to a community's need.

Remote mental health services

As in other Australian jurisdictions, mental health services are guided by various policies and standards at local and national levels. These include the recently published response to the Australian Government's Mental Health Review. It forms part of new recommendations for mental health service planning (National Mental Health Commission, 2015). Key priorities of the report identified are:

- the prevention, early detection and treatment of mental illness
- the prevention of suicide
- mental health research, workforce development and training
- the reduction of the burden of disease caused by mental illness.

In all, the response outlines twenty-five recommendations that build the framework for service planning for the next decade.

The report contains a section specific to addressing the poorer state of mental health and well-being of Aboriginal and Torres Strait Islander people (National Mental Health Commission, 2014). It makes Aboriginal and Torres Strait Islander mental health a national priority and envisages a dedicated Aboriginal and Torres Strait Islander Mental Health Plan, ensuring policy, services and programs are developed in a culturally appropriate manner.

Specifically, the recommended intentions are to embed social and emotional well-being teams into primary health care organisations, strengthen the Aboriginal and Torres Strait Islander workforce, stimulate mainstream mental health services and improve the journey of Aboriginal and Torres Strait Islander specific mental health services at a local primary health level.

The National Standards for Mental Health Services (Australian Government, 2010) provide guidance on implementing ongoing improvement in mental health service delivery though a periodic accreditation process.

On a more local level, Commonwealth-funded Primary Health Networks are currently negotiating various services with agencies that offer mental health programs. Non-government organisations provide non-clinical support services focusing that assist access to various agencies for people from remote areas. These services include sub-acute step-up and step-down and other supported accommodation options, as well as alcohol and other drugs services. In remote communities, the availability of these vary between locations, and generally no psychological or AOD services are available.

Aboriginal Health Practitioners and Aboriginal Mental Health Workers are invaluable. They are trained at various levels, and through their extensive cultural knowledge are able to form important links between Western and Aboriginal treatments. Often, Aboriginal people are wary of 'clinics' and for various reasons have little trust in Western medicine. For example, a loved one may have passed away at the clinic and family may not have understood why this happened and they may fear a similar demise for others, and so avoid seeking treatment at the health centre. Aboriginal Health Practitioners are in an ideal position to assist in breaking down such concerns with their knowledge of 'both sides'. These practitioners are often residents of the local community and high expectations are placed on them. They are often called by family or community residents at all hours of the night and asked to provide intervention even when employed in daytime hours only. In the long term, this is difficult to sustain and some burn out if not supported strongly by their employers.

Pleasingly, in the past years, consumers' voices are more and more taken into consideration in many aspects of mental health service planning. Invaluable views and recommendations based on lived experience are provided and contribute to service development.

Much has been written about the history and reasons that have led to the current state and gaps in health outcomes in mental health (Meadows et al., 2012). While this is important and interesting reading, it is beyond the scope of this chapter. Traditional owners and elders in remote communities encourage self-determination in the younger generations, which increases confidence and well-being among people, and encourages moving forward and taking ownership of their culture and lives. The recovery-focused approach in mental health treatments fits well with Aboriginal and Torres Strait Islander people who traditionally hold quite different worldviews, but increasingly are being encouraged to adjust to and move forward in today's milieu, and be able to meet the demands of both government policies and traditional customs.

Due to the vast distances between communities and urban centres, much time is spent by clinicians on travelling to and from remote areas. It is not uncommon for clinicians to travel many hours by bitumen and unsealed roads in 4WD vehicles, taking up a large chunks of time driving and, sadly, cutting short direct clinical services. Clinicians eventually get used to this reality and most probably have adapted to the travel demands of the job.

Mental health and Aboriginal cultural and spiritual beliefs

While most Australians have some understanding that Aboriginal people's views on life, health and belonging differ significantly from Western culture, some inaccurate views persist. For example, some remote residents of the Northern Territory travel to Darwin for a break, or a hospital appointment. Some take the opportunity to go 'long grassing', which means drinking significant amounts of alcohol while in town. This gives a rather misleading picture of Aboriginal people's ordinary lives in remote communities. Only by living in, or regularly visiting, remote communities will one get a greater understanding of traditional Aboriginal living. In many communities, alcohol is prohibited or its use limited to drinks containing lower levels of ethanol.

Another important aspect of remote living is the deep spiritual connection to people's 'Country'. Even remote communities are 'regional hubs' and a lot of people find it difficult to regularly spend time on Country or at outstations where they culturally and traditionally belong. Spending time on Country provides strength and healing. For many people it is necessary to stay on Country as it is in places with services such as schools, shops and health centres. During school holidays, in times of high need for healing or when people simply want to get away from problems, Aboriginal residents go 'bush' or back to Country to connect to their traditional and spiritual roots. There are some programs that aim to facilitate transport for families to go to Country, which is a great help—especially for those families who are socio-economically most disadvantaged. As a visiting clinician it was fascinating to observe the positive and strengthening effects on well-being a visit to Country can provide.

Further, it is important to have some understanding of family relationships. Aboriginal people are firmly placed within family in a system of kinship. This provides for guidance for roles and expectations of a person's behaviours. Although different people hold certain places in the family, compared to the Western view of family structure, Aboriginal people do not see themselves as individuals in the same way. Rather, the family is a unit of which a person is a part. In our practice as mental health nurses, this can be seen when the consumer does not speak to the clinician directly. In this case, a relative will speak on their behalf and this is considered perfectly normal. The consumer believes that the responsible relative is the proper person to speak on their behalf and the conviction with which this practice is undertaken can seem strange to the Western clinician. With this custom, it is difficult to maintain the confidentiality most of us are used to. It is not uncommon for several family members to attend a mental health nurse consultation, from young children to grandparents, especially if consumers are visited at home. It is considered perfectly normal for everyone to be involved in the care of the person.

The strength of the extended family has can be experienced when a 'family meeting' is called. To have many family representatives present to resolve a 'problem' can be impressive and powerful for clinicians to see. If senior members of the family decide on a particular course of action, other family members generally comply.

Mental health nursing in the remote context can be quite different from mainstream models of care. It is particularly important to be aware that the views on health and illness vary significantly from that of Western medicine. Health literacy must not be taken for granted by non-Aboriginal clinicians. Remote Aboriginal people often speak English as a second, third or fourth language. Also, many will readily agree to what is being discussed with the clinician, giving the impression the material discussed has been understood. Only if the person can relay what was discussed can the clinician be sure that the conversation was correctly interpreted and understood. Interpreters must be used wherever possible.

It has been the author's experience that people with a mental disorder are often not referred for treatment unless traditional intervention has failed to have the desired outcome or the illness becomes so acute that non-traditional services such as police and crisis health services are required to intervene urgently for safety reasons. Families and consumers have provided traditional explanations for one's illness that have nothing to do with Western understanding of mental illness and disorders. For example, black magic is commonly believed to be the cause of physical illness or mental health problems, as is an event that results in a change in someone's behaviour or health status; for example, a person having had a vision of a spiritual animal or being, or being in the wrong place at the wrong time. The possibilities of spiritually explaining something that has gone wrong are countless.

When new to a community or unknown to the people of a community, clinicians are treated with caution. It takes time to establish trust in a community, as aptly described by Westerman (2004):

> Indigenous people determine the appropriateness of the practitioner through being able to see and judge them. This often occurs through a spiritual dimension—that is, a sense of the person's strength and goodness of spirit is often the basis upon which engagement will occur.

The turnover of non-Indigenous nurses and others working in remote communities is high (Mahood, 2012) which impedes the development of trusting relationships. People take up positions in remote towns for various reasons, including expectations of life in the bush. If such expectations are unfulfilled, people tend to move away sooner than anticipated.

On the upside, there are advantages of the Aboriginal views on well-being and illness. Through strong family relationships, mental illness is generally well accepted with little associated stigma. The experience of this author suggests consumers may exhibit symptoms of mental illness (such as a psychosis) for an extended period of time before coming to the attention of visiting mental health clinicians. Often, family and consumers do not engage in questioning the person about their illness experience or attempt to find reasons for the their condition; and information about prognosis is rarely asked. The attitude taken by the consumer and family is one of optimism and acceptance—'That's just how he or she is'. The mental health clinician nevertheless provides ongoing psycho-education and treatment interventions based on individual need.

Some valuable and culturally validated resources have been developed and are widely available and used. They include the I-Bobbly App developed by the Black Dog Institute, which is used with people with depression and at risk of suicide (E-Mental Health in Practice, 2017). The Stay Strong Plan is a strengths-based treatment modality in electronic form, which is especially popular with the younger generation who often have smartphones and are more tech-savvy than the older age group (E-Mental Health in Practice, 2017). The Stay Strong Plan can be completed in paper form also and is recommended as a therapist-assisted instrument.

ABOUT THE CONSUMER   Jessie's Story

Jessie is a 21-year-old Aboriginal man who frequently moves between two communities, with or without his parents. One community is very remote and the other is remote but has a higher proportion of non-Aboriginal people in its population. The two communities fall under different geographical primary health-care jurisdictions and subsequently contact with health services can be easily interrupted when the person moves between communities without any notice given. Most health-care centres lack staff resources to ensure proactive outreach for 'non-acute' consumers.

Jessie attended the local GP clinic with his father reporting complaints of hearing voices when nobody was around, lying awake most of the night and not able to concentrate enough to focus on even simple tasks. The doctor visit was prompted by Jessie's parents, who had held concerns about his mental health for some time, but Jessie had refused to see a doctor. He was a frequent consumer of cannabis, but otherwise had been a well-functioning young man up until about a year ago.

At Jessie's request, the family decided to seek the help of a traditional healer before seeing the GP, but this resulted in only partial benefit. Following a thorough physical examination, baseline pathology investigations, CT head and ECG to exclude any organic causes for Jessie's symptoms, the doctor prescribed a low dose first-line antipsychotic tablet. Jessie refused to take the medication and requested another visit to a different traditional healer, which the family were happy to accept. He stopped smoking cannabis for some months and on further review by the GP, Jessie's symptoms were reported as improved but not resolved completely.

A few months later, the family moved to the more remote community and made contact with the local health centre as renewed concerns were apparent to the family—the symptoms had recurred. Jessie was referred to the visiting mental health nurse and a face-to-face assessment at the family's house was arranged. During the visit, Jessie made it quite clear that he wanted nothing to do with 'that white mob' and that there was nothing wrong with him. His family reported that at night-time they could sometimes hear him praying and asking for 'the thing in my head to be taken away'. While Jessie's behaviour was considered odd and family wished for Jessie to gain better functioning in the community—such as being able to hold down a job— the risk assessment identified no need to warrant involuntary treatment.

Much effort was made in the following weeks to build a therapeutic relationship with Jessie and his family, and information about possible treatments was provided. His parents were agreeable to a renewed trial of antipsychotic tablets, but Jessie again decided he did not want to try them. Eventually, attempts to see Jessie again proved fruitless; he refused to have anything to do with Western health professionals. Jessie had resumed smoking cannabis and within a week he expressed paranoid ideas, which led to him walking around the community with a weapon. Police had to be called to maintain a safe environment and to help facilitate an admission to the mental health inpatient facility via ambulance plane. While in hospital, Jessie had a swift response to treatment with psycho-social intervention and pharmacotherapy. Since returning to his community, his mental health has steadily improved and he is well engaged with health service providers. He is now employed at the local council and has maintained his well-being in the past few months.

REFLECTION QUESTIONS

1   When there are obvious signs and symptoms of psychotic illness, at what point do you think the Mental Health Act should be used to facilitate treatment? What are some of the considerations and criteria of your state or territory's Mental Health Act?

2   How would you involve the family in planning Jessie's care?

3   When developing a treatment plan with Jessie, what needs to be considered with regards to bio-psycho-socio-cultural aspects for this young man?

BOX 21.3 TAKE-HOME MESSAGES

- Break the ice—provide an opportunity for consumers and family to understand who you are.
- Establish rapport.
- Use family strengths.

- Be aware of language and literacy barriers, especially in urban settings; for example, when a consumer is required to travel interstate for an operation.
- Most of all, respect local customs—be aware that you are a guest in their community.

SECTION 3 INFLUENCES OF TRADITIONAL CULTURAL VALUES BELIEFS AND THE INTEGRATION OF TE TIRITI O WAITANGI WITHIN NURSING

GRAEME THOMPSON

BOX 21.4 PAPAKUPU: GLOSSARY

Aotearoa: New Zealand
Hauora: health
Hapu: subtribe
Iwi: nation
Kaioranga Hauora Māori: Māori Health Worker
Kaiwhakaruruhau: cultural safety
Karakia: prayer; or cleansing the way
Kaupapa Māori: a philosophical doctrine
Kia tu kia puawai: stand tall with confidence
Koha: a New Zealand Māori custom which means offering a gift
Māori: People of the land; Aotearoa, New Zealand
Mihi whakatau: informal ceremony
Pakeha: Non-Māori
Pou: supports
Pōutama: steps
Pōwhiri: formal ceremony
Rōpū: team
Tāngata whaiora: one seeking health

Tāngata whānau: Māori family
Tāngata whenua: people of the land/Earth
Te ao Māori: all things Māori
Te oranga tonu tanga: ongoing wellness for people; name of Māori mental health service for a District Health Board in New Zealand
Te Reo: Māori language
Te whare tapa wha: four cornerstones of health
Te Tiriti O Waitangi: The Treaty of Waitangi; the founding document of New Zealand, signed by Māori and pakeha in 1840
Tikanga Māori: Māori customs
Tikanga whakaaro: cultural assessment
Tino rangatiratanga: Māori self-determination
Whakapapa: history, stories or genealogy
Whakataukī: proverb
Whānau: family
Whānau ora: government policy document

This section discusses the cultural considerations that have shaped the provision of Māori mental health services within **Aotearoa**/New Zealand to date. It identifies historical factors that have led to the implementation of cultural practice within nursing and the development of Māori mental health services. It includes many terms and phrases that relate specifically to Māori and their cultural values and beliefs as supported by current legislation governing health-care delivery in Aotearoa. A glossary for these appears at the beginning of this section. **Te Reo Māori** is an official language of New Zealand (O'Brien, Boddy & Hardy, 2007).

Te Tiriti o Waitangi and cultural safety

Te Tiriti o Waitangi (1840) is the founding document of New Zealand, underpinning legislation and initiatives relating to New Zealand health services. The principles of partnership, participation and protection are incorporated into all aspects of health services (Health Practitioners Competency Assurance Act, 2003; Ministry of Health, 2008; Nursing Council of New Zealand, 2012). This document identifies duties and obligations of the Crown. Health and education providers are viewed as agents of the Crown and therefore uphold the concept of **tino rangatiratanga** (Nursing Council of New Zealand, 2011).

Irihapeti Ramsden (2002) developed the concept of kaiwhakaruruhau (cultural safety) in nursing. **Kaiwhakaruruhau** is a mechanism that allows the consumer to say whether or not a service is safe for them to approach and use. Safety is a subjective word deliberately chosen to give the power to the consumer. Designed as an educational process by Māori, it is given as a **koha** to all people who are different from the service providers, whether by gender, sexual orientation, economic and educational status, age or ethnicity. It is about the analysis of power and not the customs and habits of anybody. It also asserts that it must be the consumer who makes the final statement about the quality of care which they receive. Ramsden believed that being regardful of the differences and viewing each nurse/**tāngata whaiora** contact as a unique bicultural interaction, a relationship can be formed in a partnership of trust. This allows power to be transferred to the **tāngata whaiora**, enabling self-determination in times of ill health. The concept of cultural safety is considered to have changed the profile of nursing in New Zealand, particularly impacting on nurse education (Thompson, 2001). Of importance was Ramsden's work with educational facilities, research and the Nursing Council of New Zealand (Ramsden, 2000; Bunker, 2001), resulting in clear expectations that nurses demonstrate culturally safe practice to meet professional competencies in order to practise nursing in New Zealand (Nursing Council of New Zealand, 2012).

History of the development of Māori mental health services

A ministerial inquiry into mental health services in 1987 resulted in a document commonly referred to as the Mason Report (Ministry of Health, 1988). This report identified that mental health services had failed to provide care in a manner that incorporated the principles of *Te Tiriti O Waitangi*. A subsequent inquiry (Ministry of Health, 1996) showed there had been little or no movement to address the concerns highlighted in the Mason Report. The 1996 report was scathing in its critique of past mental health services, identifying that there were no appropriate community services and that Māori lived in an environment that was hostile to addressing their needs in a manner that acknowledged their rights as **tāngata whenua** (Ministry of Health, 1996).

Following the adoption of the *Blueprint for Mental Health Services in New Zealand* (Mental Health Commission, 1998), a strategy to address the needs of Māori was implemented. *Kia Tu Kia Puawai* (Health Funding Authority, 1999) was a signal for long-term strategies to address the mental health wellness of Māori in Aotearoa. Subsequent directives from the Mental Health Commission and Ministry of Health clearly indicated that Māori were to be consulted and involved with all aspects of health and workforce development (Ministry of Health, 2002a, 2002b, 2005, 2006, 2012; Mental Health Commission, 2001a, 2007, 2012), resulting in the development of **kaupapa** services that were underpinned by Māori models of care and included **tikanga whakaaro**.

Māori models of health care

Mason Durie (1998, 2011) provided a model for the foundation of the development of Māori mental health services: **te whare tapa wha** comprises four pou, which when in balance provides and sustains positive health and well-being (see Figure 21.1).

Te Oranga Tonu Tanga

Te Oranga Tonu Tanga, part of a Māori health directorate, is a specialist service that provides interventions and processes that acknowledge the needs of Māori who are seeking health with a kaupapa. It seeks to:

- enhance the well-being of **whānau, hapu** and **iwi** through **tikanga Māori** and restoring balance of **hauora Māori**
- restore the dreams, aspirations and hopes of **tāngata whaiora** and **whānau** through **whakapapa**.

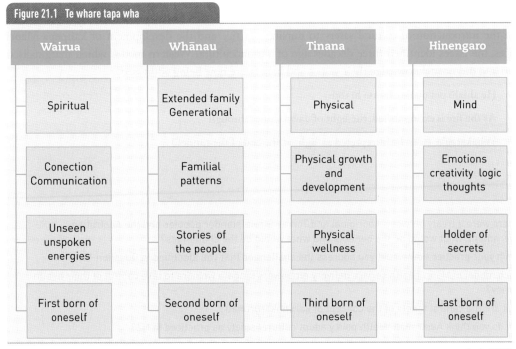

Figure 21.1 Te whare tapa wha

Wairua	Whānau	Tinana	Hinengaro
Spiritual	Extended family Generational	Physical	Mind
Conection Communication	Familial patterns	Physical growth and development	Emotions creativity logic thoughts
Unseen unspoken energies	Stories of the people	Physical wellness	Holder of secrets
First born of oneself	Second born of oneself	Third born of oneself	Last born of oneself

Durie (1998)

Cultural assessments

Tikanga whakaaro allow the **rōpū** to follow through on contributing cultural factors that **tāngata whaiora** may present with. This assists **tāngata whaiora** and **tāngata whānau** to identify and define the imbalance in their lives that contribute to their contact with mental health services (Mental Health Commission, 1998, 2001b). It is important to consider the communication between **whānau** and the multidisciplinary care team to ensure that interpretation of speech, behaviours and beliefs are not misunderstood or misinterpreted.

The **tikanga whakaaro** format highlights the **te whare tapa wha** model (Durie, 1998), which allows us to see the cultural strengths and needs of individuals and their **whānau**. A **pōutama** process such as **pōwhiri mihi whakatau** and **karakia** allows the **rōpū** to determine when **tāngata whaiora/whānau** are able to move to the next stage of assessment. It is essential to have **kaioranga hauora Māori** that can interpret and understand **te ao Māori**.

Future directions

Since 1980, significant progress has been made towards meeting the obligations of *Te Tiriti O Waitangi*, with Māori influencing health polices, education and service delivery (Durie, 2011; Gunther, 2011; Ramsden, 2002). However, it is still concerning that Māori continue to experience a higher prevalence of mental illness than non-Māori, along with delayed presentation to services, higher youth suicide rates and higher utilisation of interventions such as restraint and seclusion (Fortune et al., 2010; Mental Health Commission, 2012; Ministry of Health, 2012, 2015). The *Blueprint II* and the current service development plan (Ministry of Health, 2012) aim to consolidate the progress of the past decades with services to focus on early intervention, mental health education and more community involvement to promote self-management of mental health (Office of the Auditor-General, 2015; Te Puni Kokiri, 2015).

From the founding document *Te Tiriti O Waitangi* to present-day legislation, mental health services within Aotearoa have undergone significant restructure in relation to the provision of care for Māori. With the introduction of cultural safety to nursing practice and the development of **kaupapa Māori** services, the issues identified three decades ago of a monocultural Western model, which marginalised Māori and did not acknowledge their values and beliefs, are now being addressed.

> He ahiahi pokopoko, he ata hi tore
>
> As the fire is extinguished, the light of dawn shines through
>
> Whakataukī: (Can be interpreted as 'light at the end of the tunnel')

DISCUSSION QUESTIONS

1   If there were a treaty between Aboriginal and Torres Strait Islander peoples and the Australian Government, what would be the benefits and what would be the challenges?

2   Within your practice how would you address the challenges that you identified in Question 1?

3   Which model of Māori health service delivery empowers tāngata whaiora to take control of their health journey?

4   What are the central tenets of the concept of kaiwhakaruruhau?

5   How do you think Australian health policy adopt cultural safety as practiced in NZ?

6   Do you think a ministerial inquiry into mental health service provision is required in Australia to assess culturally safe practice in mental health?

TEST YOURSELF

1 Te Tiriti o Waitangi (1840) is the founding document of New Zealand and
   a underpins legislation and initiatives relating to New Zealand health services
   b underpins policy and procedures in health services in general
   c underpins policy and procedures in health services only in New Zealand
   d underpins health education in New Zealand

2 Irihapeti Ramsden (2002) developed the concept of cultural safety in New Zealand in
   a healthcare
   b medical care
   c nursing
   d allied health care

3 The New Zealand Mason Report (1996) showed
   a great progress in mental health services from the 1988 Manson Report
   b led to mainstreaming of services in New Zealand
   c no change on concerns identified in the 1988 Manson Report
   d created more jobs in healthcare in New Zealand

USEFUL WEBSITES

New Zealand Ministry of Health: www.health.govt.nz

Sharing the true stories: www.cdu.edu.au/centres/stts

Social Policy Evaluation and Research Unit, New Zealand: www.superu.govt.nz

Te Pou o te Whakaaro Nui: www.tepou.co.nz/

Te Rau Matatini: www.teraumatatini.com

The Treaty of Waitangi in brief: www.nzhistory.net.nz/politics/treaty/the-treaty-in-brief

REFERENCES

Australian Bureau of Statistics (2009). Causes of death, Australia: Suicides 2007. ABS Cat. No. 3303.0. Canberra: Commonwealth of Australia.

Australian Bureau of Statistics (2012). Australian Demographic Statistics, March Quarter 2012. ABS Cat. No. 3101.0. Canberra: Commonwealth of Australia.

Australian Bureau of Statistics (2013a). *Australian Aboriginal and Torres Strait Islander Health Survey: First Results, Australia, 2012–13* [Online]. Canberra. Available: www.abs.gov.au/ausstats/abs@.nsf/Lookup/4727.0.55.001main+features802012–13.

Australian Bureau of Statistics (2013b). *Estimates of Aboriginal and Torres Strait Islander Australians*, June 2011. Canberra.

Australian Bureau of Statistics (2014). *Causes of Death, Australia, 2014* [Online]. Canberra. Available: www.abs.gov.au/ausstats/abs@.nsf/Lookup/by%20Subject/3303.0~2014~Main%20 Features~Leading%20Causes%20of%20 Death~10001 [Accessed 31/07/2016 2016].

Australian Government (2010). *National Standards for Mental Health Services*. Retrieved from www.health.gov.au/internet/main/publishing.nsf/content/mental-pubs-n-servst10.

Australian Health Ministers' Advisory Council (2004a). A national strategic framework for Aboriginal and Torres Strait Islander Peoples' mental health and social emotional well-being. Canberra: Commonwealth of Australia.

Australian Health Ministers' Advisory Council (2004b). Cultural respect framework for Aboriginal and Torres Strait Islander health 2004–2009. Adelaide: Department of Health.

Australian Institute of Health and Welfare (2008). The health and welfare of Australia's Aboriginal and Torres Strait Islander peoples 2008. Canberra: AIHW.

Baxter, J., Hayes, A. & Gray, M. (2011). *Families in regional, rural and remote Australia* (Facts Sheet).

Melbourne: Australian Institute of Family Studies.

Beyondblue (2009). Mental health first aid guidelines for Aboriginal and Torres Strait Islander people. Melbourne: Beyondblue. Retrieved from www.beyondblue.org.au/index.aspx?link_id=7.102&tmp=FileDownload&fid=1344.

Bunker, W. (2001). 'Integrating cultural safety into practice'. *Kai Tiaki Nursing New Zealand*, 7(1), 18.

Cooperative Research Centre for Aboriginal Health (2008). CRC for Aboriginal Health Annual Report 2007–08. Darwin: CRCAH.

Council of Australian Governments (2008). National action plan on mental health 2006–2011: Progress report 2006–2007. Canberra: Commonwealth of Australia.

DeCrespigny, C., Kowanko, I., Murray, H., Wilson, S., Kit, J. A. & Mills, D. (2006). 'A nursing partnership for better outcomes in Aboriginal mental health, including substance use'. *Contemporary Nurse*, 22(2), 275–287.

Department of Health and Ageing (2009). *Bringing them home.* Retrieved 18 June 2009 from www. health.gov.au/internet/main/publishing.nsf/ Content/bringing-them-home-lp.

Dudgeon, P., Milroy, H., & Walker, R. (2014). *Working together: Aboriginal and Torres Strait Islander mental health and wellbeing principles and practice*, [West Perth, WA, Kulunga Research Network].

Durie, M. (1998). *Whaiora teiho Māori mental health training programme.* Retrieved from: www.teiho.org/MaoriHealthPerspective/ TirohangaMaoriByMasonDurie.aspx.

Durie, M. (2011). 'Indigenizing mental health services: New Zealand experience'. *Transcultural Psychiatry*, 48(1–2), 24–36.

E-Mental Health in Practice (2017). *eMH Services.* Retrieved from www.emhprac.org.au/services/.

Fortune, S., Watson, P., Robinson, E., Fleming, T., Merry, S., & Denny, S. (2010).*Youth '07: The health and wellbeing of secondary school students in New Zealand: Suicide behaviours and mental health in 2001 and 2007.* Auckland: The University of Auckland.

Gunther, S. (2011). 'Disparity in mental health provision for Māori and Pacific: A nursing response'. *Whitireia Nursing Journal*, 18, 39–43.

Hart, L. M., Jorm, A. F., Kanowski, L. G., Kelly, C. M. & Langlands, R. L. (2009). 'Mental health first aid for Indigenous Australians: Using Delphi consensus studies to develop guidelines for culturally appropriate responses to mental health problems'. *BMC Psychiatry*, 9(1), 47. doi:10.1186/1471-244x-9-47.

Haswell, M., Hunter, E., Wargent, R., Hall, B., O'Higgins, C. & West, R. (2009). Protocols for the delivery of social and emotional well-being and mental health services in Indigenous communities: Guidelines for health workers, clinicians, consumers and carers. Cairns: University of Queensland and Queensland Health.

Health Funding Authority (1999). Kia Tu Kia Puawai. Health Practitioner Competency Assurance Act 2003. Wellington: Government of New Zealand.

Health Practitioners Competency Assurance Act 2003 (NZ)

Henderson, S., Andrews, G. & Hall, W. (2000). 'Australia's mental health: an overview of the general population survey'. *Australian and New Zealand Journal of Psychiatry*, 34(2), 197–205.

Indigenous Health Infonet (2009). Australian Indigenous mental health: Key issues. Retrieved from http://indigenous.ranzcp.org/index2. php?option=com_content&task=view&id=12&p.

Mahood, K. (2012). 'Kartiya are like Toyotas: White workers on Australia's cultural frontier'. *Griffith Review*, 36, 43–59.

Meadows, G., Farhall, J., Fossey, E., Grigg, M. & Mcdermott, F. & Singh, B. 2012. *Mental Health in Australia– Collaborative Community Practice*, Melbourne, Oxford.

Mental Health Commission (1998). *Blueprint for mental health services in New Zealand.* Wellington: Author.

Mental Health Commission (2001a). *Recovery competencies for New Zealand mental health workers.* Wellington: Author.

Mental Health Commission (2001b). *Cultural assessment processes for Maori.* Wellington: Author.

Mental Health Commission (2007). *Te Haererenga Mo te Whakaoranga 1996–2006: The journey of recovery for the New Zealand health sector.* Wellington: Author.

Mental Health Commission (2012). *Blueprint II: How things need to be.* Wellington: Author.

Mental Health Directorate 2015. NT Suicide Prevention Action Plan 2015–2018. Darwin: Department of Health.

Ministry of Health (1988). *Report of the committee of inquiry into procedures used in certain psychiatric hospitals in relation to admission, discharge or release on leave of certain classes of patients.* Wellington: Author.

Ministry of Health (1996). *Report of a ministerial inquiry to the Minister of Health Hon. Jenny Shipley. Inquiry under section 47 of the Health and Disability Services Act 1993 in respect of certain mental health services.* Wellington: Author.

Ministry of Health (2002a). *Te Puawaitanga: Maori mental health national strategic framework.* Wellington: Author.

Ministry of Health (2002b). *Maori health strategy.* Wellington: Author.

Ministry of Health (2005). *Te Tahuhu: Improving mental health 2005–2015.* Wellington: Author.

Ministry of Health (2006). *Te Kokiri: The mental health and addiction action plan 2006–2015.* Wellington: Author.

Ministry of Health (2008). *New Zealand Standard: Health and Disability standards.* Wellington: Hutcheson Bowman & Stewart.

Ministry of Health (2012). *Rising to the challenge: The mental health and addiction service development plan 2012–2017.* Wellington: Author.

Ministry of Health (2015). *Office of the Director of mental health annual report 2014.* Wellington: Author. Retrieved from: www. health.govt.nz.

National Mental Health Commission (2014). Specific Challenges for Aboriginal and Torres Strait Islander People: A Summary of the National Review of Mental Health Programmes and Services. Sydney: National Mental Health Commission.

National Mental Health Commission (2015). Response to the Commission's mental health review: Contributing Lives, Thriving Communities.

National Public Health Partnership (2004). The National Aboriginal and Torres Strait Islander Safety Promotion Strategy. Canberra: NPHP.

Nursing Council of New Zealand (2011). *Guidelines for cultural safety, the Treaty of Waitangi and Māori health in nursing education and practice.* Wellington: Author. Retrieved from www. nursingcouncil.org.nz.

Nursing Council of New Zealand (2012). *Competencies for registered nurses.* Wellington: Author. Retrieved from http:// www.nursingcouncil.org.nz.

O'Brien, A. P., Boddy, J. M. & Hardy, D. J. (2007). 'Culturally specific process measures to improve mental health clinical practice: Indigenous focus'. *Australian and New Zealand Journal of Psychiatry*, 41, 667–674.

Office of the Auditor-General (2015). *Whānau Ora: The first four Years.* Wellington, New Zealand. Retrieved from: htpp://www.oag.govt.nz.

Ramsden, I. (2000). Cultural safety/Kawawharuruhau ten years on: A personal overview. *Nursing Praxis in New Zealand*, 15(1), 2000, 4–12.

Ramsden, I. (2001). 'Improving practice through research'. Kai Tiaki Nursing New Zealand, 7(1), 23–26.

Ramsden, I. (2002). *Cultural safety and nursing education in Aotearoa and Te Waipounamu.* (Unpublished doctoral thesis). Victoria University of Wellington.

Raphael, B. & Swan, P. (1997). 'The mental health of Aboriginal and Torres Strait Islander People'. *International Journal of Mental Health*, 26(3), 9–22.

Slade, T., Johnston, A., Teesson, M., Whiteford, H., Burgess, P., Pirkis, J., & Saw, S., (2009). The Mental Health of Australians: 2, Report on the 2007 National Survey of Mental Health and Wellbeing. Canberra: Commonwealth of Australia.

Te Puni Kokiri (2015). *Understanding whānau-centred approaches: Analysis of Phase One Whānau Ora research and monitoring results.* Wellington, New Zealand: Author. Retrieved from: htpp:// www.tpk.govt.nz.

Thompson, S. (2001). 'Developing a cultural safety curriculum'. Kai Tiaki Nursing New Zealand, 7(1), 14–5.

Usher, K., Foster, K. & Bullock, S. (2009). *Psychopharmacology for health professionals.* Chatswood: Elsevier.

Vicary, D. A. & Westerman, T. G. (2004). "That's just the way he is': Some implications of Aboriginal mental health beliefs'. *Australian e-Journal for the Advancement of Mental Health*, 3(3), 1–10: Retrieved from www.auseinet.co/ journal/vol3iss3/vicarywesterman.pdf.

Westerman, T. G. (2003). Development of an inventory to assess the moderating effects of cultural resilience with Aboriginal youth at risk of depression, anxiety and suicidal behaviours. Unpublished PhD thesis. Perth: Curtin University, School of Psychology.

Westerman, T. G. (2004). Engagement of Indigenous clients in mental health services: What role do cultural differences play? *Australia e-journal for the Advancement of Mental Health*, 3, 1–7.

CHAPTER 22

Cultural and Linguistic Diversity

DON GORMAN,
WENDY CROSS AND
SUZANNE WILLEY

Acknowledgment

The authors would like to acknowledge the contribution of Philippa Duell-Piening who co-wrote this chapter in the second edition.

KEY OUTCOMES

AFTER READING THIS CHAPTER, YOU SHOULD BE ABLE TO:

- describe the cultural issues that influence mental health and health care
- discuss different cultural beliefs related to mental health and health care
- explore the application of cultural safety to mental health nursing practice
- identify appropriate strategies for mental health nurses to work with consumers from a cultural background other than their own
- define and describe the unique characteristics of the refugee experience and how these may impact on a person's mental health
- analyse practice approaches within the mental health-care sector when working with people from refugee backgrounds

KEY TERMS

- acculturation
- asylum seeker
- cross-cultural practice
- culturally and linguistically diverse (CALD)
- ethnic
- ethnocentrism
- internally displaced persons
- refugee
- resettlement
- somatisation
- stigma
- torture
- trauma

Introduction

This chapter introduces you to the importance of culturally based health beliefs and practices to mental health and well-being, and to health care delivered by mental health nurses. There is a need for mental health professionals to incorporate knowledge about these beliefs and to develop the skills to work with consumers from cultures other than their own if they are to care for them effectively (Australian College of Mental Health Nurses, 2010).

A significant number of people from culturally and linguistically diverse (CALD) backgrounds are also asylum seekers or refugees who often experience additional trauma and losses, and this chapter will devote a section specifically to their needs.

Culture

Although most people would say that they know what *culture* is, most would have difficulty defining it, and few are aware of their own culture or the degree to which it affects their perception or expectations of other people. Culture is a major determinant of beliefs, morals and customs, and consequently behaviour. We live by thousands of rules, most of which we are not conscious of until we meet someone who breaks them, and then we commonly experience an emotional reaction that can range from discomfort to revulsion.

Baldwin and colleagues (2006) discuss the complexity of defining culture and provide a reference list of 313 definitions, arguing that the term is used in many different ways, while acknowledging that it is important to ensure that there is an agreed understanding about what we mean by the term.

Sadock and Sadock (2007), taking a mental health focus, describe culture as:

> a vast, complex concept that is used to encompass the behaviour patterns and lifestyle of the society ... Culture consists of shared symbols, artefacts, beliefs, values, and attitudes. It is manifested in rituals, customs, and laws and is perpetuated and reflected in share sayings, legions, literature, art, diet, costume, religion, making preferences, child-rearing practices, entertainment, recreation, philosophical thought, and government.

Whether the group is an ethnic group or group of people with a common set of beliefs—for example, those based on sexual preferences, age or gender—the culture of the members of this group can be described as their worldview.

Much of culture is learned unconsciously through interaction with others in the cultural group, especially family, friends and school. Because cultural values are largely unconscious, expectations of other people's behaviour are also unconscious. This means that our reaction to other people breaching those expectations tends to be emotional and judgmental. For example, in Anglo-Celtic cultures, failure to look someone in the eye when speaking can create suspicion that the person is dishonest. Conversely, in many other cultures direct eye contact is considered rude, disrespectful or even aggressive.

The unconscious nature of cultural values and beliefs tends to make us think that they are universal, so there is an expectation that all people, regardless of culture, will hold the same beliefs and values. This gives rise to ethnocentrism, where others' behaviour is judged by the cultural rules of the observer. The tendency to believe that our own beliefs and values are universally right can lead us to judge other cultures as morally inferior to our own.

An important aspect of culture is that of the roles that individuals undertake in society, and how those rights and responsibilities interact with each other. For example, in the Anglo-Celtic culture, gender roles have traditionally relegated responsibility for providing food and disciplining children to males, while caring for the children and looking after the house have been the responsibility of females. Today these roles have changed, with many couples sharing or reversing these roles, reflecting a broad change towards valuing equality; thus cultural values and beliefs are not static but change over time.

Symbolism is another aspect of culture that develops over time, and results in concepts becoming value laden, with the present members of the society not necessarily understanding their origins. An example of a powerful symbol in Anglo-Celtic cultures is that of Christmas. While Christmas originated in the Christian religion, most Anglo-Celtic Australians, regardless of their religious beliefs, consider it an important time that's laden with non-religious positive values, and often associated with family rituals.

As a multicultural society, Australia has many different cultural groups of people. It would be a mistake to stereotype these groups, suggesting that all members of a group hold identical values and beliefs to the same degree, or to imply that the groups are radically different from each other. In reality, these cultural groups have more in common with each other than they have differences, and while members of a group have much in common, there are individual differences, and considerable variation can occur within groups.

Society needs its members to work together for the common good of all. In a multicultural society, that means that the different cultures need to meet and function together. For this meeting to be fruitful, the covert cultural values, beliefs, rules, behaviours and symbols that can create barriers to understanding and acceptance need to be addressed. There is no area of society where this is more important than in relation to health and health care. Cross-cultural research in the area of mental illness has concentrated on differential definitions, symptomatology and the treatment of a variety of illnesses.

Mental health services must be accessible and appropriate to all, and should address specific culture-related needs. Ideally, there would be adequate bilingual health professionals who are culturally sensitive and competent. But because it is impossible to match all clinicians ethnically with consumers, it is important for all mental health professionals to have a culturally appropriate approach to caring for culturally and linguistically diverse (CALD) people. Moreover, it is important that appropriately translated information packages are available to inform people from CALD backgrounds about availability of mental health services.

CRITICAL THINKING OPPORTUNITY

1   What are the main reasons why you need to be culturally appropriate in your approach to caring for those from a CALD background?

2   How do your attitudes, beliefs and behaviours compare to those described in the literature concerning CALD appropriate care practices?

Culture and health

As with all values and beliefs, those relating to health and health care are culturally derived and vary between cultures. Some examples of beliefs relevant to health include:

- the impact of external forces such as weather, spirits or supernatural forces, karma and luck
- the relative importance of the individual as opposed to community
- the role of emotions in illness, either causative or symptomatic
- the role of the family in care, ranging from virtually none to expecting that the family or the head of the family will make all decisions about care and treatment.

Different cultures define health differently. Anglo-Celtic culture classifies health and illness into quite specific categories, commonly based on physiological systems. There is a major division, for example, between mental health and physical health. This categorisation is alien to a number of cultures, which can, for example, view health as a broad, holistic concept that not only does not distinguish between mental health and physical health, but also incorporates the idea of health and well-being of the entire community and of the land to which that community is attached.

Specific health beliefs

Beliefs about the causes of illness have an obvious relationship to beliefs about appropriate treatments. For instance, if you believe that an illness is caused by a cancerous growth, the removal of that growth can seem a logical treatment. If, however, you believe that the illness is caused by inappropriate diet, then the logical treatment is to change the diet. The following are examples of a variety of beliefs about what illness or health may be attributed to:

- *yin and yang*—which permeate all of nature; yang represents the positive, male energy that produces light, warmth and fullness; and yin represents the female, negative energy, the force of darkness, coldness and emptiness

- *hot and cold*—foods are classified as 'hot', 'cold' or 'neutral', not in terms of temperature or spiciness but on other grounds: if a person complains of being 'hot', he or she does not necessarily have a fever but may have a symptom, such as constipation, dark urine or hoarseness, believed to be caused by an imbalance of heat in the body
- *good luck* or *leading a good life*—either in the past or the present
- illness caused by *evil spirits* or exposure to *polluting sources*, such as blood, sick people and dead bodies; treatment is through purification rituals such as hot spring baths and herbal infusions
- *possession* by a demon, or the 'evil eye'
- *air* (wind) or *water*—which may be good or bad; a bad wind can act quickly to induce high fever, convulsion and even sudden death; whereas bad water is believed to have a slower effect on health, causing chronic fever, anaemia or muscle wasting
- *ghost possession or sorcerery.*

Such illnessness may be treated by:

- *tiger balm*—a mentholated ointment used for a variety of conditions, including colds, upset stomach, bruises and insect bites
- *tonics*—such as ginseng
- *coining*—creating small bruises on the body, commonly effected by rubbing the body with a coin or a spoon
- *a cloth wrapped around the abdomen*—to provide protection, especially for children, aged people and pregnant women
- *herbal medicine*
- *acupuncture*—the Chinese method of placing sharpened thin sticks or needles into particular places on the skin
- *moxibustion*—the burning of small balls of moxa or dried mugwort on appropriate pressure points
- *ayurvedic medicine*—the ancient Indian medical system
- *cupping*—placing a hot cup on the body and letting it cool until the air contracts and draws the skin upward.

Ill-health is usually associated with suffering in some form. Suffering is also defined by culture, how it is perceived, and the meaning attributed to it. The experience of suffering varies between cultural groups. Culture determines how a person should expect to tolerate suffering in a given situation, and how to behave. In some cultures, for example, labour pain is experienced as suffering, while in others it is more likely to be seen as normal. The degree to which pain should be expressed also varies considerably between cultures.

The response to pain by others is also culturally determined, so that judgments about and interpretations of people's suffering by nurses are influenced by their cultural background. Anglo-Celtic cultures, for example, tend to endorse the attitude of 'stiff upper lip', denying the right of people to express suffering. Overt expression of pain may be labelled as 'attention seeking'. This can lead to negative judgments about consumers from other cultures, and even a resentment of the demands on the nurse's time when asked to respond to complaints. This leads us into discussion about the impact of culture on the provision of health care.

ABOUT THE CONSUMER Bogdan's story

Bogdan is a 50-year-old Romanian man with a preliminary diagnosis of paranoid schizophrenia. He is admitted suffering from hallucinations and delusions that people are trying to harm him. English is not his first language, but he does speak broken English, and appears to understand everything that is said to him.

When his nurse approaches him to encourage him with activities of daily living, he becomes aggressive towards her, and orders her to leave him alone. He then tries to abscond, and when he is stopped he says that the nurse wants to harm him, and that he must leave the hospital before she succeeds. Given his aggressive behaviour and his apparent incorporation of the nurse into his delusions, he is kept in for assessment, resulting in him becoming highly distressed and aggressive. Consequently he is placed in seclusion and sedated.

Eventually it is determined that he is not suffering a mental illness. Communication difficulties and a failure to understand his cultural background meant that his behaviour was misunderstood.

Many people from Eastern European cultures believe in the ability of some people to cause harm to others through curses. This is sometimes called the Evil Eye. Bogdan had been experiencing pains and general ill health since having an argument with an elderly female neighbour and his nurse reminded him of her. He believed that the nurse was acting in his neighbour's interests and trying to harm him.

REFLECTION QUESTIONS

1 Cultural safety requires that the consumer feels that his or her culture is respected, and that the person is not judged by the values of another culture. What steps could have been taken to ensure that Bogdan's cultural values were taken into consideration?

2 Given that he only spoke broken English, what steps could have been taken to minimise communication barriers?

Somatisation: symptom expression

Many people migrate to Australia under traumatic circumstances. Therefore, it would be reasonable to assume that mental health service utilisation would be high. However, this is not the case. Many researchers have found that service access by CALD groups is significantly low (Lindert et al., 2009; Minas et al., 2013; Steel et al., 2006). One needs to examine the belief systems of a cultural group to glean an understanding of the reasons for this lack of utilisation of services. It has been noted that some adults do not willingly self-disclose mental illness symptoms, and view mental illness as stigmatising, both for themselves and for their family. People may be feeling wretched within but be outwardly smiling. Some researchers support the custom of somatisation (discussed below) as a means of expressing psychological difficulties. This, however, is also seen in Western cultures. We could assume, therefore, that CALD consumers might not meet criteria for some mental illnesses because of a failure to report some of the psychological symptoms (Kiropoulos, Blashki & Klimidis, 2005; Minas et al., 2013).

Somatisation refers to the expression of physical symptoms that are not explained by observable organic pathology, and may be a result of hypochondriasis or as somatic manifestations of anxiety and other disorders. Early researchers deduced that somatisation is more likely to be observed in non-Western societies than in Western societies, but non-Western writers have suggested that much of the research into physical complaints exhibited by non-Western people have been conducted using a Western framework, and as such lose validity because cultural conditions have been ignored. Moreover, cultural stereotypes have contributed to the assumption that the non-expression of emotions is an expected feature for certain cultural groups (for example, Asian). Perhaps the presentation of physical symptoms satisfies the twofold objective of gaining entry into the service system and to maintain social acceptance and support among communities where mental illness is strongly stigmatised.

Somatisation has been described as a universal phenomenon. In Britain, more that 50 per cent of people with a mental illness had solicited help for physical problems, and in the USA up to 70 per cent of those with diagnosable mental illnesses present with somatic symptoms. Many studies of mental disorders found high correlations between observable psychological problems and somatisation (Sadock & Sadock, 2007).

Although it has been traditionally believed that somatisation occurs predominantly in non-Western countries, the reasons offered to explain these beliefs have varied. Some claim that people from low socio-economic status and who are illiterate have inadequate language skills to communicate their emotions verbally, and therefore express their psychological distress through physical symptoms. In a few cultures there is no language equivalent for certain psychological problems, and overt expression of feelings is seen as a sign of weakness and is socially undesirable. The harmful social consequences of mental illness and the associated stigma may prevent the reporting of psychological distress in these cultures.

The *International Classification of Diseases* (ICD) and the *Diagnostic and Statistical Manual of Mental Disorders* (DSM) include somatisation under the axiom of somatoform disorders, whereby people have constant physical complaints despite reassurances that there is no organic pathology to explain them. These ongoing symptoms result in impaired social and familial functioning.

Acculturation

Acculturation is the process whereby migrants acquire the values and behavioural norms of the host country. Simple acculturation occurs when new residents become more like host residents over time (Sam & Berry, 2010).

Often there are major differences between pre-migration cultural values and attitudes and host country values and attitudes. Assimilation has been associated with poorer mental health among migrants (Gee et al., 2006). The partially acculturated individual may also be marginalised from both cultural groups, and may experience discrimination, which has been shown to be associated with poorer mental health status.

The acculturation literature is mixed. Not only does it lack clear evidence for any of the theoretical perspectives, but the evidence that exists is also contradictory. Almost equal numbers of studies support either a positive or negative relationship between acculturation and mental health. Acculturation is different with different populations, and varies with the instrument used to measure it. A meta-analysis by Yoon and colleagues (2012) confirm these mixed results.

Measuring acculturation is achieved conceptually, using scales that address the adoption of dominant culture values as well as those that measure linguistic fluency as a means of accessing the dominant society. There is a strong relationship between mental health service use and level of acculturation, whereby those being more acculturated have greater service use. In addition, socioeconomic status is an important issue that needs to be addressed when discussing relationships between ethnicity and psychological distress

(Cross & Singh, 2012). Further, the influence of socioeconomic status is related to whether the population is more urban or more rural in nature. Crockett and colleagues (2007) showed that higher acculturative stress was linked to higher levels of anxiety and depression among Mexican-American college students. They also showed there was a buffering effect from social support from parents. A few studies examining acculturation and depression among Latino populations have shown that higher levels of acculturation are associated with higher levels of depression (Davilla, McFall & Cheng, 2009).

ABOUT THE CONSUMER Jay's story

Jay is a 50-year-old Malaysian man who has been working in Australia managing his own small business. He speaks some English, but his wife speaks very little. He is admitted suffering from depression, and tends to sit in his room and avoid interacting with anyone except his wife when she visits. He refuses to eat the food provided to him, and staff are not sure if this is because of a lack of energy and appetite or if he is trying to starve himself. Attempts to encourage him to eat result in aggressive verbal responses, and when a nurse tries to spoon-feed him he knocks the food from her hand.

Staff have become increasingly frustrated by his behaviour, and it is decided to begin tube feeding, when one of the staff discovers his wife smuggling in food to him. Initially, staff are quite angry at what they perceive as an attempt to feign starvation. It is decided to call in an interpreter to discuss this with him and his wife. Only then is it discovered that they are Muslims, and he has been refusing to eat any food not prepared by his wife as he is concerned that it is not *halal* (prepared according to Muslim law). If staff were practising cultural safety, this should not have happened.

REFLECTION QUESTIONS

1 What culturally safe practices could have discovered the dietary requirements earlier?

2 How could the misunderstanding of his behaviour have been avoided?

3 What are some of the reasons why cultural groups do not access mental health services?

4 How would you integrate cultural behaviours and practices into your nursing assessment of consumers?

5 How can symptom expression differ between cultural groups?

Migration, health and being a member of a minority group

Although immigration requirements ensure that migrants have a high standard of health, many minority groups, including ethnic minorities, are commonly disadvantaged in society. Cultural and linguistic barriers to utilising a health-care system that they are unfamiliar with can have an accumulative effect on top of a reduction in socioeconomic status and in support systems such as family, friends and carers. Compounding the above, many migrants experience culture shock, discrimination and racism, all of which can result in a mistrust of the health-care system and make them reluctant to participate in health care.

Pernice and colleagues (2009) state that post-migration factors are more likely to be related to depression and anxiety than to demographic characteristics. Such factors include host country discrimination, isolation and loneliness, unemployment and the detachment of ethnic enclaves affected by anxiety and depression. Immigrants who had arrived within six months expressed symptoms either of anxiety, depression or both. Those who had been residing in the host country for longer than six years appeared to experience lower levels of depression, suggesting that mental health may improve over time. Religion and gender mitigate the effects to some extent. For example, Buddhists are less like to express depression or anxiety than other religious groups among migrants, and males are also less likely to experience anxiety than females.

Much of the research regarding ethnicity and mental illness has been descriptive. Moreover, this research has depended on treatment rates and case identification to estimate rates of illness. They do not address the untreated population, and are therefore limited for identifying causality. They often express different pathways to treatment rather than illness per se, and the attitudes expressed are embedded in Western psychiatry, so fail to explain any potential cultural differences in either expression or experience of illness.

CRITICAL THINKING OPPORTUNITY

1   What factors do you think would lead to migrant mistrust of the health-care system?

2   How would you enhance access to and utilisation of health-care services for migrant groups?

3   What further research is required to explain the potential cultural differences in relation to expression and experience of mental illness?

Culture and health care

Australia's health-care system is based on Anglo-Celtic cultural beliefs about health, health-related behaviours and health care. When consumers from non Anglo-Celtic cultures need to access health-care services, the differences between their cultural beliefs and values and those of the health-care service provider can create barriers to them receiving appropriate care (Cross & Singh, 2012; Gorman, Nielsen & Best, 2006).

Health care in Australia is based on scientific knowledge. Treatment regimes are formulated on the basis of what is believed to be scientifically proven data about cause and effect. Belief in the scientific method is very strong, and this increases the ethnocentric tendency to believe that the care is unquestionably correct. Even if this belief is correct, the success of treatment is highly dependent on the consumer believing in both the treatment and the health professional. Without this belief, the treatment is less likely to be effective and some consumers are less likely to participate in it.

Australian government policies emphasise equity for all cultural groups (Commonwealth of Australia, 2012), but to meet this requirement for equity, staff need to be able to understand their consumers' needs and their cultural perspective of those needs. If this is not the case, consumers can be seriously disadvantaged in terms of the care they receive.

Nursing and communication

One fundamental requirement for meeting a consumer's needs is effective communication between the consumer and the health-care professional. Cultural differences can impede communication, and this can be exacerbated if the consumer comes from a non-English-speaking background. Lack of information about treatment has been identified as being a major disadvantage non-Anglo-Celtic mental health consumers in Australia (Cross & Bloomer, 2010). A failure in communication can result in:

- the consumer's lack of knowledge of the purpose or side effects of drugs
- admission without knowledge of the treatment to be given
- treatment without consent
- misidentification of consumer
- inappropriate discharge
- culturally inappropriate treatment; for example, the administration of a blood transfusion to a consumer whose religious beliefs forbid it, or the administration of oral medications that contain alcohol to a consumer whose culture forbids the intake of alcohol.

Utilisation of services

Collecting information about patterns of service use by migrants is achieved using a variety of criteria. Unfortunately, these criteria are not uniform, which means that comparisons cannot be made. Other limitations in the research surrounding service utilisation have made interpretation of the results difficult. Limitations relate to: information gathered on treated populations only; the unreliability of cross-cultural diagnosis; incomplete records; cultural reliability and validity of standardised instruments; problems with self-reports; and the costs associated with large sample sizes. What we do know is that CALD groups generally underutilise mental health services. Factors associated with low utilisation rates include stigma, limited proficiency in English language, traditional health beliefs (Chan & Parker, 2004; Hsiao et al., 2006), lack of cultural sensitivity, inappropriateness of treatment models; and lack of cultural competency (Chui, Wei & Lee, 2006; Snowden & Yamada, 2005).

Anikeeva and colleagues (2010) indicate that while migrants to Australia were mentally healthy when they arrived, this deteriorated within one year, with higher rates of a range of mental disorders. They also had lower hospitalisation rates than people of the broader community. They attributed this in part to a lack of knowledge about available services, stigma about mental health and difficulty in communication. Consequently, when these consumers were admitted it was often involuntary and at an advanced stage of illness. In addition, CALD people tend to have longer average lengths of stay in the public system, especially for depression and schizophrenia and their related disorders. Furthermore, they are inclined to stay until they are considered well enough for discharge by clinicians, and have lower twenty-eight-day readmission rates. There are no significant differences in the numbers of occasions of service for community service provision.

Although overall hospitalisation rates are lower than average, the proportion of those hospitalised involuntarily is up to three times higher, which suggests that people from CALD backgrounds do not voluntarily seek admission. Moreover, they are more likely to be placed on a community treatment order. They are also overrepresented in the forensic population (Cross & Singh, 2012).

Stigma

The word 'stigma' has its origins in Greek. It means 'to mark the body with a burn or cut to signify that the person is shameful'. With time, its meaning has evolved to refer to a mark of social disgrace. It is more than just a negative connotation; it also invokes rejection, stereotyping and discrimination (SANE Australia, 2013). In Australia today, most forms of discrimination have slowly weakened, although there remains room for improvement in some areas. It is now socially and legally intolerable to discriminate against or ridicule someone (that is, stigmatise them) on the basis of their sex, disability, race, age, sexual preference, criminal record, trade union activity, political opinion, religion or social origin.

Mental illness still creates confusion, prejudice and fear. Some people with mental illness state that the stigma can be worse than the illness itself. According to SANE Australia (2013), stigma against people with a mental illness often involves inaccurate and hurtful representations of them as violent, comical or incompetent—dehumanising and making people an object of fear or ridicule. People may be less prepared to offer support and empathy to someone with a mental illness than a person with a physical one. Some people with a mental illness have found that others become awkward or suspicious around them, and that they lose connections with family and friends. The stigma surrounding mental illness is not confined to Western cultures.

While stigma is a significant problem in mental health, there are additional implications in relation to CALD communities. Knifton and colleagues (2010) found variations in patterns of stigma between communities which suggested were due to cultural conceptualisations of mental health. While it would seem logical that these differences exist the underlying reasons for stigma be taken into account when trying to reduce it as there is little evidence that programs to address stigma address cultural factors.

However, the post-migration experience has positively influenced their attitudes, so that the mentally ill have become more visible, positive treatment outcomes are being observed, and greater tolerance and understanding in Australia has developed towards the mentally ill. However, mental illness is still viewed as a family responsibility, and generally hidden from the community. Help-seeking is lessened because people will not acknowledge that mental illness exists; they also fear stigma and being 'locked up' for life. Men are more likely to indulge in alcohol to cope with their problems, because help-seeking is seen as a threat to their masculinity. Women avoid help because of social isolation, the dual burden of work and family responsibilities and the consequences of varying forms of abuse they have endured throughout their lives (Meadows, Singh, & Grigg, 2007).

CRITICAL THINKING OPPORTUNITY

1　What do you believe are some of the reasons for community confusion, prejudice and fear of those who experience mental illness?

2　In your capacity as a nurse, how can you work towards minimising the negative impact of confusion, prejudice and fear related to mental illness?

Working with people from CALD backgrounds

When clinicians show respect for cultural differences and attempt to demonstrate cultural understanding, as well as use appropriate cultural resources, the therapeutic alliance is enhanced (DeRosa & Kochurka, 2006).

An important point of clarification needs to be made. There is a great difference between cultural competence and cultural sensitivity. Although many clinicians are sensitive to the cultural issues and needs involved with mentally ill consumers, they may not be competent to deliver culturally compatible care. Many clinicians develop their own unique ways of incorporating cultural sensitivity into their practice. However, few have completed formal cultural studies, and most learn about cultural differences through interactions with people from other cultures. Whether the care they provide to consumers is actually culturally competent or not is cause for question.

Cultural competency

Culturally competent health care is a multilevel responsibility of the individual, organisation and system, and 'is a set of congruent behaviours, attitudes, and policies that come together in a system, agency or among professionals and enable that system, agency or those professions to work effectively in cross-cultural situations' (Cross et al., 1989).

Working cross-culturally is not just developing an understanding of the different cultural groups that access your service, but, rather, is an integrated and holistic approach to consumer care. Nurses who are effective and develop culturally competent nursing care are encouraged to acknowledge their own culture, by means of:

- making sense of one's self, including one's view of life and understanding the underlying patterns of thinking, feeling and acting
- making sense of one's surroundings to include attitudes, behaviour, assumptions and values
- making sense of how one interacts between language, social structure, religion, worldview, environment, economy, technology, beliefs and values
- making sense of what one takes for granted (Benson & Thistlethwaite, 2009).

Other attributes of the culturally competent nurse are knowledge, attitude and skill (Suurmond et al., 2010). Nurses are advised to develop a knowledge of the political and humanitarian situation of the person's country of origin and the effects of the refugee experience; have an attitude that demonstrates self-awareness of the nurse's own individual behaviour, thinking and prejudices; and mix this with the skill and ability to develop trusting relationships and sensitively ask difficult questions (Suurmond et al., 2010).

Nurses who have the capacity for cultural self-assessment and the ability to provide advocacy within organisations and the health system begin to improve the health and well-being of people from diverse cultural backgrounds by creating environments of inclusiveness and trust. Improving access to services reduces health disparity and improves the health and well-being of individuals, families and communities from refugee backgrounds.

CRITICAL THINKING OPPORTUNITY

1 Do you know other people who have different customs and beliefs from your own? When you visit or they visit you, what customs are observed?

- Do you bring a gift, food or drinks to share?
- Do you make a time to see each other or just drop by to their house?
- Do you accept an invitation after they have invited you only once?
- Do you remove your shoes before you enter their house?
- Does it matter to you if they have cleaned their house before you visit?
- What beliefs underpin these customs and behaviours?

2 How can you integrate culturally competent practices into your nursing practice? What are some of the ways you are able to improve your ability to practise self-awareness and improve your knowledge, attitude and skill in working with people from refugee backgrounds?

Working with interpreters

Essential to working with people from refugee backgrounds is the use of interpreters, for without effective communication a clinical interaction is not meaningful and may result in gross miscommunications. Using interpreters is known to:

- improve quality of care
- have better health outcomes as the health practitioner is able to better understand the consumer's health concerns
- result in greater consumer satisfaction
- enable informed decision-making and consent to take place
- promote adherence to treatment and medication management (Victorian Foundation for Survivors of Torture, 2013).

Interpreters should be used in all interactions with consumers who have limited ability to speak the same language as the nurse, and have the added benefit of acting as a 'cultural conduit' between the nurse and consumer.

When working with interpreters it is important to brief them about the nature of the visit, and instruct them to interpret everything you ask accurately and not to paraphrase. For example, a mental health nurse may have a way of leading into sensitive questions such as those around a consumer's safety, so it is important that an interpreter does not skip the lead-up questions and directly ask, 'Do you feel suicidal?' Likewise, it is important to brief the interpreter about accurately translating what the consumer is saying and not trying to paraphrase the content so 'it makes sense'. In order to gain a sense of a person's mental state it is important to have an accurate picture of what they are saying. Where it is appropriate and possible, using the same interpreter for consecutive appointments is recommended.

When booking an interpreter, consider the consumer's preference for gender and age in light of cultural protocols; for example, younger people may defer to older people, or there may be taboos about speaking about certain topics in front of the opposite gender. Choice of interpreter may greatly alter the quality of the interaction. Especially important with refugee communities is consideration for the ethnicity of the interpreter—some consumers may not want someone from their own community due to fear of gossip about a very personal matter; others may not want an interpreter from the ethnic group that had been oppressing them in their homeland. When you first meet a consumer, respectfully enquire if they have any preferences about choice of interpreter. Remember that phone interpreters may also be used without disclosing the consumer's name if sensitive matters are being discussed.

Also consider that the interpreter also may have come from a refugee or asylum-seeker background and the content they are hearing may trigger traumatic memories for them. Providing time at the end of a consultation to appropriately debrief with the interpreter may be useful for both of your learnings. Asking the interpreter if there is anything they would recommend to assist the interaction in the next consultation may provide a means to build rapport with the consumer.

Ethnic similarity

Being able to enter into the world of the consumer from a common framework enables the clinician to make sense of the consumer's distress and work towards a mutual understanding of the psychological problems (Gorman, Brough & Ramirez, 2003). Others have explored the importance of clinicians and consumers experiencing similar languages, thought processes and beliefs about the nature of the world and the causation of mental illness, and conclude that sharing a worldview is inherently therapeutic. Many other writers have explicated the benefit of a shared worldview when assisting with the acceptance of diagnosis, treatment and expectation for change. The empathic resonance and degree of consensual understanding predicts the therapeutic outcome. Importantly, within the literature regarding a shared worldview, the issues of clinician credibility arise. Clinicians are seen as more credible when the consumer has considerable similarity to the clinician, leading to greater satisfaction levels for both consumer and clinician, higher levels of self-disclosure and reduced likelihood of discontinuance with treatment. However, some consumers are culturally matched with their clinician; and some clinicians are also from CALD groups, and have consumers from other CALD groups. The nature of these dyads increases the complexity of the relationship.

When clinicians engage in culturally responsive interactions—such as showing interest and appreciation, and demonstrating knowledge of culture and ethnicity, as well as contextualising the consumer's problems—they are seen as highly credible (Griffiths, 2006). The US Center for Substance Abuse Treatment (2014) advocates the use of the RESPECT mnemonic when working with consumers from different cultural backgrounds. To be effective the counsellor should demonstrate the attitude of:

- *respect*
- seek to understand the consumer's *explanatory* model
- recognise how their *sociocultural context* affects their care
- acknowledge the *power* differential in the relationship
- express *empathy*
- elicit their *concerns and fears*
- commit to enhancing the *therapeutic alliance/trust*.

People from refugee backgrounds

People from refugee backgrounds often experience great losses, persecution, displacement and difficulties accessing the essentials to maintain life such as food, health care and clean water, frequently over a prolonged period of time. For those who access resettlement, further challenges are faced as they adjust to their new environment, and process the trauma from their pre-migration experience. Mental health nurses in resettlement countries who have knowledge of the refugee experience can play an invaluable advocacy role, as well as contributing to the development of appropriate health systems that provide collaborative relationships and culturally competent practices to their consumers. Doing so will encourage improved access to mental health care and thus enhanced mental health and well-being for these consumers and their communities.

Humanitarian protection

Humanitarian protection is a growing issue of global concern as the world comes to realise that the absence of protection for vulnerables groups is at the centre of humanitarian crisis. Particular areas of concern are refugees, asylum seekers, internally displaced persons, unaccompanied minors, women and girls and issues of rights deprivation.

Refugees

The United Nations (UN) *Convention Relating to the Status of Refugees* was ratified in Geneva in 1951, in response to the forcible displacement of many European people following the Second World War. In 1967, the United Nations removed the limitations of the 1951 convention to include refugees from any country in the world. The 1951 Refugee Convention and the subsequent 1967 Protocol remain the two defining documents that offer protection for refugees worldwide.

The Convention defines a refugee as:

> [a]ny person who owing to well-founded fear of being persecuted for reasons of race, religion, nationality, membership of a particular social group or political opinion, is outside their country of his nationality and is unable or, owing to such fear, is unwilling to avail himself of the protection of that country; or who, not having a nationality and being outside the country of his former habitual residence as a result of such events, is unable or, owing to such fear, is unwilling to return to it.

United Nations High Commissioner for Refugees (UNHCR, 1951)

Of the 196 member countries of the UN, 142 are signatories to both the Convention and the Protocol (UNHCR, 2016). All are bound by the legal and moral obligations of these documents.

Asylum seekers

Asylum seekers are those who are seeking protection under the Convention. Until a person's claim for protection is determined, a person's status is referred to as 'asylum seeker' (UNHCR, n.d.). The *Universal Declaration of Human Rights* (1948) recognises that everyone has the right to seek asylum from persecution. Article 14.1 of this document states that '[e]veryone has the right to seek and to enjoy in other countries asylum from persecution'.

Most countries and regions have processes in place to manage asylum seekers. The complexity and ever-changing nature of asylum seeker trends and responses is beyond the scope of this chapter; however, keeping abreast of the local developments is important for mental health nurses. Commonly, asylum seekers lack access to services, risk being detained and often do not have the right to work while their application is being processed.

Internally displaced persons

Internally displaced persons are fleeing persecution, but are unable to cross a border, and cannot seek protection under the Convention.

Unaccompanied minors

An unaccompanied minor is any child aged under 18 years who has travelled alone or is without a biological parent. Unaccompanied minors may or may not have a relative over the age of 21 years to care for them.

The literature suggests unaccompanied minors have increased risk of mental health issues such as post-traumatic stress disorder, depression and anxiety disorders due to separation from parents, exposure to violence and post-migration experiences (Department of Education and Early Childhood Development, 2011). Unaccompanied minors are a vulnerable group of young people who may be more frequently referred to mental health services, yet research shows they have higher rates of missed appointments (Colucci et al., 2012).

Women and girls

Women and girls are particularly vulnerable to victimisation throughout conflict. Sexual violence during conflict can be arbitrary, but is often more prevalent due to the breakdown of traditional protection measures. It can also be a systematic weapon with a wide variety of aims, including attacking what the enemy holds sacred—'womanhood', 'purity' or 'future generations'—or providing sex as a reward to the troops (Zannettino, 2013).

Gender-based violence and rape are also endemic in protracted refugee situations. Often makeshift accommodation does not have lockable doors, and women and children are targeted while completing everyday tasks, such as collecting firewood or water from the communal tap. Women who have been raped or sexually assaulted often suffer from discrimination, racism and ostracism. They almost never receive counselling or support for sexual assault, because services are not available or, if available, are not accessed for fear of a breach in confidentiality (Cremonese, van Horssen & Riera, 2011).

Rights deprivation

People from a refugee background often have a long history of rights deprivation. In their homeland they are generally members of a persecuted minority, and during flight they are often exploited at border crossing and other points where they come into contact with people in power. In prolonged refugee and asylum seeker contexts, they continue to live in a situation of rights deprivation, sometimes for decades. Generally countries of first asylum are overwhelmed with huge numbers of people, and establishing law and order is almost impossible, even with the assistance of the UNHCR and other non-government organisations (Cremonese, van Horssen & Riera, 2011).

The differences between a refugee and migrant

While there are some similarities in the migrant and refugee experiences, there are also significant differences. All people found to be refugees meet the Convention and so are fleeing their country of origin due to a well-founded fear of being persecuted. Refugees are forced to leave their home for survival and to find safety. Removing choice removes the opportunity for people to farewell family and friends, and plan for transitions to the culture, language and environment of the country of migration. Ongoing precarious situations may also prevent people from returning home. By contrast, migrants have made a choice. They are able to make plans and have the ongoing advantage of maintaining contact with relatives and friends post-migration.

The refugee journey and living with uncertainty

Decisions to flee one's homeland are often made quickly, with people frequently only taking what they can carry. Refugees and asylum seekers must often evade authorities or opposing forces to find a route to safety, a journey that is generally characterised by anxiety, uncertainty, chaos, insecurity and impossible choices (Victorian Foundation for Survivors of Torture, 1998). Crossing borders can be difficult and dangerous; people often rely on word of mouth from others in the same situation and mistrust authority. Further, it is not guaranteed that the country of first asylum is a signatory to the Convention (for example, Thailand or Pakistan); and even if that country is a signatory, it may not have the capacity to provide protection (for example, Sudan or Afghanistan). Although refugee camps may provide a level of safety from persecutory forces, refugee camps are often not safe and peaceful places for refuge.

Asylum seekers and refugees will often experience long periods of 'living in limbo' with the uncertainty of not knowing if permanent protection will be granted; this impacts enormously on the mental health of many people, with lifelong consequences. Even if asylum seekers are recognised as refugees, they can live for many decades in precarious situations waiting for resettlement; for example, Afghan refugees living in Pakistan and refugees from Burma living in Thailand. People living in these situations are very vulnerable: they may be indiscriminately detained, forced by authorities to pay bribes, unable to work or forced to work in unsafe jobs to provide for their families, sexually exploited, and without access to the basics to sustain life, such as food, health care and clean water.

Some asylum seekers may live for prolonged periods in detention, which causes long-lasting adverse mental health outcomes for years after release into the community (Coffey et al., 2010; Newman, Dudley & Steel, 2008).

Regardless of how a refugee or asylum seeker arrives in their resettlement country, the perilous journeys these individuals undertake often leave emotional and psychological marks, and many have extremely complex physical and mental health issues at resettlement (Victorian Foundation for Survivors of Torture, 2012a). Many will have had limited access to health care, both in their country of origin and in the country of first asylum, where infrastructure and preventative health-care services may be limited or non-existent (Victorian Foundation for Survivors of Torture, 2012a). Due to this limited access to health care, refugee and asylum seeker resettlement requires sensitive and timely health checks to manage and treat physical and psychological health problems.

Global trends

In 2015, an average of 34,000 people per day became refugees, and by the end of 2015 more than 65.3 million people had been forcibly displaced worldwide (UNHCR, 2015). A majority of the world's refugees are hosted by developing countries, and this can create added social and economic burdens on these countries. In 2015, Turkey hosted the largest number of refugees; Pakistan and Lebanon ran second and third, respectively (UNHCR, 2015). Finding safety is not without its challenges as often entire regions can be unstable, making it difficult for refugees to find safety in neighbouring countries.

The UNHCR identifies three durable solutions for people who are refugees:

1   *Voluntary repatriation.* People choose to return to their homeland when a conflict has finished or a political regime has changed.
2   *Local integration.* People are able to establish a new life in the country in which they sought asylum, where they are afforded opportunities and rights similar to those who live in the country.
3   *Third country resettlement.* Where the first two options are not possible, people who are identified as vulnerable may be offered resettlement. This is a complex processes that involves UNHCR assessment and a resettlement country accepting the person based on the resettlement country's criteria.

As for previous years, resettlement needs in 2015 exceeded the number of places available with thirty-three states resettling a total number of 107,100 refugees (UNHCR, 2015). Efforts to expand opportunities for resettlement through alternative programs such as private sponsorship, family reunification and labour schemes aim to provide solutions to refugees at risk and offer more resettlement places (UNHCR, 2015). Given the sheer numbers of people seeking protection, the process of resettlement is a difficult and fraught one, which is not as orderly as the definitions may suggest.

The impact of resettlement

> Most refugees want to return home to live a peaceful and safe life in their country; resettlement is for those refugees who have no other option.
>
> UNHCR (2010, p. 2)

Resettlement is not without its challenges and mental health professionals must be cognisant of the many issues that are likely to affect a person's psychological health (Giger, 2013). Many people from refugee backgrounds struggle with issues such as separation from family, cultural differences, negotiating new and complex systems, language barriers (Victorian Foundation for Survivors of Torture, 2012a), social isolation and racism (Gardiner & Walker, 2010).

Refugees present to their primary health-care provider with psychological illnesses including anxiety, depression and rates of post-traumatic stress disorder significantly higher than other immigrants (Spike, Smith & Harris, 2011). Both physical and psychological health and well-being are directly related to how well a person from a refugee background will resettle (see Table 22.1).

TABLE 22.1 FACTORS THAT AFFECT REFUGEE MENTAL HEALTH AND RESETTLEMENT

Pre-refugee status	Living as a refugee	Resettlement
• Social status: education, employment, gender and political involvement • Exposure to violence, torture and trauma • No choice in migration; need to flee home • Age at time of exposure to violence and fleeing	• Dangers and impossible choices faced during fleeing • Length of time in refugee camp or detention centre • Ongoing exposure to harsh living conditions and violence • Living in a developing country with minimal access to health services • Uncertainty about future • Loss of, or separation from, family members • Disrupted education	• Initial honeymoon period, followed by period of transition and reality • Cultural differences • Language barriers • Intergenerational differences in acculturation; traditional versus new culture • Loss of, or separation from, family members • Access to education, employment and health care • Disruption of community networks • Loss of identity • Discrimination • Unemployment or underemployment • Less control over social determinants of health: income, housing and food security

Imagine that you are a person from a refugee background living in a foreign country after resettlement.

1   How do you think you would feel?

2   What support do you think you would need?

3   What support would not be helpful?

※ CRITICAL THINKING OPPORTUNITY

Mental health consequences of the refugee experience

The refugee experience creates many complexities in diagnosing and treating mental health issues. Mental health nurses must consider undiagnosed disorders that may be present due to lack of previous health care, the impacts or sequelae of lack of early intervention, unhelpful or dangerous treatments that people may have had previously, brain trauma that a person may have received during conflict or torture, and the complex social situations that a person exists within.

Mental health prevalence data for people from refugee backgrounds are contentious for several reasons: cross-culturally validated tools are rare; clinicians that are skilled in conducting cross-cultural assessments are also rare; and there are large variations in prevalence according to ethnic group (Bhugra, Craig & Bhui, 2010). However, broadly speaking risk factors for mental illness include migration, trauma and having a parent or grandparent who has experienced trauma. Furthermore, the resettled refugee cohort has attended pre-settlement interviews and passed basic medical exams suggesting their level of functioning pre-departure may have been moderate or high. People with significant mental illnesses may be screened out during this process.

CRITICAL THINKING OPPORTUNITY Given what you have learnt about the refugee experience in this chapter and what you have learnt about mental health models from previous practice and study, what could be some of the strengths and some of the concerns with the models of practice when working with people from refugee backgrounds? Consider trauma-informed care, family-based therapies, stress-vulnerability model, recovery model, involuntary treatment, strengths-based approach and consumer-led care.

Survivors of torture

Torture is 'a strategy used by oppressive regimes and groups to destroy communities' (Victorian Foundation for Survivors of Torture, 2012a, p. 47). Some of the most common methods of physical torture include beating, electric shocks, stretching, submersion, suffocation, burns, rape and sexual assault (IRCT, n.d.). Physical torture can often leave physical scars that lead to difficult, often painful recounts of how the injury occurred. Psychological forms of torture and ill-treatment often has the most long-lasting consequences for victims and commonly include isolation, threats, humiliation, mock executions, mock amputations and witnessing the torture of others (International Reabilitation Council for Torture Victims, n.d.). Nobody is immune from torture: men, women and children all may be tortured. Torture is perpetrated by people in power, including police, armed forces, prison guards and health professionals (International Rehabilitation Council for Torture Victims, n.d.). The effects of torture are intended to be felt long after the acts (see Table 22.2).

It is estimated that up to 35 per cent of the world's refugees have experienced at least one incidence of torture (Victorian Foundation for Survivors of Torture, 2012a). Approximately 80 per cent of refugee women are estimated to have experienced sexual abuse and torture, and children are often witness to horrific events or are used as targets for torture (Victorian Foundation for Survivors of Torture, 2012a). Recent studies indicate survivors of torture have 'prevalence rates for PTSD of between 32 per cent and 100 per cent' (Victorian Foundation for Survivors of Torture, 2012a, p. 49) and rates of depression in refugee and political detainees are between 47 per cent and 72 per cent (Victorian Foundation for Survivors of Torture, 2012a). Survivors of torture have a right to rehabilitation according to Article 14(1) of the *Convention Against Torture and Other Cruel, Inhuman or Degrading Treatment or Punishment*. Rehabilitation approaches are generally holistic; a framework for recovery is presented later in the chapter.

Survivors of other refugee-related trauma

Trauma is an emotional response to a terrible event (American Psychological Association, 2013b) and will have different meanings to different individuals, families and communities (Victorian Foundation

TABLE 22.2 COMMON PHYSICAL AND PSYCHOLOGICAL EFFECTS OF TORTURE	
Physical	**Psychological**
• Brain damage • Cardiopulmonary complications • Scars and disfigurement from burns • Mutilation of body parts • Limited mobility • Muscle swelling and muscle atrophy • Chronic pain • Headaches • Deafness • Blindness • Loss of teeth • Internal injuries	• Problems with concentration and memory • Anxiety • Depression • Grief • Relationship problems • Intrusive memories and images • Lack of sleep • Nightmares • Numbing and anhedonia • Irritability • Adjustment disorders • Sexual dysfunction • Feelings of powerlessness • Shame and guilt • Shattered assumptions of human existence—security, trust, meaning

Victorian Foundation for Survivors for Torture (2007, p. 29)

for Survivors of Torture, 2012a). Many refugees will experience trauma associated with forced separation from family; being subjected to or witnessing torture, physical or emotional abuse (Gardiner & Walker, 2010); exposure to war-related conflict; the perilous escape and refugee journey; and living with extreme deprivation and poverty (Victorian Foundation for Survivors of Torture, 2012a). The cumulative effect of torture and trauma is often compounded by the resettlement process (Gardiner & Walker, 2010). As a result, refugees can be left to feel humiliated, isolated, helpless and degraded (Victorian Foundation for Survivors of Torture, 2012a) and suffer from symptoms of sleeplessness, poor concentration, family dysfunction and emotional disturbance (Gardiner & Walker, 2010). Somatisation of psychological stress is not uncommon for refugees (Victorian Foundation for Survivors of Torture, 2012a).

Perinatal mental health

Promoting maternal mental health has a number of well-known benefits for families, with clear associations between maternal health and well-being and the health and well-being of families. Conversely, maternal mental health disorder directly correlates with poorer developmental and cognitive outcomes in children who have a mother with a mental illness (Harvey, Fisher & Green, 2012; Rintoul, 2010). The impact of the refugee experience often results in women being separated from loved ones, resulting in feelings of isolation and vulnerability in the perinatal period. Resettlement can result in a lack of belonging to a community and the loss of cultural rituals associated with the birth of a baby (Rintoul, 2010). In many societies, female relatives provide care and support to the mother during the perinatal period; following resettlement this often becomes the role of the baby's father due to the lack of an extended family. This can potentially lead to tensions in the spousal relationship due to unexpected changes in the role of men within the family (Rintoul, 2010). Caring for a newborn is demanding and may enhance the feeling of being unable to cope in a new country.

Women from a refugee background are more likely to have experienced the death of an infant or child, inadequate care in previous pregnancies and traumatic birth experiences, which may significantly affect their mental health during the perinatal period (Beyondblue, 2013). Missing children are very common, and separation or loss may have occurred due to conflict, during flight or during protracted waiting time for resolution. Consequently, the perinatal period is a time of added stress and emotional upheaval that can result in newly diagnosed or worsening mental health disorders.

Children and adolescents

Children and adolescents are not immune to the horrors of torture and trauma, and commonly present with mental health problems such as learning and behavioural difficulties, poor appetite and sleep, psychosomatic symptoms, enuresis and encopresis, low self-esteem and guilt (Gardiner & Walker, 2010). Mental health nurses need to consider the impact traumatic experiences may have on development, how children may have made sense of the traumatic event(s) at a given developmental stage, and the ongoing impact of a family system affected by traumatic experiences. Parents may be experiencing their own mental health problems, which can make them less available to their children. Each member of the family has their own resettlement experience and will acculturate at different rates.

ABOUT THE CONSUMER Maria's story

Maria is a 40-year-old South American woman admitted unconscious to an emergency department as a result of a car accident. She has a fractured skull caused by the accident. She regains consciousness shortly after admission, and becomes increasingly agitated. The treating team decides to give her some sedation to calm her down. When the nurse approaches her with the medication she starts screaming and jumps out of the bed, knocking down the nurse and a doctor in the process.

When staff approach her she becomes even more hysterical and attacks them, scratching their faces and attempting to gouge their eyes. She is restrained, and a psychiatric evaluation is carried out. After some time it is discovered that she is a refugee who suffered torture and abuse, which were carried out with the aid of health-care staff. As a consequence, she was suffering from post-traumatic stress disorder triggered by finding herself in the hospital environment, which she associates with the previous traumatic experiences.

It is not uncommon for refugees to have had horrific experiences, often inflicted by government officials. In countries where torture is considered a legitimate means of interrogating prisoners, medical and nursing staff can be involved to ensure that the prisoner survives the experience. In this particular scenario, it would have been very difficult for staff to have anticipated the possible reaction, but in situations involving refugees, the likelihood of highly traumatic life experiences should be anticipated.

REFLECTION QUESTIONS

1 What sorts of things should you consider when working with consumers who may be refugees?

2 What sorts of strategies could you implement when working with refugee consumers to minimise the risks?

Clinical considerations when working with people from refugee backgrounds

People from refugee backgrounds have distinctive and diverse needs. They face many barriers when accessing mental health services; however, mental health nurses and organisations can modify practices and processes that will facilitate more equitable access to services, including cultural competency and working with interpreters.

Barriers and facilitators to mental health services

In many instances, barriers to health services are a primary reason for poor health outcomes in populations from refugee backgrounds. Gaps and issues identified by people from refugee backgrounds when accessing mental health care include:

- stigma associated with and acceptance of mental health issues
- different health-seeking behaviour, with services only accessed when health issues become severe
- long waiting periods for mental health services
- poor interpreter usage, with some interpreters unfamiliar with mental health terminology and concepts
- lack of affordability of services
- service providers that lack trauma-informed approaches to care, and therefore are unable to respond appropriately
- co-morbidities such as substance abuse and differences in cultural understandings
- clinic-based approaches to mental health care that are often not appropriate for newly arrived refugees, in particular young people (Department of Health, 2013).

Nurses are one of the first points of contact for these vulnerable people. Acknowledging these gaps and issues and being prepared to develop and implement health care that meets the needs of the consumer is critical in improving health access and equity. Accessible organisations require careful planning to implement, and are reliant on culturally responsive health professionals and systems. Mental health services can implement a range of initiatives to provide greater access for refugees, such as the following.

- Accessibility and flexibility can be increased by locating services near the residences and schools of people from a refugee background, or close to public transport. This may require planning and implementing an outreach service, rather than expecting the consumer to come to a clinic-based service.
- Coordination involving collaborative relationships, partnerships and networks between all agencies involved in care can minimise appointments and reduce duplication in assessment, treatment and management.
- Professional development for staff is important, including:
  - culturally competent health care
  - education about refugee experiences
  - culture and refugee health
  - how the social determinants of health impact upon resettlement.
- Use of interpreters and bilingual workers minimises communication errors and assists in understanding cultural differences (Department of Education and Early Childhood Development, 2011).

Achieving good physical and mental health and well-being outcomes for people from refugee backgrounds occurs when frameworks that recognise the broader determinants of health and social outcomes are developed. Consideration of housing insecurity and affordability, employment, poverty, education levels, changing social status, adapting to a new culture and environment, family separation, discrimination and the ability to access health services all impact enormously on health outcomes for this population group (Department of Health, 2013).

Other nursing considerations when working with people from a refugee background are listed in Table 22.3.

TABLE 22.3 NURSING CONSIDERATIONS WHEN WORKING WITH PEOPLE FROM A REFUGEE BACKGROUND

Nursing intervention	Outcome and benefits
Develop trusting relationships based on mutual respect.	• Take the time to establish trust; once established the refugee or asylum seeker client has a greater opportunity to trust the health system to seek health assessment and treatment. • A trusting relationship improves health outcomes for individuals and communities. • Refugee communities are small, and when a service offers what the community want, 'word of mouth' travels quickly.
Consider health beliefs and health literacy.	• Practise client-centred health care. • Enquire and build an understanding of an individual's beliefs on health, and work together to develop a culturally and individually appropriate care plan. • Recognise that people who have had limited exposure to Western health systems will probably have a low level of health literacy; develop appropriate communication skills and resources that facilitate improved understanding of the health issue—that is, avoid medical jargon, use simple and plain language and ask the client to repeat back their understanding of the health issue and treatment. • Use other community members as trusted sources of information, bearing in mind people's previous experience of 'official' information. • Do not dismiss the health beliefs of people from refugee backgrounds; rather, explore their beliefs to see if there is any point of intersection, and work together to build a consensus. • Allow plenty of time for understanding to be established. • Provide examples familiar to the client. • Remember that people from refugee backgrounds are diverse; some people may be highly trained health professionals in their own country so do not assume all people from refugee backgrounds have low health literacy.
Communal versus individual—many cultures will want to include family in discussion about health care.	• Consider family systems and social networks (Kirmayer et al., 2011). • Discuss privacy and confidentiality laws.
The demands of resettlement conflicting with the refugee or asylum seeker client accessing health care	• Consider whether the client is experiencing issues that impact on their control over the social determinants of health; that is, unstable housing, financial stressors, legal issues relating to seeking asylum and limited language skills or education. • Consider some of the supports you could implement to support your client; that is, referral to local migrant support services, community organisations and places of worship. • Support your client with mutually agreed goals of care that are within a realistic time frame. • Provide outreach services rather than expecting clients to always attend your service. • Home visiting might be appropriate.
Taking care of self	• Be mindful of how you are feeling, reacting and responding. • Participate in formal debriefing sessions. • Utilise the team around you for case reviews; continue to engage in ongoing professional development.

Adapted from Victorian Foundation for Survivors of Torture (2012a)

ABOUT THE CONSUMER   Satkunam's story

Satkunam is a 35-year-old Tamil man from Sri Lanka who lives with his parents and is being treated by a community assertive outreach team. He has been diagnosed with schizophrenia and the administration of his medication is supervised by clinicians every evening. His parents are distressed about this intrusion into their home every dinner time; however, previously when the consumer's medication was not monitored, he did not adhere to the regimen and relapsed. This occurred a number of times, resulting in multiple acute inpatient admission. The consumer's parents do not speak English and rely on the consumer to translate.

One day, the assertive outreach team received a phone call from a minister of faith who knew the family. He wanted to arrange a meeting to discuss the son's treatment. The minister reported that the consumer repeatedly told his parents that he was not unwell. The parents believed their son. The assertive outreach team were surprised, and agreed to meet with the minister, the consumer and his parents, with the consumer's consent.

The meeting was held attended by the psychiatric nurse, consultant psychiatrist, a Tamil interpreter, the consumer, his parents and the minister. The minister questioned the presence of the interpreter, so the clinical staff explained the role of the interpreter was to ensure everyone understood the conversation and outcomes.

The minister explained his understanding of the family's situation, explaining the evening visits were intrusive. The parents understood that their son was 'a little odd', but did not believe he was unwell and believed he could stop doing the odd things when directed by the family.

The clinical team listened and provided some psycho-education via the interpreter. They reminded the family of the critical incidents that had brought their son to psychiatric services' attention, and explained that this is a normal part of his illness. They explained that the consumer remains well when he takes his medicine as instructed.

The family had low levels of health literacy, so the minister provided some further explanations and examples, providing culturally relevant reference points for the family to understand the disorder.

The family expressed concerns about how tired the consumer became after taking his medicine. The clinical team acknowledged this and agreed that after a period of stability they would trial a reduction in the medication.

The clinical team also acknowledged that it is very intrusive to visit the family every evening and asked the family if they could suggest other ways to ensure that the consumer took his medication. The father offered to supervise the medicine every second night, which was agreed upon by everyone. The consumer and clinical team agreed that they would monitor medication compliance through a monthly blood test. The consumer was provided time to talk about his anger at receiving medicine that made him tired, when he believed he was not unwell. The psychiatric nurse and psychiatrist listened to the consumer speak about his concerns. They then explained their perspective to the consumer, mentioning he was on a community treatment order and must adhere to the treatment. They helped him to understand the differences in his mental health when he didn't take the medicine and provided references to previous times he stopped the medication and became unwell.

The meeting took one hour and provided an opportunity for everyone to raise their concerns and develop a collaborative plan for the medication management.

REFLECTION QUESTIONS

1   What impact do you think having an involuntary or community treatment order would have on a person from a refugee background and their family?

2   What was the role of the minister in this case study?

3   What extra difficulties do you think carers with low English proficiency experience having a family member with a mental illness? What strategies could mental health nurses use with carers with low English proficiency to support them in their role as carers?

DON GORMAN, WENDY CROSS AND SUZANNE WILLEY

Framework for recovery

The Victorian Foundation for Survivors of Torture uses a Framework for Recovery (see Figure 22.1), which is useful to consider when working with people from refugee backgrounds. The framework illustrates the relationship between violence and persecution associated with the refugee experience, the consequent social and psychological effects—both short and long term—and then presents goals for recovery. It can assist in determining a focus for intervention, developing a greater ability to understand how the trauma presents and providing a basis for developing appropriate recovery goals within a care plan. All interventions can take this framework into account, no matter how brief or complex. For example, enhancing safety, control and dignity should be part of every interaction—whether at a triage counter in an emergency department or as part of an ongoing treatment plan in the community. This

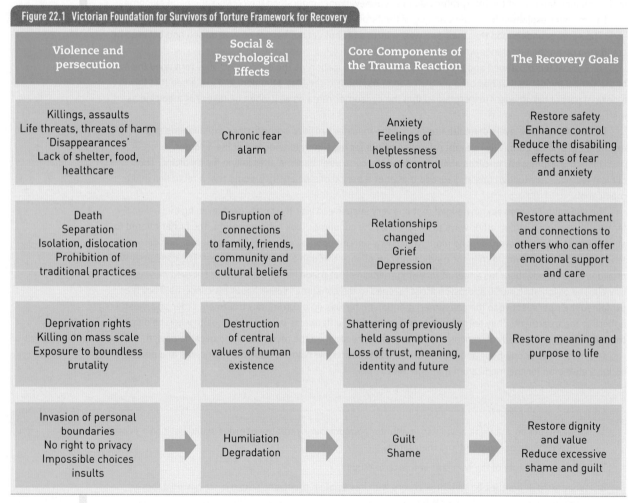

Figure 22.1 Victorian Foundation for Survivors of Torture Framework for Recovery

Violence and persecution	Social & Psychological Effects	Core Components of the Trauma Reaction	The Recovery Goals
Killings, assaults Life threats, threats of harm 'Disappearances' Lack of shelter, food, healthcare	Chronic fear alarm	Anxiety Feelings of helplessness Loss of control	Restore safety Enhance control Reduce the disabling effects of fear and anxiety
Death Separation Isolation, dislocation Prohibition of traditional practices	Disruption of connections to family, friends, community and cultural beliefs	Relationships changed Grief Depression	Restore attachment and connections to others who can offer emotional support and care
Deprivation rights Killing on mass scale Exposure to boundless brutality	Destruction of central values of human existence	Shattering of previously held assumptions Loss of trust, meaning, identity and future	Restore meaning and purpose to life
Invasion of personal boundaries No right to privacy Impossible choices insults	Humiliation Degradation	Guilt Shame	Restore dignity and value Reduce excessive shame and guilt

Victorian Foundation for Survivors of Torture (2012b)

may be achieved by providing information about your role, about what they can expect from treatment, providing interpreters, arriving for appointments on time and, if circumstances change, providing an explanation as to why they have changed.

Mental health nurses have a vital role to play in the recovery of people from refugee backgrounds with mental illnesses. The complexities in mental, psychological, social, environmental and cultural circumstances warrant that the mental health nurse pays special attention to understanding the unique needs of people from refugee backgrounds. Current mental health frameworks of practice that place the consumer as the expert of their own experience have a lot to offer in the recovery of people from refugee backgrounds. Cross-cultural practice, working with interpreters, active listening skills and respectful enquiry will be useful tools for mental health nurses working with people from refugee backgrounds.

Conclusion

A consumer's worldview is the sum total of his or her values, beliefs and perspectives about human nature, social relationships, nature, time and activity. It is influenced by the consumer's socio-political history and cultural and gender identity. Nurses need to explore the consumer's frame of reference with a view to facilitating therapeutic engagement (Center for Substance Abuse Treatment, 2014). Nurses should use an approach to assessment and interactions with people from CALD communities that acknowledges the divergent attitudes, values and behaviours embedded in specific cultures. This serves as a basis for assigning meaning to concepts either across or within cultures. Through the understanding of such meanings, specific information relevant to the individual and diagnosis will be encouraged.

Establishing credibility with the consumer can be achieved in a number of ways (Hwa-Froelich & Vigil, 2004). They include the display of professional qualifications, taking time to listen to consumers' stories from their perspective, giving understanding, advice and treatment, and respecting difference. Provided that the consumer does not perceive a power imbalance and reject the relationship because of professional displays, the other interpersonal skills will assist with establishing credibility (Griffiths, 2006). Nurses should learn to enhance their credibility with a variety of different cultural groups rather than attempt to learn the specific healing remedies and techniques of individual cultures. Therefore, broad principle-based interactive skills are more important than amassing discrete knowledge about individual cultures.

Cultural belief systems about mental health and illness will influence the consumer's response to the psychiatric interview and expectations for treatment. Therefore, careful explanation of the purpose of the procedure is crucial to avoid misunderstanding and potentiate accurate diagnosis. Thorough explanations and assurances of confidentiality also increase the likelihood of engagement. Modifying and using diverse treatment modalities that are compatible with the consumer's expectations will ensure greater follow-up and compliance. Moreover, it will encourage disclosure from the consumer about troubling issues related to treatment; for example, disclosing medication side effects leading to adjustment of dose or replacing it with another medication rather than simply deciding not to continue to take the medication.

The DSM 5 (American Psychiatric Association, 2013a) allows for clinicians to identify culture-specific disorders and other manifestations such as acculturation difficulties in relation to minorities and provides useful guidelines for implementing cross-cultural assessment and appraisal.

Nurses need to expand the boundaries of their professional interactions (Cross & Bloomer, 2010). This demonstrates commitment and interest in the individual when they conduct their work in the environment of the consumer. It provides a common ground to establish a shared worldview, and advances the prospect that clinicians can assist them (Gorman, Brough & Ramirez, 2003).

Obtaining cultural knowledge is a continuous process. Nurses need to consult with and be supervised by knowledgeable colleagues to ensure that cultural knowledge is applied in a competent way and that consumers are seen as individuals first and members of a specific cultural group second.

If values, beliefs and behaviours differ between cultures, it stands to reason that to understand and deal with these differences you need to be aware of your own values, beliefs and behaviours. Take the time to consider the rules that you live by—these will give you an insight into your values and beliefs and help you to become conscious of them. That way it becomes easier to see them as cultural rather than universal, and therefore to be less judgmental.

ABOUT THE CONSUMER   Meng's story

Meng is a 65-year-old Chinese woman who has been readmitted to hospital in a psychotic state. She has been admitted periodically over many years, with her stays followed by treatment in the community, but has a history of noncompliance with her antipsychotic medication, resulting in her readmission. Her English is poor, and she relies on her son to communicate for her. Meng responds to medication and her psychotic symptoms subside.

REFLECTION QUESTIONS

1   Given that Meng comes from a Chinese culture, what might be some of the reasons for her noncompliance?

2   What strategies could you implement to try to bridge the gap between her worldview and that of the treating team?

3   What information would you want to acquire to enable you to provide culturally appropriate care?

4   What strategies would you implement to ensure appropriate communication with Meng?

Care planning

The following is an example care plan for Jay. This plan only addresses the cultural issues that may arise. All areas of daily living would also need to be considered. Remember, the success is in the detail, so be specific about who, when and what in the collaborative plan; and never include someone in the plan if they were not consulted in the planning process.

Date: [Today's date]

Consumer's name: Jay | Case manager: Mental health nurse

Areas of daily living	Assessment of current situation	Goal	Plan (undertaken with consumer)	Implementation	Who is responsible (include only those who have been consulted in the planning process)	Evaluation/ review date
Language	English language limited; he speaks Bahasa Malaysia	Maximise communication	Utilise face-to-face qualified interpreters when possible, or telephone interpreters when not. Minimise the use of family members as interpreters. Staff to learn some basic Bahasa Malaysia words to not only improve communication but also to demonstrate respect for the consumer's culture.	Ensure that interpreter contacts are readily available to staff. Ensure that a list of common Bahasa Malaysia words and phrases is readily available to staff.	Mental health nurse	Ongoing
Cultural and religious differences	Muslim religious practice requirements	Minimise disruption to his cultural and religious practices.	Explore his preferences through a cultural assessment and accommodate wherever possible.	Provide access to a Muslim cleric. Ensure a halal diet can be provided. If this is not available then facilitate his wife's ability to provide meals. Ensure that where possible intimate procedures are carried out by male staff.	Mental health nurse, Jay and his wife	Ongoing

SUMMARY

Our beliefs, morals, customs and the rules we live by, and consequently our behaviour, are largely determined by our culture. As these are mostly unconscious, we have a tendency to think of them as universal, and therefore to expect others to fit our expectations. This leads to ethnocentricity and the risk of judging others by our rules. When working with people from cultures other than our own, we need to be aware of our rules and expectations, and the fact that these are not universal but cultural, to enable us to undertake culturally safe practice.

Most people who are not from the dominant mainstream culture are migrants, and some of them are refugees. Migration and refugee experiences can have significant implications for mental health, which can be complicated by culturally unsafe practices on the part of health professionals. We as mental health professionals have an obligation to ensure that our consumers are not disadvantaged by our practices.

DON GORMAN, WENDY CROSS AND SUZANNE WILLEY

The UN *Convention Relating to the Status of Refugees* defines who may have protection. Most refugees want to go home—resettlement is for those who have no other choice. Culturally competent nurses play a critical role in improving access to services by integrating a holistic approach to consumer care that is underpinned by knowledge, an attitude of self-awareness of their own behaviour and the skill to develop trusting relationships. Interpreters must be utilised in all communication where two people do not speak the same language. The evidence-based Victorian Foundation for Survivors of Torture Framework for Recovery offers structure to develop appropriate interventions for treatment and recovery goals

DISCUSSION QUESTIONS

1   What are your values and beliefs about health?

2   How might you engage with consumers who have different cultural backgrounds and beliefs from your own?

3   Given the need to be culturally safe, what would you do when you found yourself in a conflict about health values?

4   Having read this chapter, what would you now do differently when working with consumers from a culture other than your own?

5   What are the legal criteria that people have to meet to gain refugee status according to the 1951 Convention?

TEST YOURSELF

1   The most significant difference between a person from a refugee background and a migrant is a refugee will:

a   maintain contact with loved ones post-migration

b   prepare for the migration experience in advance

c   have no choice when leaving their country of origin

d   be able to return home freely

2   To work effectively with people from refugee and CALD backgrounds, mental health nurses must do all the following *except*:

a   make sense of their own attitudes, behaviour, assumptions and values

b   provide an integrated and holistic approach to consumer care

c   utilise interpreting services at all times an interpreter is deemed necessary

d   ensure the person adopts the Western view of health and well-being

3   Which of the following statements is incorrect about the influence of culture on health:

a   Ill-health and suffering are defined by a person's cultural background

b   Culture determines how a person should expect to tolerate suffering in a given situation

c   The response to pain by others is not culturally determined

d   Over expression of pain may be labelled as 'attention seeking'

4   Which of the following statements is incorrect in relation to acculturation:

a   Acculturation is the process whereby migrants acquire the values and behavioural norms of the host country.

b   Acculturation occurs when new residents become more like host residents over time

c   Acculturation is the same with different populations

d   The partially acculturated individual may also be marginalised from both cultural groups

USEFUL WEBSITES

Centre for Culture, Ethnicity & Helath: www.ceh.org.au

International Rehabilitation Council for Torture Victims: www.irct.org

Mental Health in Multicultural Australia: www.mhima.org.au/

Queensland Transcultural Mental Health Centre: www.health.qld.gov.au/metrosouthmentalhealth/qtmhc/default.asp

United Nations High Commissioner for Refugees: www.unhcr.org

Victorian Foundation for Survivors of Torture: www.foundationhouse.org.au

World Federation for Mental Health: www.wfmh.global

REFERENCES

American Psychiatric Association (2013a). *Diagnostic and statistical manual of mental disorders 5th Ed.; DSM 5* (5th ed.). Washington: American Psychiatric Publishing.

American Psychological Association (2013b). *Trauma.* Retrieved from www.apa.org/topics/trauma.

Anikeeva, O., Bi, P., Hiller, J. E., Ryan, P., Roder, D. & Han, G.-S. (2010). 'The health status of migrants in Australia: A review'. *Asia-Pacific Journal of Public Health*, 22(2), 159–93. doi:10.1177/1010539509358193.

Australian College of Mental Health Nurses (2010). *Standards of practice for Australian mental health nurses.* Canberra: ACMHN.

Baldwin, J., Faulkner, S., Hecht, M. & Lindsley, S. (eds) (2006). *Redefining culture perspectives across the disciplines.* London: Lawrence Erlbaum Associates, Publishers.

Benson, J. & Thistlethwaite, J. (2009). *Mental health across cultures: A practical guide for health professionals.* United Kingdom: Radcliffe Publishing Ltd.

Beyondblue (2013). *Perinatal mental health of women from culturally and linguistically diverse (CALD) backgrounds: A guide for primary care health professionals.* Retrieved from https://www.bspg.com.au/dam/bsg/product?client=BEYONDBLUE&prodid=BL/1082&type=file.

Bhugra, D., Craig, T. & Bhui, K. (eds) (2010). *Mental health of refugees and asylum seekers.* New York: Oxford University Press.

Center for Substance Abuse Treatment (2014). *Improving Cultural Competence.* Rockville: Substance Abuse and Mental Health Services Administration (US).

Chan, B. & Parker, G. (2004). 'Some recommendations to assess depression in Chinese people in Australasia'. *Australian and New Zealand Journal of Psychiatry*, 38(3), 141–7.

Chui, M., Wei, G. & Lee, S. (2006). 'Personal tragedy or system failure: A qualitative analysis of narratives of caregivers of people with a severe mental illness in Hong Kong and Taiwan'. *International Journal of Social Psychiatry*, 52(5), 413–23.

Coffey, G. J., Kaplan, I., Sampson, R. C. & Tucci, M. M. (2010). 'The meaning and mental health consequences of long-term immigration detention for people seeking asylum'. Social Science & Medicine, 70(12), 2070–9. doi:10.1016/j.socscimed.2010.02.042.

Colucci, E. J., Swarc, J., Minas, H., Paxton, G. & Guerra, C. (2012). 'The utilization of mental health services by children and young people from a refugee background: A systematic literature review'. *International Journal of Culture and Mental Health*. doi:10.1080/17542863.2012.713371.

Commonwealth of Australia (2012). *Mental health statement of rights and responsibilities 2012.* Canberra: Department of Health and Ageing.

Cremonese, L., van Horssen, I. & Riera, J. (2011). *Survivors, protectors, providers: Refugee women speak out.* UNHCR: Geneva.

Crockett, L. J., Iturbide, M. I., Stone, R. A. T., McGinley, M. & Raffaelli, M. (2007). *Acculturative stress, social support, and coping: Relations to psychological adjustment among Mexican American college students:* Faculty Publications, Department of Psychology.

Cross, T. L., Bazron, B. J., Dennis, K. W. & Isaacs, M. R. (1989). *Towards a culturally competent system of care* (vol. 1). Washington: National Technical Assistance Center for Children's Mental Health, Georgetown University Child Development Center.

Cross, W. & Bloomer, M. (2010). *Extending boundaries: Clinical communication with culturally and linguistically diverse mental health clients and carers.* International Journal of Mental Health Nursing. 19(4), 268–277.

Cross, W. M. & Singh, C. (2012). 'Dual vulnerabilities: Mental illness in a culturally and linguistically diverse society'. *Contemporary Nurse*, 42(2), 156–66.

Davilla, M., McFall, S. L. & Cheng, D. (2009). 'Acculturation and depressive symptoms among pregnant and postpartum Latinas'. *Maternal and Child Health Journal*, 13(3), 318–25.

Department of Education and Early Childhood Development (2011). *Refugee status report: A report on how refugee children and young people in Victoria are faring.* Melbourne: DEECD.

Department of Health (2013). *Consultation summary: Victorian refugee health and wellbeing action plan.* Retrieved from http://docs.health.vic.gov.au/docs/doc/Consultation-Summary-Victorian-refugee-health-and-wellbeing-strategy.

DeRosa, N. & Kochurka, K. (2006). 'Implement culturally competent healthcare in your workplace'. *Nursing Management*, 37(10), 18–26.

Gardiner, J. & Walker, K. (2010). 'Compassionate listening; Managing psychological trauma in refugees'. *Australian Family Physician*, 39(4), 198–203.

Gee, G. C., Ryan, A., Laflamme, D. J. & Holt, J. (2006). 'Self-Reported Discrimination and Mental Health Status Among African Descendants, Mexican Americans, and Other Latinos in the New Hampshire REACH 2010 Initiative: The Added Dimension of Immigration'. *American Journal of Public Health*, 96(10), 1821–8. doi:10.2105/AJPH.2005.080085.

Giger, J. (2013). *Transcultural nursing: Assessment and intervention* (6th ed.). St Louis: Elsevier.

Gorman, D., Brough, M. & Ramirez, E. (2003). 'How young people from linguistically diverse backgrounds experience mental health: Some insights for mental health nurses'. *International Journal of Mental Health Nursing*, 12(3), 194–202.

Gorman, D., Nielsen, A. & Best, O. (2006). 'Western medicine and Australian Indigenous healing practices'. *Aboriginal and Islander Health Worker Journal*, 30(1), 28–9.

Griffiths, M. (2006). 'Moving multicultural mental health to mainstream: Building capacity and facilitating partnerships'. *Australian e-Journal for the Advancement of Mental Health*, 5(2), 1–4: http://ausnet.com/journal/vol5iss2/griffithseditorial.pdf.

Harvey, S. T., Fisher, L. J. & Green, V. M. (2012). 'Evaluating the clinical efficacy of a primary care-focused, nurse-led, consultation liaison model for perinatal mental health'. *International Journal of Mental Health Nursing*, 21(1), 75–81. doi:10.1111/j.1447-0349.2011.00766.x.

Hsiao, F. H., Klimidis, S., Minas, H. & Tan, E. S. (2006). 'Cultural attribution of mental health suffering in Chinese societies: The views of Chinese patients with mental illness and their caregivers'. *Journal of Clinical Nursing*, 15(8), 998–1006.

Hwa-Froelich, D. & Vigil, D. (2004). 'Three aspects of cultural influence on communication: A literature review'. *Communication Disorders Quarterly*, 25(3), 107–18.

International Reabilitation Council for Torture Victims (n.d). *Defining torture.* Retrieved 15 August 2013 from www.irct.org.

Kirmayer, L. J. M. D., Narasiah, L., Munoz, M., Rashid, M., Ryder, A. G. P., Guzder, J., et al. (2011). 'Common mental health problems in immigrants and refugees: General approach in primary care'. *Canadian Medical Association Journal*, 183(12), E959–67.

Kiropoulos, L., Blashki, G. & Klimidis, S. (2005). 'Managing mental illness in patients from CALD backgrounds'. *Australian Family Physician*, 34(4), 259–64.

Knifton, L., Gervais, M., Newbigging, K., Mirza, N., Quinn, N., Wilson, N. & Hunkins-Hutchison, E. (2010). 'Community conversation: addressing mental health stigma in ethnic minority communities'. *Social Psychiatry and Psychiatric Epidemiology*, 45, 497–504. doi:10.1007/s00127–009–0095–4.

Lindert, J., Ehrenstein, S., Priebe, S., Mielck, A. & Brähler, E. (2009). 'Depression and anxiety in labor migrants and refugees: A systematic review and meta-analysis'. *Social Science & Medicine*, 69(2), 246–57.

Meadows, G., Singh, B. & Grigg, M. (eds) (2007). *Mental health in Australia: Collaborative community practice.* Melbourne: Oxford University Press.

Minas, H., Kakuma, R., Too, L, S., Vayani, H., Orapeleng, S., Prasad-IIdes, R., Turner, G., Procter, N., Oehm, D. (2013). *Mental health research and evaluation in multicultural Australia: developing a culture of inclusion.* International Journal of Mental Health Systems, 7:23. doi: 10.1186/1752-4458-7-23.

Newman, L. K., Dudley, M. & Steel, Z. (2008). 'Asylum, detention and mental health in Australia'. *Refugee Survey Quarterly*, 27(3). doi:10.1093/rsq/hdn034.

Pernice, R., Trlin, A., Henderson, A., North, N. & Skinner, M. (2009). 'Employment status, duration of residence and mental health among skilled migrants to New Zealand: Results of a longitudinal study'. *International Journal of Social Psychiatry*, 55(3), 272–87.

Rintoul, A. (2010). *Understanding the mental health and wellbeing of Afghan women in South East Melbourne.* Retrieved from http://refugeehealthnetwork.org.au/understanding-the-mental-health-and-wellbeing-of-afghan-women-in-se-melbourne/

Sadock, B. & Sadock, V. (2007). *Kaplan and Sadock's synopsis of psychiatry: Behavioural sciences clinical psychiatry* (10th ed.). Baltimore: Lippincott Williams and Wilkins.

Sam, D,L.. & Berry, J.W. (2010). *Acculturation: When Individuals and Groups of Different Backgrounds Meet.* Perspectives of Psychological Science. July (4):472-81. doi: 10.1177/1745691610373075.

SANE Australia. (2013). What is stigma? www.sane.org/stigmawatch/what-is-stigma.

Snowden, L. R. & Yamada, A. M. (2005). 'Cultural differences in access to care'. *Annual Review of Clinical Psychology*, 1, 143–66.

Spike, E. A., Smith, M. M. & Harris, M. F. (2011). 'Access to primary health care services by community-based asylum seekers'. *Medical Journal of Australia*, 195(4), 188–91.

Steel, Z., McDonald, R., Silove, D., Bauman, A., Sandford, P., Herron, J. & Minas, I. H. (2006). 'Pathways to the first contact with specialist mental health care'. *Australian and New Zealand Journal of Psychiatry*, 40(4), 347–54.

Suurmond, J., Seeleman, C., Rupp, I., Goosen, S. & Stronks, K. (2010). 'Cultural competence among nurse practitioners working with asylum seekers'. *Nurse Education Today*, 30(8), 821–6. doi:10.1016/j.nedt.2010.03.006.

United Nations High Commissioner for Refugees (1951). *Convention and protocol relating to the status of refugees.* Retrieved from www.unhcr.org.au/pdfs/convention.pdf.

United Nations High Commissioner for Refugees (2010). *UNHCR projected global resettlement needs 2011.* Retrieved from www.unhcr.org/4c31e3716.html.

United Nations High Commissioner for Refugees (2015). *Global trends: Forced displacement in 2015.* Retrieved from www.unhcr.org/statistics/unhcrstats/576408cd7/unhcr-global-trends-2015.html?query=global%20trends%202015.

United Nations High Commissioner for Refugees (2016). *States Parties to the 1951 Convention relating to the Status of Refugees and the 1967 Protocol,* Retrieved from www.unhcr.org/protection/basic/3b73b0d63/states-parties-1951-convention-its-1967-protocol.html.

United Nations High Commissioner for Refugees (n.d.). *Asylum-seekers.* Retrieved from www.unhcr.org/pages/49c3646c137.html.

Universal Declaration of Human Rights (1948). *Home page,* Retrieved from www.un.org/en/documents/udhr/index.shtml.

Victorian Foundation for Survivors of Torture (1998). *Rebuilding shattered lives.* Retrieved from www.foundationhouse.org.au/rebuilding-shattered-lives-2/

Victorian Foundation for Survivors of Torture (2012a). *Promoting refugee health: A guide for doctors and other health professionals caring for people from refugee backgrounds* (3rd ed.). Retrieved from http://refugeehealthnetwork.org.au/wp-content/uploads/PRH-online-edition_July2012.pdf.

Victorian Foundation for Survivors of Torture (2012b). *Refugee experience course material.* Melbourne: VFST.

Victorian Foundation for Survivors of Torture (2013). *Promoting the engagement of interpreters in Victorian health services.* Melbourne: Victorian Foundation for Survivors of Torture.

Yoon, E., Chang, C. T., Kim, S., Clawson, A., Cleary, S. E., Hansen, M., et al. (2012). 'A meta-analysis of acculturation/enculturation and mental health'. *Journal of Counseling Psychology*, 60(1), 15–30.

Zannettino, L. (2013). Refugees, sexual and domestic violence and prior experiences of trauma: introduction and context. In *Practice monograph: Improving responses to refugee with backgrounds of multiple trauma: Pointers for practitioners in domestic and family violence, sexual assault and settlement services.* Sydney: Australian Domestic & Family Violence Clearing House.

CHAPTER 23

Forensic Mental Health Nursing

JO RYAN AND
CHRIS QUINN

Acknowledgment

The authors would like to acknowledge the contribution of Trish Martin who co-wrote this chapter in the second edition.

KEY OUTCOMES

AFTER READING THIS CHAPTER, YOU SHOULD BE ABLE TO:

- explain the legal framework that applies to the consumer who has offended
- describe the components of a forensic mental health service
- identify common factors involved in mental illness and offending
- discuss the skills of the mental health nurse in a forensic mental health context

KEY TERMS

- diminished responsibility
- forensic mental health services
- forensic mental health nursing
- forensic mental health team
- mental health courts
- mentally disordered offenders

Introduction

This chapter introduces you to the field of forensic mental health nursing and the skills that forensic mental health nurses require to assess and deliver care to people experiencing mental illness who have also been charged with a criminal offence. In Australia, the consumer of most forensic mental health services would be an offender, or alleged offender, who is experiencing mental illness, is being assessed for mental illness or is exhibiting at risk behaviours such as property damage, which may lead the person to offending.

The term 'forensic' is derived from the Latin word *forensis*, which means 'public debate'. In Ancient Rome, public debate took place in the Forum, and today one place where public debate takes place is in the court of law. A contemporary definition of forensic is 'pertaining to the court'; therefore, it is applied to civil and criminal legal proceedings. On the civil side, for example, a mental health professional may provide evidence about a person's mental capacity to write a will or have custody of a child, or about a person's psychological damage in a case of negligence. On the criminal side, a mental health professional may provide evidence about a person's mental state, and how their compromised mental health may have contributed to their offending behaviour.

The fact that a person has a mental illness may be relevant at different stages of their movement through the criminal justice system. At any of the following points, the person may be assessed and treated by a mental health nurse from an area mental health service team or a specialist forensic mental health team:

- At the time of apprehension by the police, a person experiencing mental illness may be too unwell to be interviewed by the police and may be referred to a mental health service to have treatment before the interview takes place. For minor charges, the police can exercise some discretion about whether to lay charges, and in light of the person's mental illness may decide that if the person is receiving treatment there are no additional benefits to any party to charge the person.

- In court, it needs to be determined whether a person is fit to stand trial; if the person is deemed unfit to stand trial due to the experience of mental illness, the trial may be postponed until a later date.
- Also in court, it needs to be determined whether a person, as a result of their mental illness, should be held responsible for their actions while unwell. In most jurisdictions, there is provision to divert the person for treatment and/or find the person not guilty.
- While a person is undergoing a sentence of imprisonment, they may become mentally unwell. The illness may have existed before imprisonment, or may be a consequence of the stressors associated with imprisonment, such as depression or anxiety. The person who is assessed as being mentally ill within the prison may be treated in the prison (if resources are available and the prisoner consents) or transferred to a forensic mental health hospital for treatment.
- People on orders (for example bail, parole or community-based orders) may also experience mental illness and will require assessment and treatment or may be ordered to attend treatment as part of their order.

The term 'consumer' is used in this chapter to identify the person experiencing mental illness or being assessed for mental illness, who has been charged with an offence and is subject to court dispositions (defined below), or is a person who because of offending behaviours has been identified at risk to others and requires specialist forensic mental health services. This person is also likely to be receiving treatment from a forensic mental health service.

ABOUT THE CONSUMER Thomas's story

Thomas is a 24-year-old man. He is married and has no children. Six months ago, Thomas became paranoid about his wife Sandra, believing that she was reading his thoughts and using a form of telepathy to poison his mind. Thomas believed that he was receiving 'special' messages from the radio and television confirming this belief. As a consequence of this, Thomas began spending more time alone listening to the radio in his car. He was beginning to find it difficult to sleep at night, and also found it difficult to get up in the mornings, which led to him losing his job as a plumber.

Thomas's friends and family noticed his bizarre behaviour. Thomas did visit a GP and was prescribed medication, but he secretly flushed it down the toilet every night. Two days before committing the offence, Thomas presented to his local police station and demanded that his wife be arrested. Thomas was adamant that his mind was being telepathically poisoned, and that his death was imminent. One night, Thomas approached his wife and told her to 'stop poisoning him', which led to an argument that ended in Thomas striking Sandra several times with a garden spade and subsequently killing her.

REFLECTION QUESTIONS

1 What is your assessment of Thomas's mental state?

2 What type of interventions may well have assisted Thomas and his wife before the argument?

3 How do you feel about providing care for Thomas? Outline your reasons.

The context of forensic mental health

Forensic mental health is a complex area involving a number of important considerations in determining the mental status of a person when considering prosecution.

The legal framework

Each state and territory in Australia has legislation that sets out the laws of sentencing, defines the behaviour that is against the law and establishes the sentencing rules. The Office of Public Prosecutions (or equivalent body) on behalf of the Director of Public Prosecutions, prepares and presents prosecutions against people accused of serious offences, through the county and supreme courts on behalf of the public.

As the decision to prosecute can affect people's lives in an extreme way, it is considered the most important decision in the prosecution process. (Director of Public Prosecutions Victoria, Directors Policy, 2014). When considering whether a prosecution should go ahead in the public interest, consideration is also given to the age of an offender as well as whether they have any intellectual disability or mental illness.

Sentencing principles form the basis of sentencing decisions so as to provide due process and are expected to be fair and just, with judges relied on to protect the human rights of individuals. The sentencing principles of parsimony, proportionality, parity and totality form the basis of all sentencing decisions in criminal law (Sentencing Advisory Council, 2016).

Two lines of defence for people experiencing mental illness are whether they are fit to stand trial, and whether they are mentally ill at the time of the offence.

Fitness to stand trial

A defendant appearing before a court must be fit to plead. To be fit to stand trial, a defendant must be able to:

- understand the nature of the charge
- enter a plea to the charge and to exercise the right to challenge jurors or the jury
- understand the nature of the trial (that it is an inquiry as to whether they committed the offence)
- follow the course of the trial
- understand the substantial effect of any evidence that may be given in support of the prosecution
- give instructions to their legal practitioner.

If the defendant is unable to meet the above criteria, a magistrate or judge can adjourn the case, and it may not proceed (van der Wolf et al., 2010). A defendant experiencing mental illness may be found unfit to stand trial. All Australian jurisdictions have legislation that allows the person to be detained and treated for their mental illness exists.

CRITICAL THINKING OPPORTUNITY

1   Do you believe Thomas is fit to be interviewed by the police?
2   Who do you think should assist in making this decision?

JO RYAN AND CHRIS QUINN

Mental illness at the time of the offence

In addition to fitness to stand trial, there are also special conditions that are applied to defendants who were mentally ill at the time of the offence. In Australia, the requirements for determining mental impairment have been developed from the McNaughton Rules, which were formulated in England in 1843 (Soothill, Rogers & Dolan, 2008).

Daniel McNaughton held a paranoid delusion about the British prime minister, and mistakenly and fatally shot the prime minister's private secretary. The court found McNaughton 'not guilty on the ground of insanity'. Public outcry following this and other contemporary high-profile cases led to the UK Parliament debating the issue and formulating the rules of diminished responsibility for people committing serious crimes when mentally ill.

The McNaughton Rules (Bennett, 2009) are founded on Lord Tindal's report from the Parliamentary debate into the case stating that:

> [I]t must be clearly proved that, at the time of the committing of the act, the party accused was labouring under such a defect of reason, from disease of the mind, as not to know the nature and quality of the act he was doing; or, if he did know it, that he did not know he was doing what was wrong.

To which he added a further consideration:

> … that he labours under such partial delusion only, and is not in other respects insane, we think he must be considered in the same situation as to responsibility as if the facts with respect to which the delusion exists were real.

The substance of these rules continues to be preserved in legislation. This defence only applies if, at the time of engaging in conduct constituting the offence, the person was suffering from a mental illness or other form of impairment, such as intellectual disability or dementia. While options for disposition from court vary, in most cases the person is subject to compulsory treatment. This person is then detained under a custodial or community order for a considerable period of time while receiving mental health treatment. Other dispositions that are available to courts include a referral to a mental health service for assessment or diversion to a mental health service or mental health clinician for treatment. Conditions related to these orders vary across jurisdictions.

CRITICAL THINKING OPPORTUNITY

1   Do you think that the McNaughton Rules should apply to Thomas?

2   Why or why not?

Forensic mental health services

The previous section identified the main target populations for forensic mental health services:

- people who have appeared before the courts and have been found unfit to plead, or who are found not guilty because they were mentally ill at the time of the offence
- prisoners and detainees with severe mental illness requiring mental health assessment and treatment
- people who are referred by the courts to mental health services for assessment and treatment.

Forensic mental health services aim to treat the consumer's mental illness, ameliorate the factors that decrease a consumer's quality of life and prevent their successful integration into the community, and ultimately to reduce the likelihood of further offending. This treatment approach to addressing the person's mental health needs along with the issues that contributed to their offending is crucial in supporting the recovery journey of consumers (Drennan & Wooldridge, 2014). Forensic mental health nurses undertake assessment and deliver treatment to these consumers in a range of settings. These settings include police custody centres, courts, prisons, forensic mental health hospitals and the community.

Police custody centres

The process of entering the criminal justice system begins with a person being charged with an offence and possibly being detained in a police custody centre. During this period in detention, the person's impaired mental state may come to the attention of police officers, who can call upon a nurse. The nurse may be employed by the police or another service providing an *inreach program*. The main roles of the nurse are screening detainees for general health issues, and identifying evidence of mental illness and substance use as soon as possible. Following the assessment, the nurse may be required to provide, or make a referral for, health care. Police detainees often have medical complaints, and/or present with mental disorders, and/or have substance use problems. Nursing intervention typically focuses on substance intoxication, withdrawal and overdose, acute symptoms of mental illness, self-harm and suicidal behaviour.

Courts

The mental health nurses who work in courts provide on-site specialist mental health assessment and advice to magistrates and judges. The nurse may be employed by a forensic mental health service, an area mental health service, or the court. The role may be one of diverting people with mental illness away from prison to a hospital for treatment, or providing assessment and advice to the court. The nurse may take referrals from the court or from other sources, including legal representatives, family, court services, police and the alleged offender. Mental health courts and mental health diversion programs are a recent addition to the judicial system. These courts aim to work more closely with mental health services to improve the quality of life of people with mental illness and to provide supportive treatment-based alternatives to imprisonment (Frailing, 2011).

The nurse undertaking a mental health assessment of a consumer will interview the consumer and possibly others, who can include the legal representative, case manager and family. The court nurse may have access to databases (mental health, corrections, police or court) that can provide further information. When the assessment is complete, the nurse provides a verbal and/or written report to the court. The report will include recommendations based on the nurse's assessment. If required, the nurse might make arrangements for follow-up care and support by mental health services and/or other agencies.

Prisons

Nurses may work within a specialist mental health unit in a prison, and/or provide services across the prison, or they may work in an area mental health service providing inreach services to a prison. A significant proportion of prisoners have pre-existing mental health concerns, and/or experience mental health difficulties as a result of incarceration. The estimated risk of imprisonment for mental health consumers is estimated at up to 25 times greater than the incidence experienced by persons of the general population (Barrenger & Draine, 2013; Huxter, 2013). The experience of imprisonment for this overrepresented group of people increases the risk of mental health decline once imprisoned (Goomany & Dickinson, 2015). As such, prisoners experiencing mental illness are a concern to prison management: their disorganised behaviour can threaten the good order of the prison, they commit more infractions and they are often victimised by other prisoners (O'Connor, Lovell & Brown, 2002).

Nursing in an environment designed for punishment, retribution and deterrence requires a more conscious commitment towards maintaining an ethical caring practice (Maeve & Vaughn, 2001). Nurses have a key role in many of the processes that are required for an effective mental health service in a prison. These processes include:

- screening for mental illness at the time of reception to identify mental illness and begin treatment planning
- ongoing assessment, monitoring and treatment of prisoners through mental health outpatient clinics
- crisis intervention
- provision of acute care or rehabilitation in a prison mental health unit
- identification, treatment and supervision of prisoners at risk of suicide and self-harm
- planning for transfer to a forensic mental health hospital or release (Ogloff, 2002; Weiskopf, 2005).

Forensic mental health hospitals

Forensic mental health hospitals take a range of forms that are dependent on local legislative frameworks, political ideologies and other services that are available. Some are standalone facilities, some are co-located with prisons and some are programs within larger mental health services. Consumers are admitted to forensic mental health hospitals for acute treatment and rehabilitation under a range of legislative options: referred by the courts; transferred from prison (transfer is needed when medication cannot be administered involuntarily in a prison); or transferred from mainstream mental health services when their needs cannot be met in a less secure setting (Jansman-Hart et al., 2011).

Nurses in a forensic mental health hospital must come to terms with integrating security with therapeutic goals. Central to the idea of security is that public safety is maintained by ensuring that consumers do not escape from the hospital or abscond from approved leave (Tilt, 2000). Effective rehabilitation requires that consumers are given the opportunity to practise and test their progress in real-life situations. Leave from the hospital is therefore an important component of hospital treatment for many consumers, but approval of leave is dependent on factors such as legal status, whether the safety of the consumer or the public will be seriously endangered, and whether the leave will contribute to the consumer's rehabilitation goals. Leave is also pivotal in assisting the consumer regain community confidence and develop their sense of citizenship, which are important aspects in supporting recovery (Drennan & Wooldridge, 2014). Leave from the hospital remains an Achilles heel for forensic mental health services, as political and media reactions when a consumer escapes or absconds from leave are generally extreme. Nurses are generally the escorts for consumers on leave, and while this is a security function, there are ample opportunities for therapeutic work while off the secure unit and away from the presence of other consumers.

Nurses in forensic mental health hospitals require an understanding of the importance of maintaining security, and must adhere to numerous, often intrusive, procedures. Security has been described as having physical, procedural and relational components (Collins & Davies, 2005). These components are:

- *physical security*—that is, the structural features of the facility, including the walls, keys, alarms, scanning on entering and exiting, cameras, doors and lighting
- *procedural security*—the procedures used by staff to maintain security, including counting consumers; searching of units, consumers and their belongings; storage of tools and implements; management of visitors, consumer mail and telephone calls; and escorting on approved leave
- *relational security*—which arises out of the therapeutic relationship between staff and consumers, and involves knowing and understanding the consumers and the circumstances in which there is a security risk. Nurses must know the consumers: their history, risk potential, current health state, behaviour and stressors.

A number of early research projects that have examined incidents of escaping and absconding from security hospitals in the UK found that most events were impulsive or opportunistic acts (Dolan & Snowden, 1994; Huws & Shubsachs, 1993; Moore & Hammond, 2000). The findings are significant because many fears and commonly held beliefs related to consumer escapes and absconds are dispelled. The findings show that there are few clear precipitants, the absconder rarely uses violence and very few offences are committed. The focus has been on nursing roles in preventing absconding through the use of locked doors and increased observation. Grotto and colleagues (2015) explored the perceptions of nurses regarding absconding and identified the need for further research to ascertain alternative approaches, such as specific absconding assessment tools and management strategies to improve outcomes for consumers and for nurses.

The need for safety in the forensic mental health hospital is crucial. The consumers generally have a mental illness, a history of offending, and personality attributes and ways of acting and reacting that heighten their potential for risk of harm to self and others. While consumer violence may be a common event, the skills of the nurses, the increased nurse–consumer ratio, and policies and purpose-designed environments contribute to effective management of violence.

Forensic mental health hospitals have clear objectives: to be secure, safe and therapeutic. The therapeutic objectives include providing therapy for consumers so that their illness can be treated and other risk issues dealt with so that their behaviour becomes less dangerous for others and themselves. Consumers present with a range of needs—mental health, psychological, physical, social, cultural and spiritual—that require comprehensive and specialist nursing assessment and care (Glorney et al., 2010; Nicholls et al., 2011).

Community

A consumer can be referred to a forensic mental health community service for assessment, consultation, ongoing treatment or shared care. There are numerous sources of referral to a community forensic mental health service. The sources of referral include forensic hospitals, justice agencies (prisons, Community Corrections or the Adult Parole Board) and legal aid centres. A past history of violence and other offending; high levels of anger, suspicion or hostility; poor response or non-adherence to treatment; failure to maintain contact with the service; or substance use are reasons why consumers are often not accepted by mainstream community mental health services, and are referred to forensic community services (Gilmour & Edment, 2001).

As case manager, the mental health nurse coordinates necessary services (including health, legal, social, vocation, finance and accommodation) in order to facilitate the transition to the community and treat or manage the mental illness, substance use, offending and other case specific concerns. Community care of consumers also requires working with families and carers. At times, other agencies or clinicians will be brought in on complex cases, necessitating agreements about collaborative arrangements so there are no gaps or duplication in services or passing of responsibility.

1 Do you think that the forensic area of nursing might be of interest to you? Outline your arguments both for and against.

2 What do you perceive to be the barriers in working with people who have offended?

The mentally disordered offender

The relationship between offending and mental illness is complex, and varies between individuals. Knowledge of this relationship informs risk, treatment needs and clinical nursing care. It is evident that consumers are defined by clinical, legal and political considerations. Many consumers move back and forth between the mental health and criminal justice systems. Police and court tolerance and willingness to divert from the criminal justice system, and availability of mental health services that are able to treat the consumer, are significant factors (Müller-Isberner & Hodgins, 2000; Rice & Harris, 1997).

There is growing evidence of increased numbers of mentally ill people in prisons and increased numbers of people with forensic histories in mainstream mental health services (Hodgins & Müller-Isberner, 2004; Nicholls, Ogloff & Douglas, 2004; Walsh et al., 2001). In the USA, there are three times as many mentally ill people in prisons than in psychiatric hospitals (Berzins & Trestman, 2005), and although international figures vary, the reported rates of mentally ill people in prison vary between 5 per cent and 40 per cent (Welsh & Ogloff, 2003).

Australian research (Mullen, 2006; Mullen et al., 2000; Wallace, Mullen & Burgess, 2004) compared criminal records of mental health consumers and community comparison subjects, and found that male and female subjects in the schizophrenia cohorts had significantly more convictions for violent offences than the community comparison cohorts. They also found that the increased rates of offending were consistent with the change in the pattern of offending in the general community. The authors do, however, caution that 'the results do not support theories that attempt to explain the mediation of offending behaviours in schizophrenia by single factors, such as substance abuse, active symptoms, or characteristics of systems of care, but suggest that offending reflects a range of factors that are operative before, during, and after periods of active illness' (Wallace, Mullen & Burgess, 2004, p. 716).

BOX 23.1 ASSOCIATION BETWEEN MENTAL ILLNESS AND OFFENDING

International research on the association between mental illness and offending started in the 1990s and include the following:

■ Hodgins (1992), using a birth cohort in Sweden, found that subjects who had been treated for mental illness were more likely to be convicted for a violent offence than those without mental illness.

■ Wessley, Castle and Douglas (1994), undertaking a case linkage study in the UK, found males and females with a diagnosis of schizophrenia were at significantly greater risk of conviction for a violent offence than matched subjects. A further UK study by Kooyman and colleagues (2012) reports that 60 per cent of those convicted had offending histories prior to the onset of their mental illness.

■ DeHart and colleagues (2014) conducted interviews with 115 women in prisons across five states in the USA and established high rates of mental disorder: 50 per cent of the women met the diagnostic criteria for serious mental illness, 51 per cent for post-traumatic stress disorder and 85 per cent for a substance use disorder.

■ Link, Andrews and Cullen (1992) compared former mental health consumers and a control group in New York, and found an association between mental illness and violence, although demographic factors were also found to be significant.

■ In Finland, Tiihonen and colleagues (1997), using a birth cohort, found that people with mental illness were more likely to have a record for criminal violence than the community cohort.

■ The results of a longitudinal study by Linqvist and Allebeck (1990) in Sweden also found an association between schizophrenia and violent offences.

■ The first Spanish study by Vicens and colleagues (2011) explored this relationship with 707 male prisoners and found that 84.4 per cent of these men had a lifetime prevalence of mental disorder.

■ A recent study in Chile (Mundt et al., 2016), assessing mental disorder in a sample of 229 male and 198 female prisoners, revealed high prevalence of illicit substance use prior to imprisonment, and high current occurrence of major depression and current non-affective psychotic disorders. The results of the study challenged the previous underestimated extent of mental health problems experienced by prisoners in Chile.

Hodgins and colleagues (2007) reported that these findings of increased criminal and violent behaviour by mentally ill people were robust; however, there is no evidence that mental illness causes criminal behaviour—only that a number of factors have been identified as mediators of mental illness and offending. Most studies have found not only an association between mental illness and increased rates of offending, but also complex associations between each of the mediating factors. Each of these factors—demographic characteristics, acute symptoms, substance abuse, cognitive and social skills, early social adversity, social disadvantage, and the treatment of mentally ill people and mentally disordered offenders—is discussed below.

CRITICAL THINKING OPPORTUNITY

1 After you have taken into consideration what has been outlined above, what are your feelings about working with consumers who have the potential for violence?

2 Based on best evidence, what risk-reduction strategies do you think need to be in place in order to provide a safe environment for both the health-care staff and the consumers in the area of forensic psychiatry?

Demographic characteristics

Studies examining consumers generally describe a similar population in terms of demographical characteristics: young, male, never married, low socioeconomic status, unemployed and itinerant prior to conviction (Douglas et al., 1999; Kaliski, 2002; Ogloff, Lemphers & Dwyer, 2004; Silver & Teasedale,

2004; Williams et al., 1999). Monahan (2002) found that mentally ill men were no more likely to be violent than mentally ill women, although there were gender differences where men were more likely to harm strangers than their partners or children.

Acute symptoms

The nature of the relationship between the various mental disorders and criminal behaviour is complex. People with major mental illness who offend present with multiple problems: positive and negative symptoms, impoverished life skills and social skills, severe affective and cognitive deficits, substance abuse and a lifestyle conducive to deviant behaviour (Müller-Isberner & Hodgins, 2000). Most people with schizophrenia do not commit criminal offences, but of those who do, their offending reflects a range of factors that are present before, during and after periods of acute illness (Hodgins, 2002; Wallace, Mullen & Burgess, 2004). There may be different subgroups of offenders with schizophrenia.

Taylor (2004) attributed more serious violence to delusions (when people are frightened or depressed by delusions or when challenged on their belief in them). Mullen (1997a, p. 7) allowed that 'fear-inducing preoccupations with a subjective sense of decreased control is particularly productive of violent outburst'. Monahan (2002) stated that voices that commanded violent acts increased the likelihood of violence, although Mullen (1997b, p. 170) suggested that these voices are rarely acted upon, but when they 'reinforce delusional preoccupations, particularly fear of imminent attack' the risk may be greater. The study by Swanson and colleagues (2006) found that positive symptoms increased the risk of minor and serious violence, while negative symptoms lowered the risk of serious violence.

Substance abuse

There is clear evidence that substance abuse is common in psychiatric populations (Gournay, 2000), offender populations and the community generally (Mullen et al., 2000). Consumers have high rates of substance abuse, and consumers who meet the criteria for dual diagnosis have more extensive criminal histories and higher level of risks and needs than those with just mental illness (Hodgins, 2002; Ogloff, Lemphers & Dwyer, 2004; Short et al., 2013). Moreover, the presence of co-occurring substance use has been associated with an increased history of both youth and adult imprisonment and greater severity in offending (Ogloff et al., 2015). Again, it must be noted that the majority of mainstream dual-diagnosis consumers and people experiencing schizophrenia do not offend, but are four to five times more likely to be violent when substance abuse is implicated. The relationship may be immediate or mediated, or there may be some common cause (Hodgins, 2002; Taylor, 2004). One observation was that substance abuse may be an indicator of general antisocial and deviant behaviour rather than a cause of offending (Scott et al., 2004; Wright et al., 2002). Others have also indicated that a dual diagnosis was found to be a key factor in the occurrence of violence (Bloom & Wilson, 2000; Monahan, 2002; Silver & Teasedale, 2004). Schizophrenia and substance abuse magnified violence, but a significant amount of violence was also perpetrated in the absence of substance use (Arseneault et al., 2000).

Cognitive and social skills

Cognitive and social skills have increasingly received attention as a mediator between mental disorder and offending, based on the premise that diminished skills will adversely affect insight and successful social performance, and lead to increased offending (Welsh & Ogloff, 2003; Woods, Reed & Collins, 2004). Offenders lack some of the cognitive and social skills that are necessary for pro-social adaptation, and frequently show deficits in interpersonal problem-solving skills, impulsivity, perspective taking, assertiveness, self-regulation, moral and critical reasoning, empathic understanding and interpersonal communication (Day & Howells, 2002; Polaschek & Reynolds, 2001; Robinson & Porporino, 2001). Anger is a frequently considered emotion preceding violence; however, anger is not the mediation of all violence. Davey, Day and Howells (2005) concluded that offenders are a heterogeneous group in terms of the functional antecedents of their violent acts, and high inhibition of anger may be as problematic as the more recognised deficiencies in controlling anger.

Individual differences in social cognitive skills are influenced by neurophysiology, but are primarily learnt in the context of the family, environment and culture. Harsh or inconsistent parenting and delinquent peer associations can limit the development of pro-social cognitive skills. Deficits in cognitive ability are not causes but mediators between risk factors and delinquent behaviour (Bennett, Farrington & Huesmann, 2005; Blud & Travers, 2001). It is unclear in the population of consumers to what extent the skills deficits are a consequence of the mental illness (positive and negative symptoms) or of criminogenic thinking (avoiding gainful employment, parasitic lifestyle, lack of realistic goals, impulsivity and poor behavioural controls) (Rice & Harris, 1997).

Early social adversity

Studies have found an association between the hereditary, obstetrical and problematic childhood–parenting context and adult offending. These developmental aspects may contribute to childhood cognitive, behavioural and emotional vulnerabilities that may be antecedents of violent behaviour. A significant proportion of consumers admitted to forensic mental health hospitals have histories that include traumatic childhood experiences (Heads, Taylor & Leese, 1997). In addition, a consequence of inadequate parenting may be that many of the cognitive skills needed for pro-social adjustment are not acquired in childhood (Robinson & Porporino, 2001).

The results of the birth cohort study by Arseneault and colleagues (2000) implied that the link between adult mental disorders and violence is often rooted in childhood and adolescent conduct problems. Childhood variables (early childhood maladjustment) have proved to be a powerful predictor of violence (Blumenthal, 2000; Webster & Bailes, 2001; Williams et al., 1999). Monahan (2002) found that physical abuse as a child was associated with violence but that sexual abuse was not, and that deviant behaviours (such as excessive substance use) by parents was strongly associated with increased violence.

Social disadvantage

The social context and socioeconomic status and influences on minority disadvantaged groups are important (Blumenthal, 2000). Violence may be a function of the high-crime neighbourhoods where mentally ill people live (Monahan, 2002). The downward drift hypothesis suggests that mentally ill people move into, or fail to rise out of, a low socioeconomic group because of the impact of the illness (Sadock & Sadock, 2003). The stigma, symptoms and course of the illness may prevent people experiencing mental illness from acquiring vocational qualifications and from securing stable employment. Subsisting on social security payments can result in accommodation in lower socioeconomic status areas, where local community norms may be more supportive of offending and where there is likely to be increased contact with others who are offenders. The immediate and larger social environments (that is, the strains, events, situations and people) must intervene for severe mental illness, even active psychosis, to lead to violence (Mullen, 2006).

Treatment of mentally ill people and mentally disordered offenders

Hodgins (2001) identified that recent issues related to the treatment of mental health consumers—that is, the criteria for involuntary treatment being strengthened, short inpatient stays, consumer rights to refuse treatment and the limiting of professionals' powers to impose treatment—may influence criminality among people with mental illness. Hodgins suggests that criminality in mentally ill people is affected by the quality, type and intensity of the treatment and services they receive. Evidence suggests that community mental health consumers under supervision are less likely to reoffend (Mullen, 1997a; Swanson et al., 2000).

Therefore, it can be concluded that consumers make up a heterogeneous population presenting with multiple disorders (including substance use disorders and personality disorders), and that violence may also be associated with features of the larger social environment, and/or related to vulnerabilities resulting from childhood experiences and the mental disorder itself (Hodgins, 2002). Many people shift between prison and hospital as the two systems compete to offload difficult individuals, and the lack of relevant treatment should not be overlooked as a contextual factor (Mullen, 2006).

Assessment of risk

In recent years there has been greater emphasis placed on the need to assess risk in a systematic evidenced based way utilising a structured professional judgment (SPJ) approach. The SPJ approach assists nurses in forensic mental health settings to gather information about the consumer, which is evaluated by combining a structured approach with their judgment. The goal of this approach is to enhance and support their clinical decisions to assist in making a prediction about the risk of aggression and violence, and other risks such as self-harm or substance use. Two commonly used SPJ tools are the Dynamic Appraisal of Situational Aggression (DASA; Ogloff & Daffern, 2006) and the Short-Term Assessment of Risk and Treatability (START; Webster et al., 2004).

The DASA is used by nurses on a daily basis and rates the consumers on the following seven items: negative attitudes, impulsivity, irritability, verbal threats, sensitive to perceived provocation, easily angered when requests are denied, and unwillingness to follow directions. The score provides a good prediction to violence for the next 24 hours and assists the nurse to identify the need to provide increased support for the person in distress.

The START is used to evaluate a range of protective factors or personal strengths and vulnerabilities along with additional other risks: self-harm, suicide, unauthorised leave, substance abuse, self-neglect, being victimised and case-specific items. The START is completed fortnightly, or less frequently for more settled consumers, and is considered to be a useful tool not only for predicting violence and the other risks mentioned above, but also for supporting recovery-focused forensic mental health nursing care by identifying protective factors that nurses can work on with the consumer to help them towards positive change (Doyle & Jones, 2013).

CRITICAL THINKING OPPORTUNITY

The nature of the relationship between the various mental disorders and criminal behaviour is complex. Discuss with reference to best evidence.

Skills and attitudes for practice with mentally disordered offenders

Mental health nurses working in the forensic setting require the core knowledge, skills and attitudes of nursing, plus the specialist knowledge and skills of mental health nursing. Additional skills have been identified as being necessary to work effectively in the forensic context, and must be considered as building on the nursing standards, competencies and codes of practice and ethics that are common to all nurses, and further as building on mental health nursing standards. Box 23.2 lists skills for mental health nurses in forensic settings that were written by senior nurses at the Forensicare (Martin et al., 2013), based on their practice and existing evidence. Each of these skills is further discussed below.

BOX 23.2 NURSING SKILLS IN THE FORENSIC MENTAL HEALTH CONTEXT

In the forensic mental health context, the mental health nurse:

- structures the treatment environment to integrate security with therapeutic goals
- applies knowledge of the legal framework to service delivery and individual care
- conducts forensic mental health nursing practice ethically
- practises within an interdisciplinary team that may include criminal justice staff
- establishes, maintains and terminates therapeutic relationships with consumers using the nursing process
- integrates assessment and management of offence issues into nursing care processes
- assesses for the impact of trauma and engages in strategies to minimise the effects of trauma
- assesses and manages the risk potential of consumers
- manages the containment and transition process of consumers
- promotes optimal physical health of consumers
- minimises potential harm from substance use by consumers
- practises respectfully with families and carers of consumers
- advocates for the mental health needs of consumers in a prison or police custodial setting
- supports and encourages optimal functioning of consumers in long-term care
- demonstrates professional integrity in response to challenging behaviours
- engages in strategies that minimise the experience of stigma and discrimination for consumers.

Martin et al. (2013)

Structures the treatment environment to integrate security with therapeutic goals

In secure settings, the nurse maintains an attitude of vigilance and adheres to the security policies and procedures that are in place to prevent consumers escaping from the facility or absconding from approved leave. There are implications for public safety should the consumer offend while absent without leave. The repercussions for the consumer who escapes or absconds can also be serious, as leave may be discontinued, and discharge or release can be delayed. The nurse can distinguish between the requisites for security and safety, and identify strategies and outcomes that are common to maintaining security and ensuring safety. Clinical intervention must be consistent with security requirements. Integrating therapeutic goals with security requirements needs constant appraisal of organisational processes and nurse–consumer relationships to ensure that opportunities for therapeutic practice are maximised. Nurses in forensic mental health hospitals require an understanding of the importance of maintaining security, and must adhere to numerous, often intrusive, procedures (Martin et al., 2012).

Applies knowledge of the legal framework to service delivery and individual care

The nurse requires knowledge of legislation and the processes of the agencies within the criminal justice system to provide nursing assessment and treatment that is congruent with the consumer's legal status (Martin et al., 2012).

Conducts forensic mental health nursing practice ethically

Practising in custodial settings where the values and policies potentially conflict with the principles of mental health nursing practice and caring for consumers in all settings can result in nurses experiencing ethical dilemmas and problems. The nurse needs to refer to professional codes of conduct and ethics to solve ethical dilemmas and problems. A commitment to professionalism, transparency and team communication provides an important safeguard for accountability (Martin et al., 2012).

Practices within an interdisciplinary team that may include criminal justice staff

TOPIC LINK

See Chapter 19 for more on case management.

An interdisciplinary approach allows a broad theoretical base that draws on the knowledge and skills of each discipline to enhance assessment, formulation, implementation and evaluation of treatment and care. The nurse practises as a member of an interdisciplinary team at the interface of the criminal justice system and mental health system to deliver nursing care that meets the needs of the consumer. In a secure setting, the interdisciplinary team can include custodial officers, community corrections officers, police officers, security officers and court staff (Martin et al., 2012).

Establishes, maintains and terminates therapeutic relationships with consumers using the nursing process

The therapeutic relationship is the fundamental interpersonal process of assessment, collaborative goal setting, intervention and evaluation. There are inherent tensions in the therapeutic relationship with consumers. The security requirements of custodial environments are grounded in distrust rather than trust, the legal status of consumers challenges notions of voluntary treatment, and the experience of consumers can result in attitudes of suspicion, hostility and subversion to treatment goals. The nurse's therapeutic optimism is integrated with vigilant assessment of the consumer's risk potential. The nurse recognises these tensions and makes prudent use of self and interpersonal therapeutic skills. Knowledge of the developmental, social, cultural and environmental influences on patterns of relating—including trust and power relations that have an impact on the therapeutic relationship—will assist the nurse to maintain professional boundaries in the therapeutic relationship (Martin et al., 2012).

Integrates assessment and management of offence issues into nursing care processes

It is the alleged or proven offending behaviour that differentiates the consumers of the forensic mental health nurse. Knowledge of the contribution of mental illness and other factors to offending behaviour, and the circumstances, nature and consequences of the consumer's offending, is integrated within the comprehensive nursing process that promotes personal recovery. The nurse works in partnership with consumers and their families, carers and significant supports to facilitate an understanding of offending behaviour and mental illness through individual and group programs that address offending behaviour (Martin et al., 2012).

Assesses for the impact of trauma and engages in strategies to minimise the effects of trauma

Exposure to trauma is a common experience for consumers and their families and carers. Exposure to trauma can have profound neurological, biological, psychological and social effects on the individual. The main areas related to consumers and trauma are:

- exposure to traumatic experience (such as being a victim of or witness to abuse or neglect)
- trauma related to committing the index offence
- trauma related to detention (including isolation from supports, and community role loss)
- trauma related to experiencing coercion in secure settings
- trauma related to the impact of the secure environment (such as locked doors and loss of privacy).

Appreciating the high prevalence of trauma and understanding the impact that trauma and violence can have on an individual, the nurse must assess for impact of trauma, implement appropriate treatment and avoid inadvertently re-traumatising consumers. The nurse also recognises that the traumatic experiences of the consumer, family and carers can be experienced vicariously by the nurse, and that nurses can become desensitised by constant exposure to trauma. Nurses actively seek and utilise a range of professional and organisational strategies to maintain professional integrity, including education, consultation, reflective practice, clinical supervision and critical incident stress management (Martin et al., 2012).

■ TOPIC LINK
See Chapter 7 for more on nurses' self-care.

Assesses and manages the risk potential of consumers

The nurse works with mental health and criminal justice processes to assess and manage risk at individual, interpersonal, organisational and community levels. Using recognised risk assessment tools and knowledge of the factors that place each consumer at personal risk and at risk to others, the nurse implements evidence-based interventions to manage risk and assist consumers to deal with their own risk behaviours. This dynamic process requires ongoing risk assessment and adaptation of the level of intervention, monitoring and supervision, according to the consumer's changing risk status. The nurse needs to demonstrate sensitivity when imposing controls or restrictions as part of the risk management plan. Transparency is achieved through communication and documentation of all matters related to the consumer's risk assessment and management (Martin et al., 2012).

Manages the containment and transition process of consumers

Transition between environments such as from the community, between higher and lower security environments, and returning to the community are potentially stressful events for the consumer. Critical life events for consumers, such as arrest, incarceration, sentencing and release, are also stressful. This stress can result in decompensation of mental state, which may lead to behaviours such as deliberate self-harm, harm to others or absconding, which can compromise the transition. Care and treatment planning for consumers incorporates judgment about risks, protective factors, available resources and therapeutic objectives. The nurse has a duty of care to make recommendations that do not compromise the safety of the consumer or others, while having regard for human rights. Arrest, incarceration, sentencing and release all require nursing care that supports adaptation. The nurse works with the interdisciplinary team, family, carers and other agencies to plan and implement strategies to manage the transition (Martin et al., 2012).

Promotes optimal physical health of consumers

The community and custodial lifestyle of many consumers renders them vulnerable to poor physical health. Incarceration also imposes potential threats to physical health. These threats include mental state disturbance, substance use, unsafe sexual behaviour, victimisation, trauma and interpersonal violence. Access to physical health care may also be compromised in custodial settings and by itinerant lifestyles. The nurse contributes to a treatment environment that promotes a healthy lifestyle and works with the consumer, family, carers and the interdisciplinary team to deliver health education and health-enhancing activities (Martin et al., 2012).

Minimises potential harm from substance use by consumers

Substance use is common in the community and in custodial settings. The association between substance use and offending behaviour for people with mental illness makes this an important issue for nurses to address in order to reduce risk to the consumer's health and to minimise reoffending. The nurse uses recognised tools to undertake a comprehensive substance use assessment of the consumer, and ensures that consumers have access to specialist dual-diagnosis education, counselling and health promotion programs (Martin et al., 2012).

Practises respectfully with families and carers of consumers

Families can provide important links to the community and promote the well-being of consumers through supportive relationships. Mental illness and the nature of the offence and its consequences have an impact on the family and their relationship with the consumer. The nurse appreciates the experience of the family as victim, or potential victim, and assesses and manages ongoing risk of the consumer to family members. The detention of the consumer can have an impact on family function (emotional, financial or social), and the nurse works with the family to address these concerns and make appropriate referrals when specialist support is needed for them. The nurse needs to demonstrate skill and sensitivity in working with the family around these significant issues (Martin et al., 2012).

Advocates for the mental health needs of consumers in a prison or police custodial setting

A significant proportion of prisoners and detainees have pre-existing mental health or substance use problems. Detention can impact on the consumer's mental health and access to treatment. Provision of health care is not the primary focus in a prison or police custodial setting, and nurses are uniquely positioned to advocate for the mental health needs of consumers. The nurse must negotiate for appropriate and timely health care for the consumer, advocating systemic processes that promote humane and effective approaches to prisoner and detainee health care (Martin et al., 2012).

Supports and encourages optimal functioning of consumers in long-term care

Legal status and enduring mental illness can result in long-term care of consumers in secure settings and the community. Special needs of consumers in long-term care arise from a range of factors, including loss of hope, institutionalisation and separation from usual supports. The nurse maintains therapeutic optimism and promotes 'a life worth living', using an open, flexible and transparent approach (Martin et al., 2012).

Demonstrates professional integrity in response to challenging behaviours

Consumers can demonstrate maladaptive styles of relating and behaving that threaten the physical and emotional safety of themselves and others. The nurse will encounter adverse incidents, some extreme in their consequences, including deliberate self-harm, violence, protest behaviour and offending behaviour. Theoretical understanding of causative factors, empathic and flexible limit setting, consistent treatment planning and monitoring of emotional responses to consumers with challenging behaviours are necessary to maintain therapeutic effectiveness (Martin et al., 2012).

Engages in strategies that minimise the experience of stigma and discrimination for consumers

Community attitudes towards mental illness and offending behaviour are influenced by misinformation, ignorance, fear and sensationalist representation in the media. Consumers are disadvantaged through negative appraisal by others and by internalised impacts on identity, self-concept and personal recovery related to forensic status and mental illness. The forensic mental health nurse is aware of this and demonstrates that understanding, support, education and advocacy are necessary to combat stigma and discrimination. Acting as an advocate for consumers, the nurse consults and negotiates with agencies such as health, legal, housing, education and employment services to ensure the consumer has fair and reasonable access to these (Martin et al., 2012).

The competence, knowledge and skills required of a nurse working in forensic mental health services are more easily defined than the attitudes, values and morals that the role demands (Bowring-Lossock, 2006). A skill required by all mental health nurses, and particularly the forensic mental health nurse, is the ability to not be influenced by bias and negative views of the consumer. The media coverage of the mentally ill—and in particular those who have offended—portrays them in a negative light, sensationalising their cases and creating stereotypes that further contribute to the stigma around mental illness (McKenna, Thom & Simpson, 2007).

It is the alleged or proven offending—and other challenging, antisocial behaviour—that distinguish the consumer within a forensic mental health setting. As identified earlier, the role of the nurses in forensic mental health settings is to minimise the experience of stigma and discrimination for consumer. It is therefore important that nurses manage their own personal values, judgments and feelings. Moral judgment can compromise the delivery of quality nursing care.

Prisons are designed to provide punishment and deterrence. It requires nurses to make a conscious commitment to ensure they remain detached from the criminal justice values, while remaining attached to mental health nursing standards, professional values and ethical practice.

Nurses are at risk of cognitive biases that can derail and influence the care that is provided. Influences on the way we think come about not only through the media but also what the nurse has already experienced. Clinical judgment can be influenced by information that is readily available, more recent or evokes strong emotions, but does not take into account the broader history and knowledge of the consumer.

The work of Amos Tversky and Daniel Kahneman in the early 1970s has been influential in identifying heuristic and biases. Their focus of interest was with cognitive biases that stem from the reliance on judgmental heuristics (Tversky & Kahneman, 1974) Heuristic biases are thinking shortcuts that lead to a judgment error. They are more common when the cognitive system is under stress from demanding problems and the need for quick decisions (Fine, 2006). Although it may be a reasonable perception that consumers in a forensic mental health service are dangerous, when this judgment is applied to all consumers it leads to a judgment error and contributes to stigma (Glendinning & O'Keeffe, 2015; Lammie et al., 2010). To manage personal response and maintain therapeutic optimism, the nurse must engage in professional strategies of clinical supervision, self-reflection and professional development.

CRITICAL THINKING OPPORTUNITY

1   What is the importance of the therapeutic relationship in working with consumers?

2   What are some of the barriers to engaging in a therapeutic relationship with consumers?

3   What are the ethico-legal implications for you as a nurse working with people who have offended and have a mental illness?

ABOUT THE CONSUMER Thomas's story (continued)

Thomas himself phoned the police and stated that he had killed his wife. He was arrested, taken to his local police station and charged with murder. Thomas's impaired mental state was immediately obvious to the police, and subsequently his interview was postponed until after he received psychiatric treatment. Thomas was taken to the reception prison where all newly received prisoners are assessed to identify mental illness and those who may be 'at risk'. The nurse on reception identified that Thomas was experiencing acute symptoms of mental illness. Three days later, Thomas was transferred to the forensic mental health hospital, where his psychiatric assessment and treatment began.

Three months later, Thomas was required to attend a committal hearing at the Magistrates' Court. At the committal hearing, the magistrate heard all the evidence in order to determine if there was enough to support a conviction at the Supreme Court. The judge decided that the case should proceed, and Thomas was re-remanded to appear again in four months' time.

Thomas's trial at the Supreme Court began over a year after his offence was committed. His treating psychiatrist at the hospital had written a psychiatric report in his defence. The report outlined Thomas's mental state at the time of the offence and at the time of his admission; how he had responded well to treatment in the last 13 months; and how his illness had been in stable remission for five months. The report identified that Thomas's mental state was significantly impaired at the time the offence was committed. Both the prosecution and the defence agreed that Thomas should be found 'not guilty on the terms of mental impairment'. Thomas was indeed found 'not guilty on the ground of mental impairment', and was returned to the hospital to continue his recovery.

REFLECTION
QUESTIONS

1   Now that the court proceedings have been finalised, what issues do you think Thomas will have to deal with?

2   What interventions might you as a nurse carry out to help Thomas cope with his current proceedings?

3   What might Thomas's family be thinking, feeling and experiencing?

4   What might Sandra's family be thinking, feeling and experiencing?

5   What would be your response if a friend of yours read about Thomas's court case in the newspaper, and commented that Thomas was getting off easy at the hospital and he should be locked up forever in a prison?

6   Should you be discussing Thomas's case?

7   What are the ethical considerations that would inform your decision?

SUMMARY

This chapter has provided some information about an area of mental health nursing where practitioners have only recently identified its therapeutic contribution to the treatment and care of consumers. The justice context (court, police cells and prison) is concerned with punishment and containment, and nurses who practise in these settings are confronted with clinical and ethical dilemmas. The nurses working in this context learn to cultivate strategies that build a professional resilience that supports them as they continue to attend to health and caring.

The research demonstrates that the needs of consumers are complex, and that considerably more research is necessary for a reasonable understanding of the experience of the consumers. The relationship with their consumer is crucial to nurses' work, and there is recognition that mentally disordered offenders often come to the relationship with a history of trauma, distrust and cynicism. Breaking through such barriers is possible when the nurse can maintain therapeutic optimism and an ethical approach to care.

DISCUSSION
QUESTIONS

1   What does the term 'consumer' in a forensic context mean?

2   What are some of the factors involved in mental illness and offending?

3   What knowledge, skills and attitudes are necessary for nurses when working with consumers?

4   What would be your response to undertaking a placement in a forensic mental health service setting?

5   What are the components that make up a forensic service for people with a mental illness?

TEST YOURSELF

1 A consumer of a forensic mental health service may be:

  a unfit to stand trial

  b not guilty by reasons of mental impairment

  c serving a parole or community-based order

  d all of the above

2 Security is described as:

  a healing, relational and therapeutic

  b physical, containing and corrective

  c physical, procedural and relational

  d technical, procedural and punishing

3 It is important for a nurse who works in forensic mental health to:

  a allow their own experience to influence and direct the care they provide

  b ensure they follow the principles of punishment

  c manage their own personal values, judgments and feelings

  d focus on what the media portray about the mentally ill who offend

4 Forensic mental health services aim to:

  a treat the consumer's mental illness

  b assist consumers towards successful integration into the community

  c reduce the likelihood of further offending for the consumer

  d all the above

USEFUL WEBSITES

Australian Institute of Criminology: www.aic.gov.au

Forensic Mental Health Services Managed Care Network, Scotland: www.forensicnetwork.scot.nhs.uk

Forensicare: www.forensicare.vic.gov.au

Justice Health & Forensic Mental Health Network NSW: www.justicehealth.nsw.gov.au

REFERENCES

Arseneault, L., Moffitt, T. E., Caspi, A., Taylor, P. J., & Silva, P. A. (2000). Mental disorders and violence in a total birth cohort. *Archives of General Psychiatry, 57*(10), 979–986.

Barrenger, S. L., & Draine, J. (2013). 'You Don't Get No Help': The role of community context in effectiveness of evidence-based treatments for people with mental illness leaving prison for high risk environments. *American Journal of Psychiatric Rehabilitation, 16*(2), 154–178.

Bennett, A. O. M. (2009). Criminal law as it pertains to 'mentally incompetent defendants': A McNaughton rule in the light of cognitive neuroscience. *Australian & New Zealand Journal of Psychiatry, 43*(4), 289–299. doi: 10.1080/00048670902721137.

Bennett, S., Farrington, D. P., & Huesmann, L. R. (2005). Explaining gender differences in crime and violence: The importance of social cognitive skills. *Aggression and Violent Behavior, 10*(3), 263–288.

Berzins, L. G., & Trestman, R. L. (2005). The development and implementation of dialectical behaviour therapy in forensic settings. *International Journal of Forensic Mental Health, 3*(1), 93–103.

Bloom, J. D., & Wilson, W. H. (2000). Offenders with schizophrenia. In S. Hodgins & R. Müller-Isberner (Eds.), *Violence, crime and mentally disordered offenders* (pp. 113–29). Chichester: John Wiley & Sons.

Blud, L., & Travers, R. (2001). Interpersonal problem-solving skills training: A comparison of R&R and ETS. *Criminal Behaviour and Mental Health, 11*(4), 251–261.

Blumenthal, S. (2000). Developmental aspects of violence and the institutional response. *Criminal Behaviour and Mental Health, 10*(3), 185–198.

Bowring-Lossock, E. (2006). The forensic mental health nurse: A literature review. *Journal of Psychiatric and Mental Health Nursing, 13,* 780–785.

Collins, M., & Davies, S. (2005). The security needs assessment profile: A multidimensional approach to measuring security needs. *International Journal of Forensic Mental Health, 4*(1), 39–52.

Davey, L., Day, A., & Howells, K. (2005). Anger, over-control and serious violent offending. *Aggression and Violent Behavior, 10*(5), 624–635.

Day, A., & Howells, K. (2002). Psychological treatments for rehabilitating offenders: Evidence-based practice comes of age. *Australian Psychologist, 37*(1), 39–47.

DeHart, D., Lynch, S., Belknap, J., Dass-Brailsford, P., & Green, B. (2014). Life history models of female offending: The roles of serious mental illness and trauma in women's pathways to jail. *Psychology of Women Quarterly, 38*(1), 138–151.

Director of Public Prosecutions Victoria, Directors Policy (2014). *The prosecution process.* Retrieved from www.opp.vic.gov.au/Resources/Publications.

Dolan, M., & Snowden, P. (1994). Escapes from a medium secure unit. *Journal of Forensic Psychiatry, 5*(2), 275–286.

Douglas, K. S., Ogloff, J. R. P., Nicholls, T., & Grant, I. (1999). Assessing risk for violence among psychiatric patients: The HCR-20 violence risk assessment scheme and the psychopathy checklist: Screening version. *Journal of Consulting and Clinical Psychology, 67*(6), 917–930.

Doyle, M., & Jones, P. (2013). Hodges' health career model and its role and potential application in forensic mental health nursing. *Journal of Psychiatric and Mental Health Nursing, 20*, 631–640.

Drennan, G., & Wooldridge, J. (2014). *Making recovery a reality in forensic settings* (Centre for Mental Health & Mental health Network NHS Confederation, Trans.).

Fine, C. (2006). *A mind of its own: How your brain distorts and deceives.* New York: W.W. Norton & Co.

Frailing, K. (2011). Referrals to the Washoe County mental health court. *International Journal of Forensic Mental Health, 10*(4), 314–325.

Gilmour, A., & Edment, H. (2001). Supervising the rehabilitated patient in the community. In C. Dale, T. Thompson & P. Woods (Eds.), *Forensic mental health* (pp. 243–250). London: Harcourt.

Glendinning, A. L., & O'Keeffe, C. (2015). Attitudes towards offenders with mental health problems scale. *Journal of Mental Health Training, Education and Practice, 10*(2), 73–84.

Glorney, E., Perkins, D., Adshead, G., McGauley, G., Murray, K., Noak, J., & Sichau, G. (2010). Domains of need in a high secure hospital setting: A model for streamlining care and reducing length of stay. *International Journal of Forensic Mental Health, 9*(2), 138–148.

Goomany, A., & Dickinson, T. (2015). The influence of prison climate on the mental health of adult prisoners: A literature review. *Journal of Psychiatric & Mental Health Nursing, 22*(6), 413–422.

Gournay, K. (2000). Schizophrenia. In R. Newell & K. Gournay (Eds.), *Mental health nursing: An evidence based approach* (pp. 147–163). Edinburgh: Churchill Livingstone.

Grotto, J., Gerace, A., O'Kane, D., Simpson, A., Oster, C., & Muir-Cochrane, E. (2015). Risk assessment and absconding: Perceptions, understandings and responses of mental health nurses. *Journal of Clinical Nursing, 24*(5–6), 855–865.

Heads, T. C., Taylor, P. J., & Leese, M. (1997). Childhood experiences of patients with schizophrenia and a history of violence: A special hospital sample. *Criminal Behaviour and Mental Health, 7*(2), 117–130.

Hodgins, S. (1992). Mental disorder, intellectual deficiency and crime: Evidence from a birth cohort. *Archives of General Psychiatry, 49*(6), 476–483.

Hodgins, S. (2001). Offenders with major disorders. In C. R. Hollin (Ed.), *Handbook of offender assessment and treatment* (pp. 433–451). Chichester: John Wiley & Sons.

Hodgins, S. (2002). Research priorities in forensic mental health. *International Journal of Forensic Mental Health, 1*(1), 7–23.

Hodgins, S., & Müller-Isberner, R. (2004). Preventing crime by people with schizophrenic disorders: The role of psychiatric services. *British Journal of Psychiatry, 185*(3), 245–250.

Hodgins, S., Müller-Isberner, R., Freese, R., Tiihonen, J., Repo-Tiihonen, W., Eronen, M., Kronstrand, R. (2007). A comparison of general adult and forensic patients with schizophrenia living in the community. *International Journal of Forensic Mental Health, 6*(1), 65–77.

Huws, R., & Shubsachs, A. (1993). A study of absconding by special hospital patients: 1976 to 1988. *Journal of Forensic Psychiatry, 4*(1), 45–58.

Huxter, M. J. (2013). Prisons: The psychiatric institution of last resort? *Journal of Psychiatric & Mental Health Nursing, 20*(8), 735–743.

Jansman-Hart, E. M., Seto, M. C., Crocker, A. G., Nicholls, T. L., & Cote, G. (2011). International trends in demand for forensic mental health services. *International Journal of Forensic Mental Health, 10*(4), 326–336.

Kaliski, S. Z. (2002). A comparison of risk factors for habitual violence in pre-trial subjects. *Acta Psychiatrica Scandinavica, 106*(412), 58–61.

Kooyman, I., Walsh, E., Stevens, H., Burns, T., Tyrer, P., Tatten., T., & Dean, K. (2012). Criminal offending before and after the onset of psychosis: Examination of an offender typology, *Schizophrenia Research, 140*(1–3), 198–203.

Lammie, C., Harrison, T. E., Macmahon, K., & Knifton, L. (2010). Practitioner attitudes towards patients in forensic mental health settings. *Journal of Psychiatric and Mental Health Nursing, 17*(8), 706–714.

Link, B. G., Andrews, H. A., & Cullen, F. T. (1992). The violent and illegal behaviour of mental patients reconsidered. *American Sociological Review, 57,* 275–292.

Linqvist, P., & Allebeck, P. (1990). Schizophrenia and crime: A longitudinal follow-up of 644 schizophrenics in Stockholm. *British Journal of Psychiatry, 157*(3), 345–350.

Maeve, M. K., & Vaughn, M. S. (2001). Nursing with prisoners: The practice of caring, forensic nursing or penal harm nursing? *Advances in Nursing Science, 24*(2), 47–64.

Martin, T., Maguire, T., Quinn, C., Ryan, J., Bawden, L., & Summers, M. (2013). Standards of practice for forensic mental health nurses: Identifying contemporary practice. *Journal of Forensic Nursing, 9*(3), 171–178. doi: 10.1097/JFN.0b013e31827a593a.

Martin, T., Ryan, J., Bawden, L., Maguire, T., Quinn, C., & Summers, M. (2012). *Forensic mental health nursing standards of practice.* Melbourne: Victorian Institute of Forensic Mental Health.

McKenna, B., Thom, K., & Simpson, A. (2007). Media coverage of homicide involving mentally disordered offenders: A matched comparison study. *International Journal of Forensic Mental Health, 6*(1), 57–63.

Monahan, J. (2002). The MacArthur studies of violence risk. *Criminal Behaviour and Mental Health, 12*(1), S67–S72.

Moore, E., & Hammond, S. (2000). When statistical models fail: Problems in the prediction of escape and absconding behaviour from high-security hospitals. *Journal of Forensic Psychiatry, 11*(2), 359–371.

Mullen, P. E. (1997a). A reassessment of the link between mental disorder and violent behaviour, and its implications for clinical practice. *Australian and New Zealand Journal of Psychiatry, 31*(1), 3–11.

Mullen, P. E. (1997b). Assessing risk of interpersonal violence in the mentally ill. *Advances in Psychiatric Treatment, 3*(3), 166–173.

Mullen, P. E. (2006). Schizophrenia and violence: From correlations to preventive strategies. *Advances in Psychiatric Treatment, 12*(4), 239–248.

Mullen, P. E., Burgess, P., Wallace, C., Palmer, S., & Ruschena, D. (2000). Community care and criminal offending in schizophrenia. *Lancet, 355*(9204), 614–617.

Müller-Isberner, R., & Hodgins, S. (2000). Evidence-based treatment for mentally disordered offenders: Violence. In S. Hodgins & R. Müller-Isberner (Eds.), *Crime and mentally disordered offenders* (pp. 7–37). Chichester: John Wiley & Sons.

Mundt, A. P., Kastner, S., Larraín, S., Fritsch, R., & Priebe, S. (2016). Prevalence of mental disorders at admission to the penal justice system in emerging countries: A study from Chile. *Epidemiology and Psychiatric Sciences, 25*(5), 441–449.

Nicholls, T. L., Ogloff, J. R. P., & Douglas, K. S. (2004). Assessing risk for violence among male and female civil psychiatric patients: The HCR-20, PCL:SV and VSC. *Behavioural Sciences and the Law, 22*(1), 127–158.

Nicholls, T. L., Petersen, K., Brink, J., & Webster, C. (2011). A clinical and risk profile of forensic psychiatric patients: Treatment team STARTs in a Canadian service. *International Journal of Forensic Mental Health, 10*(3), 187–199.

O'Connor, F. W., Lovell, D., & Brown, L. (2002). Implementing residential treatment for prison inmates with mental illness. *Archives of Psychiatric Nursing, 16*(5), 232–238.

Ogloff, J. R. P. (2002). Identifying and accommodating the needs of mentally ill people in gaols and prisons. *Psychiatry, Psychology and Law, 9*(1), 1–33.

Ogloff, J. R. P., & Daffern, M. (2006). The dynamic appraisal of situational aggression: An instrument to assess risk for imminent aggression in psychiatric inpatients. *Behavioral Sciences and the Law, 24*(6), 799–813.

Ogloff, J. R. P., Lemphers, A., & Dwyer, C. (2004). Dual diagnosis in an Australian forensic psychiatric hospital: Prevalence and implications for services. *Behavioural Sciences and the Law, 22*(4), 543–562.

Ogloff, J. R. P., Talevski, D., Lemphers, A., Wood, M., & Simmons, M. (2015). Co-occurring mental illness, substance use disorders, and antisocial personality disorder among clients of forensic mental health services. *Psychiatric Rehabilitation Journal, 38*(1), 16–23. doi: 10.1037/prj0000088.

Polaschek, D. L. L., & Reynolds, N. (2001). Assessment and treatment of violent offenders. In C. R. Hollin (Ed.), *Handbook of offender assessment and treatment* (pp. 415–431). Chichester: John Wiley & Sons.

Rice, M. E., & Harris, G. T. (1997). The treatment of mentally disordered offenders. *Psychology, Public Policy, and Law, 3*(1), 126–183.

Robinson, D., & Porporino, F. J. (2001). Programming in cognitive skills: The reasoning and rehabilitation programme. In C. R. Hollin (Ed.), *Handbook of offender assessment and treatment* (pp. 179–193). Chichester: John Wiley & Sons.

Sadock, B. J., & Sadock, V. A. (2003). *Synopsis of psychiatry* (9th ed.). Philadelphia: Lippincott Williams & Wilkins.

Scott, F., Whyte, S., Burnett, R., Hawley, C., & Maden, T. (2004). A national survey of substance misuse and treatment outcome on psychiatric patients in medium security. *Journal of Forensic Psychiatry and Psychology, 15*(4), 595–605.

Sentencing Advisory Council (2016). *A quick guide to sentencing*. Retrieved from https://www.sentencingcouncil.vic.gov.au/sites/default/files/publication-documents/A%20Quick%20Guide%20to%20Sentencing%202016_0.pdf

Short, T., Thomas, S., Mullen, P., & Ogloff, J. R. P. (2013). Comparing violence in schizophrenia patients with and without comorbid substance-use disorders to community controls. *Acta Psychiatrica Scandinavica, 128*(4), 306–313. doi: 10.1111/acps.12066.

Silver, E., & Teasedale, B. (2004). Mental disorder and violence: An examination of stressful life events and impaired social support. *Social Problems, 52*(1), 62–78.

Soothill, K., Rogers, P., & Dolan, M (2008). *Handbook of forensic mental health*. Devon: Willan Publishing.

Swanson, J. W., Swartz, M. S., Borum, R., Hiday, V. A., Wagner, H. R., & Burns, B. J. (2000). Involuntary out-patient commitment and reduction of violent behaviour in persons with severe mental illness. *British Journal of Psychiatry, 176*(4), 324–331.

Swanson, J. W., Swartz, M. S., Van Dorn, R. A., Elbogen, E. B., Wagner, H. R., Rosenheck, R. A., Stroup, T. S., McEvoy, J. P., & Leiberman, J. A. (2006). A national study of violent behavior in persons with schizophrenia. *Archives of General Psychiatry, 63*(5), 490–499.

Taylor, P. J. (2004). Mental disorder and crime. *Criminal Behaviour and Mental Health, 14*, S31–S36.

Tiihonen, J., Isohanni, M., Raesaenen, P., Koiranen, M., & Moring, J. (1997). Specific major mental disorders and criminality: A 26-year prospective study of the 1996 northern Finland birth cohort. *American Journal of Psychiatry, 154*(6), 840–845.

Tilt, R. (2000). *Report of the review of security at the high security hospitals*. London: National Health Service Executive.

Tversky, A., & Kahneman, D. (1974). Judgment under uncertainty: Heuristics and biases. *Science, 185*(4157), 1124–1131.

van der Wolf, M., van Marle, H., Mevis, P., & Roesch, R. (2010). Understanding and evaluating contrasting unfitness to stand trial practices: A comparison between Canada and the Netherlands. *International Journal of Forensic Mental Health, 9*(3), 245–258.

Vicens, E., V., Tort, R. M., Dueñas, Á., Muro, F., Pérez-Arnau, J., Arroyo, M. Sarda, P. (2011). The prevalence of mental disorders in Spanish prisons. *Criminal Behaviour & Mental Health, 21*(5), 321–332.

Wallace, C., Mullen, P. E., & Burgess, P. (2004). Criminal offending in schizophrenia over a 25-year period marked by deinstitutionalisation and increasing prevalence of comorbid substance use disorders. *American Journal of Psychiatry, 161*(4), 716–727.

Walsh, E., Gilvarry, C., Samele, C., Harvey, K., Manley, C., Tyrer, P., Creed, F., Murray, R., & Fahy, T. (2001). Reducing violence in severe mental illness: Randomised control trial of intensive case management compared with standard care. *British Medical Journal, 323*(7321), 1–5.

Webster, C. D., & Bailes, G. (2001). Assessing violence risk in mentally and personality disordered individuals. In C. R. Hollin (Ed.), *Handbook of offender assessment and treatment* (pp. 71–83). Chichester: John Wiley & Sons.

Webster, C. D., Martin, M. L., Brink, J. H., Nicholls, T. L., & Middleton, C. (2004). *Short-Term Assessment Risk and Treatability (START)*. Coquitlam, Canada: Forensic Psychiatric Services Commission.

Weiskopf, C. (2005). Nurses' experience of caring for inmate patients. *Journal of Advanced Nursing, 49*(4), 336–343.

Welsh, A., & Ogloff, J. R. P. (2003). The development of a Canadian prison based program for offenders with mental illness. *International Journal of Forensic Mental Health, 2*(1), 59–71.

Wessley, S., Castle, D., & Douglas, A. J. (1994). The criminal careers of incident cases of schizophrenia. *Psychological Medicine, 24*(2), 483–502.

Williams, P., Badger, D., Nursten, J., & Woodward, M. (1999). A review of recent academic literature on the characteristics of patients in British special hospitals. *Criminal Behaviour and Mental Health, 9*(4), 296–314.

Woods, P., Reed, V., & Collins, M. (2004). Relationships among risk, and communication and social skills in a high security forensic setting. *Issues in Mental Health Nursing, 25*(8), 769–782.

Wright, S., Gournay, K., Glorney, E., & Thornicroft, G. (2002). Mental illness, substance abuse, demographics and offending: Dual diagnosis in the suburbs. *Journal of Forensic Psychiatry, 13*(1), 35–52.

ANSWERS TO TEST YOURSELF

Chapter 1
1D; 2A; 3B; 4D

Chapter 2
1D; 2D; 3D; 4A

Chapter 3
1C; 2D; 3A; 4A

Chapter 4
1A; 2B; 3D; 4A

Chapter 5
1A; 2D; 3A; 4B

Chapter 6
1A; 2C; 3B; 4D

Chapter 7
1F; 2D; 3F; 4D

Chapter 8
1C; 2B; 3B; 4D

Chapter 9
1D; 2D; 3A; 4C

Chapter 10
1B; 2D; 3A; 4D

Chapter 11
1C; 2B; 3D; 4A

Chapter 12
1C; 2E; 3B; 4D

Chapter 13
1B; 2D; 3C; 4A

Chapter 14
1D; 2D; 3D; 4A

Chapter 15
1C; 2A; 3B; 4D

Chapter 16
1A; 2C; 3C; 4B

Chapter 17
1D; 2A; 3C

Chapter 18
1A; 2D; 3E; 4B

Chapter 19
1B; 2D; 3A; 4A

Chapter 20
1D; 2D; 3B; 4E

Chapter 21
1A; 2C; 3C

Chapter 22
1C; 2D; 3C; 4C

Chapter 23
1D; 2B; 3C; 4D

GLOSSARY

acculturation
The process of socialisation by which an individual or society absorbs cultural elements and traits from the host culture

addiction
Compulsive engagement in behaviours (e.g., taking drugs alcohol or gambling) despite experiencing adverse consequences as a result of the behaviour.

adherence
The extent to which clients take medications as prescribed by their health-care providers

adolescence
The period of human development from puberty to maturity

affect
The external manifestation of emotion

aggression
Forceful, hostile or attacking behaviour or disposition

alexithymia
A specific disturbance of psychological functioning characterised by difficulties in giving words to emotions

amenorrhea
the absence of menstrual periods

anhedonia
The inability to gain pleasure from experiences

anorexia nervosa
A complex eating disorder characterised by low body weight and body image distortion; a severe, debilitating mental illness, it has significant mortality rates over the long term

anxiety
A major motivating force in life; to be a disorder, it must be experienced out of proportion to the actual threat

assault
Through words or actions, the creation in the mind of another of the belief that he or she will be physically harmed or coerced without consent

assertive case management
Care coordination provided to clients in receipt of mental health services in the community setting, usually by a health-care professional

asylum
A hospital specialising in the treatment of people with mental illness, such as schizophrenia, anxiety, mania and depression

asylum seeker
A person seeking protection under the UN Refugee Convention; until a person's claim for protection is determined, a person's status is referred to as 'asylum seeker'.

attachment
Emotional ties and reciprocal relationships that infants and toddlers develop with significant people in their lives

autonomy
Relationships between an individual and other individuals and institutions that give genuine opportunities for choice

battery
Touching, or other physical constraint, without a person's consent; there is no need for injury to be sustained for battery to take place

behavioural and psychological symptoms of dementia
A range of symptoms that are associated with disturbed perception, thought content, behaviour or mood

beneficence
The principle that requires health practitioners to do good, prevent evil or harm, and remove evil or harm

binge eating disorder
An eating disorder characterised by excessive eating unusually large amounts of food and feel unable to stop

biopsychosocial
An approach that systematically considers biological, psychological, and social factors and their complex interactions in understanding health, illness and health-care delivery

bipolar disorder
A serious disorder that causes sudden shifts in a person's mood and energy between depression and hypomania

body mass index
The physical measurement used to assess total body fat and is calculated by your weight (kg) by the square of your height (m^2)

borderline personality disorder (BPD)
A diagnostic category describing people suffering a pattern of unregulated emotions, impulsivity, unstable identity, high levels of anxiety (particularly when alone), chronic suicidal ideas, high risk-taking behaviours, self-harm and poor capacity to manage and maintain social relationships

boundaries
Limits within professional relationships that allow safe connections based on the needs of individuals

brokerage model
A case manager-specific approach linking appropriate mental health services

bulimia nervosa
An eating disorder characterised by frequent episodes of binge eating followed by inappropriate behaviours such as self-induced vomiting to avoid weight gain

bullying
When people repeatedly and intentionally use words or actions against someone or a group of people to cause distress and risk to their well-being

capacity
A legal concept that describes the level of intellectual functioning a person requires to make and accept responsibility for important decisions that often have legal consequences concerning themselves

care recipient
A person who lives with some form of chronic condition or illness that causes difficulties in completing the tasks of daily living

carer/caregiver
A person who assumes responsibility for ensuring that the client is adequately cared for

carer burden
The stress that caregivers feel due to the situation at home when caring for a family member; such a burden is subjective and is one of the most important predictors of adverse consequences of the care situation—for carers and consumers alike

case management
A multidisciplinary approach to coordinating the care of those experiencing serious mental illness

categorical approach
Personality dysfunction viewed through a symptom checklist in which a designated number of symptoms denotes the diagnosis

childhood
The period of human development from birth until puberty

CHIME
A framework that identifies five recovery processes: Connectedness; Hope and optimism about the future; Identity; Meaning in life; and Empowerment (giving the acronym CHIME)

clinical case management model
A type of case management that facilitates clients' physical well-being, personal growth, community participation and recovery from, or adaptation to, mental illness

clinical staging
A diagnostic model commonly used in medicine that has the benefit of offering different treatments depending on the stage of a person's disorder

clinical supervision
The process of two or more professionals formally meeting to reflect and review clinical situations, with the aim of supporting the clinician in their professional environment.

code of conduct
A statement identifying mandatory standards of practice

code of ethics
A statement of values to which a profession is committed and is expected to uphold

cognition
The aspect of mental functioning that takes up belief-desire reasoning and perspective taking

cognitive behaviour therapy (CBT)
Non-medical therapy that attempts to teach people to control their own behaviour by means of self-developed problem-solving skills; it is often referred to as 'talking therapy'

collaborative care
The process by which two or more health-care professionals and health-care organisations work together to provide health care to clients

co-morbidity
Where one or more disease or disorder is present in addition to a primary disease or disorder

communication skills
The processes through which we share ideas with one another

compassion fatigue
A gradual lessening of compassion over time due to continued exposure to clients' demands for help; it's directly related to their level of pain and suffering

competency standards
Performance standards that reflect the complex nature of a nurse's roles, skills and knowledge

complementary alternative medicine (CAM)
the use by patients/clients of alternative medicines to those prescribed by their treating health-care worker

comprehensive psychiatric assessment
The process necessary to diagnose any number of emotional, behavioral or developmental disorders

concordance
Ensuring the involvement of the person in their care and treatment goals; goals are set out together by the client and practitioner towards better adherence to medications and treatment interventions.

confidentiality
The ethical and legal obligation to keep patients' information private

consent
Agreement to undergo treatment, which is lawful or ethical, if it meets certain conditions

consultation–liaison nurse (CLN)
An advanced practice psychiatric mental health nurse who consults to nurses and other health-care professionals within non-psychiatric settings, most commonly but not exclusively general hospital wards, emergency departments and nursing homes

consumer
A person who has experienced mental illness and has been a recipient of mental health care by professionals

consumer advocate
A person who listens to and acts on behalf of mental health consumers about what is wrong with the mental health system

consumer participation
A process of quality improvement for service delivery that increases consumer satisfaction through offering the opportunity to be influential in decision-making processes across policy and development, including training and evaluation

co-occuring disorders
The presence of both a substance use disorder and mental health disorder

coping
To face and deal with problems or difficulties

counter-transference
Where a therapist forms an emotional attachment toward a client based on a perceived connection to the client

craving
An intense desire for some particular thing

credentialed mental health nurse
A mental health nurse who has successfully met a particular standard and is authorised to practise as an accredited mental health nurse (MHN)

critical appraisal
The identification of methodological flaws in research and provision of the opportunity to make informed decisions about the quality of research evidence

cross-cultural practice
Two or more cultures working together to incorporate awareness and knowledge of other cultures, critical reflective practice, culturally safe responses to another culture and commitment to anti-racist practice and social justice

cultural competence
The ability to interact effectively with people of different cultures and socio-economic backgrounds, particularly in the context of human resources, non-profit organisations and government agencies whose employees work with persons from different cultural and/or ethnic backgrounds

cultural formulation
Beginning with a review of the individual's cultural identity, it includes the patient's self-construal of identity over time

cultural safety
A health professional's understanding of her own personal culture and how these personal cultural values may impact on the provision of care to the person, regardless of race or ethnicity

cultural sensitivity
The understanding that cultural differences as well as similarities exist, without assigning values (for example, better or worse, right or wrong) to those cultural differences

culturally and linguistically diverse (CALD)
The characteristics of a society that make it multicultural; the support for a wide variety of cultural beliefs within a society

culture
A major construct that describes the total body of beliefs, behaviours, sanctions, values and goals that marks the way of life of any people

deinstitutionalisation
The worldwide mental health policy change that took place between 1960 and 1990, when institutions were closed and the care of mental health clients was shifted to community settings

delirium
An acute and debilitating decline in the ability to focus attention, perception and cognition that produces an altered conscious state

delusion
A firmly held, false belief that is not supported by social reality

dementia
Progressive deterioration in a person's mental functioning

deontology
The study of social duties or moral obligations

dependence
Severe substance use disorder characterised by increased tolerance to a substance, and can include the experience of withdrawal upon cessation of use.

depression
A mood disorder that includes such symptoms as a lowered mood, feelings of sadness and tearfulness

development
The mental growth and adaptation or a human being in order to maintain the self and social relationships within society

diagnostic overshadowing
the tendency for clinicians to attribute symptoms or behaviours of a person with a learning disability or SMI to their underlying cognitive deficits

Diagnostic and Statistical Manual of Mental Disorders (DSM)
A multi-axial classification system of mental disorders published by the American Psychiatric Association

dialectical behavioural therapy (DBT)
A form of psychological therapy developed by Linehan that has been shown to be an effective intervention for people with significant emotional and relationship problems

dimensional approach
Personality dysfunction seen through the dimensions of the intrapsychic, the interpersonal and the social

diminished responsibility
A legal defence under which a person experiencing mental illness at the time of an offence is considered not to be criminally liable

disability
Includes temporary and permanent disabilities; physical, intellectual, sensory and psychiatric disabilities, diseases or illnesses; medical conditions; work-related injuries; past, present and future disabilities; and association with a person with a disability

dramatherapy
A technique used by creative arts therapists to bring about socially oriented change

Dreaming (or Dreamtime)
In Australian Aboriginal mythology, a sacred era in which ancestral totemic spirit beings created the world. In this worldview, every event leaves a record in the land and everything is a result of the past.

drug dependence
The body's physical need, or addiction, to a specific chemical agent; the dependent person often feels the need to ingest ever greater quantities of the drug in order to attain the original effect

drug interaction
The phenomenon whereby the effects of one drug are altered by the concurrent administration of another

dual diagnosis
Used to describe the situation where a person has both a co-occurring mental illness and a substance use problem

duty of care
A legal duty to avoid harming another or others by one's act/s or omission of act/s

dysthymia
A mild form of depression, characterised by persistent depressive symptoms of at least two years' duration

eating disorders
A disturbance of normal eating behaviours, including anorexia nervosa, bulimia nervosa and eating disorders not otherwise specified

engagement
Becoming involved and invested emotionally and cognitively in interpersonal processes

ethics of care
Emotional commitment to and willingness to act on behalf of people for whose care we take responsibility

ethnic
A population and/or language group that maintains its identity within a wider society

ethnocentrism
A belief in the inherent superiority of one's own group and culture, accompanied by feelings of contempt for other groups and cultures

evidence-based practice (EBP)
The application of best evidence to inform decision-making about professional practice and patient care

extrapyramidal
Relating to spinal fibres that coordinate and maintain posture as well as support locomotion

facilitation
The process of helping groups or individuals to learn, find a solution or reach a consensus, without imposing or dictating an outcome

false imprisonment
The holding or restraint of a person against his or her will, in order to prevent the person from leaving or moving freely

family
Personal relationships—formalised through marriage, same sex partners or close friends, de facto relationships or single parents—identified by a person with mental illness as the next of kin

flight of ideas
Cognitive incoherence and disorganisation characterised by rapid speech; grandiosity that may be so extreme that the person loses contact with reality

forensic mental health nurses
Professional nurses who have undertaken a course of study in forensic psychiatry and are working in the area

forensic mental health team
Mental health service team, either within a secure forensic mental health hospital or an area mental health service, for prisoners with serious mental illness

genogram
A pictorial display of family and relationships used in a comprehensive psychiatric assessment

guardianship
Authority to represent or stand in for a person who is without legal capacity herself or himself

guided imagery
Mind stimuli that can provoke responses such as stress reduction and relaxation

hallucination
A perceptual experience that occurs without external sensory stimuli

hard paternalism
The assumed right of one person to make decisions that override informed, voluntary and autonomous actions of the other person

healing
Restoration of balance and well-being to the client

health assessment
Holistic assessment of health and well-being, not just systemic assessment of signs and symptoms of disease

health promotion
Action directed towards changing social, environmental and economic conditions to promote the health of individuals and societies, based on research, policy and community action

hoarding
Persistent difficulty discarding or parting with possessions, regardless of their actual value

holistic
From the noun holism, which is the idea that things, in particular people, can have properties as a whole that are not entirely explained by understanding the properties of their parts

hope
A way of thinking that focuses on the positive aspects, expectations and outcomes of an experience

hypomania
A condition similar to mania but less severe

iatrogenic
A problem that is caused by, rather than relieved by, a physician's or other medical treatment

identity
Ideas that define the self

illicit drugs
Drugs that have been made unlawful because of the social perception that they are too dangerous to self-administer

imagination
The capacity to form mental images, leading to the ability to mould experience into something new, and to find creative expression of those images and experiences

infancy
The period between birth and the acquisition of language; infants develop at differing levels depending on factors including their emotional and physical health

internally displaced person
A person who is fleeing persecution but is unable to cross a border, and cannot seek protection under the UN Convention for Refugees

International Classification of Diseases (ICD)
A system of diagnosis and classification of mental illness produced by the World Health Organization

interventions
Therapeutic actions on behalf of another

intimacy
A sense of psychological and physical closeness or connectedness with another where deep personal sharing can take place

justice
The social principle that supports rights claims to redress past wrongs, remove discrimination or focus on fair resource allocation

Kaiwhakaruruhau
A Māori concept of cultural safety; a mechanism that allows the consumer to say whether or not a service is safe for them to approach and use.

Koha
A New Zealand Māori custom which means offering a gift

leadership
Ability to create and communicate a vision of actions and ideas for oneself and colleagues

legislation
Acts of Parliament, which are the basis for statutory law

liaison
Linking the knowledge base of mental health nursing to the care of patients with physical health problems through the professional relationship that develops between the CLN and the staff/organisation. Integral to liaison activity

is the promotion of holistic care and capacity-building of general hospital staff in patients' mental health care through regular contact with and education of staff. It incorporates understanding patients, relatives and staff from a systems perspective and the culture of the hospital/organisation

lifestyle choices
Factors that increase or decrease health well-being, including diet, exercise, and alcohol and drug intake

mainstreaming
The fundamental shift of psychiatric services from psychiatric institutions to more general health-care settings; it was intended to increase consumers' access to quality, comprehensive health-care services and to reduce the stigmatisation of and discrimination against people experiencing mental illnesses

major depressive disorder
Two or more major depressive episodes including depressed mood for most of the day, significant weight loss or gain, insomnia or sleeping too much, agitation noticed by others, fatigue, feelings of worthlessness or excessive guilt, diminished cognitive function, and/or recurrent thoughts of death

mania
Persistent and pervasive elevated or irritable mood

masculinity
A term constructed by a society to refer to the characteristics or key elements of what constitutes being a man

medical model
The school of psychological thought whose basis is that mental disorders are the product of physiological factors

mental disorders
The full range of mental health, neurological and substance use disorders that make up 14 per cent of the total global burden of disease

mental health
A state of well-being in which the individual realises his or her own potential and can cope with the normal stressors of life

mental health court
A specialist court within the judicial system established to take into consideration the circumstances of the mental illness and its contribution to offending

mental health nurse practitioner (MHNP)
A mental health nurse who practises at an advanced level in the delivery of psychiatric nursing interventions

mental health nursing
A field of nursing in which the nurse cares for patients who are experiencing a mental illness, dysfunction or disorder

mental health promotion
Action taken towards improving the mental health status of individuals and populations, based on research, policy and community action

mental illness
A diagnosable disorder that significantly interferes with an individual's cognitive, emotional and/or social abilities

mental status examination (MSE)
A system of making an objective assessment of the neurological and psychological status of a client

mentalisation
The understanding arising from the act of focusing on the mental states of oneself and others. It is a developmental ability

meta-analysis
A method used to compare and contrast findings from different studies using statistical means

mindfulness
The practice of bringing awareness to the present moment in an attitude of openness, interest and receptivity

mood
A subjective feeling state

narrative therapy
A form of psychological therapy developed in the 1970s that uses a collaborative and non-blaming approach

negative symptoms
Symptoms that reflect a decrease in the person's normal functioning, such as anhedonia or amotivation

negligence
In a legal sense, when it can be shown that a duty of care is owed, the duty has been breached and the breach caused harm

non-maleficence
The principle or moral obligation to do no harm

nurse practitioner
A registered nurse, educated and authorised to function autonomously and collaboratively in an advanced and extended clinical role

organisational culture
A system whereby relationships are governed by tacit and manifest norms of behaviour and values

parenting
Performance of critical roles that parents must take in order to meet children's needs for safety, care, control and intellectual stimulation

paternalism
The presumed right of one person to act as parent or authority figure over another, overriding autonomy, for the possible benefit of the person being controlled

person-centred care
A collaborative therapy consisting of the efforts of patients, patients' families, friends, general practitioners and other health professionals

pharmacodynamics
The scientific discipline used as a basis to understand the effects of drugs in the body, including the mechanisms by which a drug produces any pharmacological action, either therapeutic or harmful, as well as the effects produced by the concurrent administration of more than one drug

pharmacokinetics
The pharmacological science addressing the disposition of drugs and their metabolites in the human body

pharmacological management
Care intervention aimed at reducing the number of or rationalising the use of as many medications as possible

pharmacotherapy
The use of medicinal drug therapy for therapeutic purposes in the treatment or prevention of disease

plasticity of symptoms
Changes in symptoms due to events

play
Any activity that opens imaginative reality to the client within a creative arts therapy construct

positive symptoms
Symptoms that are an excess or distortion of a person's normal functioning, such as formal thought disorder, hallucinations or delusions

post-traumatic stress disorder (PTSD)
A history of exposure to a traumatic event that meets specific conditions and symptoms from each of four symptom clusters: intrusion, avoidance, negative alterations in cognitions and mood, and alterations in arousal and reactivity

praxis
The practical application of a theory

premorbid
The normal state that can precede psychotic symptoms

primary health-care team
A team made up of professional practitioners who practise from the general practice setting

primary prevention
The support and promotion of good health; examples of successful primary prevention program include reducing

smoking, improving cardiovascular disease and reducing road trauma

prodrome
Early symptoms of mental illness that precede the manifestation of the acute phase of mental illness

professional boundaries
Used to distinguish between personal and professional relationships, whereby professionals, due to the power associated with their roles, could exploit or damage consumers unless professionals maintain appropriate boundaries between themselves and their clients

psychiatric advance directive (PAD)
A document completed by a person when they are well that stipulates their wishes about treatment they wish to receive or refuse during a future episode of severe mental illness, when they may not be competent to make these decisions

psychiatry
A medical speciality devoted to the study, diagnosis, treatment and prevention of mental disorders

psychoeducation
The education presented to people with mental health disorders and their families to support and empower them and manage and cope with their condition in ideal ways

psychosis
A condition in which a person experiences a misinterpretation of reality as a result of impaired cognition and emotional, social and communicative behaviours

psychotropic drug
Any medication capable of affecting the mind, emotions and behaviour

primary treating team (PTT)
The multidisciplinary team primarily responsible for the patient in the non-psychiatric setting

public health
Action taken to improve the health of the population as a whole

quality use of medicines
A framework used to describe strategies to achieve safe, effective, judicious and cost-effective medicinal drug use, involving input from all stakeholders including consumers

randomised controlled trial
An experimental method of research that compares a set of individuals who are randomly selected to receive treatment with a group of equal numbers who do not receive the treatment, with the aim of evaluating the long-term effectiveness of a treatment or intervention

rechallenge
A medical testing protocol where drugs are administered, withdrawn then readministered

reciprocity
Mutual action or exchange of ideas between individuals or groups for mutual benefit

reconnection
The point of the recovery process where individuals can re-engage with significant others and the community at large

recovery
The state of functioning characterised by regaining symptom management, returning to an optimal level of functioning and quality of life

recovery approach
A philosophical position that focuses on the capacity and capabilities of consumers to experience a meaningful and satisfying life; adopting a recovery approach suggests all people have value, and can contribute to society regardless of symptoms or illness

recovery model
A case management model that challenges the traditional view of caring (disease management) in favour of facilitating personal recovery by working with consumers' abilities to grow, utilising their strengths, community-focused interventions and the strength of the case manager–consumer relationship

reflection
Any concentrated activity that links thought and action

refractory
Of drugs, resistant to usual therapeutic interventions

refugee
Any person who owing to well-founded fear of being persecuted for reasons of race, religion, nationality, membership of a particular social group or political opinion, is outside their country of his nationality and is unable or, owing to such fear, is unwilling to avail himself of the protection of that country; or who, not having a nationality and being outside the country of his former habitual residence as a result of such events, is unable or, owing to such fear, is unwilling to return to it (UNHCR)

registration
Statutory recognition of qualification and capacity to practise a profession

relapse
The recurrence of symptoms after a period of recovery from mental illness

remission
A reduction in symptoms such that the diagnosis does not apply

resettlement
The selection and transfer of refugees from a state in which they have sought protection to a third state which has agreed to admit them – as refugees – with permanent residence status. The status provided ensures protection against refoulement and provides a resettled refugee and his/her family or dependants with access to rights similar to those enjoyed by nationals. Resettlement also carries with it the opportunity to eventually become a naturalized citizen of the resettlement country (UNHCR).

resilience
The ability to recover and rebound from the effects of adverse events

respect for autonomy
Respect for personal and national self-government and hence respect for people's choices about their lives and perhaps deaths

restraint
Limiting a person's freedom of movement by chemical or physical means

rights-based theory
The theory that society should provide certain universal and impartial guarantees to individuals, such as the right to free speech or the right to happiness

risk
The potential for an undesirable outcome or loss

risk assessment
A clinical assessment of a client's risk in relation to risk to self (the client), risk to others (including aggression and violence) and risk to property

risk management
The assessment and subsequent prioritisation of risk

risk plan
The documentation of risk assessment, risk management and evaluation

safety plan
An individualised, proactive intervention plan developed collaboratively between clinical staff and the client to help the client with their safety needs and preferences for care

screening tools
Generally reliable and valid tools or instruments used to measure a behaviour or a particular situation

seclusion
Confinement to a room, designed to isolate a person considered to be otherwise at risk of harming herself or himself or others

self-care
Decisions and actions undertaken by an individual in order to cope with a health problem or to improve his or her health

self-efficacy
Belief in one's own ability to succeed in specific situations

self-talk
Learning how to challenge and replace any irrational thoughts that feed anxiety

severe mental illness (SMI)
Mental illness judged by the type of illness, intensity of symptoms, length of illness (chronicity) and the degree of disability caused; its rating of severe can be compared with mild and moderate

social and emotional well-being
The preferred term for 'mental health' by Australia's Aboriginal and Torres Strait Islander peoples because it offers a more holistic view

social determinants of health
The social conditions in which people live and work as considerations to the underlying reasons why people experience poor health

social capital
The network of social connections that exist between people, and their shared values and norms of behaviour, enabling and encouraging mutually advantageous social cooperation

soft paternalism
Making decisions on behalf of people whose agency is limited

somatic
relating to the physical body, as distinct from the mind

somatisation
The expression of physical symptoms that are not explained by observable organic pathology, which may be a result of hypochondriasis or as manifestations of anxiety and other disorders

splitting
An unconscious dynamic arising from unrecognised polarities in the client with BPD that is enacted divisively between workers in the system around that client.

stigma
Mark of disgrace; stain, as on one's reputation or a sign of defect; degeneration; or disease

strengths model
A model developed by Rapp and Chamberlain in the 1980s that is based on goal-oriented behaviour and promotes less dependence on the hospital

stress
A psychological response to a situation or stressor; the response, which can be positive (motivation) or negative (distress), can be experienced differently by individuals

substance use disorders
A condition in which the use of one or more substances leads to a clinically significant impairment or distress (when an individual experiences physical, psychological, social, or interpersonal problems as a result of their substance use)

systematic review
An appraisal and synthesis of primary research papers on a specific topic, using a systematic and rigorous search strategy to locate the papers.

Te Tiriti o Waitangi (Treaty of Waitangi)
A treaty signed by Māori leaders and white settlers in 1840; a foundation document of New Zealand that underpins many aspects of legislation, and its principles are incorporated into all aspects of health services.

therapeutic alliance
Goals and conditions for treatment that may affect the therapeutic path adhered to by the bond between client and clinician

therapeutic optimism
The clinician's expectation of a positive outcome for the consumer. Therapeutic optimism contains elements of self-efficacy, hope and belief in the consumer's capacity to recover from illness, set realistic goals and overcome and transcend obstacles

thought disorder
A disturbance in the structure, form, content and logic of thought

torture
Any act by which severe pain or suffering, whether physical or mental, is intentionally inflicted on a person for such purposes as obtaining from him or a third person information or a confession, punishing him for an act he or a third person has committed or is suspected of having committed, or intimidating or coercing him or a third person or, for any reason based on discrimination of any kind, when such pain or suffering is inflicted by or at the instigation of or with the consent or acquiescence of a public official or other person acting in an official capacity. It does not include pain or suffering arising only from, inherent in or incidental to lawful sanctions (UNHCR).

transference
Where an individual receiving care through a therapeutic process attaches to their care giver feelings formerly held towards other significant people who have held past emotional importance

trauma
Psychological injury interfering with a child's capacity during growth to integrate sensory, emotional and cognitive information; terms of the refuge experience, an emotional response to a terrible event and one that will have different meanings to different individuals, families and communities.

treatment plan
A plan devised by all health workers that sets out a therapeutic path and rationale for treatment

utilitarianism (consequentialism)
An ethical theory that judges the correctness of personal actions by the consequences of those actions

validation
A therapeutic statement in response to the client's pain, which offers an attuned understanding of the client

validity
The degree to which a research study measures what it intends to measure

violence
The use of physical force against self or others to intimidate or to cause actual harm

virtue ethics
An ethical theory based on the moral character of individuals and societies; a person or society with the required virtues will act ethically

vulnerability
The potential susceptibility of a person to a health deviation

well-being
A state of contentment and satisfaction with self and fulfillment with life, resulting in positive functioning

worldview
The overall perspective from which one sees and interprets the world